Two week

NEPHROTOXICITY

Assessment and Pathogenesis

Monographs in Applied Toxicology No.1 1982

Editors: M. R. Greenwood, R. von Burg and L. Magos

NEPHROTOXICITY

Assessment and Pathogenesis

Proceedings of the International Symposium on
Nephrotoxicity

University of Surrey, UK
7- 11 September 1981

Editors: **P. H. BACH**
F. W. BONNER
J. W. BRIDGES
E.A. LOCK

A Wiley Heyden Publication

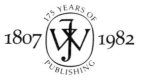

1807   1982

JOHN WILEY & SONS
Chichester · New York · Brisbane · Toronto · Singapore

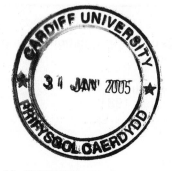

Copyright © 1982 Wiley Heyden Ltd.

British Library Cataloguing in Publication Data:

International Symposium on Nephrotoxicity
  (1981: University of Surrey)
  Nephrotoxicity.—(Monographs in applied toxicology; 1)
  1. Kidneys—Diseases—Congresses
  2. Chemicals—Toxicology—Congresses
  I. Title   II. Bach, P. H.   III. Series
  616.6'1   RC902.A2

  ISBN 0 471 26212 9

Printed in Great Britain by
St Edmundsbury Press,
Bury St Edmunds, Suffolk

CONTENTS

FOREWORD

I may, of course, be biased, but it seems to me entirely reasonable that a series of monographs on applied toxicology should start with one devoted to the kidney. The only other possible contender would, of course, be the liver, through which must pass the whole of any poison entering via the alimentary tract. But some potentially toxic agents are ingested in an inert form, and become poisonous only after metabolic transformation. The liver both engenders toxicity from harmless precursors and neutralises it by conjugation to less toxic compounds. But, at the end of the day, the only effective means of eliminating the final product from the body is renal excretion (sweating and alimentary losses being negligible in this context).

The kidneys are well equipped for this task. They receive a fifth of the cardiac output; in addition, they have the capacity to produce urine with several times the osmolality of blood, even in man, and in the desert animals, urine of still greater concentration. The hairpin medullary concentrating mechanism which adds to excretory efficiency is likely also to increase the vulnerability to toxic agents which will, in the deeper medulla, attain a concentration much greater than in the other tissues of the body. This theoretical possibility is, no doubt, reflected structurally in the syndrome of papillary necrosis.

As a dedicated nephrophile, admittedly somewhat emeritus, it gives me great pleasure to contribute this foreword, and to commend the initiative of the organisers of the International Nephrotoxicity Symposium, held by the Robens Institute of Industrial and Environmental Health and Safety and the Department of Biochemistry at the University of Surrey.

London
April 1982

Professor Sir Douglas Black MD, DSc
President of the Royal College of Physicians

PREFACE

The kidney plays a major role in health and disease; however, efforts to understand its function and malfunction continue to present one of the most challenging areas of research to the biological sciences.

Over the years, renal function has most often been assessed by measuring substances in blood and urine, but these have generally given only a gross measure of what functional abnormalities have already developed. Attempts to assess more subtle changes, such as those which precede irreversible functional change, are blurred by the heterogeneity both along and between nephrons, by the cycling of metabolic components within and between cells and between different areas within the kidney, by the functional reserve that the kidney possesses, and by the immense technical difficulties associated with gaining access to all of the morphological and functional regions of the kidney.

Thus, the dichotomy of renal structure and function provides an *imbroglio,* particularly for the toxicologist who is attempting to evaluate the safety of substances to which humans will be exposed. The clinician must also assess renal malfunction in humans before a suitable therapy can be instituted, a task made more difficult by the nephrotoxic potential of many drugs.

This Symposium was convened to provide a forum in which the clinician, morphologist, physiologist, biochemist, toxicologist and pathologist could combine to approach the fundamental question of assessing renal function and understanding the processes leading to malfunction. Only through multidisciplinary studies will the pathomorphological changes associated with chemical insults to the kidney be understood at a physiological and biochemical level. Indeed, until the molecular processes underlying the development of a chemically induced lesion are understood, there will be no rational basis for clinical management, nor for therapeutic intervention to prevent or limit the pathophysiological changes. Furthermore, the nephrotoxic potential of all chemicals can only be properly assessed when more is known about renal function and malfunction.

Some authors of abstracts submitted to the Poster Session (published in the *Journal of Applied Toxicology* 1(4), v–xxv, 1981) were invited to contribute expanded papers for the proceedings. These are included in the text.

We are indebted to those of our colleagues who advised us on the scientific programme, to the participants for providing the critical multidisciplinary forum in which ideas were exchanged and discussion took place, and particularly to the many people who helped organize the Symposium. The Symposium could not have been run, nor the final proceedings published, without the continued assistance of Jan McCall, Janet Williams and Carole Barlow, the extensive advice from the publishers, and Christopher Powell for compiling the extensive index.

Guildford
March 1982

Peter H. Bach
Frank W. Bonner
Edward A. Lock
James W. Bridges

INDEX TO CONTRIBUTORS

Alt, J. M. *Hannover Medical School, Department of Physiology, Laboratory of Experimental Nephrology, Hannover, FRG* (p.102)

Bach, P. H. *Robens Institute of Industrial and Environmental Health and Safety, University of Surrey, Guildford, Surrey GU2 5XH, UK* (pp. 27, 128, 182, 437)

Balazs, T. *Food and Drug Administration, Washington, DC, USA* (p. 487)

Beaton, E. M. *Robens Institute of Industrial and Environmental Health and Safety, University of Surrey, Guildford, Surrey GU2 5XH, UK* (p. 182)

Bellon, B. *Hôpital Broussais, 96 rue Didot, 75674 Paris Cedex 14, France* (p. 206)

Bernard, A. *Unite de Toxicologie Industrielle et Médicale, Faculté de Médecine, Université de Louvain, 30.54 Clos Chapelle-aux-Champs, 1200 Bruxelles, Belgium* (p. 371)

Berndt, W. O. *Department of Pharmacology and Toxicology, University of Mississippi Medical Center, Jackson, Mississippi 39216, USA* (pp. 54, 378)

Bonner, F. W. *Robens Institute of Industrial and Environmental Health and Safety, University of Surrey, Guildford, Surrey GU2 5XH, UK* (pp. 27, 182, 310, 320)

Bremner, I. *Rowett Research Institute, Bucksburn, Aberdeen AB2 9SB, UK* (p. 280)

Bridges, J. W. *Robens Institute of Industrial and Environmental Health and Safety, University of Surrey, Guildford, Surrey GU2 5XH, UK* (pp. 182, 437)

Brod, J. *Division of Nephrology, Medical School, Hannover, FRG* (p. 1)

Burnett, R. *The Boots Co. Ltd, Pathology Department, Biological Research R3, Pennyfoot Street, Nottingham NG2 3AA, UK* (p. 98)

Carter, B. A. *Department of Biochemistry, University of Surrey, Guildford, Surrey GU2 5XH, UK* (pp. 310, 320)

Cattell, W. R. *Departments of Chemical Pathology and Nephrology, St Bartholomew's Hospital, London EC1, UK* (p. 78)

Chin, T. Y. *Department of Pharmacology, University of Minnesota, Minneapolis, Minnesota 55455, USA* (p. 113)

Clarkson, T. W. *Division of Toxicology, University of Rochester School of Medicine, Rochester, New York 14642, USA* (p. 263)

Daley-Yates, P. T. *Biochemistry Department, School of Biological Sciences, Brunel University, Uxbridge, Middlesex, UK* (p. 356)

Dawnay, A. B. St.J. *Departments of Chemical Pathology and Nephrology, St Bartholomew's Hospital, London EC1, UK* (p. 78)

Dees, J. H. *Biochemistry Department, University of Texas Health Center at Dallas, Dallas, Texas 75235, USA* (p. 246)

The organizers wish to acknowledge the support received from the following:

The National Kidney Research Fund
The Royal Society
The Wellcome Trust

The Boots Co. Ltd.
Ciba-Geigy Pharmaceuticals Division
Glaxo-Holdings Ltd.
Shell Research Ltd.
Pfizer Central Research

Abbott Laboratories Ltd.
Ames Division Miles Laboratories
Banton & Kingman Ltd.
Beecham Pharmaceuticals
Boehringer Ingelheim
The British Petroleum Co. Ltd.

Fisons Ltd.
Imperial Chemical Industries Ltd.
Johnson Matthey Ltd.
May & Baker Ltd.
Ortho Pharmaceutical Ltd.
Reckitt & Colman Ltd.
Richardson-Merrell Ltd.
Roche Products Ltd.
R.T.Z. Services Ltd.
Riker Laboratories
Smith Kline & French Research Ltd.
WB Pharmaceuticals Ltd.
The Wellcome Research Laboratories
    Ltd.

Heyden & Sons Ltd.

TOXIC NEPHROPATHIES IN MAN

J. Brod

Division of Nephrology, Medical School Hannover, FRG

It was known as early as the beginning of the last century that the kidney can be acutely damaged by poisoning, the best known instance being that of mercury chloride intoxication producing anuria. This was mainly due to the fact that the increasing use of mercury chloride as an antiseptic agent made it easily accessible, especially to the hospital personnel. Early in this century instances of chronic renal disease among printers and people exposed to lead were frequently reported.

Spühler and Zollinger [1] published the first report of cases of chronic renal nephropathy due to analgesic abuse. At the same time Oliver et al [2] carried out a thorough morphological study of 23 cases of acute poisoning with renal involvement, the toxic agent being mercury chloride in 7 cases and sulphonamides in 10 cases (Table 1).

Table 1.   Causes of Toxic Renal Injury in
           Oliver's et al. Statistic

Sulfonamides	10
Mercuric chloride	7
Di-ethylene glycol	2
Carbon tetrachloride	2
Potassium chlorate	1
Mushroom poisoning	1
	23

Already from this it is obvious that the kidney can be affected
by a multitude of substances used as drugs or by injected, ingested
or inhaled toxic agents. With the exponentially increasing number
of chemicals or biologic substances used in medicine, in food production, households transportation or in industry man is daily
exposed to agents which may be potentially poisonous, either acutely
or chronically. It is, therefore, very appropriate that the University
of Surrey has taken the initiative and organised a Symposium devoted
to the problems of nephrotoxicity and I consider it as a very great
honour to have been asked to open it.

Due to a rich blood supply, which per unit weight, is over 100
times that of a resting muscle, the potentially nephrotoxic substances
are brought preferentially to the kidney and here they may act in
several ways (Table 2):

Table 2.   Mechanisms of Nephrotoxicity

    1)   Effect on Renal Blood Flow

    2)   Toxic Action on Tubular Cells

    3)   Immunologically Mediated Injury
         (glomerular or tubulo-interstitial)

    4)   Obstruction of Tubuli or Ureters

    5)   Cancerogenic

1.   They may exert their toxic action by affecting the renal vessels,
jeopardizing the renal blood flow and decreasing the glomerular
filtration rate (GFR) directly e.g. indomethacin, analgesics (by
blocking the intrarenal production of vasodilating prostaglandins) or
indirectly by a combination of toxic action and dehydration.

2.   They come into an intimate contact with the tubular cells and
they may pass through them in the process of secretion or of
reabsorption. During this they may affect the brush-border, the
various cell organelles, they may inactivate cellular enzymes and lead
to a functional damage or even to cellular death (aminoglycosides,
cephaloridin, old tetracyclines, mycotoxins, aflatoxin, ochratoxin A,
heavy metals, cadmium, carbon tetrachloride etc.).

3.   Acting as haptens, they may produce an immunologically mediated
injury both to the glomeruli and, even more frequently, to the renal
interstitium and start a reversible or progressive glomerular or
tubulo-interstitial disease (some antibiotics, e.g. methicillin,
rifampicin etc.).

4.   They may fall out of solution during the concentration of
urine or change of pH of the tubular fluid and block the tubuli
with crystals (sulphonamides, contrast dyes?). The same thing
can be caused by detritus of the necrotic tubular cells and,
perhaps, by casts.

5.   Also the ureters can be blocked from the inside by crystals
or by necrotic renal tissue (necrotic papillae) or constricted
from the outside by retroperitoneal periureteric fibrosis
(radiation-injury, methysergide).

6.   The toxic substances themselves or their metabolites may be
carcinogenic (paracetamol etc.).

    It is obvious, that the mechanism of action of the steadily
increasing heterogeneous group of toxic agents is variegated.
Equally variegated may be the clinical pattern of the intoxication.
With small exceptions the clinical picture is not specific and only
a thorough past history and enquiry into the possible acute
or chronic exposure to any such agent may give a clue to the correct
diagnosis. The following syndromes can be encountered:

1.   The best known is the clinical picture of mercury poisoning
illustrated in Fig. 1 by the case of a 50 years old female who
ingested with suicidal intentions, 2,5 g of mercury oxycyanate.
The ingestion of poison left behind a metallic taste in her mouth
and shortly afterwards she started vomiting profusely, got diarrhoea
and abdominal pain. Next day she was admitted to the hospital having
been completely anuric since the previous day. Her subsequent course
is obvious from Fig. 1: the anuria persisted for 4 weeks (which
is unusually long) during which she was maintained alive by
haemodialysis. The recovery was heralded by a polyuric phase during

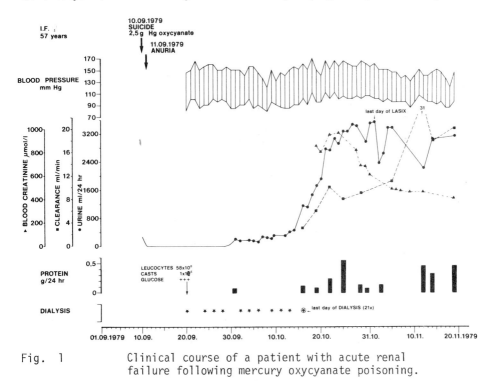

Fig.   1   Clinical course of a patient with acute renal
                      failure following mercury oxycyanate poisoning.

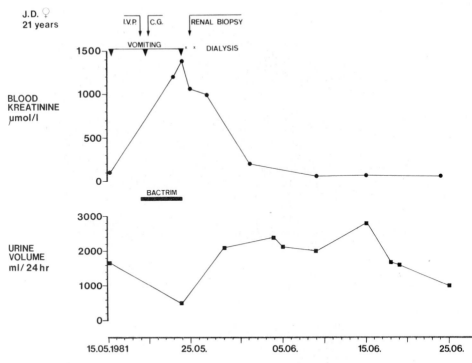

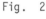

Fig. 2   A case of acute renal failure following
                cholecystoradiography.   (IVP = intravenous
                pyelography;   CG = Cholecystoradiography)

which the glomerular filtration rate rose from 1 ml/min to
20 ml/min 2 months later. At this time she was free from uraemic
symptoms and could be discharged.

2.   Quite frequently during the last 10 years we have encountered
patients in whom, following the administration of certain antibiotics,
iodinated contrast agents etc. the plasma urea and creatinine started
to rise wihin a day or two. The patient may not be feeling well and
may develop uraemic symptoms. There is, however, no dramatic
change of the urine volume, proteinuria is absent or only slight, very
often of a tubular type, and the only striking abnormality is a
severe drop of the urinary osmolality, which may overlast the acute
episode by weeks or months. This is shown by the clinical course
of an 18 years old girl (Fig. 2), who fell sick with an acute
gastrointestinal upset with vomiting, diarrhoea and severe abdominal
pain and was admitted to a peripheral hospital. Because of her
symptoms an IVP and the next day an oral cholecystoradiography
were carried out. After the second procedure the vomiting
intensified for 2 days. 5 days later, a laboratory screening was
carried out which showed her plasma creatinine to be raised at
1100 µM/1 and blood urea at 35,8 mM/1. Urine was free from protein
and contained only a few erythrocytes. The patient was transferred
to our department. The urine output on the first day amounted to
500 ml but rose immediately afterwards. The initial GFR after

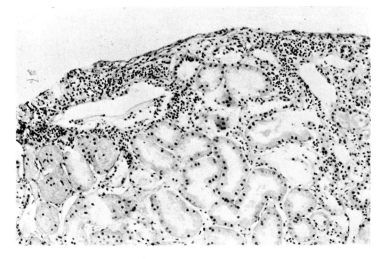

Fig. 3   Renal biopsy of case in fig. 2.

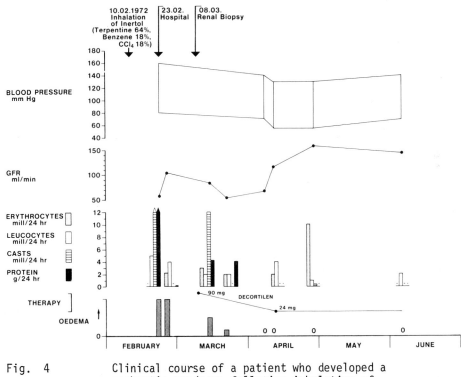

Fig. 4   Clinical course of a patient who developed a
                nephrotic syndrome following inhalation of
                turpentine, benzene and carbon tetrachloride.

admission was 4 ml/min but rose within 4 weeks to 115
ml/min and in the concentration test a specific gravity of 1030
was reached at this time. Renal biopsy (Fig.3) carried out
during the oliguric phase showed a marked interstitial
infiltration with lymphocytes and plasma cells.

3. The patient may develop a renal glycosuria phosphaturia
and aminoaciduria resembling a Fanconi-syndrome. This pattern
is best known after the use of out-dated tetracyclines but
may also follow other agents damaging the function of the
proximal tubular cells, e.g. lead.

4. The patient may develop a glomerular disease with severe
proteinuria leading to a nephrotic syndrome, with decreased
GFR, as documented by Fig. 4. In this case of a 40 years old
male the toxic agent was possibly an inhaled mixture of carbon
tetrachloride, turpentine and benzene, the oedema developed
36 hours later and a prompt permanent recovery followed a
6 weeks course of prednisone. Renal biopsy revealed minimal
proliferative changes in the glomeruli and interstitial
lymphocytic infiltration.   The best known aetiological factor
of such a toxic nephropathy appears to be heroin which leads to
a focal glomerulosclerosis with IgM, IgA, IgG and complement
deposition in the glomeruli, nephrotic syndrome and other typical
features as reported recently by Schreiner [3] (Table 3).

5.   A chronic exposure to a variety of agents, of which the
analgesic combinations are the best known examples, will
produce a pattern of a tubulointerstitial disease which may
be difficult to differentiate from chronic pyelonephritis.
A discontinuation of the exposure may affect a partial or

Table 3   Drug-related heroin nephropathy: pathogenetic mechanisms

1. Rhabdomyolysis and myoglobinuria producing acute tubular
        necrosis

            Coma crush syndrome

            Acute limb myositis

2. Vasculitis

3. Nephrotic syndrome segmental hyalinosis (immunofluorescent-
        positive for IgM, IgA, IgG and complement)

4. S. aureus septicemia

5. Diluent nephropathy (Lead? Quinine? Fungus?)

6. Australia-antigen-positive immune-complex nephritis

Schreiner, [3]

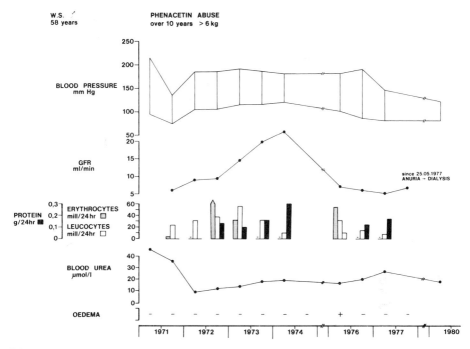

Fig. 5   Clinical course of a parient who had a
phenacetin abuse exceeding 6 kgs in 10 years.

complete restitution. This is illustrated by the course of
a 58 years old male (Fig. 5) who was taking 6 to 8 headache
tablets a day over 10 years (a total phenacetin intake
amounting to almost 6kg). He was well and even playing tennis
until 2 months prior to the admission. Then, he became increasingly tired, short of breath and anorexic and was admitted
to our department almost suffocated and comatose. Because
of a fluid lung haemodialysis was started immediately. His
initial urine volume was 500 ml/min, urine contained only
traces of protein and no cellular elements and the GFR was
below 5 ml/min. Three days later the urine flow rate fell to
2450 - 3130 ml/min. Uraemic symptoms subsided, haemodialysis
could be discontinued and the patient, who lost his headaches,
stopped his analgesic abuse. Later the GFR stabilised at 9 - 12
and eventually, after 2 years, at 20 - 24 ml/min and the patient
was symptom free. Unfortunately, he later took to alcohol,
got a reversible acute liver failure but during that episode
his GFR dropped to 7 ml/min and since 4 years he lives on a
haemodialysis. On the other hand chronic drug abusers of this
kind were until recently among the most frequent candidates of
chronic haemodialysis.

6. In an area round the bend of the Danube in Yugoslavia,
Roumania and Bulgaria, a massing of instances of uraemia was
discovered when improving the health-care after the war. The
patients have strikingly small kidneys, and a typical

functional pattern of interstitial nephropathy. They are restricted to villages and to people who have dwelled in this area for at least 10 years. Recently mycotoxins from the grain kept in these village houses under the roof and possibly getting wet during the rainy seasons, were identified as possible etiologic agents [4,5,6].

7. In the past, when sulfonamides were introduced into therapy and the knowledge of their solubility was not adequate, frequent cases of acute blockage of ureters with acute anuria and renal colic may have been produced by their improper administration. Such a picture is presently encountered in patients with analgesic nephropathy shedding necrotic papillae.

8. A chronic administration of sulfonamides and possibly of other agents can lead to a kidney disease on a vascular immunological basis such as periarteritis nodosa [7].

Many of these syndromes are transient, some of them may be introduced by fever and eosinophilia, in some the toxic agent or its metabolites (lead, paracetamol) may be discovered in the blood or urine. However, as stressed above, the recognition of the proper cause depends on the history. This is all the more important that in the majority of instances, the renal damage is reversible and may heal, if the exposure to the toxic agent is discontinued and if, whenever possible, its excretion from the body can be enhanced (e.g. lead by EDTA).

The possibility of a toxic injury to the kidney has to be considered with any potentially nephrotoxic drug, particularly in the case of combined preparation, or in patients whose kidneys are already damaged, or who are dehydrated.
One has to think of the possibility of a toxic renal pathology in any case of unclear nephropathy. And it may even be that, in the not too distant a future, with a steadily improving control of infection and blood pressure and with an increasing exposure to new chemicals and drugs, the toxic etiology of renal disease will gradually move to the center of interest of the nephrologist.

REFERENCES

1) Spühler O and Zollinger H U, Helv Med Acta 17:564-567, 1950.

2) Oliver, J et al. J Clin Invest 30: 1305-1438, 1951.

3) Schreiner G E, Contr Nephrol 10, 30-41, 1978.

4) Dimitrov M, In Endemic Nephritis in Bulgaria (Puchlev, P ed.) Bulgarian Academy of Sciences, Sofia, 1960, pp.201-207 .

5) Austwick P K C, et al. Contr Nephrol 16: 154-160, 1979.

6)   Krogh P et al. Acta Path Microbiol Scand 85B: 238-240, 1977.

7)   Rich A R et al. Bull Johns Hopkins Hosp 87: 549-568, 1950.

MORPHOLOGY OF THE KIDNEY IN RELATION TO NEPHROTOXICITY —
PORTAE RENALES

D. B. Moffat

Department of Anatomy, University College, Cardiff CF1 1XL, UK

The kidney is made up of four main compartments - vascular, intratubular, intracellular and interstitial. The concentration of substances within these compartments depends upon the unique permeability properties of the various barriers that separate them and there may be large concentration gradients across the barriers. The routes from the vascular to the other compartments - the "portae renales" - are affected by the morphological and biochemical make-up of the barriers. Entrance to the intratubular compartment is mainly via the glomerular filtration membrane and depends upon molecular size, shape and charge, and upon haemodynamic factors. From the tubular lumen filtered substances may enter the tubular cells by specific transport mechanisms or by endocytosis. Transepithelial transport into the interstitium or into the peritubular capillaries varies in different parts of the nephron and may be transcellular or paracellular. Transport in the reverse direction is also possible. The cortical capillaries are permeable to many large molecules and these may appear in the lymph. In the medulla the contents of all four compartments become concentrated but not necessarily to the same degree. The countercurrent exchange mechanism of the vascular bundles may effect trapping of substances in the medulla or may exclude them from it. The fenestrated vessels of the medulla are permeable to many large molecules and in the absence of lymphatics, these are removed from the interstitium by phagocytic cells. It seems likely that exchanges are possible between the pelvic urine and the papillae.

Kidney; morphology; permselectivity; transport mechanisms; concentrating mechanisms; nephrotoxicity.

From the point of view of nephrotoxicity, the main interest in morphological studies lies in the information they can give concerning the routes by which nephrotoxic agents, delivered in the arterial blood, can reach the cells and interstitial tissues of the kidney and the mechanisms by which they may be concentrated in one or more of the compartments. Such routes may perhaps be described as the *portae renales* - the gateways to the kidney substance. Essentially, the kidney can be divided into four compartments - intravascular, intratubular, intracellular and interstitial, the latter draining, at least in part, via a fifth component, the lymphatic system. The kidney differs from other organs in a number of important ways. Firstly, it can really be considered as two organs - the cortex and the medulla. These have a different development, a different blood supply, different functions and different reactions to injury. It will therefore sometimes be necessary, in the account that follows, to treat these two regions separately.

The kidney has a very high blood flow, taking about 25% of the cardiac output, because this blood is not only meant for the nutrition of the organ itself but is also passing through to be processed. For this reason, a relatively large amount of any substance carried by the blood is delivered to the kidney in unit time but a more important consideration than this is the degree to which such substances undergo concentration or dilution in various parts of the kidney parenchyma. The concentration of a substance in the various compartments depends on the unique permeability properties of the barriers between them and there may be very steep concentration gradients across these barriers. Although the contents of the intratubular compartment finally pass to the exterior as the urine, the concentration of any substance in the urine may be quite different from that in the other compartments so that a high urinary concentration of, say, an antibiotic does not necessarily reflect its concentration in the parenchyma. Finally, one must consider the extraordinary *milieu* of the renal medulla where the osmolality of all the compartments may be well over 1000 mOsm, where the pO_2 is much lower than that of the blood in the renal vein (as is that of the urine), where there are no lymphatics although the blood vessels are very permeable to large molecules, and where there is a high turnover of interstitial water that must be removed if the high osmolality is to be maintained.

Figure 1 shows diagrammatically the four principal compartments and the main routes, direct or indirect, between the vascular compartment and the others. These, and other possible routes will now be considered in more detail. It should, perhaps, be stressed that the pathways will be described from a morphological viewpoint and that other physiological factors that may affect the toxicity of drugs, such as the degree of protein binding and the effects of pH and osmolality of the urine have to be considered in addition.

THE GLOMERULUS

As can be seen from Figure 1, the principal route between the vascular and the intratubular compartments is via the glomerular filter. The filtrate consists of the main constituents of the plasma except for the larger molecules, whose possible passage into Bowman's capsule and the tubules depends upon the properties of the filtering membrane which therefore merits detailed consideration. The components of the membrane are shown in Figure 2.

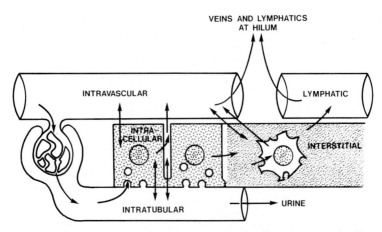

Figure 1.   Diagram to show the "portae renales".

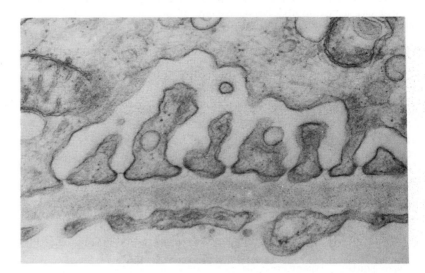

Figure 2.   The glomerular filter. The fenestrated
                             endothelium is at the bottom. Above this
                             is the GBM and then the foot processes.
                             Part of a trabecula is seen above. X 43,200.

Endothelium. The capillary endothelium is thin and fenestrated
so that the blood comes directly into contact with the glomerular
basement membrane(GBM) through the fenestrations. The diameter of
these is 50-100 nm so that they are very much larger than the
physiological "pores" that are described in the glomerular filter.
The endothelial cells have an anionic cell coat that will be discussed
later.

Glomerular basement membrane. The GBM is between 250 and 350 nm
in thickness in the normal human glomerulus but there are species

differences and the thickness increases with age. In electron micrographs it is seen to be composed of three layers, a central darkly stained lamina densa with, on either side of it, a lamina rara interna (nearest to the endothelium) and a lamina densa externa (nearest to the epithelial cell layer). It has a fibrillar structure and biochemically it consists of collagenous and non-collagenous elements. It has important carbohydrate components including certain glycosaminoglycans such as sialic acid and heparan sulphate. These give it its most important physical characteristic - its strongly anionic nature - and this, in turn, accounts for its characteristic staining properties such as its affinity for cationic reagents like Alcian blue and colloidal iron. The anionic sites have been clearly visualised by Kanwar & Farquhar (1) using cationised ferritin. Digestion by heparinase and other techniques have shown that an important contribution to these anionic sites is made by the heparan sulphate along with a small amount of hyaluronic acid (2, 3). Biochemical analysis of the GBM by Parthasarathy and Spiro (4) has confirmed this. They have identified various types of polysaccharide including heparan sulphate - like polysaccharide chains forming part of a proteoglycan, linked by disulphide bonds to a collagenous component.

Epithelial cells. Applied to the external surface of the GBM are the visceral epithelial cells (podocytes). These are highly complicated cells with numerous long processes (trabeculae) which, in turn, give rise to smaller side branches, the foot processes. These are partially embedded in the lamina rara externa of the GBM (Fig. 2). The space between the bases of the foot processes is known as the filtration slit and is 20 - 30 nm in width. It is closed by a thin membrane - the slit diaphragm - which can be seen as a dark line in sections cut at right angles to its plane. In sections that happen to be tangential to the slit diaphragm, when an appropriate fixative is used, the membrane is seen to have a zipper-like appearance with a central dark line running longitudinally and dark and light areas on either side of it (5). The light areas may represent "pores" and are approximately 4 by 14 nm - about the size of the albumin molecule. The podocytes have a strongly anionic cell coat that fills the filtration slit completely. Under certain conditions of fixation the foot processes are seen to be close together all the way along their adjacent edges so that the cell coat fills the whole space between them and the glomerular filtrate has to percolate through it before reaching the urinary space.

Permselectivity of the glomerular filter. Since the endothelial fenestrations are so large compared to the size of the macromolecules that have to be retained in the blood, they offer no barrier, except for the effect of the anionic cell coat which will be discussed later. The glomerular filter therefore consists of the GBM, the slit diaphragm and the space between the foot processes, together with the electrostatic barrier provided by the glomerular polyanion. Prior to 1975, investigation of the permselectivity of the barrier was mainly based upon the perfusion of the kidney with a whole spectrum of molecules of different sizes and either studying their clearance values or trying to visualize them with the light or electron microscope. Such experiments showed that while some large

molecules are held up by the GBM, other smaller molecules are able
to penetrate as far as the slit diaphragm or into the urinary space
of Bowman's capsule. In view of the strongly anionic nature of the
filtering membrane, Chang et al. (6) compared clearance values for
dextran and dextran sulphate while Rennke et al. (7) examined
the filtration of ferritins having different isoelectric points.
The results of these studies, and those of a number of later workers,
showed that the charge of the molecules is as important as molecular
size (or shape) on the filtration properties; cationic molecules
penetrate the membrane more freely than anionic molecules of a similar
size, which are repelled by the fixed negative charges of the glomerular
filter.

The contribution of the glycosaminoglycans of the GBM to the charge
effect has been demonstrated by Kanwar and his colleagues (8, 9).
They removed the heparan sulphate with heparinase and found that native
ferritin was then able to traverse the GBM freely and enter the
urinary space, whereas in control animals it only reached the lamina
rara interna. It was also shown that the regularly spaced anionic
sites, demonstrated by labelling with cationized ferritin, could no
longer be seen after the enzyme treatment.

As well as molecular size, shape and charge, haemodynamic effects
in the glomerular capillaries play an important role in determining
the filtration properties of the glomerulus. Ryan & Karnovsky (10)
studied the filtration of endogenous albumin in Munich-Wistar rats
which have a number of glomeruli on the surface of the kidney. When
the glomeruli were fixed in vivo by dripping fixative directly onto
them, it was found that albumin was held up at, or just beyond, the
endothelial fenestrations. If, however, the circulation was
interrupted before fixation, albumin was found in the GBM and the
urinary space. Different results, however, have been obtained by
Olivietti et al. (11), also using Munich-Wistar rats. They found
that even when fixed under normal haemodynamic conditions, albumin
penetrated to the urinary space in over 70% of the 35 glomeruli they
examined. They also showed that after the administration of
angiotensin II to raise the blood pressure, all the glomeruli examined
showed large amounts of albumin in the urinary space and it was also
found in enlarged mesangial channels. IgG leaked into Bowman's space
in over 80% of glomeruli. The increased permeability in the hypertensive
animals may have been due to the raised blood pressure in the
capillaries or to the binding of angiotensin II to some of the
negative sites in the filtration membrane.

Other functions of glomerular polyanion. It has been suggested
that the foot processes are held apart by the mutual repulsion of
their negative charges. When the anionic sites are blocked, or
removed, by perfusion with cations such as protamine sulphate (12),
treatment with neuraminidase which removes sialic acid (13) or by
culturing isolated glomeruli in the presence of polycations (14), the
epithelial cells undergo changes similar to those in the experimental
and human nephroses with cell swelling, 'fusion' of foot processes and
changes in the slit diaphragm.

As might be expected, proteinuria is also a feature but attempts
to demonstrate the loss of anionic sites in the GBM has given
equivocal results. Caulfield & Farquhar (15) using lysozyme
as a cationic marker, found that in the later stages of puromycin

aminonucleoside nephrosis, lysozyme no longer bound to epithelial cells or the GBM in most of the animals and, where it did bind, the periodicity of the binding sites was lost. Kanwar et al. (9) however, found that while the aminonucleoside produced a nephrotic syndrome, there was no change in the pattern of distribution or the density of the anionic sites when cationized ferritin or cationized cytochrome C were used as markers. They suggested that proteinuria may not only be due to changes in the GBM but also to a disruption of other components of the glomerular capillary walls as well.

Recently Hunsicker et al. (16) have been able to demonstrate all the features produced by neutralization of polyanion in vivo by using the polycation hexadimethrine (HDM). Infusion of this into rats produced a heavy proteinuria after 30 - 50 minutes which was reversible by stopping the infusion. The urine contained not only albumin but also intact IgG, suggesting that the proteinuria was the result of size-related as well as charge-related permselectivity. Electron microscopy showed the HDM to be bound to the laminae rarae of the GBM and to the cell coat of the podocytes. Scanning electron microscopy showed swelling of the foot processes with narrowing of the filtration slits and, in the most heavily proteinuric animals, complete loss of the foot process pattern. The morphological changes, like the proteinuria, were rapidly reversible.

Another sialoglycoprotein in the glomerulus, namely fibronectin, may play an important part in maintaining the normal architecture. Fibronectin appears to act as a tissue adhesive, binding cells to each other or to adjacent structures. Its distribution in human and rat glomeruli has been examined by Dixon et al. by light microscopy (17) and by Courtoy et al. by electron microscopy (18). Both groups of investigators found fibronectin in the mesangium and in the GBM (in the laminae rarae). Kanwar & Farquhar (19) perfused rats with neuraminidase for $\frac{1}{2}$ to 1 hour and found that both endothelial cells and foot processes became detached from the GBM and lost their normal staining properties. Free sialic acid was found in the urine.

The mesangium. This consists of a central core of tissue in the glomerulus, comprising mesangial cells and matrix, around which the glomerular capillaries are closely arranged. Part of the circumference of each capillary is, therefore, not covered by foot processes but has a 'bare area' that is directly in contact with mesangial tissue. Thus there is only a fenestrated endothelium and a thin capillary basement membrane between the blood and the mesangium. The mesangial cells contain microfilaments which are probably contractile and the cells appear to be phagocytic. The mesangial cells are continuous with the lacis cells of the juxtaglomerular apparatus and some authors (20) therefore prefer to call the latter 'extraglomerular mesangial cells'.

The mesangium is of interest in relation to nephrotoxicity on account of its ability to take up large molecules including immune complexes. This property has been studied with a number of tracers including colloidal gold, ferritin and dextrans. All these are able to pass into the mesangial matrix and some, at least, are taken up by the mesangial cells. There is some evidence that the distribution of foreign materials between matrix and cells depends on the size of the molecules, the larger molecules tending to remain in the matrix. Lee and Vernier (21) have recently studied the processes involved in some detail by investigating the fate of aggregated human albumin in mouse kidneys. It was found in the mesangial matrix within 40 minutes of its injection and reached maximum concentration in 8 hours, mainly in the mesangial matrix but with some uptake by the cells. It was later found between the lacis cells, in the walls of arterioles and in the interstitial spaces. The ultimate fate of such materials in the mesangium is unknown but it is possible that they enter the lymphatic system. Albertine and O'Morchoe (22) have shown that small lymphatic vessels come into close relationship with the juxtaglomerular apparatus, which may, incidentally, explain the high concentration of renin in the lymph.

There are still a number of other problems to be solved in connection with the mesangium. Karnovsky and Kreisberg (23) have cultured glomeruli, which produced three types of cells. One of these contained bundles of filaments but they were unable to culture any phagocytic cells. It was suggested that the phagocytic cells in the mesangium might not be resident mesangial cells but cells, perhaps monocytes, that have entered the mesangium from the blood. The differing fate of foreign particles has yet to be explained and it seems probably that this, like the ability of molecules to penetrate the glomerular filter, depends on the charge. Several workers have produced evidence that the mesangial tissue carries negative charges and recently Reale et al (24) using a glutaraldehyde-Alcian blue fixative, have demonstrated polygonal, darkly staining particles, close to the mesangial cells, that were similar in appearance to particles found by previous workers using the same fixative, in the laminae rarae of the GBM.

Another possible route to the mesangium is from the distal tubule via the macula densa. During the course of another investigation (Moffat, unpublished data) Imferon, an iron dextran solution, was injected in a retrogade fashion into a single collecting duct at the tip of the rat papilla.   In a number of experiments the iron particles were consistently found to have passed between the cells of the corresponding distal tubules, particularly in the region of the macula densa. Here it passed into the lacis region and thence into the mesangium where it was taken up by the mesangial cells (Figs. 3 and 4). It is, perhaps, of interest that a glomerular disto-tubular shunt has been described by Biava et al. (25) in Bartter's syndrome in which anastomotic channels developed between the glomerular capillaries and the distal tubule at the vascular pole. It has long been known that the tubular basement membrane of the macula densa is thin and splits up to form a network and cytoplasmic processes extend from the bases of the macula densa cells so that this region may represent a weak spot in the distal tubules. The normal hydrostatic pressure in the distal tubule is approximately 7 mm Hg and that in the glomerular capillaries about 50 mm Hg (with considerable species differences) and it may be that the distal tubule-mesangium pathway could be important when this gradient is reversed for any reason.

THE PROXIMAL TUBULE

The proximal tubule is probably the most important part of the nephron as far as nephrotoxicity is concerned and it will be described in rather more detail than the other parts. Its essential function is the isosmotic reabsorption of salt and water, along with other solutes, and of most of the protein that escapes the glomerular filtering process.

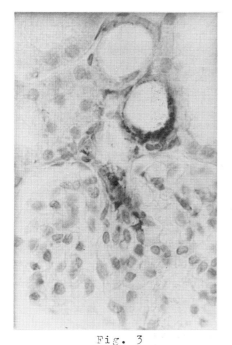 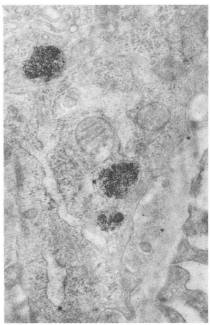

Fig. 3   Fig. 4

Figure 3.   The vascular pole of a glomerulus after the
                   retrograde injection of Imferon into a
                   collecting duct. The darkly staining iron can
                   be seen in the macula densa of the distal tubule
                   and in the mesangium, Prussian Blue, X 600.
Figure 4.   Electron micrograph showing accumulation of iron
                   in a mesangial cell. X 27600.

The structure of the cells is therefore modified to this end and,
in particular, the surface area of both apical and basal surfaces
is increased by the presence of a brush border and of basal
infoldings respectively, while the enzymatic make-up of the two
surfaces is quite different. The morphology and functional
characteristics of the proximal tubule are not identical along its
length, and it has been subdivided in various ways (26). For the
present purpose however it will be sufficient to recognise only the
convoluted part and the deeper straight part, the latter leading
into the loop of Henle.
    The brush border consists of closely packed microvilli which
increase the surface area of the cell 36-fold in the convoluted
part of the tubule and 15-fold in the straight part (27). The
microvilli are covered by a negatively charged cell coat and
between their bases are invaginations of the cell membrane into
the cytoplasm, indicating that endocytosis is taking place in this
region. The cell membrane carries a number of important enzymes
including alkaline phosphatase. This enzyme is present in relatively
large amounts and is released into the urine when the cells are
damaged. The amount of alkaline phosphatase present in the proximal
tubule cells has recently been used to quantify renal damage by
Wachsmuth (28) who studied the optical density of appropriately

stained frozen sections of rabbit kidney after the administration of
cephaloridine.

In the cytoplasm, apical vesicles are plentiful and deeper in the
cells there are a number of other prominent organelles including
peroxisomes and lysosomes. At the base of the cell, the cell membrane
shows a large number of invaginations, each of which is occupied
by a process from an adjacent cell so that the interlocking
processes form a complicated basal labyrinth. The space between
the 'tramlines' of the basal invaginations is therefore intercellular
space and the cell membranes here, as well as those at the lateral
borders of the cells, carry $Na^+ K^+$ ATPase and are closely related
to the large mitochondria that are found in this region. It is into
these intercellular spaces that the active extrusion of sodium
occurs, a process mediated by the enzyme. The relative proportion
of intracellular to extracellular space in various parts of the
tubule wall has recently been calculated by Beck et al. (29). Using
a technique which must surely become one of the most important tools
in the study of nephrotoxicity, namely electron microprobe analysis,
they found that in scanning fields where extracellular space was
present, the concentrations of sodium and chloride were higher than
those in the nucleus, and those of potassium and phosphorus lower.
It was calculated that at the base of the cell, 20% of the scanning
area represented extracellular space.

Transport processes. Reference to Figure 1 will show that there are
two routes from the intratubular to the intracellular compartment,
namely via the cell membrane by specific transport mechanisms, and by
endocytosis. The former route will not be dicusssed in detail because
at the present state of our knowledge it bears little relationship
to morphology except that the distribution of enzymes can be studied
by histochemical methods. Sodium entry is passive, down an electrochemical gradient and is coupled with the entry of other solutes such
as glucose and amino acids. There is also transport of certain
substances such as organic acids in the reverse direction.

Of more interest to the morphologist is the process of
endocytosis by which proteins and large polypeptides are taken
up by the cell. Smaller peptides are probably degraded by
brush border enzymes before absorption (30). Endocytosis has
been studied by using labelled albumin, ferritin, horseradish
peroxidase and other identifiable tracers and it appears that the
first stage is the taking up of the protein into small endocytic
vacuoles between the bases of the microvilli. There is some
evidence, however, that this is often preceded by binding of
protein molecules to the cell membrane. Christensen et al. (31)
examined the effect of molecular charge on protein reabsorption in
the rat, and found that the endocytic uptake of cationized
ferritin was eight to nine times greater than that of anionic
ferritin. Mogensen and Sølling (32) showed that in normal human
subjects, protein reabsorption was inhibited by the simultaneous
intravenous injection of amino acids with a terminal positively
charged group which might be expected to block fixed negative
charges on the cell coat. More to the point of the current topic
is the possibility that nephrotoxic agents bearing positive charges
may be bound in this way and thus be taken into the cell. This
possibility was suggested by Silverblatt & Kuehn (33) as an

explanation of their finding that labelled gentamycin is taken up
by proximal tubule cells.

Once within the cell, the endocytic vesicles (phagosomes) fuse with
the lysosomes of the cell so that the protein within them is exposed
to the digestive action of the lysosomal enzymes. Digestion then
proceeds, at least in part, to amino acid level(34). There is no
convincing evidence for the transepithelial transport of intact
proteins under normal conditions and although uptake through the
contraluminal aspect of the cells can certainly occur, it has not
been directly visualized by tracer methods.

Paracellular transport. The transport of solute and water from
the lumen to the interior of the cell and from the cell to the
interstitial tissue has already been briefly mentioned and part
of this route is paracellular in the sense that sodium, for example,
is primarily extruded into the intercellular spaces. The main
interest of morphologists in recent years has been directed to a
true paracellular route that does not involve the intracellular compartment
at all. When the junctional complex that holds cells together at their
lumenal aspect was first described in detail, it was thought that
the zonula occludens was a continuous impenetrable barrier between
the lumen and the intercellular space, hence its name and its more
commonly used informal name of 'tight junction'. It then became
apparent that this was a misnomer. Electron microscopical studies
have shown that the depth of tight junction can vary in different parts
of the nephron and in some regions colloidal lanthanum can penetrate
the junctions. Electrophysiological studies, too, have demonstrated
a pathway through which the transepithelial resistance is very much
less than the sum of the resistances across two cell membranes (see
(35) for review). Frömter (36) after demonstrating the existence
of such a pathway in *Necturus* gall bladder was able elegantly to show
that the pathway involved the cell junctions by passing a current
from lumen to interstitium and then searching the lumenal surface
with a microelectrode. Whenever the tip of this passed over a cell
border it indicated a negative pulse deflection significantly greater
than that given when it was over the middle of a cell.

Finally, the structure of tight junctions has been displayed
by the technique of freeze fracturing in which the frozen tissue
is split, the fracture sometimes passing through cell junctions and
demonstrating the internal structure of the cell membrane at this
point. This technique shows a series of anastomosing strands in the
tight junctions, indicated by ridges on the P face (the face nearest
to the Protoplasm) and corresponding grooves on the E face (that facing
the Extracellular tissues). Some of the strands may be discontinuous.
The number of strands present correlates well with other morphological
and physiological studies and with the permeability of epithelia and
so the concept of 'tight' and 'leaky' tight junctions has arisen. In
the case of the proximal tubule, the convoluted part is a leaky
epithelium in which the depth of the tight junction is only 20 - 40
nm, the junction is permeable to colloidal lanthanum, has only one or
two strands in freeze fracture preparations and has a low transepithelial
resistance. The straight part, on the other hand, has more elaborate
tight junctions and Roesinger et al. (37) in a study of six species,
have shown that there is an increased number of strands (a mean of
3.8 in the rat, for example), although in the rabbit there was little
difference between the straight and the convoluted parts.

A number of experiments have been designed to attempt to show morphological changes in the intercellular spaces under different transport conditions (38). Tisher and Kokko (39), for example, have shown widening of the intercellular spaces of isolated proximal tubules when sodium and water flux is increased in response to an increase in extratubular oncotic pressure. A number of other workers have shown similar results in various epithelia in response to other stimuli to increased permeability. However, Maunsbach and Boulpaep (38) have recently sounded a note of caution in this respect, having shown that, in the proximal tubules of *Necturus* kidneys, the width of the intercellular spaces was dependant upon the hydrostatic pressure gradient across the epithelium, a steep gradient leading to a decrease in width and vice versa. The decrease in width correlated with the increase in electrical resistance that occurs when the intratubular pressure is increased but there was no correlation between the width of the spaces and the transepithelial water flux. Schiller et al. (40) have also pointed out that in attempting to correlate transepithelial resistance with the structure of intercellular spaces one must also take into account the length of the spaces as influenced by the height of the cells and the relative tortuosity of spaces. In such experiments, too, the conditions of fixation must be rigidly controlled since imperfect fixation may lead to marked changes in the width and configuration of the spaces.

THE REMAINDER OF THE NEPHRON

The straight portion of the proximal tubule gives way abruptly to the thin-walled descending limb of the loop of Henle which, after a long or a short course returns as a thin ascending limb. At the junction between inner and outer medulla another abrupt change in the height of the epithelium indicates the beginning of the thick ascending limb (often known as the medullary straight part of the distal tubule). This leads on into the distal convoluted tubule proper which begins a short distance beyond the macula densa, then into a connecting tubule and finally into a cortical collecting duct. The structural and functional characteristics of the various parts of the distal nephron have been clarified in the last few years as a result of the morphological studies of Kaissling and Kriz (41) and the functional studies of Imai (42), Morel (43) and their colleagues, so it is worth giving here a brief description of the segments.

The thick ascending limb is obviously an actively transporting epithelium with tall cells, numerous large mitochondria, deep basal invaginations and high Na^+ K^+ ATPase activity.
The transepithelial potential difference is about 7 mV lumen positive and an active Cl pump here leads to salt reabsorption without water, thus producing dilution of the tubular contents. Morel (43) has suggested that the salt reabsorption is possibly regulated by vasopressin activity since in the rat, (but not in man), adenylate cyclase activity is stimulated by this hormone. The distal convoluted tubule has a similar structure to that of the thick ascending limb. This changes gradually (abruptly in the rabbit) to a connecting tubule the cells of which have simple basal invaginations and some mitochondria but are otherwise rather pale in appearance. Interspersed with these are some intercalated 'dark' cells. The principal cells of the cortical collecting duct have a still less complicated structure but intercalated cells are still present. In general, the tight

junctions increase in depth and in the number of strands present, reaching their greatest complexity in the collecting ducts (40).

Some uptake of ferritin by endocytosis has been observed in the distal nephron (31), and personal observations) but otherwise the detailed structure and physiological transport processes in this region are too complex to be described here, particularly as there are very marked species differences. It must be mentioned, however, that two properties traditionally associated with the distal convoluted tubule are now suspected not to occur in this segment, namely its permeability to water in response to vasopressin and its secretion of potassium. Morel and his colleagues (43) have shown that this portion of the nephron does not respond to vasopressin stimulation by high adenylate cyclase activity while Stanton et al., (44) showed that potassium adapted rats did not secrete potassium into the distal tubule although the principal cells in the connecting tubule and initial collecting duct responded by a great increase in the extent of their basal invaginations. The intercalated cells were not affected.

THE CORTICAL INTERSTITIAL TISSUE

The interstitial tissue in the cortex is rather more scanty than that in the medulla but is, nevertheless, extremely important since most, if not all of the enormous volume of fluid and solute that is exchanged in the cortex must pass through it (Fig. 1). Kriz and Napiwotzky (45) have estimated that only 26% of the total outer tubular surface is directly related to capillaries while 53.9% of total outer capillary surface is directly related to tubules. Most of the tubular reabsorbate must therefore pass into the interstitium. The interstitial tissue is extremely sparse between the closely opposed tubular and capillary walls but in the angular intervals between them, the interstitium is more copious and contains interstitial cells. The cells themselves are of two main types, one resembling fibroblasts and the other being small round mononuclear cells (46).

The peritubular capillaries are extremely thin-walled (except in that part of the cell that contains the nucleus and other organelles) and, like the glomerular capillaries, are fenestrated. The fenestrations differ from those in the glomerulus, however, since they are small (about 70 nm), more regular in shape, and are closed by a thin membrane. They are, however, highly permeable and ferritin molecules, for instance, can pass through them. Pinter and his colleagues (47) have investigated the size and turnover rate of the interstitial albumin pool using a double injection technique of ^{131}I and ^{125}I albumin and found that the volume of distribution in the cortex of young rats was 1.7 ml/100 g tissue and calculated that this might be contained in 5-10 ml/100 g of tissue.

Lymphatic vessels are found in the interstitial tissue, recognised in electron micrographs by their thin but non-fenestrated endothelium and the absence of a basement membrane. Several authors have found open gaps in the endothelium (45) but Albertine and O'Morchoe (48), who studied the cortical lymphatics of the dog, came to the conclusion that the primary pathway for the uptake of poorly diffusible substances was via cytoplasmic vesicles and the normal intercellular channels.

THE MEDULLA

The medulla, which includes the papilla, contains the loops of
Henle, the collecting ducts, descending and ascending vasa recta and
their associated capillary plexus, and a large amount of interstitial
tissue. Since one of the features of the medulla is the concentration
of the contents of all compartments, the morphological basis of the
concentration process will now be briefly discussed.

Concentration of urine in the medulla. The final stage in the
concentrating process is the reabsorption of water from the collecting
duct, made permeable by the effect of vasopressin, as it passes through
the hyperosmotic medulla. The mechanism by which the medullary
osmotic gradient is developed, however, is still controversial. The
original idea of countercurrent multiplication conceived by Kuhn and
his colleagues involved the active transport of salt out of the
water-impermeable ascending limb of the loop of Henle, which was the
'single effect' to be multiplied throughout the medulla by the
countercurrent flow in the two limbs of the loop. This theory has now
been modified, mainly because the thin ascending limb (TAL) has a very
simple structure and because the active transport of salt out of the
limb cannot be demonstrated. New theories are based on the active
transport of salt out of the thick ascending limb (ThAL) by means of
a chloride pump (leaving only a passive role for the TAL) and they also
include the participation of urea in the process. The ThAL is
morphologically suitable for such active transport; it contains a very
high concentration of $Na^+ K^+$ ATPase, and the existence of a chloride pump
can be demonstrated. Kokko and Rector (49) brought these factors
together by suggesting that the active reabsorption of salt from the
ThAL dilutes the tubular fluid while increasing the osmolality of the
outer medulla. In the cortical and outer medullary collecting ducts,
water is reabsorbed from this hypotonic fluid, producing an increased
intratubular concentration of urea. In the inner medulla this urea
enters the interstitium where it has the effect of extracting water
from the descending thin limb (DTL) causing a rise in salt
concentration in its lumen. The salt leaves the TAL passively and
contributes to the interstitial osmolality. Various modifications
of the basic idea have been published (50), most recently by Bonventre
and Lechene (51). Their hypothesis differs from previous ideas in
that instead of the fluid leaving the inner medulla in the TAL being
hypotonic, the fluid in the DTL is hypertonic to the fluid leaving
the inner medulla via the interstitial - vasa recta compartment. This
could be effected by equilibration of the DTL fluid with the hypertonic
outer medulla or to the active secretion of solute into the DTL. All
these rather complex theories depend upon precise and differing
permeability properties of the various parts of the nephron and, so
far, no theory has been produced that is compatible with all the
experimental findings.

The vascular supply of the medulla. A full account of the vascular
supply of the human kidney has been given by Moffat (52) and only a
brief description need be given here. The blood supply comes mainly
from the efferent arterioles of the juxtamedullary glomeruli. In
addition, the outer surface of the papilla receives a number of
branches from the plexus of vessels in the caliceal wall, which
arch over the caliceal fornix. The efferent arterioles (Fig. 5)

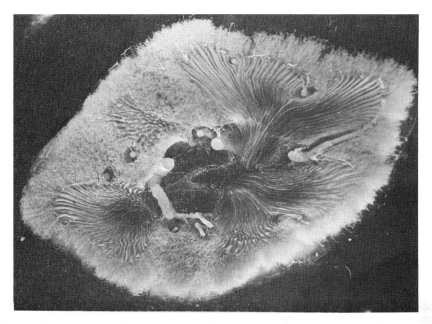

Figure 5.   Human kidney, Microfil injection. Note the
                             vascular bundles, some of which can be seen cut
                             in cross section in the lobe at 10 o'clock.

break up into a bundle of 12-25 descending vasa recta (DVR). The
efferent arteriole and the upper parts of the DVR have smooth muscle
in their walls and are accompanied by nerve fibres. The DVR break
up in turn to form the dense capillary plexus of the outer medulla
and the elongated plexus of the inner medulla. These plexuses are
drained by ascending vasa recta (AVR) which, in the outer medulla,
form vascular bundles together with the DVR. In the bundles the DVR
and AVR come into very close contact with each other, thus forming a
countercurrent exchange system. The AVR end by joining the arcuate
or interlobular veins. In some species there is also a mingling of
some of the DTLs with the vascular components of the bundles (41)
but this probably does not occur in the human kidney.
    Interest in the vascular system of the medulla resides mainly in
two functional aspects. Firstly, the removal of water, which has
entered the interstitium from the collecting duct and from the DTL,
in order to preserve the osmotic gradient. In the absence of lymphatics
this process must be carried out by the AVR. Secondly, in the
possibility of countercurrent exchanges in the vascular bundles.
Transport of solute from the AVR to the DVR would result in recycling
and trapping of the solute in the inner medulla while transport from
DVR to AVR would result in at least a partial exclusion of the solute.
There is a good deal of evidence that such exchanges do occur but
research is hampered by the inaccessibility of the vascular bundles.
    The interstitial tissue.   The interstitial tissue of the medulla
consists of a number of medullary interstitial cells embedded in a
voluminous matrix. The cells are characterized by their content of
lipid droplets and by their well developed and sometimes dilated

granular endoplasmic reticulum. A number of authors have reported
changes in the content of lipid droplets in various conditions such as
hypertension, potassium deficiency and changes in salt and water balance,
but it is difficult to correlate all these effects to produce an idea
of the function of the cells. The most widely accepted notion is, or
was, that the cells are involved in prostaglandin synthesis. The
droplets contain some arachidonic acid, a prostaglandin precursor,
but only a small quantity of prostaglandin synthetase is present, most
of it being in the collecting ducts. Bohman (53) was able to remove
almost all the collecting ducts from kidney slices and found that nearly
half of the total medullary prostaglandin synthetase was in the
collecting duct fraction. The true function of the interstitial cells
must therefore remain in doubt for the present.

Another challenging feature of the interstitium is its high content
of acidic glycosaminoglycans which give it its characteristic staining
reactions with colloidal iron, Alcian blue and Azure A (54). Such stains
show a gradient of colour intensity in the medulla, the deepest stain
being towards the tip of the papilla. Various workers have studied the
effects of diuresis and antidiuresis with equivocal results, but the
balance of opinion favours the idea that in dehydration the intensity
of staining decreases. It is of interest that in an early stage of
papillary necrosis produced in rats treated with analgesics, staining
with Alcian blue was totally lost (55).

It is possible that the cells are connected in some way with the
production of the interstitial ground substance but there is no
convincing evidence for this.

The capillaries and AVR have a fenestrated endothelium and are
highly permeable; protein rapidly leaks out from them into the
interstitium . Such leakage is more marked in diuretic states, at
least in the mature rat (56) and the protein disappears from the
interstitium more rapidly when water diuresis is checked by vasopressin
(57). It is possible that the extravascular protein plays a part
in the maintenance of the osmotic gradient by its water-holding
properties when combined with the glycosaminoglycans. Be that as it
may, the presence of extravascular protein in the medulla and the
absence of lymphatics in this region must raise the question of its
removal. This has been investigated by the injection of small
quantities of ferritin or Imferon into the interstitium of rats
(58). These particles are taken up by phagocytic cells which can
be seen, after Prussian blue staining, to be arranged in long
columns between the tubules of the inner medulla. In the outer
medulla they are found in relation to distended blood vessels and
many of the cells seem to pass through the vessel wall into the
lumen. Whether these cells are modified interstitial cells or
whether they are derived from the blood in response to the foreign
material is, at present, unknown.

TRANSPORT FROM PELVIC URINE TO MEDULLA

The final 'porta', not shown in Figure 1, must be mentioned, namely
the possible pathways between the pelvic urine and the medulla. In
the human kidney, the papillary tissue is separated from the urine in
the calix only by the papillary epithelium while in many animals and
in the immature human kidney (59) the outer medulla is separated from
the urine by an even thinner epithelium. Changes in the intercellular

spaces in these epithelia during diuresis suggest the transport of water, and/or solute across them (60). The perfusion of the intact pelvic cavity with solutions of urea of appropriate concentration increases the osmolality of the urine (61) while, conversely, it is well known that exposing the papilla and so preventing its contact with pelvic urine causes a fall in osmolality. There is thus a possibility that the recycling of urea from the urine to the papillary tissue may be important in maintaining the osmotic gradient. However, Marsh and Martin (62) have produced some evidence against this idea. In hydropenic hamsters they found that slightly more urea reached the ureter than left the collecting ducts, instead of less which would be the case if recycling had occurred.

I should like to express my thanks to Mrs. Diana Hayman, who provided the expert technical assistance for much of my own work which is quoted here.

REFERENCES

1. Kanwar YS and Farquhar MG, J Cell Biol 81: 137-153, 1979.
2. Kanwar YS and Farquhar MG, Proc natn Acad Sci USA 76: 1303-1307, 1979.
3. Kanwar YS and Farquhar MG, Proc natn Acad Sci USA 76: 4493-4497, 1979.
4. Parthasarathy N and Spiro RG, J Biol Chem 256: 507-513, 1981.
5. Rodewald R and Karnovsky MJ, J Cell Biol 60: 423-433, 1974.
6. Chang RLS, et al. Kidney International 8: 212-218, 1975.
7. Renke HG, et al. J Cell Biol 67: 638-646, 1975.
8. Kanwar YS, et al. J Cell Biol 86: 688-693, 1980.
9. Kanwar YS, et al. Renal Physiol Basel 4: 121-130, 1981.
10. Ryan GB and Karnovsky MJ, Kidney International 9: 36-45, 1976.
11. Olivietti G, et al. Lab Invest 44: 127-137, 1981.
12. Seiler MW, et al. Lab Invest 36: 48-61, 1977.
13. Andrews PM, Kidney International 15: 376-385, 1979.
14. Norgaard JOR, Lab Invest 41: 224-236, 1979.
15. Caulfield JP and Farquhar MG, Lab Invest 39: 505-512, 1978.
16. Hunsicker LG, et al. Kidney International 20: 7-17, 1981.
17. Dixon AJ, et al. J Clin Path 33: 1021-1028, 1980.
18. Courtoy PJ, et al. J Cell Biol 87: 691-696, 1980.
19. Kanwar YS and Farquhar MG, Lab Invest 42: 375-384, 1980.
20. Barajas L, Am J Physiol 237: F333-F343, 1979.
21. Lee S and Vernier RL, Lab Invest 42: 44-58, 1980.
22. Albertine KH and O'Morchoe CCC, Kidney International 16: 470-480, 1979.
23. Karnovsky MJ and Kreisberg JI, in Functional Ultrastructure of the
        kidney. (AB Maunsbach, TS Olsen and EI Christensen, eds). Academic
        Press, London, 1980, pp 119-132. ISBN 0-12-481250-3.
24. Reale E, et al. Renal Physiol Basel 4: 85-89, 1981.
25. Biava C et al. Lab Invest 20: 575, 1969.
26. Maunsbach AB, J Ultrastr Res 16: 239-258, 1966.
27. Welling LW and Welling DJ, Kidney International 8: 343-348, 1975.
28. Wachsmuth ED, Histochemistry 71: 235-238, 1981.
29. Beck F, et al. Kidney International 17: 756-763, 1980.
30. Carone FA, et al. Kidney International 16: 271-278, 1979.
31. Christensen EI, et al. Lab Invest 44: 351-358, 1981.
32. Mogensen CE and Sølling K, Scand J clin Lab Invest 37: 477-486, 1976.

33. Silverblatt FJ and Kuehn C, Kidney International 15: 335-345, 1979.
34. Christensen EI and Maunsbach AB, in Functional Ultrastructure of
      the Kidney. (AB Maunsbach, TS Olsen and EI Christensen, eds).
      Academic Press, London, 1980. pp 341-359. ISBN 0-12-481250-3.
35. Tisher CC in Functional Ultrastructure of the Kidney. (AB Maunsbach,
      TS Olsen and EI Christensen, eds). Academic Press, London, 1980.
      pp 191-206. ISBN 0-12-481250-3.
36. Frömter E, J Membr Biol 8: 259-301, 1972.
37. Roesinger B, et al. Cell Tissue Res 186: 121-133, 1978.
38. Maunsbach AB and Boulpaep EL, Kidney International 17: 732-748, 1980.
39. Tisher CC and Kokko JP, Kidney International 6: 146-156, 1974.
40. Schiller A, et al. Cell Tissue Res 212: 395-413, 1980.
41. Kaissling B and Kriz W, Structural Analysis of the Rabbit Kidney.
      Springer-Verlag, Berlin Heidelberg New York, 1979. ISBN 3-540-09145-9.
42. Imai M, Kidney International 15: 346-356, 1979.
43. Morel F Am J Physiol 240: F159-F164, 1981.
44. Stanton BA, Kidney International 19: 36-48, 1981.
45. Kriz W and Napiwotzky P, Contr Nephrol 16: 104-108, 1979.
46. Bulger RE and Nagle RB, Am J Anat 136: 183-204, 1973.
47. Pinter GG, et al. in Functional Ultrastructure of the Kidney.(AB
      Maunsbach, TS Olsen and EI Christensen, eds). Academic Press,
      London, 1980. pp411-422. ISBN 0-12-481250-3.
48. Albertine KH and O'Morchoe CCC, Micro Vascular Res 19: 338-351, 1980.
49. Kokko JP and Rector FC Jr, Kidney International 2: 214-223, 1972.
50. Jamison RL and Robertson CR, Kidney International 16: 537-545, 1979.
51. Bonventre JV and Lechene C, Am J Physiol 239: F578-F588, 1980.
52. Moffat DB, in Renal Disease, 4th edit. (DAK Black and NF Jones, eds)
      Blackwell, Oxford, 1979, pp 3-29. ISBN 0-632-00349-9.
53. Bohman S-O, Prostaglandins 14: 729-744, 1977.
54. Moffat DB The Mammalian Kidney, Cambridge University Press,
      Cambridge, 1975. ISBN 0-521-20599-9.
55. Molland EA, Kidney International 13: 5-14, 1978.
56. Williams MMM , et al. Quart J exp Physiol 56: 250-256, 1971.
57. Moffat DB and Williams MMM, Experientia 30: 556-557, 1974.
58. Moffat DB J Clin Path, 1981 (In the Press).
59. Moffat DB and Laurence KM, Nephron 16: 205-212, 1976.
60. Bonventre JV et al. Am J Physiol 235: F69-F76, 1978.
61. Bonventre JV et al. Am J Physiol 239: F609-F618, 1980.
62. Marsh DJ and Martin CM, Mineral Electrolyte Metab 3: 81-86, 1980.

THE BIOCHEMISTRY OF THE KIDNEY

F. W. Bonner, P. H. Bach and M. Dobrota

Robens Institute of Industrial and Environmental Health and Safety, University of Surrey, Guildford, Surrey GU2 5XH, UK

ABSTRACT

The kidney is characterised by a disproportionately high oxygen consumption in relation to its mass. The energy generated by renal metabolic processes is required to support the many active transport phenomena such as glucose, amino acid, inorganic and organic acid reabsorption and secretion, that contribute to the capacity of the kidney to maintain a relatively constant internal environment. It is also apparent that the kidney is a highly heterogeneous organ, being composed of many cell types. The biochemical properties of the kidney are closely related to anatomical regions. This paper emphasises the need to relate biochemical function to the various cell populations and dicusses intermediary metabolism in relation to the distribution of enzymes along the nephron.

Keywords: kidney; biochemistry; intermediary metabolism; enzyme
             distribution.

INTRODUCTION

The kidney has the capacity to perform many complex and diverse functions simultaneously, such as filtration, concentration and secretion, in order to fulfil the primary purpose of maintaining homeostasis. A discussion of the functional anatomy of the kidney has been presented by Moffat (this volume). In the same way that specialised functions can be attributed to particular anatomical regions of the kidney, so too can specific biochemical processes be related to functional differences both along and between nephrons. This 'heterogeneite des nephrons' as opposed to 'heterogeneite du nephron' has been discussed [1]. The maintenance of normal renal function necessitates a dynamic biochemical status which is reflected by the high renal blood flow and oxygen uptake. It is not

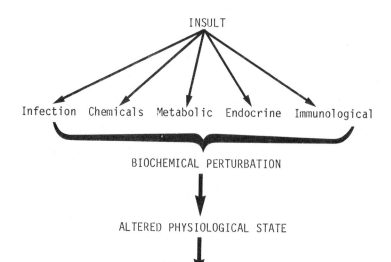

Figure 1.   The events underlying the origin of renal damage.

surprising, therefore, that the kidney is a common target organ for toxic chemicals.   A potentially toxic agent is delivered in high concentrations via the systemic circulation and, due to the filtration and concentrating capacity of the kidney, may accumulate to critical cellular concentrations.   The kidneys are also sensitive to extra-renal factors such as changes in blood flow or neural activity, and thus biochemical processes are susceptible to disruption by a variety of factors.   The events underlying the origin of renal damage are represented schematically in Figure 1.

An understanding of renal diseases and the mechanisms of action of nephrotoxic substances requires a thorough knowledge, not only of renal morphology, but also of the molecular processes underlying renal function and the biochemical inter-relationships and inter-dependences of its various cell populations.   It is not the purpose of this article to provide a detailed discussion of the various pathways of intermediary metabolism since such processes, as they occur in other organs, are well documented elsewhere, and have been discussed in more detail in relation to the kidney [2].

BIOCHEMICAL CHARACTERISTICS OF RENAL CORTEX AND MEDULLA

The kidney must be regarded as a highly heterogeneous tissue from anatomical, physiological and biochemical considerations.   Thus the interpretation of biochemical data derived from whole organ studies is complicated, and may be misleading.   Any approach to understand the complex array of metabolic processes that occur in the kidney must recognise this, and attempts to investigate the problem of metabolic heterogeneity using a variety of experimental techniques (such as microdissection) should be further developed [1]. However, at present

Table 1. Biochemical processes occurring predominantly in the renal cortex or medulla.

CORTEX	MEDULLA
Gluconeogenesis	Glycolysis
Fatty acid utilisation	Lipogenesis
Prostaglandin catabolism	Prostaglandin synthesis
Cytochrome P450 drug	Co-oxygenation of
metabolim	xenobiotica
Vitamin D metabolism	
Deamination	

there is a lack of information regarding the biochemistry of individual nephron segments and a paucity of data on individual cell types.

The significant involvement of the kidney in metabolic processes is reflected by the high rate of oxygen uptake and Table 1 summarises some of the biochemical pathways that can be attributed to either cortex or medulla. Each of these two regions has distinctive metabolic features.   For instance, the cortex has a considerably higher blood flow and correspondingly higher rate of oxygen utilisation.   It has been estimated that the inner medulla of the dog, whilst contributing 10% of total kidney weight, receives only 1% of the renal blood flow [3] but oxygen utilisation corresponds to less than 5% of that used by the cortex [4].   The medulla is also deficient in mitochondria compared with the cortex [5], and respiratory enzymes for oxidative metabolism are less plentiful [6] e.g. histological staining techniques have failed to demonstrate the presence of succinic dehydrogenase in the inner medulla [7].   However, all the enzymes directly involved in the oxidation of citrate or isocitrate are more active in the medulla than in the cortex [8].   The distribution of a number of enzymes in various segments of the human kidney is described below and in Figure 2.

The predominant metabolic process in the medulla is glycolysis, while gluconeogenesis is characteristic of the cortex.   It has, therefore, been assumed that the medulla depends mainly on anaerobic metabolism.   The cortex is certainly capable of considerable substrate uptake and utilisation via aerobic processes and in vitro the capacity of mammalian renal cortex to utilise oxidative pathways far exceeds that of the medulla [9].   This infers that active solute transport by nephron segments in the renal cortex derive energy from oxidative pathways whereas those segments located in the medulla depend upon non-oxidative.   Such results have been used to emphasise the dependency of the cortex on a continuous oxygen supply in contrast to the medulla where oxygen demands appear to be less critical. However, aerobic metabolism is only limited at pO_2 of less than 1 mm Hg (compared to a medullary pO_2 of 5-15 mm Hg and cortical pO_2 of 75 mm Hg) and this together with recent metabolic studies, may suggest that glycolysis in the inner medulla is not obliged to be anaerobic.

INTERMEDIARY METABOLISM IN THE KIDNEY

Carbohydrates   It has been commonly assumed that gluconeogenesis is characteristic of the renal cortex while glycolysis is the sole

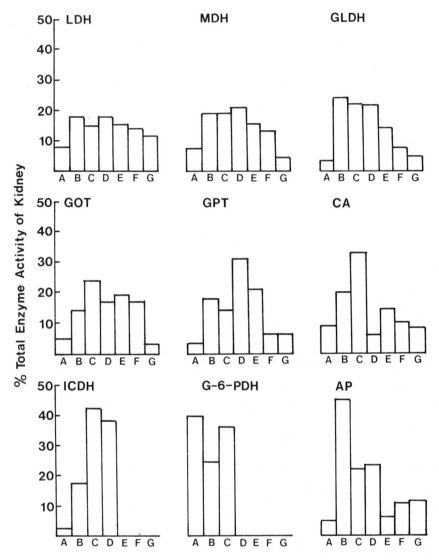

Figure 2.   The distribution of enzymes along the nephron   of the
             normal human kidney (from Mattenheimer, [10]).

Expressed as % of total activity.   Regions of the nephron correspond
as follows: A: glomeruli;   B: proximal convolutions;   C: distal
convolutions; D: medullary ray; E: outer medulla; F: inner medulla;
G: papilla.

LDH - Lactate dehydrogenase; MDH - malate dehydrogenase; GLDH -
glutamate dehydrogenase;   GOT - glutamate oxatoacetate transaminase;
GPT - glutamate pyruvate transaminase; CA - carbonic anhydrase;
ICDH - isocitrate dehydrogenase; G-6-PDH - glucose-6-phosphate
dehydrogenase; AP - alkaline phosphatase.

metabolic function of the medulla.   Renal gluconeogenesis from lactate, pyruvate, amino acids and the intermediate products of the citric acid cycle was first demonstrated by Benoy and Elliott [11] using tissue slices.   The liver must be regarded as the major site of gluconeoenesis but the kidney normally contributes some 20% of the total production of glucose.   During prolonged starvation or acidosis, hepatic gluconeogenesis decreases while that of the kidney increases such that the two organs contribute almost equally to the formation of glucose [12].   The effects of renal gluconeogenesis include:-

1.   The provision of glucose and maintenance of energy production,
2.   The production of ammonia in order to counteract acidosis,
3.   The metabolism of amino acids,and
4.   The utilisation of lactate, glycerol etc.

   The end product of renal gluconeogenesis tends to be glucose rather than glycogen because the capacity of the kidney to store glycogen is limited [13].   The overall rate of gluconeogenesis in the kidney is sensitive and adaptive to changes, for instance in diet.   A low carbohydrate intake has been shown to increase the activities of some enzymes such as glucose-6-phosphatase [14, 15].
   The metabolism of carbohydrate in the renal medulla has been reported to be anaerobic [16] i.e. glycolytic (see previous section),based upon the early observations of Gyorgy et al [17] and confirmed by others [18].   However, Cohen has pointed out that there is significant aerobic glycolysis in the papilla and inner medulla [16]: the rate of aerobic metabolism by inner medulla slices was, in fact, considerable in the early experiments.   It has been shown by Holmes and Di Scala [19] using renal slice techniques, that the rat inner medulla exhibited a greater rate of glycolysis (compared to the cortex) but the outer medulla has a significant capacity for both aerobic and anaerobic metabolism.
   The utilisation of glucose in relation to renal function has been discussed. Frega et al [20], have shown that the addition of glucose to a perfusate, containing fatty acid as the only metabolic substrate,produced an increased fractional reabsorption of sodium, and increased glomerular filtration rate.   Such observations did not appear to be explained by sodium/glucose co-transport and it was concluded that oxidative processes were responsible for the effects since glucose is rapidly oxidised by perfused kidneys.   The results of Gregg et al [21],using isolated rat kidneys have also been used to relate sodium reabsorption to the energy production from renal glucose oxidation.
   There is little information on the oxidative metabolism in the medulla, but results [8] indicate that medullary mitochondria are capable of efficient oxidation of most citric acid cycle inter-mediates, as well as pyruvate and glutamate.   There appear to be no differences in the rate of oxidation of such substrates by the medulla or by the cortex.   On the basis of the work of Mikulski et al [8], and others [22],it appears that the synthesis of energy rich compounds in the medulla may be derived from either glycolysis or the oxidative metabolism of the citric acid cycle intermediates, but the greater efficiency means that more energy is produced via the oxidative processes.
   Most investigations of medullary biochemistry have used slices or homogenates, thus the exact contribution of the different cell types

to functional energy dynamics and the changes that underly, for example diuresis or anti-diuresis, have yet to be related to the phosphorylation and redox states within these individual cell types. Until these investigations have been undertaken, the exact role of altered intermediate metabolism must remain a matter for speculation.

Finally, carbohydrates are stored in the medulla as glycogen or glycosaminoglycan, the former in the collecting ducts and epithelia, and the latter as the major constituent of the interstitial ground substance. There is evidence to suggest that both of these polysaccharides may be metabolised to provide either an energy source or the "sugar" units for the synthesis of other macromolecular carbohydrates [23].

Fatty Acids The exact contribution of fatty acids to the fuel of respiration is subject to debate, but is known to be greatly influenced by the acid-base status of the organism. The renal cortex has one of the highest rates of oxygen consumption of any tissue, but its respiratory quotient is very low. This suggests extensive oxidation of fatty acids. Both in vivo and in vitro experiments have demonstrated a rapid utilisation of fatty acids in the cortex [24-26]. Whereas Pitts [27] has suggested that 16-22% of renal oxidative metabolism is supported by fatty acids. Hohenleitner and Spitzer [24] have put the contribution of fatty oxidation acids as high as 60-80% of the fuel of respiration. Similar evidence may also be derived from the data of Lee et al [28] who studied the in vitro metabolism of ^{14}C-labelled substrates using rabbit kidney cortex and medulla slices. Weidemann and Krebs [29] studied the contributions of a variety of substrates (including glucose, lactate, acetoacetate, butyrate, oleate and endogenous substances) to cortical respiration. They concluded that fatty acids and acetoacetate would be the main exogenous substrates when they were available in physiological concentrations. When exogenous fatty acids are not available the main source of respiratory energy is fatty acids derived from endogenous tri-acylglycerols [29]. During periods of starvation the kidney takes up more fatty acid than can be utilised on the basis of oxygen consumption [30]. It is not clear why this occurs, but for every four fatty acid molecules taken up, three appear as tri-acylglycerols which may suggest storage especially since, in the kidney, tri-acylglycerols are precursors for fatty acids whilst the capacity for fatty acid de novo synthesis is very low. Glycerol oxidation is even more active in the cortex than liver, but it is apparently not metabolised by the medulla [28]. Glycerokinase activity has been demonstrated in rat kidney [32] thus glycerol oxidation is thought to occur by phosphorylation to L-α-glycerophosphate.

It is well known that liver microsomes catalyse the hydroxylation of various fatty acids to ω-and (ω-1)-hydroxy derivatives [33, 34], and that cytochrome P-450 is the oxygen activating component [35]. Cytochrome P-450 of rat kidney cortex microsomes has also been shown to be involved in the hydroxylation of fatty acids [36]. The hydroxlyation of laurate in renal cortex occurs at similar rates to the liver but the substrate specificity for the two systems is different. The kidney microsomes do not appear to hydroxylate testosterone to any measurable extent [37]. Ellin et al have suggested a more specific role for kidney cortex Cytochrome P-450 in fatty acid oxidation compared to the liver indicated by the size of

Table 2. Comparison of the fatty acid composition of the medullary
interstitial cell lipid inclusion bodies isolated from papillary
slices and plasma tri-aclylglycerols in the rat.

FATTY ACIDS Trival name (carbon number: number of double bonds)		PERCENTAGE Medullary Interstital Cell Droplets	Plasma
Saturated:-			
Myristic acid	(14:0)	< 5	< 5
Palmitic acid	(16:0)	±15	±30
Stearic acid	(18:0)	±15	± 5
Arachidic acid	(20:0)	< 5	-
Unsaturated:-			
Palmitoleic acid	(16:1)	< 5	-
Oleic acid	(18:1)	±15	±30
Linoleic acid	(18:2)	±15	±30
Linolenic acid	(18:3)	< 5	< 5
Cis-11-eicosenoic acid*	(20:1)	< 5	-
Cis-11,14-eicosa- dienoic acid*	(20:2)	< 5	-
Homo-γ-linolenic acid	(20:3)	± 5	-
Arachidonic acid	(20:4)	±15	-
Adrenic acid	(22:4)	±15	-

* Non-trival names. After data published by Bojsen[38,39,41].

the Type I spectral change produced on the addition of laurate to
isolated microsomes.

On the other hand, lipogenesis appears to be a most important
function of renal medulla. The numerous lipid droplets in the
interstitial cells (see Moffat, this volume) have been found to
contain traces of cholesterol esters and a few · percent of
phospholipids, mainly phosphatidyl-choline, and rarely, trace amounts
of phosphatidyl-ethanolamine. A few percent of free fatty acids and
tri-acylglycerols make up the remaining 80-90%; the composition of
which varies in different species and is shown for the rat in Table 2.
The most striking features are the large amounts of various types of
unsaturated fatty acids; most notably those of 20 or more carbon
atoms such as arachidonic acid and especially adrenic acid. The
large amount of arachidonic acid suggests that the interstitial lipid
droplets may be an important pool for prostaglandin (PG) synthesis
(see below) in the kidney [38, 39].

Using rat kidney medulla slices and eviscerated anaesthetised rats
Bojesen et al [40, 39] have shown that [1-^{14}C] acetate was
incorporated into tri-acylglycerols and phospholipids (only a few
percent was found in free fatty acids) where adrenic acid (docosa-
7,10,13,16-tetraenoic acid) accounted for 40% of the tri-acylglyerol
and 20% of the phospholipid fatty acids. Acetate was incorporated
into myristic, palmitic, stearic and adrenic acids, but only myristic
and palmitic acids were synthesised de novo . Fatty acids with 18 or
more carbon atoms were found to be labelled predominantly on the

carboxyl group, suggesting chain elongation of some prevalent fatty acid, such as arachidonic to adrenic acid.   Label was, however, absent from arachidonic acid suggesting that it was not synthesised from linoleic acid in this tissue.

Radiolabelled glucose has also been shown to be a lipogenic precursor [39, 41] which provided 70% and 80% of the glycerol backbone to renal interstitial tri-acylglycerol and phospholipids respectively. The remaining ^{14}C activity was found in the bound fatty acids, with 40 to 60% in saturated molecules and most of the remainder in adrenic acid, as was the case for acetate lipogenesis.   This suggested that both glucose and acetate shared a common acetyl-CoA pool from which lipogenesis proceeds.   Glucose also contributed more to fatty acid chain elongation than to de novo synthesis, but, in common with acetate, no labelled arachidonic acid was formed.

Bojesen [39, 41] also estimated the rate of renewal of the different fatty acids into phospholipids and tri-acylglycerols, and concluded that the hydrolytic release of fatty acids and their reincorporation (after de novo synthesis or chain elongation) into glycerolipids either phospholipid or tri-acylglycerol) was rapid enough to account for pathophysiological changes in the number and size of lipid droplets.   Bojesen [41] estimated a half-life of 25h for membrane phospholipids, while lipid droplet tri-acylglycerols had a half-life of 11h.

The spectrum of fatty acid synthesis varied in vitro (medulla slices) compared to the in vivo (anaesthetised, eviscerated rat) situation, probably due to the contribution of plasma free fatty acids which could act as substrates for chain elongation [38, 39, 41].

An increased osmolality (in vitro) depressed lipogenesis overall from both acetate and glucose and also altered the distribution of incorporated label from glucose, providing more of the glycerol backbone and proportionately less to the fatty acids [39, 41, 42].

Short term (4 day) dietary loading with linoleic acid had pronounced effects on plasma fatty acids, but caused only a slight change in the papillary tri-acylglycerol fatty acids.   Long term (12 week) feeding also failed to produce dramatic changes in the papillary lipids.   Bojesen [41] suggested that the fatty acid profile of the renal papilla was species- and tissue-specific rather than dependent on diet.

INTEGRATION OF RENAL INTERMEDIATE METABOLISM

In view of the complexity and diversity of biochemical functions in pathways of degradation and synthesis occur in controlled relationship to one another, and in different "anatomical" regions of the kidney. Since glycolysis and gluconeogenesis have a number of enzymes in common, it is reasonable to assume that regulation of the activity of these enzymes will control both the rate and direction of glucose metabolism.   Such control mechanisms   have been discussed in detail [12,43-44], and there is evidence that pyruvate carboxylase, fructose-1,6-diphosphatase, phosphofructokinase, and phosphoenolpyruvate carboxykinase function in a regulatory capacity.   In addition hexokinase and glucose-6-phosphatase may be regulatory for the kidney [43]. Gluconeogenesis in the cortex can be stimulated by catecholamines and it has been demonstrated that this occurs through an α-type adreno-receptor [45].

Fatty acid oxidation/gluconeogenesis/ketogenesis   The concentration of acetyl-CoA may be envisaged as playing a central role in the
integration of several metabolic pathways in the kidney.   Acetyl-CoA
is a common regulatory factor for gluconeogenesis and ketogenesis from
lactate.   Fatty acid oxidation in kidney cortex can also lead to
increased concentrations of acetyl-CoA, thus the regulation of all
three pathways is linked.   Whenever acetyl-CoA accumulates, a
proportion is converted to acetoacetyl-CoA.   However, the mechanism
of ketogenesis appears to be different in the kidney compared to the
liver.   In the liver ketone body formation normally proceeds via the
β-hydroxy-β-methylglutaryl-CoA pathway, but the kidney only has very
low activity of β-hydroxy-β-methylglutaryl-CoA synthetase which is a
vital enzyme.   Instead 3-oxo acid CoA-transferase is present and most
likely accounts for the rates of ketogenesis from fatty acids [29].

BIOCHEMISTRY OF THE KIDNEY IN RELATION TO ENZYME DISTRIBUTION

The mammalian kidney contains at least 12 readily identifiable cell
types [46].   It is thus not surprising that such a heterogeneous
complement of cells possesses such a diverse complement of enzymes.
Kidney enzymes have been studied by classical histochemical and subfractionation methods.   However, the most useful information on the
distribution of enzymes amongst the various cell types has come from
the very elegant microdissection studies in which the whole nephron
has been segmented into distinct regions [47].
The following brief survey of kidney enzymes is rather loosely
classified on the basis of their biochemical function.

ENZYMES INVOLVED IN ENERGY PRODUCTION

Glycolysis and Krebs cycle.   The kidney has the highest oxygen
consumption of any mammalian organ and it is therefore rich in various
oxido-reductases and other enzymes involved in the generation of ATP.
The activity of these enzymes is high in tubular regions, lower in the
glomerular and lowest in the papilla [48].   The high activity of
these respiratory enzymes is now thought to be associated with sodium
transport [49].
There is also morphological evidence for the distribution of these
enzymes;   there are numerous large, branched mitochondria [50] in
tubular cells, but fewer mitochondria are present in other cell types.
Oxygen consumption of the different regions follows the distribution
of respiratory enzymes very closely [6].   The cortex contains the
enzymes of the citric acid cycle, whilst the medulla and papilla are
essentially glycolytic in parallel with regional oxygen consumption.
A typicial citric acid cycle enzyme, succinic dehydrogenase, has the
highest activity, taken as 100%, in the thick ascending loop, with 30%
in the proximal convoluted tubule, 60% in the straight proximal
tubule, 43% in the distal convoluted tubule, 14% in glomeruli and 9%
in the collecting ducts [51].
Gluconeogenesis   The kidney is capable of significant glucose
production.   A key enzyme of gluconeogenesis, phosphoenolpyruvate
carboxykinase is reported to be found only in the proximal convulted
tubule [52].   Gluconeogenesis of the kidney is in fact ascribed to
this region [49].
Ammoniagenesis   Glutamine, which is avidly taken up by the
kidney, is broken down to ammonia and thus contributes to the urinary

acid/base balance [53]. The enzymes, glutaminase, glutamate deaminase
and glutamate dehydrogenase catalyse the major steps of
ammoniagenesis.   These enzymes are found in the mitochondria of the
convoluted and straight proximal tubule cells [54].   Ammoniagenesis
and gluconeogenesis are closely linked since the enzymes of the two
pathways have similar distributions [55] and glutaminase has been
reported to contribute to gluconeogenesis [54].

    Fatty acid metabolism   Oxidation of fatty acids is an important
source of energy in the kidney [56]. Total fatty acid metabolism is
three times greater in the renal cortex than in the medulla and twice
that of the liver [28]. The kidney differs from the liver and derives
energy from either long chain fatty acids or ketone bodies.

    Virtually no data is available on the distributions of individual
enzymes of renal fatty acid metabolism.   Little is known about the
enzymes of the different forms of fatty acid oxidation or the
contribution made by peroxisomal β-oxidation.   Although peroxisomes
of the kidney have not been comprehensively studied, the presence of
fairly active catalase in kidneys [57] indicates functional
peroxisomes.

ENZYMES INVOLVED IN CATION TRANSPORT

    Na/K-ATPase plays an essential role in the transport of sodium
(possibly other cations) across the renal cell membranes.   The
highest activity of this enzyme is found in the distal and is lowest
in the proximal tubule [58]. Thus the distribution of Na reabsorption
is quite opposite to that of fluid and macromolecule reabsorption.
Na/K-ATPase appears to be regulated by aldosterone levels [59].
Because of its plasma membrane (PM) location the enzyme has often been
used in subfractionation studies as a marker enzyme when it exhibits a
subcellular distribution identical with other PM markers such as
alkaline, phosphatase, maltase etc.   However, the latter enzymes
originate from the proximal tubule PM whilst Na/K-ATPase is found in
the distal tubule.

    Sodium transport is apparently driven by ATP, which may be
generated from glucose and lactate, but not fatty acids.   Thus the
"type" or perhaps the location of the ATP that has been generated may
influence the transport of Na.   The transport of Na may also have a
role in the transport of other small molecules since, in the absence
of intra-luminal Na, the transport of amino acids and hexoses is
virtually eliminated [60].

    Calcium ATPase is found uniformly distributed throughout the
nephron [61], both in the plasma membrane and in the mitochondrial
membrane.   Its function is to maintain low intracellular Ca
levels and high levels within the mitochondria [62]. Two forms of the
enzyme, a low and a high affinity may be found in the kidney [63] but
the reasons for this dichotomy are not understood.

ACID HYDROLASES

    The kidney contains an abundance of lysosomal hydrolases [64].
Isolated glomerular and tubular fractions from rabbit kidney cortex
have very different acid hydrolase distributions [65]; acid
phosphatase [assayed with p-nitrophenol(pNP)-phosphate] is 5 times
more active in glomeruli than in tubules, whilst β-galactosidase is 4

times greater in tubules than in glomeruli and aryl sulphatase (A, B) is 2-3 times greater in glomeruli.   Similar acid phosphatase distribution in the human kidney has been reported [66].   However, acid hydrolases assayed (using 4 methylumbelliferone substrates)   in segmented isolated single nephrons [47] exhibit a different pattern. Acid phosphatase is highest in the proximal tubule, somewhat lower in the glomerulus and lowest in the distal tubule.   pNPphosphate is not an ideal substrate for acid phosphatase, and the results of Helwig et al [65] may not be as reliable as those of Le Hir et al [47].   Other enzymes measured by Le Hir et al showed that β-galactosidase was very low in glomeruli, high in the convoluted proximal tubule and highest in the first part of the straight proximal, but then gradually decreased down the length of the tubule. N-acetyl β-glucosaminidase (NAG) is extremely low in glomeruli, has a distinct peak   in the convoluted proximal tubule, has high activity in the collecting duct but is low elsewhere in the tubule.   This high activity of NAG in the collecting duct might be involved in glycosaminoglycan metabolism. These results in general agree with the biochemical data of Taylor et al [67] and the histochemical data of Lansdown and Ellaby [68].   In conclusion most renal acid hydrolases are involved in handling reabsorbed macromolecules in the proximal tubule: acid phosphatase may also exhibit a glomerular function.

Subfractionation studies on kidney cortical lysosomes [64,69,70,71] have revealed two (or possibly more) enzymically and morphologically heterogenous populations. The kidney possesses specific large granules (protein droplets) which are found in the proximal tubule cells, which contain the full complement of hydrolytic enzymes and are involved in the breakdown of reabsorbed plasma proteins [72].   The protein droplets are found mainly in the proximal tubule cells thus indicating that acid proteinases, such as the cathepsins, are also found in these cells. In addition the kidney also has a heterogeneous mixture of small lysosomes which have a heterogeneous acid hydrolase content [70, 71,73,74].   The acid proteinases [75] and acid glycosidases [76] which are localised in the glomerulus, are thought to be associated with the catabolism of the glomerular basement membrane.   The cellular origin of the small lysosomes is not known but they may be in specific cell types (i.e. glomerulus, juxtaglomerular complex, epithelial) or they may be present together with the large granules in the proximal tube cell.

Some lysosomal enzymes are also found in other organelles.   β - Glucosidase [70], NAG [77] and acid phosphatase are also present in the cytosol.   NAG has also been associated with the "microsomal" fraction [70]. These are all probably multiple forms of the lysosomal enzymes,   which   may   contain   different   glyco-residues   and phosphomannosyl recognition markers.

Acid and neutral phospholipase, which are possibly involved in membrane fusion, have been found in the lysosomal membrane of the rat kidney   [78].   Phospholipase may also affect membrane permeability and hence transport and secretion of many different molecules. Phospholipase A_2 degrades membranous phospholipids to produce arachidonic acid which may serve as a precursor to prostaglandins [79].

OTHER HYDROLASES AND SPECIFIC PROTEASES

The mammalian kidney specifically contains renin, a highly specific protease which is localised, in its active form, in lysosomal granules [80] in the epithelial cells of the juxtaglomerular complex. An inactive, high molecular weight form of renin is found in the cytosol of the same cells. Cytochemically renin granules have been shown to contain acid phosphatase, β-glucuronidase, NAG and aryl sulphatase [81]. Renin increase (induced by artery clip-hypertension) is accompanied by increases in some acid hydrolases [82] suggesting that renin granules may be specific types of, or related to lysosomes. Although at present the "distinct renin granule-lysosome" controversy is unresolved, it is clear that renin-associated acid hydrolases are involved in the secretion of renin.

Renin releases angiotensin I from circulatory kinins. The conversion of angiotensin I to the powerful vasoconstrictor angiotensin II is accomplished by another specific kidney located enzyme, "converting enzyme" or kininase II. Converting enzyme is reported to be located on the outer (luminal) plasma membrane (brush border) of the proximal tubule cells [83]. This location is somewhat puzzling, since it suggests that angiotensin I, and the vasoactive product angiotensin II, are present and active in the filtrate.

Glandular kallikrein is yet another renal protease involved in the control of blood pressure. The action of kallikrein is to convert circulating kininogens into kinins, which are active vasodilators. Renal kallikrein is localised in the convoluted distal tubule from the macua densa to the collecting tubules [84]. Intracellularly it is associated with endoplasmic reticulum and plasma membranes and appears to have ectoenzyme activity, thus releasing kinins without being secreted. The physiological role of kallikrein has been discussed in detail [85]. A detailed survey of mechanisms controlling blood pressure has been presented (see Thurston, this volume).

The vasoactive action of kinins is terminated by very active and abundant neutral ectoproteinases which are found on the brush border of the proximal tubule [86]. Thus those active kinins which enter the glomerular filtrate are destroyed. Kinins may appear in urine, together with kallikrein, but only when they have been secreted from cells distal to the proximal tubule.

Other proteases, which may be found in the kidney, in cases of glomerulonephritis, may be of extrarenal origin. Davis et al [75] have demonstrated that elastase and cathepsins may be released from invading polymorphs in the glomerulus.

DRUG METABOLISING ENZYMES

Two of the kidney's mechanisms for detoxifying xenobiotics, the P-450 system of the cortex and the prostaglandin endoperoxide synthetase of the medulla and papilla, are comprehensively discussed by Rush and Hook (this volume). It is noteworthy to emphasise that the kidney contains considerably less P-450 than the liver. However, Lake et al [87] have reported that 3-methylcholanthrene induced benzpyrene hydroxylase in the kidney was activated 20-fold whilst the liver enzyme was activated only 5-fold. All other enzymes were induced more significantly in the liver.

The kidney is also capable of detoxifying and excreting foreign compounds by conjugation reactions. However, its capacity, like the

P-450 system, is considerably lower than that of the liver.   The activity of UDP glucuronyltransferase, found in the cortical 'microsomal' fraction, is about 1.4-fold lower than that of the liver in the glucuronidation of aromatic drugs and 16 to 41-fold lower for steroids [88]. The kidney is also capable of other enzyme catalysed conjugation reactions in N-acetyl [89], glycine, alanine, serine [90] aspartate [91] glutathione [92] and sulphate [93].

NUCLEASES, PHOSPHATASES AND RELATED ENZYMES

Little is known about the renal endo- and exo-nucleases which catabolise nucleic acids.   There are, however, a number of reported phosphodiesterases which attack cyclic nucleotides.   Cytochemical localisation of a cyclic AMP phosphodiesterase has been demonstrated [94] in the medullary interstitial cells with some low activity in the loop of Henle and the collecting ducts.   Biochemically the same enzymes, together with adenyl cyclase, was found in the medullary ascending loop of Henle and the collecting tubule [95].   The identical location with prostaglandin synthesis suggests that the two enzymes may be implicated with prostaglandin and therefore anti-hypertensive activity.   It has been suggested that cyclic GMP phosphodiesterase and GMP cyclase exhibit higher activity in the glomeruli than in tubules [96], but the significance of this difference is unclear.   Both enzymes are said to be in the plasma membrane [94] where they probably regulate the availability of cyclic nucleotides which are essential for binding of macromolecules to membrane receptors.   The control mechanisms are, however, clearly complex and not well understood.

Renal enzymes with high poly-phosphatidyl inositide hydrolase activity are 3 times more active in the cortex than in the medulla [97].   Their functional significance is not known.

Alkaline phosphatase is localised mainly in the brush border and has often been used as a marker enzyme for brush border plasma membrane preparations.   Considerably more of the enzyme is found in the cortex than in the outer medulla [98].   Alkaline phosphatase activity has also been measured routinely in urine as an index of renal damage.   It must, however, be stressed that alkaline phosphatase activity is due to a heterogenous group of enzymes, whose multiple forms have wide overlapping substrate specificities: some activities may even be due to completely unrelated enzymes such as the cyclic nucleotide phosphodiesterases.   The metabolic function of alkaline phosphatases of the kidney is still not clear.

The distribution of 5'-nucleotidase in the kidney appears not to have been studied, but it is fairly active and in common with alkaline phosphatase it has been routinely employed as a marker enzyme for brush border and other plasma membranes in fractionation studies.

Glucose-6-phosphatase represents the last step of gluconeogenesis and enzymic activity appears to be present in all regions of the kidney with some higher activity in the proximal tubule [49].

OTHER RENAL ENZYMES

Transaminases (GOT and GPT) of the human kidney seem to be con-siderably less active than those of the liver [99].

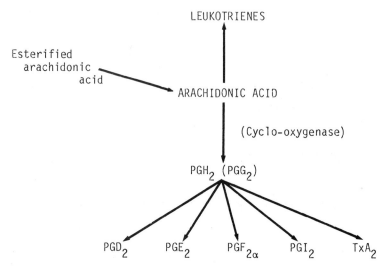

Figure 3.   Schematic representation for the bioconversion of arachidonic acid to biologically active substances.

The only disaccharidase found in the cortical brush border preparations is maltase [99] which is also a useful marker enzyme for brush border preparations. Its function in the kidney remains unexplained.

γ -Glutamyl transpeptidase, which degrades glutathione is located on the luminal side of the brush border of the straight proximal tubule   [100].(See also section on glutathione).

MISCELLANEOUS BIOCHEMICAL FUNCTIONS OF THE KIDNEY

Prostaglandins   The prostaglandins (PG) and endoperoxides are a group of ubiquitously distributed hormones with a broad spectrum of potent biological activity that shows marked receptor specificity. They are synthesised (Fig 3) from the C20:4 fatty acid arachidonic acid, by an enzyme system (which includes cyclo-oxygenases, peroxidases, isomerases and reductases) collectively called PG synthetase.   The literature on renal PG biology is vast and complex, much of it is contradictory and difficult to intepret.   Recently the topic has been reviewed [79, 101-107]. The PG are structurally similar, several are labile and undergo spontaneous chemical changes, and they are only present in minute concentrations.   PGs are not stored in renal tissue, but synthesised de novo from arachidonic acid which is released from stored phospholipid or triglyceride pools by the action of phospholipase A_2.   The factors which modulate   the release of arachidonic acid include both receptor mediated   responses (such as vasoactive peptides and biogenic amines), and non-specific stimuli (ischaemia).   Arachidonic acid (the availability of which is rate limiting) is converted to prostaglandin G_2 and thence in other prostaglandin related substances (Fig 3).

The anatomically identifiable areas of the kidney synthesise a different pattern of prostaglandins in vitro (Table 3).   The in vivo contributions of each of these areas to prostaglandin synthesis and the function of each prostaglandin remains largely a matter of

Table 3. The relative amounts of PG synthesised in vitro by different renal cell types.

CELL TYPES	PRODUCTS	LIKELY FUNCTIONAL RELATIONSHIP
Cortex		
Glomeruli	$PGF_{2\alpha} > PGE_2 > TxA_2 >$ $PGI_2 > PGD_2$	Modulating cortical function:-
Arterioles	PGI_2	e.g. renal vascular resistance, renin secretion and
Cortical tubules	Traces of PGE_2 and $PGF_{2\alpha}$	glomerular filtration rates
Medulla		
Collecting ducts	$PGE_2 > PGI_2 > PGF_{2\alpha} > PGD_2$	Modulating medullary function:-
		e.g. medullary blood flow response to anti-diuretic
Interstitial cells	$PGE_2 >> PGF_{2\alpha}$	hormone and ion absorption
Bladder	PGE_2	Contracting of the bladder smooth muscle

Data from [102,112].

educated speculation at present.   Total prostaglandin synthesis is several times higher in the medulla (where typically it is greater in the papilla) than in the cortex [79]. However, the distribution of, for example PGE_2 synthesis reflects a more complex picture, its concentration being lower in the papilla than the rest of the inner medulla [108]. Furthermore, there are marked sex related differences in the effects of cofactors on medullary PG synthetase activity. Some PGs break down spontaneously (e.g. PGI_2 to 6-keto-PGF_1), but the majority are metabolically degraded.   The enzymic conversions are mediated by a number of enzymes, including dehydrogenases, reductases, and β- and ω-oxidases.   The enzymes which degrade prostaglandins are located mainly in the cortex, but there are species differences in the corticomedullary ratio of these enzymic activities [109].

The factors regulating the biosynthesis of each type of PG are only poorly defined [110] and a large number of endogenous and exogenous substances have been reported to alter renal PG synthesis and several pathophysiological conditions have been described in which renal PG synthesis is increased.   For example, peptides including angiotensin II, bradykinin and anti-diuretic hormone: diseases such as ischaemia, unilateral ureteral obstruction, cirrhosis with ascites.   Some chemicals such as catecholamines and furosemide stimulate PG synthesis, while other substances inhibit synthesis either by binding covalently to cyclo-oxygenase (acetylsalicylic acid, salicylic acid, phenacetin) or reversibly (non-steroidal anti-inflammatory drugs e.g. Indomethacin, Meclofenamate, Phenylbutazone , Fenoproen, Paracetomol) [102].   Most attention has been focussed on the inhibition effects of the anti-inflammatory drugs.   The steroidal compounds (e.g. corticosteroids) prevent the release of arachidonic acid from its lipid pools, and the non-steroidal products (e.g. Indomethacin) inhibit cyclo-oxygenase.   It is, however, essential to be aware that

Table 4.   The actions of indomethacin.

PROSTAGLANDIN RELATED ACTIONS
 Inhibits PG synthesis
 Reduces PG degradation
 Reduces the convesion of PGE_2 to $PGF_{2\alpha}$
 Reduces arachidonic acid release
 Inhibits renal tubular transport of PG

PROSTAGLANDIN UNRELATED ACTIONS
 Inhibits cAMP degradation
 Decreases cellular efflux of cAMP
 Inhibits cAMP-stimulated protein kinase
 Competes with aldosterone for mineralocorticoid receptors
 Reduces angiotensin II binding to adrenal cells
 Inhibits calcium transport and alters smooth muscle contractility

Data from [102].

any factor which perturbates PG synthesis may act differently at different sites in the synthetic (or degradative) pathway.
   The exact physiological roles of the PGs in normal renal function and how these altered in the development of nephropathies is not clear.   Firstly, indomethacin has, for example, been shown to cause biochemical effects which may be classified as either related or unrelated to prostaglandin dynamics (Table 4).   Secondly, many attempts to define renal PG function have been based on the hypothesis that urinary PG excretion reflects de novo renal synthesis, notwithstanding analytical difficulties of measuring very low levels of various PGs and apparently ignoring the fact that de novo synthesised PGs may have undergone extensive degradation.   The measurement of urinary PGs, as an estimate of their de novo renal synthesis, remains equivocal because seminal PGE_2 is an unavoidable and variable contaminant in the urine of males [111] and recently Brown et al [112] have demonstrated that both rabbit and rat urinary bladder can synthesise PGE_2 from arachidonic acid.   Finally, the physiology of renal function is controlled by several hormonal systems the detailed functioning of which are not clearly established.   It is known that renal PGs may be altered by (or may alter) the renin - angiotensin II - aldosterone system [113-117] the kallikrein - kinin system [118-120] and the regulation of fluid balance and water reabsorption via anti-diuretic hormone [121].   Further, each of these hormonal systems may interact with the others via direct or indirect mechanisms.   It seems likely that a full understanding of the pathophysiology of the renal hormone system will take some time to crystallize.
   Despite the rather abstruse biology there is general consensus [79, 102-103] that PGSs have a central role in renal function (Table 5). It seems however, that renal PGs play little, if any, major regulatory role in basal renal blood flow to normal conscious animals.   There is evidence that PGs are released to response to ischaemic and vaso-constriction stress, where their role seems to be to provide a protective effect by maintaining glomerular dynamics.   The role of PGs (especially PGE_2) in preventing experimentally induced acute renal failure is conflicting.   Arachidonic acid does stimulate renin

Table 5. The possible role of prostaglandins in renal function.

RENAL FUNCTION	EFFECT	PROSTAGLANDIN
Renal blood flow	Vasodilatation Vasoconstriction	PGE_2, PGI_2 $TxA_2, PGF_{2\alpha}$, (weak)
Glomerular filtration rate	Increased Decreased	PGE_2, PGI_2 TxA_2
Renin secretion	Increased Decreased	PGI_2, PGE_2, PGD_2 TxA_2
Natiuretic		PGE_2, PGI_2, PGD_2
Water diuretic		PGE_2

After Dunn [79,102]

release, a response which is blocked by cyclo-oxygenase inhibitors, but it remains uncertain which of the PGs mediate this effect in vivo and the renal zone from which such mediators are synthesised and released.   Renin release may, in turn, affect PG synthesis and the kallikrein-kinin system (which in turn may modulate PG synthesis and the renin system).   Anti-diuretic hormone is assumed to stimulate PGE_2, but published data on the controlling effects of PGs on salt and water balance are very difficult to interpret.   Similarly, the mass of literature on hypertension and PGs favours the concept that the two are related, but fails to propound a unifying hypothesis.

RENAL PROTEOGLYCANS AND GLYCOSAMINOGLYCANS

The important biochemical functions of these carbohydrate or protein-carbohydrate macromolecules is beginning to receive attention. The presence of these substances in the glomerular basement membrane has been the focus of a recent symposium and will not be considered here [122].

RENAL PROTEOGLYCANS(POG) AND GLYCOSAMINOGLYCANS(GAG)

The chemistry and biology of these ubiquitously distributed molecules have been reviewed [123]. The molecules exist in vivo in their supramolecular structure, the POG, which consists of a linear protein backbone, with GAG molecules covalently bound at intervals along its length. The GAG molecules are linear anionic polysaccharides made up of repeating disaccharide units, where the combination of a hexuronic acid and hexosamine moiety, together with the type of linkage and derivatives (Table 6) defines each of the seven identifiable types in which these macromolecules occur.   There is evidence that both molecular weight and chemical heterogeneity may also occur in any specific type of GAG [124-126]. It has only been in recent years that the concept of the POG has been accepted;   before this vigorous chemical steps were taken to remove all vestiges of protein "contamination" when GAGs were isolated.   Most of the

Table 6.   The types and structures of GAGs

TYPE OF GAG   DISSACHARIDE UNIT

(Commonly used abbreviation)	Hexuronic acid moiety (derivative)	Bond	N-acetylhexosamine moiety (derivative)
Chondroitin 4-sulphate (Ch4S)*	D-Glucuronic acid	1,3 link	D-Galactosamine (N-acetylated and 4-sulphated)
Chondroitin 6-sulphate (Ch6S)*	D-Glucuronic acid	1,3 link	D-Galactosamine (N-acetylated and 6-sulphated)
Dermatan Sulphate (DS)	L-Iduronic acid**	1,3 link	D-Galactosamine (N-acetylated and 4-sulphated)
Heparin (Hep)	L-Iduronic acid (2-sulphated)	1,4 link	D-Glucosamine (N- and 6-sulphated)
Heparan Sulphate (HS)	L-Iduronic acid	1,4 link	D-Glucosamine (N-acetylated and 6-sulphated)
Hyaluronic Acid (HA)	D-Gluronic acid	1,3 link	D-Glucosamine (N-acetylated)
Keratan Sulphate (KS)	D-Galactose	1,4 link	D-Glucosamine (N-acetylated and 6-sulphated)

*   When these have not been resolved on separation they are generally referred to as chondroitin sulphates (ChS).

**   May be up to 20% D-Gluronic acid

After [123].

biochemical   data   presented   below   may   therefore   represent experimentally induced artefact, but it is the only information available to date.   The distribution of POG-PAG is morphologically most concentrated at the glomeruli and between the collecting ducts of the medulla, especially at the papilla tip.   Table 7 shows the type and quantity of GAG that have been isolated from the cortex and medulla of different species.   Depending on species etc. the amount of medullary GAG was between 2 and 13-fold greater than that in the cortex.   In humans the ratio was age related [139] and increased rapidly to the fourth decade and then declined slowly.

Table 7. Species variation in the type and distribution of GAGs in kidney.

SPECIES	TYPE AND AMOUNT OF GAG	YIELD	REF
Chicken	HA 38%,HS 50%,ChS 4%, Hep 8%[a]	2.1g/100g dry defatted tissue	[127,128]
Rat	Heparin - like and some HA. Only small amounts of galactosamine,thus small amounts of ChS[a]	*	[129]
	HS 56-64%,HA 13-17%, DS 4-13%, ChS 15%[b]	*	[130]
	HS 88%,DS 12%,ChS<2%[a]	65 µg/g dry tissue	[124]
	HS 65-70%,HA 20-25%[c,d]	*	[131]
	HS as part of glomerular basement membrane	*	[132]
	HS containing proteoglycan as part of glomerular basement membrane	*	[133]
Guinea Pig	HS 70%,DS 22%,ChS<2%[a]	192 µg/g dry tissue	[125]
	HA 20-25%,DS+ChS 50%[c,d]	*	[131]
Rabbit	HA and Ch4S[c]	*	[134]
	HA 20%,Ch4S 15%,Ch6S 15%, DS<3%, HS trace[c]	0.89% of dry defatted tissue	[135]
	HS 62%,DS 24%,ChS 12%[a]	143 µg/g dry tissue	[125]
Dog	HA 30%,ChS 30%[b,c]	100 µg/100g wet tissue	[136]
	HS 80%,HA 10%,DS 10%[b]	1mg/g dry tissue[b] 9mg/g dry tissue[c]	[137]
	HS 61%,DS 26%,ChS 13% Hep<0.5%[a]	534 µg/g dry tissue	[125]
Beef	HA and ChS[c]	1-2% dry tissue	[134]
Pig	HA 30%,ChS 30%[b,c]	100 µg/100g wet tissue	[136]
	HS 73%,DS 22%,ChS 5%, Hep<0.5%[a]	300 µg/g dry tissue	[125]
Sheep	HA 30%, ChS 30%[b,c]	100 µg/100g wet tissue	[136]
Man	HS 55%,ChS 17%,DS 15%, HA 10%[b]	2.7 mg/g dry defatted tissue	[138]
	HA 38%,HS 33%,DS 15%, ChS 14%[c]	6.6 mg/g dry defatted tissue	[138]
	HS 59%,DS 26%,ChS 15%, Hep<0.5%[a]	150 µg/g dry tissue	[125]

[a] = Whole kidney ; [b] = Cortex ; [c] = Inner medulla and
* = no data given.

The biosynthesis of renal POG and GAG.   The processes underlying and controlling the biosynthesis of POG-GAGs are complex and incompletely documented [123].   Pitcock et al [140] have reported that medullary interstitial cells synthesise POGs-GAG (both in situ and in culture) and that these macromolecules were associated with the cellular cisterns (dilated rough endoplasmic reticulum).   Darnton [23] presented data to show that glycogen, associated with the epithelial cells of the collecting duct in the rabbit, could be mobilised and incorporated in GAGs.   In addition, exogenous sulphate, glucose [I30],glucosamine and galactosamine [127, 128] are incorporated into de novo synthesised GAGs.   The pools from which these precursors are drawn, and the inter-conversion of carbohydrates between the pools is very complex.   More galactosamine than glucosamine was incorporated into fowl kidney GAGs and the time course of labelled precursor incorporation differed in the four major types of GAG that had been isolated.   There were also subtle differences in labelling kinetic depending on the type of hexosamine precursor administered [128].

Barry and Bowness [I30] showed that the specific activity of incorporated radiolabelled sulphate into both the total cortex and medullary polyanions decreased bi-exponentially, with an alpha-phase half-life of 2 days for the cortex and 2.5 days for the medulla and a beta-phase (attained after 5 days) of about 5 to 6 days for both regions.   The apex of the medulla (papilla) showed a mono-exponential decay curve with a half-life of 4 days.   Up to 80% of the radio-activity from both the ^{14}C and ^{35}S precursors was incorporated in heparan sulphate (HS) during the first 24h.   During this early time period (0-24h) there were changes in the specific activity of individual GAGs, a finding consistent with the concept that more than one metabolic pool of precursor molecules exists.   The turnover rates of individual GAGs were similar to those studies in other tissues, except for hyaluronic acid (HA) which was more rapid.

There is a paucity of data on glomerular POG-GAG metabolism. Recently, Foidart [141] showed that cultured rat glomeruli epithelial cells synthesised both HS and HA, but the mesangial cells synthesised only HA.

The function of POG-GAG deposits in the kidney   The role of POG-GAG molecules extends beyond that of being a "space filling matrix" and is unquestionably complex [123-124,142-143].   The polyanionic nature of these molecules serves to provide part of the permselectivity of glomerular filtration and may also play an essential role in the structure of the glomerular foot processes. (see Moffat, this volume for a more detailed discussion).

The role of the medullary matrix is equally poorly defined.   It most probably serves to support the delicate tubular and capillary elements within it and, through its large water binding capacity plays an essential, but still poorly understood role in the urine concentrating process.   Ginetzinsky [144] was the first to suggest that the state of polymerisation of the medullary matrix could be a controlling factor in water homeostasis.   Subsequent attempts to study these changes have given conflicting results [23,145-148]. Failure to resolve this question may relate to the method that have been used to probe the problem.   Most workers have used the changes in the intensity of histochemical straining of the medulla as their criterion of the degree of matrix polymerisation [144-145, 147-148].

GAG staining is, however, relatively non-specific and the intensity of staining assesses only the availability of dye binding sites and not the amount of macromolecule.   Biochemical approaches have also failed to resolve the problem.   Jacobsen et al [146] showed that diuresis caused both an increase in papillary hexosamine and staining, but Darnton [23], using an autoradiographic technique, found a lower incorporation of labelled glucose into the papillary matrix during diuresis and reported less intense staining.

The role of the medullary matrix in urine concentrating may depend on one or more of its physiochemical features.   For example, conformation, chain length, or the functionally available $-NH_2$, $-COOH$, N-Acetyl, N-sulphate or O-sulphate groups, factors which have not yet been investigated.   Further, the types of POG-GAG may be heterogenously distributed within the kidney.   Thus relatively subtle changes or interconversions may alter the interstitial milieu enough to cause major functional changes.   These would go undetected by the innapropriate means so far used.

The medullary ground substance may also serve two other major functions.   In addition to its role in the transition of water, this matrix can act as an ion exchange resin which will bind cations. This may, in itself, contribute "passively" to the retention of those cations which are deficient in the diet.   More importantly, it would serve to reduce the possibility of the "urinary" saturation product being exceeded when the kidney is solute loaded [149-150], and inhibit the formation of the inorganic niduses from which nephrolithiases grow.

Parsons and co-workers [151] have established an important role for bladder epithelial POG-GAG in preventing the attachment of, and urinary tract colonisation by, pathogens.   There is evidence [123] that at least part of the urinary POG, GAG or their breakdown products are derived from the kidney, probably via the medullary turnover of its ground substance.   These molecules, may, therefore also contribute to the natural defence system that protects the urothelia.

GLUTATHIONE

The renal capacity for glutathione synthesis in the rat is estimated to be several grams per day and occurs via two enzymic ATP-utilising steps involving:-

i) γ-glutamyl cysteine synthetase and
ii)   glutathione synthetase.

This first enzyme contributes some 2-5% of the total soluble protein in rat kidney [152]. Biosynthesis and utilisation of glutathione is balanced, producing steady state levels in tissues, and is facilitated by the γ-glutamyl cycle (reviewed by Meister [153]). The activities of the various enzymes involved in the breakdown of the tripeptide are higher in renal tissue than in liver, and correspondingly there is greater turnover of glutathione in the kidney [154].

The first stage in glutathione breakdown is catalysed by γ-glutamyl transpeptidase and involves the transfer of the γ-glutamyl moiety to an acceptor amino acid, thus forming a γ-glutamyl amino acid. Overall it is proposed that the γ-glutamyl cycle functions, among other things, in the membrane transport of amino acids [153].

γ-Glutamyl transpeptidase is obviously an important component of the cycle.   Histochemical studies have shown that the enzyme activity is closely associated with the brush border membrane and exhibits maximal activity in proximal straight of the tubule [155].

In addition to the transport of amino acids, glutathione is also important in the detoxication of xenobiotics via the production of mercapturic acid conjugates. Drugs possessing electrophilic centres conjugate with glutathione, the reaction being catalysed by glutathione-S-transferase, thus preventing potential interactions of the drug with vital nucleophiles in the cell such as proteins, nucleic acids etc. Quantitatively drug biotransformation in the kidney is less important than the liver, a topic considered in detail by Rush and Hook, this volume.

METABOLISM OF PLASMA PROTEINS AND PEPTIDES

The role of the kidney in the metabolism of plasma proteins and peptides such as β_2-microglobulin, lysozyme, insulin, growth hormone, glucagon, L-chain of immunoglobulins etc. is well established and has been reviewed [72, 156-158]. Absorption, transport and degradation of such substances appear to be a function of the proximal tubule and there is little evidence to suggest the involvement of other regions of the nephron. Molecular size and charge are significant factors in determining the role played by the kidneys and several mechanisms for the renal handling of such compounds are apparent.

Plasma proteins enter the nephron by way of the glomerulus [159]. The ease of passage across the filter is dependent mainly upon molecular size, glomerular clearance decreasing progressively as molecular weight and radius increase. The glomerulus is almost impenetrable to molecules with molecular weight greater than 60,000 daltons [72]. IgM for example (900,000 daltons) is completely retained by the healthy kidney and therefore does not appear in urine and is not subjected to renal catabolism. Intermediate sized proteins like albumin (69,000 daltons) are partly retained although it has been shown that more than 90% of the small amount of albumin filtered by the glomerulus is absorbed by the proximal tubule and digested [156]. Lower molecular weight proteins such as lysozyme (14,000 daltons) are readily filtered.

Morphological, cytochemical, micropuncture studies and iodine-labelled protein have been used to investigate the mode of protein re-absorption by proximal tubules [reviewed by 157,158,160]. This is thought to occur at the luminal epithelial surface and is followed by endocytosis, transfer to lysosomes and subsequent digestion. Evidence obtained from in vitro and kidney slice techniques suggests that once absorbed, proteins are digested by the lysosomal and hydrolases to varying degrees e.g. albumin is almost completely degraded to amino acids while lysozyme is only partly so, even in the presence of excess enzymes [157].

Renal catabolism is also important for polypeptides [86] such as insulin, growth hormone etc. and occurs via similar processes. Smaller peptides (8-10 amino acids) appear to be handled differently by a mechanism involving hydrolysis at the luminal surface of the proximal tubule brush border [158]. Both in vivo and in vitro microperfusion techniques have confirmed such a process for angiotensin I and II, bradykinin and oxytocin [86]. Amino acids are also reabosrbed by the proximal tubule by a carrier-mediated, energy-dependent transport mechanism at the luminal membrane [161].

VITAMINS

Significant concentrations of a number of vitamins may be found in the kidney, e.g. riboflavin as flavin mononucleotide) is indicative of the requirement of many vitamins for the normal biochemical function and structural integrity of the organ.   The vitamin content per gram of tissue tends to be higher in the kidneys than in other organs, which is consistent with the higher metabolic activity of the tissue. The rat kidney is known to contain an active system for the decarboxylation of L-ascorbic acid, and in some non-mammalian species, biosynthesis of vitamin C occurs [162-164].   With the exception of Vitamin D, however, little is known about renal vitamin metabolism.

Vitamin D.   The metabolism and function of vitamin D have been the subject of several excellent reviews [e.g. 165-166].   It has been known for some time that the absorption of calcium from the gastrointestinal tract is regulated by vitamin D_3 through the synthesis of a specific calcium-binding protein.   Vitamin D_3 (cholecalciferol) is not itself biologically active, but requires metabolic activation in order to express the required function with respect to calcium metabolism.   Cholecalciferol is rapidly removed from the plasma (where it is transported on plasma proteins) by the liver when it is hydroxylated forming 25-hydroxycholecalciferol [167]. Although one of the major circulating metabolites, 25-hydroxycholecalciferol [25(OH)D_3] requires further metabolism to 1,25-dehydroxycholecalciferol, the active metabolite.   The kidney is the sole site of 1,25-dihydroxycholecalciferol production since nephrectomised animals are unable to synthesise the metabolite [168] whereas homogenates from chick kidneys are fully capable of hydroxylating 25(OH)D_3 at the 1-carbon position.   The enzyme system responsible for the conversion, 25-(OH)D_3-1-hydroxylase is located in the inner mitochondrial membrane of the proximal tubule cells and requires molecular oxygen, NADPH and cytochrome P-450 as integral components of the system [169].

CONCLUSIONS

There are important biochemical differences not only between the various regions of the kidney, but also among the different cell types within a region.   Intermediary metabolic processes such as the opposing pathways of glucose metabolism (glycolysis-medulla; gluconeogenesis-cortex) and fatty acid metabolism (synthesis-medulla; utilisation-cortex) and hence energy production, are carefully regulated and integrated.   In addition the kidney fulfils an important role in the synthesis and catabolism of a wide variety of substances including prostaglandins, proteoglycans, vitamin D_3, glutathione etc., and possesses a miscellany of other biochemical properties such as mixed-function oxidase and co-oxygenase mediated drug metabolism.   These characteristic functions make the kidney a sensitive target organ for toxic substances and indicate a wide range of biochemical processes available for interaction.   The current methods for studying renal biochemical function are complicated by the heterogeneity of the tissue and a clearer understanding will only come about as a result of improved techniques such as microdissection, microprofusion and the culture of pure cell types.   Hopefully, this will facilitate the interpretation of data and allow specific biochemical functions to be related to single cell populations or specific anatomical regions of the kidney.

REFERENCES

1. Guder WG and Ross RD, Int J Biochem 12: 1-2, 1980.
2. Cohen JJ and Kamm DE in The Kidney, 2nd Edit.
    (BM Brenner and FC Rector, eds.),Saunders, Philadelphia, 1981.pp
    144-248.
3. Thurau K, Am J Med 36: 698-719, 1964.
4. Kramer K, et al. Arch Ges Physiol 270: 251-269, 1964.
5. Rhodin J, Am J Med 24: 661-675, 1958.
6. Kean EL, et al. Biochem Biophys Acta 64: 503-507, 1962.
7. Sternburg WH, et al. J Histochem Cytochem 4: 266-281, 1956.
8. Mikulski P, et al. Am J Physiol 223: 485-491, 1972.
9. Weinstein SW and Szyjewicz J, Am J Physiol 227: 171-177, 1974.
10. Mattenheimer H, Med Clin N Amer 55: 1493-1508, 1971.
11. Benoy MP and Elliott KAC, Biochem J 31: 1268-1275, 1937.
12. Exton, JH, Metabolism 21: 945-990, 1972.
13. Froesch ER, et al. Endocrinology 62: 614, 1958.
14. Freedland RA and Harper AE, J Biol Chem 228: 743-751, 1957.
15. Krebs HA, et al. J Biol Chem 86: 22-27, 1963.
16. Cohen, JJ, Am J Physiol 236: F423-F433, 1979.
17. Gyorgy P, et al. Biochem Z 200: 356-366, 1928.
18. Dickens F and Weil-Malherbe H, Biochem J 30: 657-660, 1936.
19. Holmes EW and Di Scala VA, Am J Physiol 221: 839-843, 1971.
20. Frega NS, et al. Am J Physiol 233: F235-F240, 1977.
21. Gregg CM, et al. Am J Physiol 235: F52-F61, 1978.
22. Bernanke D and Epstein FM, Am J Physiol 208, 541-545, 1965.
23. Darnton SJ, Z Zellforsch 102: 273-282, 1969.
24. Hohenleitner FJ and Spitzer JJ, Am J Physiol 200: 1095-1098, 1961.
25. Grafflin AL and Green DE, J Biol Chem 176: 95-115, 1948.
26. Geyer RP, et al. J Biol Chem 180: 1037-1045, 1949.
27. Pitts RF, in Physiology of the Kidney and Body Fluids. Year Book
    Medical Publishers, Chicago, 1974.
28. Lee JB, et al. Am J Physiol 203: 27-36, 1962.
29. Weidmann MJ and Krebs MA, Biochem J 112: 149-166, 1969.
30. Hohenegger M, et al. in Biochemical Nephrology (WG Guder and U
    Schmidt, eds) Huber, Bern, 1978, pp 397-404.
31. Guder WG and Winthensohn G, G Eur J Biochem 99: 577-584, 1979.
32. Wieland O and Suyter M, Biochem Z 329: 320, 1957.
33. Preiss B and Bloch K, J Biol Chem 239: 85-88, 1964.
34. Bjorkhem I and Danielsson H, Eur J Biochem 17: 450-459, 1970.
35. Lu AYH and Coon MJ, J Biol Chem 243: 1331-1332, 1968.
36. Ellin A, et al. Arch Biochem Biophys 150: 64-71, 1972.
37. Jakobsson S, et al. Biochem Biophys Res Commun 39: 1073-1080,
    1970.
38. Bojesen I, Lipids 9: 835-843, 1974.
39. Bojesen I et al, Biochim Biophys Acta 424: 8-16, 1976.
40. Bojesen IN, in The Renal Papilla and Hypertension (AK Mandal and
    SO Bohman eds). Plenum, New York, 1980, pp. 121-147.
41. Bojesen IN, Biochim Biophys Acta 619:308-317, 1980.
42. Bojesen IN, Lipids 15: 519-523, 1980.
43. Newsholme EA and Gevers W, Vitamin Hormone 25: 1-87, 1967.
44. Newsholme EA and Underwood AH, Biochem J 99: 24C-26C, 1966.
45. Saggerson ED, et al. Int J Biochem 12: 107-111, 1980.
46. Bulger RE in Histology, 4th Edit. (L Weiss and RO Greep, eds)
    McGraw Hill, New York, 1977 pp 831-879, ISBN, 0-07-069091-X.

47. Le Hir M, et al. Histochemistry 63: 245-251, 1979.
48. Dubach UC and Schmidt U, Enzyme Biol Clin 11: 32-51, 1970.
49. Schmidt U and Guder WG, Kidney Int 9: 233-242, 1976.
50. Bergeron M, et al. Kidney Int 17: 175-185, 1980.
51. Hohmann B, et al   . Pflugers Arch. 312: 110-125, 1969.
52. Guder WG and Schmidt U, Z Physiol Chem 355: 273-278, 1974.
53. Pitts RF, et al. J Clin Invest 51: 557-565, 1972.
54. Curthoys NP and Lowry OH, J Biol Chem 248: 162-168, 1973.
55. Goodman AD, et al. J Clin Invest 45: 616-619, 1966.
56. Hohenegger M, in Renal Metabolism in Relation to Renal Function
    U Schmidt and UC Dubach, eds) Huber, Bern 1976, p 99-107.
57. Masters C and Holmes R, Physiol Rev 57: 816-882,1977.
58. Schmidt U and Dubach UC, Pflugers Arch 306: 219-226, 1969.
59. Schmidt U, et al. J Clin Invest 55: 655-660, 1975.
60. Ullrich KJ, et al. Pfhigers Arch 351: 49-60, 1974.
61. Katz AI and Dencet A, Int J Biochem 12: 125-129, 1980.
62. Angielski   et al. Int J Biochem 12: 119-123. 1980.
63. Moore L, et al. Biochim Biophys Acta 345: 405-418, 1974.
64. Shibko S and Tappel AL, Biochem J 95: 731-741, 1965.
65. Helwig JJ, Int J Biochem 8: 323-327, 1977.
66. Kramer HJ, Enzyme Biol Clin 11: 435-449, 1970.
67. Taylor DG, et al. Biochem J 112: 641-645, 1971.
68. Lansdown AB and Ellaby SJ, Histochemistry 42: 111-113, 1974.
69. Straus W, J Biophys Biochem Cytol 2: 513-521, 1956.
70. Price RG and Donce N, Biochem J 105:   877-883, 1967.
71. Andersen KJ, et al. Biochem Soc Trans 8: 597-598, 1980.
72. Strober W and Waldmann TA, Nephron 13: 35-66, 1974.
73. Davies, M in Lysosomes in Biology and Pathology (JT Dingle and RT
    Dean, eds) North Holland-Elsevier, Amsterdam, 1975, pp 305-348.
74. Goldstone A, et al. Biochem J 132: 259-266, 1973.
75. Davies M, et al. Clin Sci Mol Med 54: 233-240, 1978.
76. Velosa JA, et al. in The Glomerular Basement Membrane (G Lubec
    ed.) Karger, Basel, 1980, pp 120-125.
77. Pierce RJ, et al. Biochem J 180: 673-676, 1979.
78. Seager SF, et al. Biochem Soc Trans 6: 1378-1380, 1978.
79. Dunn MJ and Hood VL, Am J Physiol 233: F169-F184, 1977.
80. Sagnella GA, et al. Clinical Science 59: 337-345, 1980.
81. Soltesz BM, et al. Experientia 35: 533-534, 1979.
82. Artizzu M, et al. Life Sci 24: 1023-1028, 1979.
83. Ward PE, et al. Biochem J 157: 643-650, 1976.
84. Ostarvik TB, et al. J Histochem Cytochem 24:   1037-1039, 1976.
85. Carretero OA and Scicli AG. Am J Physiol 238: F247-F255, 1980.
86. Carone FA and Peterson DR. Am J Physiol 238: F151-F158, 1980.
87. Lake B, et al. Drug Metab Disposition 1:   342-349, 1973.
88. Lucier GW and McDaniel OS, J Steroid Biochem 8: 867-872, 1977.
89. Hirom PC, et al. Xenobiotica 6: 55-64, 1976.
90. Gingell R, Xenobiotica 6: 15-20 , 1976.
91. Pinto JD, et al. J Biol Chem 240: 2148-2154, 1965.
92. Jones DP in Functions of Glutathione in Liver and Kidney (H Sies
    and A Wendel, eds), Springer-Verlag, Berlin, 1978, pp 194-200.
93. Fry JR, et al. Xenobiotica 8: 113-120, 1978.
94. Florendo NT, et al. J Histochem Cytochem 26: 441-451, 1978.
95. Jackson BA, et al. Endocrinol 107: 1693-1698, 1980.
96. Helwig JJ, et al. Int J Biochem 12: 209-214, 1980.
97. Cooper PH and Hawthorne JN, Biochem J 150: 537-551, 1975.
98. Kempson SA and Price RG, Int J Biochem 10: 67-73, 1979.

99. Schmidt E and Schmidt FW, Enzym Fibel Biochem Abt, CF Boehringer and Sohne GmbH, Mannheim, 1966.
100.Curthoys NP, et al. Int J Biochem 12: 219-232. 1980.
101.Samuelson B, et al. Ann Rev Biochem 47: 997-1029, 1978.
102.Dunn MJ and Zambraski EJ, Kidney Int 18: 609-622, 1980.
103.Morrison AR, Amer J Med 69: 171-173, 1980.
104.Weber PC, Contr Nephrol 23: 83-92, 1980.
105.Zusman RS, in The Renal Papilla and Hypertension (AK Mandal and SO Bohman eds) Plenum, New York, 1980, pp 187-207.
106.Dunn MJ, Kidney Int 19: 86-102, 1981.
107.Frolich JC et al, Kidney Int 19: 755-868.
108.Van Dorp D, Ann NY Acad Sci 100: 181-199, 1971.
109.Powell WS, Prostaglandins 19: 701-710, 1980.
110.Horrobin DF, Med Hypotheses 6: 687-709, 1980.
111.Suzuki S et al, Biochim Biophys Acta 428: 166-181, 1976.
112.Brown W, et al, Amer J Physiol 239: F452-F458, 1980.
113.Franco-Saenz, et al, Prostaglandins 20: 1131-1143, 1980.
114.Hackenthal E, et al, Prog Biochem Pharm 17: 98-107, 1980.
115.Lee JB, Clin Nephrol 14: 159-163, 1980.
116.Abe K et al, Kidney Int 19:869-880,1981.
117.Baer PG, Life Sciences 28: 587-593, 1981.
118.Fitzgerald GA, et al, Prostaglandins Med 5: 445-456, 1980.
119.Margolins H, Prog Biochem Pharm 17: 116-122, 1980.
120.Rockel A and Heidland A, Contr Nephrol 23: 105-124, 1980.
121.Blair-West JR, et al, Prog Biochem Pharmacol 17: 20-28, 1980..
122.Lubec G, Renal Physiol 3: 1-432, 1980.
123.Kennedy JF, Proteoglycans - Biological and Chemical Aspects in Human Life, Elsevier Scientific, Amsterdam, 1979.
124.Dietrich CP, et al, Biochem Biophys Res Commun 71: 1-10, 1976.
125.Toled OSM and Dietrich CP, Biochim Biophys Acta 498: 114-122, 1977.
126.Suzuki S, et al, Biochim Biophys Acta 428: 166-181, 1976.
127.Ng Kwai Hang KF and Anastassiadias PA, Can J Biochem 58: 319-324, 1980.
128.Ng Kwai Hang KF and Anastassiadias PA, Can J Biochem 58: 325-335, 1980.
129.Allalonf D, et al. Biochim Biophys Acta 83: 278-287, 1964.
130.Barry DN and Bownes JM, Can J Biochem 58: 713-720, 1975.
131.Lis D and Morris B, Experientia 34: 693-695, 1978.
132. Kanwar YS and Farquhar MG, Proc Nat Acad Sci (USA) 76: 1303-1307, 1979.
133. Hassell JR, et al, Proc Nat Acad Sci (USA) 77: 4494-4498, 1980.
134. Farber SJ, et al, Trans Assoc Amer Physns 75: 154-159, 1962.
135. Faber SJ and Van Praag D, Biochim Biophys Acta 208: 219-226, 1970.
136. Dicker SE and Franklin CS, J Physiol (Lond) 186: 110-120, 1966.
137. Castor CW and Green JA, J Clin Invest 47: 2125-2132, 1968.
138. Constantopoulos G et al, Med Biochem 7: 376-388, 1973.
139. Inoue G, et al. Gerontologia 16: 261-265, 1970.
140. Pitcock JA, et al. Fed Proc 37: 633, 1978.
141. Foidart JB, et al. Renal Physiol 3: 169-173, 1980.
142. Long WF and Williams FB IRCS Med Sci 7: 429-434, 1979.
143. Kjellen P, et al. Biochem Biophys Res Commun 74: 126-133, 1977.
144. Ginetzinsky AG, Nature 182: 1218-1219, 1958.
145. Merard JC and Abadie A, J Physiol (Paris) 60: 323-356, 1968.
146. Jacobson A, et al. Proc Soc Exp Biol Med 115: 1153-1156, 1964.

147. Ivanova LN and Vinagradov VV, Fed Proc 22: 931-934, 1962.
148. Boss JMN, et al. J Physiol (Lond) 157: 35P-36P, 1961.
149. Nordin BEC, in Nephrology (J Hamburger, J. Crosnier and J-P Grunfeld, eds). Wiley-Flammarion, New York-Paris, 1979, pp. 1091-1128.
150. Fleisch H, Kidney Int 13: 361-371, 1978.
151. Parsons CL, et al. Science 208: 605-607, 1980.
152. Bender DA in Amino Acid Metabolism, Wiley, Chichester, 1975, pp. 106-111.
153. Meister A in Functions of Glutathione in Liver and Kidney (H Sies and A Wende, Eds), Springer-Verlag, Berlin, 1978. pp. 43-59.
154. Sekura R and Meister A, Proc Nat Acad Sci 71: 2404-2409, 1974.
155. Albert Z, et al. Nature 191: 767-781, 1961.
156. Bourdeau JE and Carone FA, Nephron 13: 22-34, 1974.
157. Maunsbach AB, Int Rev Physiol 11: 145-167, 1976.
158. Carone FA, et al. Kidney Int 16: 271-278, 1979.
159. Farquhar MG, et al. J Exp Med 113: 47-66, 1961.
160. Christensen EI and Maunsbach AB, Kidney Int 6: 396-407, 1974.
161. Silbernagh S, et al. Rev Physiol Biochem Pharmacol 74: 105-167, 1975.
162. Burns JJ, et al. J Biol Chem 232: 107-115, 1958.
163. Roy RN and Guha BC, Nature 182: 319-320, 1958.
164. Weber F and Wiss O, in The Kidney (C Rouiller and AF Mullerr, eds.). Academic Press, New York, 1971. pp. 271-295.
165. Norman AW, et al. Vitamin D. Basic Research and its clinical application. Walter de Gruyter, Berlin, 1979.
166. Norman AW. Vitamin D. Molecular Biology and Clinical Nutrition. Marcel Dekker, New York, 1980.
167. Ponchon G, et al. J Clin Invest 48: 2032-2037, 1969.
168. Deluca HF and Schnoes HK, In ref 156. pp. 445-458.
169. Ghazarian JG, et al. Arch Biochem Biophys 184: 596-604, 1977.

RENAL TUBULAR FUNCTION

William O. Berndt

Department of Pharmacology and Toxicology, University of Mississippi Medical Center, Jackson, Mississippi 39216, USA

ABSTRACT

This article will review several aspects of renal physiology an understanding of which will be important for an appreciation of the actions of nephrotoxic substances. Where appropriate, generally used techniques for the assessment of function will be discussed. Glomerular function involves selection of molecules for passage both by size and charge. In general only small molecular weight substances reach the tubular fluid, hence the presence of protein in the urine or elevation of the blood urea nitrogen would suggest renal dysfunction. The proximal tubule possesses a large number of discreet reabsorptive and secretory mechanisms. Sodium chloride, potassium and bicarbonate all are reabsorbed as are some divalent cations. Various amino acids and sugars also undergo active reabsorption in the proximal tubule. Organic anions and organic cations are secreted by the proximal tubular cells. The distal tubule is complicated both anatomically and functionally. Movement of organic compounds out of the distal segment is passive, but several active reabsorptive processes for inorganic electrolytes occur. Potassium secretion occurs distally.

> glomerular function
> BUN
> anion and cation secretion
> glucose reabsorption
> potassium secretion
> sodium and chloride reabsorption

This presentation will be directed at an analysis of the normal physiology of the kidney. This material will not be in as great detail as can be obtained from many textbooks of physiology, but sufficient information will be given to permit a discussion of the effects of various chemicals on renal function parameters. In particular, those aspects of renal physiology will be emphasized which bear more or less directly on the actions of various nephrotoxic compounds. Hence, some aspects of renal function will not be discussed at all either because these appear to be unrelated to the production of a nephrotoxic event or are so poorly understood in relation to nephrotoxicity that nothing can be learned. In addition, assessment of some aspects of renal tubular function will be presented, particularly as these relate to the classical renal tubular functions. That is, those techniques will be presented that are involved in a classical study of renal dysfunction. Specialized techniques will be presented by others as they relate to specific renal tubular events.

Several detailed treatises should be examined for a thorough examination of renal tubular function. These will be useful for material not covered in this chapter as well as for more detail on those aspects of renal function which follow.

Brenner BM and Rector F, The Kidney, two volumes, W. B. Saunders Co., Philadelphia, 1981.

Valtin H, Renal Function: Mechanisms preserving fluid and solute balance in health. Little, Brown and Co., Boston, 1973.

Handbook of Physiology, Section 8: Renal Physiology, ed. by J Orloff and RW Berliner, Amer. Physiological Soc. Washington, DC, 1973.

GLOMERULAR FUNCTION

In the simplest terms the glomerulus (A, Fig. 1) serves as a filter permitting the passage of water and small molecules while retarding the passage of large molecules, such as the plasma proteins. The idea of ultrafiltration as the initiation of urine formation was demonstrated unequivocally by Wearn and Richards in 1924 [1]. Passage of fluid and electrolytes across capillary membranes occurs in all capillary beds. Ordinarily this fluid is returned to the vasculature. However, with the

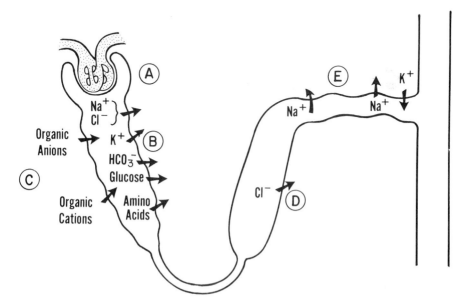

Figure 1. Schematic Representation of Nephron.

glomerular filter it is clear that part of the filtered fluid will ultimately be lost as the final urine, although normally the volume lost
constitutes only a very small fraction of that filtered. The driving
force for the filtration process is the cardiac action which results
ultimately in the final filtration pressure responsible for filtration
of the fluid and electrolytes. The final filtration pressure, however,
is a function not only of the blood pressure generated by the action of
the heart, but also the plasma colloid osmotic pressure, the
intracapsular pressure, and intratubular pressure. Normally the balance
of these will yield a net filtration pressure of the order of 15mm Hg
[2].

Quantitative estimates of glomerular filtration can be obtained with
the classical clearance equation [3]. This relationship describes that
hypothetical volume of plasma from which the substance is removed totally per unit time.

$$\text{clearance} = \frac{U \times V}{P}, \qquad ml/min = \frac{mg/ml \times ml/min}{mg/ml}$$

where U is the urinary concentration of the test substance, P the plasma
concentration and V the urinary flow rate.

In addition to filtration pressure, molecular charge is also an important determinant of how readily a substance crosses the glomerular
filter. Various studies have shown that certain negatively charged
molecules are filtered less well than their uncharged counterparts.
Dextran sulfate, for example, of a given molecular weight is always
filtered less well than neutral dextran of a comparable molecular weight
[4]. Hence, negatively charged dextran appears to interact with the
structures of the glomerulus retarding filtration. Cationic
macromolecules cross the glomerular barrier more effectively than
predicted by molecular size. The importance of charge is clear only
with macromolecules which appear to interact with the glomerular
structure. Charge is not important with small molecular weight
substances such as most drugs, xenobiotics, etc.

Routine assessment of glomerular function can be undertaken with
various procedures. In general, the extent of glomerular integrity is
inversely related to protein excretion. Those large molecular weight
(i.e., > 50000 daltons) which contribute to the colloid osmotic forces
of the plasma normally do not appear in the urine. Should large
quantities of albumin, for example, be found in the urine, one would
have to suspect that the glomerular integrity has been compromised. The
appearance of the smaller molecular weight proteins, however, may
indicate only that the reabsorptive and/or catabolic processes normally
responsible for removing such materials from the tubular fluid have
failed. For example, λ-L-chain protein may appear in the urine when
glomerular filtration is normal, suggesting that glomerular integrity is
still intact, but that reabsorptive processes have been compromised.

Assessment of the blood urea nitrogen (BUN) or plasma creatinine also
is useful in determining glomerular function. As glomerular function
fails, filtration is reduced and BUN and creatinine rise. Although
there are reasons unrelated to compromised glomerular function that
might account for elevations in the BUN or plasma creatinine, usually an
elevation of these parameters outside of the normal range indicates
glomerular dysfunction. The hyperbolic relationship between BUN or
plasma creatinine and the degree of glomerular filtration permits
accurate assessment of GFR from BUN or plasma creatinine in chronic

renal failure [5]. In the experimental laboratory, periodic assessment of BUN is a quick way of determining the degree of renal failure after administration of a nephrotoxin. This is particularly useful with high output renal failure when the classic endpoints of severe renal compromise, i.e. oliguria or anuria, are disguised.

Inulin is an effective marker of glomerular filtration because its molecular size and charge permits its free filtration at the glomerulus. It can be infused into an experimental animal and its renal clearance equated to the GFR. Inulin is not bound to plasma proteins, is not reabsorbed from the tubular fluid, has no pharmacological effects, and is filtered freely at the glomerulus. For all of these reasons, it is an ideal marker for glomerular filtration. Of course, inulin is an exogenous substance and therefore must be infused in order to perform the analysis of glomerular function. Analysis of inulin is accomplished readily either by chemical means or through radiochemical assessment.

PROXIMAL TUBULAR FUNCTION

A very large variety of reabsorptive and secretory processes occur in the various segments of the proximal tubule. Exactly which transport function occurs in which segment of the proximal tubule varies enormously from species to species. For example, although the proximal tubular secretion of p-aminohippurate (PAH) is observed predominantly in the *pars recta* of the rabbit, [6] the *pars recta* and *pars convoluta* show approximately the same magnitude of PAH transport in the rat [7] and the *pars convoluta* is much more active than the *pars recta* in the pig [8]. Despite these quantitative differences in proximal tubular function among various species, approximately the same transport functions occur in all mammalian proximal tubules, and earlier suggestions of species-independent, intratubular heterogeneity of organic anion transport probably were exaggerated. Hence, for this discussion, no further anatomical, biochemical or physiological distinction will be made concerning the proximal tubule segments and the specific transport processes located therein. Rather, the transport functions and methods of their assessment will be discussed as general events located in proximal tubular epithelia.

Inorganic electrolytes (B, Fig. 1). Although specific mechanisms of inorganic electrolyte transport vary greatly from tubule segment to tubule segment, transport of virtually every species of inorganic electrolytes occurs in the proximal tubule. For example, large quantities of sodium and chloride are reabsorbed as part of the isosmotic reabsorptive process (Table 1). Potassium, which is filtered freely at the glomerulus, is reabsorbed throughout the proximal tubule so that within the limits of the errors of measurement, all potassium that was filtered is reabsorbed before the tubular fluid enters the distal segment. Transport may also occur in the loop of Henle, but certainly the vast majority of reabsorptive potassium movement occurs in the proximal segment. Bicarbonate reabsorption also occurs in this nephron segment.

Sodium and chloride movements also occur in the proximal segment in conjunction with the movement of a large volume of fluid. The mechanisms underlying proximal tubule sodium and chloride movement involve the same mechanisms noted in electrolyte transport through a variety of leaky epithelia [9, 10]. Whatever the mechanisms of

isosmotic transport of sodium, chloride and water in the proximal
tubule, it is noteworthy that large quantities of these substances are
reabsorbed from the proximal segment. The transport mechanisms do not
work effectively against large concentration gradients, but as much as
65% of the filtered load of these electrolytes and water are reabsorbed
in the proximal tubule. This isomotic reabsorptive process is useful
for mobilizing large volumes of fluid and electrolyte, but is not an
effective device for producing large reductions in tubular fluid concentrations.

The mechanism of sodium bicarbonate reabsorption has been studied for
many years and earlier suggestions have been documented repeatedly.
Specifically, a major part, if not the total, bicarbonate reabsorption
seems to occur as free carbon dioxide and water through the mediation of
carbonic anhydrase. Furthermore, the carbonic anhydrase involved in
this reasorptive mechanism appears to be localized within the proximal

Table 1. Reabsorption of Water and Solutes by Segments of
Nephron - Percentages are Estimated Typical Values and not
Precise Values Obtained from Segmental Analyses.

	% of filtered load at end of segment		
	Na^+	K^+	H_2O
Proximal Tubule	33	30	33
Loop of Henle	8	8	--
Distal Tubule	3	30	--
Collecting Ducts	0.6	10-20	0.8

tubular lumen or on the cell membranes facing into the lumen. This is
not to suggest that there is no role for intracellular carbonic
anhydrase, but under ordinary circumstances it would seem that the
intratubular enzymes are more important quantitatively.

Potassium reabsorption must be active in the proximal tubule. Although the potassium concentration at the tip of Henle's loop indicates
significant potassium entry in the descending limb, the amount of
potassium reaching the first segment of the distal nephron is less than
that in the late proximal tubule suggesting net reabsorption has
occurred somewhere in the loop of Henle. Almost all filtered potassium
is removed completly from the tubular fluid in its passage through the
proximal tubule and loop of Henle. The potassium present in the final
urine is added by secretion in both the late distal segment and the
cortical collecting duct.

Other electrolyte reabsorptive mechanisms also occur in the proximal
tubule. Primary movement of phosphate, sulfate, etc., appear to be in
this tubule segment. The mechanisms underlying these reabsorptive
processes are poorly understood.

Organic anion transport (B, Fig. 1). A variety of amino acids are
reabsorbed by specific transport processes located in the proximal
tubule. For example, specific transport systems for neutral and basic
amino acids are present. A separate system also exists for the β-amino
acids (e.g. taurine, β-alanine) and probably for cysteine/cystine.
Others also may exist so the exact number of these transport mechanisms

is not completely certain. In general, however, the mechanisms conform to the general chemical group of amino acids [11, 12]. These transport mechanisms are reabsorptive in nature and facilitate the conservation of amino acids filtered at the glomerulus. Evidence for secretory process for amino acids has not been forthcoming.

Renal tubular secretion of a variety of organic acids (C, Fig. 1) does occur, however. The precise number of mechanisms responsible for the secretion of organic anions has been debated. Barany [13, 14, 15] has suggested that more than one process exists although some workers have proposed that the differences in transport characteristics for different acids simply reflects different affinities of the acids for a single set of carriers. In any event similar, although not identical systems exist in other organs [13, 16, 17]. This suggests the possibility that differences in renal transport of various organic anions is related to different families of transport processes. In addition, dramatic variation in the renal handling of urate emphasizes the importance of different organic anion systems. Hook and Hewitt [18] were able to differentiate three anion transport systems based on developmental patterns. For example, induction of the hippurate system occurred in the newborn when the pregnant dams were pretreated with transport substrates for that system. Transport by other systems were not induced or only minimally so (Table 2).

Whether different processes exist, or a very broad, non-specific single process, it is true that renal organic anion secretion occurs in the proximal tubule. In mammalian species it seems likely that this secretory process represents a mechanism for the accumulation of metabolizable organic anions by renal tubular cells [19, 20]. For example, α-ketoglutarate enters renal cortical cells by the same transport system as that which translocates PAH. Substances such as PAH are capable of entering the renal tubular cell by active transport and not being metabolized, are eliminated by passive mechanisms from the cytoplasm into the renal tubular fluid. Whether or not entry into the luminal fluid is by passive diffusion or a facilitated process is unclear. Evidence for mediated luminal transport is stronger in nonmammalian proximal tubules which suggests a similar possibility for the mammalian kidney. The scheme of transport for mammalian kidney was proposed by Tune et al., [6] as a result of their pioneering studies with the isolated perfused nephron techniques.

Although the organic anion secretory process does not show great specificity with respect to chemical structure of the transport substrate, there are clear characteristics of this transport system which are quite reproducible from species to species and laboratory to laboratory. In general, these transport substrates are organic anions with pKa's usually below 7. A select group of organic acids, metabolizable substrates (acetate, pyruvate, lactate, etc.) appear to stimulate the transport of these organic anions whether measured by in vitro renal slice accumulation, or by in vivo renal clearance. Further, studies with renal slices demonstrate that PAH uptake and the uptake of other organic acids is dependent upon the bathing solution electrolyte content. Sodium, potassium, and calcium are necessary for optimal transport of the organic anions such as PAH [21, 22]. Interestingly, a high potassium concentration (20 or 40 mM) seems to optimize organic anion transport, at least for some anions [23]. Whether or not the potassium effect applies to all transportable anions is uncertain.

Table 2. Organic Anion Transport Systems as Delineated
by Developmental Studies

System	Transport Substrates	Effect of Penicillin Treatment on development
I	PAH, penicillin G, Phenolsultophthalein	+
II	Uric acid, Sulfisoxazole	±
III	Chenodeoxycholate	-

The transport of organic anions is an active one as judged by the fact that metabolic inhibitors can block these accumulation and/or transport processes. In addition, specific, competitive inhibitors of transport also exist, for example, probenecid. Probenecid and related substances do not block metabolism, but apparently have a greater affinity for the renal carrier or binder than PAH and can compete effectively with PAH for membrane translocation. In addition organic anion transport demonstrates saturation kinetics as expected for a mediated transport process.

Organic cation transport (C, Fig. 1). Just as there exists a system or systems for the transport of organic anions by renal cortical tissue, there also exists a transport mechanism or mechanisms for the movement of organic cations. The cation transport processes are less well understood than those for the anions. A similar, non-specific structural requirement is involved, however, as is a similar anatomical transport site. Many drugs and other xenobiotics are eliminated by the renal cation mechanism. In general these compounds are not similar chemically except in that they contain nitrogen and a net positive charge at physiological pH. Tetraethylammonium (TEA) and N-methylnicotinamide (NMN) are prototypical of the transport substrates. The proximal tubule is the anatomical site of transport, but no evidence exists as to which proximal tubule segment is involved [2, 22, 23]. Substrate requirements are poorly defined [24]. Although a high potassium concentration does not stimulate TEA nor NMN transport, neither does high potassium reduce the transport of these organic cations [25]. These data suggest the importance of an active transport process, since the high potassium would be expected to depolarize cell membranes eliminating the negative intracellular potential which might serve as a driving force for cation accumulation. Hence accumulation is against both electrical and chemical gradients. In addition, metabolic inhibitors block the transport of these cations, demonstrating that cellular energy is needed for transport, a characteristic of active transport.

Specific competition of one cation for the transport of another can be readily demonstrated [25]. In addition, a specific inhibitor, cyanine #863 has also proven to be a specific inhibitor of cation transport. At low doses or concentrations this substance appears to act competitively, while at high doses or concentrations non-competitive inhibition occurs. Phenoxybenzamine and other alkylating agents appear to alkylate specifically the organic cation carrier and block transport irreversibly [26]. Indeed, Ross and colleagues used the irreversible tagging of the carrier as a first step in the carrier isolation procedure.

Although all of the details of organic cation transport have not been defined quite as clearly as those for organic anion transport, there seems to be little doubt that this transport process represents a separate entity from that for organic anions. Despite the demonstration by Koschier and Berndt [27] of an interaction between 2,4,5-trichlorophenoxyacetic acid (2,4,5-T) and TEA, the general rule is that organic anion-organic cation interactions do not occur. Hence, there appears to be a secretory process for organic cations in the mammalian renal tissue that parallels a similar process for organic anions. Although there has been proposed a physiological role for organic anion transport, namely, accumulation of metabolizable acids by renal tissue, no such suggestion has been forthcoming for the organic cations. Although some compounds are accumulated by the cation system and subsequently metabolized (e.g., morphine), these do not contribute to energy mechanisms within the renal cells. However, from a pharmacological or toxicological point of view, organic cation transport is very important since many drugs and other xenobiotics possess structures which allow them to be handled by this transport process.

Sugars (B, Fig. 1). Glucose is filtered freely at the glomerulus and passes into the proximal tubule. In a normal individual or animal, almost no glucose appears in the final urine. Therefore, given normal blood glucose levels, total reabsorption or virtually total reabsorption of glucose occurs in the kidney. The vast majority of this process occurs in the proximal tubule, although small amounts of glucose reabsorption do occur in distal segments. Apparently glucose transport is coupled to that for sodium. Transport of glucose alone is much less efficient than in the presence of sodium. In the vesicle models, sodium movement is down its electrochemical gradient which promotes "uphill" movement of glucose. This demonstrates that glucose transport (i.e., reabsorption) is active. Details of physiological mechanisms for reabsorption of glucose and other sugars are given elsewhere [28].

The glucose reabsorptive process appears to be quite sensitive to the effects of a variety of nephrotoxins with actions on the proximal tubule. Not uncommonly after the administration of nephrotoxins, changes in glucose excretion occur while normal blood glucose concentrations are maintained. Whether this generalized action relates to some unusual, specific affinity of nephrotoxins for the glucose carrier or whether this is an effect which reflects the ready availability of the glucose carrier to nephrotoxins in the tubular fluid is not known. However, the latter possibility is the more likely.

The assessment of proximal tubular function is managed by several techniques. If one is to examine the effects of a chemical substance on the transport of inorganic electrolytes, intact animal studies, micropuncture on isolated perfused nephrons are needed. Although renal slice data with respect to electrolyte transport are interesting and important, they describe cellular mechanisms for maintaining normal electrolyte concentrations and do not give data pertaining to nephron function. Hence, the use of the more sophisticated techniques is required.

On the other hand, the transport of xenobiotics (e.g., PAH, radiopaque substances, toxins) can be studied with all techniques. The renal slices have proven useful over the years because this technique affords a simple, straightforward evaluation of the transport of organic anions or organic cations. The technique is simple (compared to micropuncture, isolated vesicles, isolated perfused tubules) and much less complicated than whole animals. Although the data must be interpreted with care, the technique is powerful [29, 30]. Renal slices do present a problem in the study of transport of substances which are metabolized by kidney tissue, but even some approaches to that problem are possible as demonstrated with various sugars [28].

Hence, selection of the right mechanism of study to suit a specific system or process is essential. Organic anions are studied well by renal slices as well as other techniques, whereas inorganic electrolyte transport is not. From the point of view of assessment of nephrotoxicity, the highly sophisticated techniques of micropuncture and the isolated perfused tubule have not been used extensively. Probably the major reason for this is that the techniques are extremely demanding in terms of both time and money. Hence, one almost needs to learn the technique before studying a toxicological problem rather than expecting a toxicologist to learn the technique while trying to practice other aspects of his or her profession.

Classical clearance techniques can be used to assess renal tubular elimination of organic anions and cations. Calculations such as those above for inulin will yield clearance values for the test compound. Indeed routine measurement of p-aminohippurate (PAH) clearance is used to assess renal plasma flow. It is important to note, however, that since two functions are needed for proper clearance of PAH (renal cell transport and adequate blood flow to the kidney), decreased PAH clearance may not reveal which renal function has been altered.

LOOP OF HENLE: WATER BALANCE MECHANISMS

Because direct effects of toxins on renal concentrating mechanisms seem to be relatively unimportant in terms of the mechanisms of nephrotoxicity, this topic will be commented on very superficially. Detailed explanations of the renal counter current mechanism for urinary concentration are available elsewhere [31]. Suffice it to say that through a fortunate anatomical arrangement of the loops of Henle and the blood vessels which course near them (vasa recta), differential permeability characteristics of the different segments of the loop of Henle, and the ultimate role of ADH, the mammalian kidney is capable of producing a final urine of extremely high total solute concentration. Similarly blockade of ADH release will permit elaboration of a very dilute urine. Apparently the initiating event in the development of renal tubular concentration is the ejection of sodium and chloride from the thick ascending limb of Henle's loop into the interstitium (D, Fig. 1). This event coupled with a recycling of urea and the unusual differential permeability characteristics of the loop of Henle permit the attainment of very high tubular fluid concentrations at the tip of the loop of Henle and at the outflow from the collecting ducts. The overall economy of this process is striking. Despite the elaboration of a highly hyperosmotic urine, at no point along the length of the nephron does a large osmotic gradient exist. Although huge concentration differences exist between the tip of Henle's loop and the distal segment the concentration differences across the cellular barriers from interstium to tubular fluid are quite small.

Measurement of urinary concentrating or diluting ability is often done as a clearance experiment wherein total urine and solute excretion are monitored with time. For quantitative assessment, two protocols are performed, one designed to promote maximal urine concentration (ADH infusion) and a second designed to promote minimal urine concentration (water diuresis). From these, osmolar clearance and free water formation (positive or negative) can be calculated by standard procedures. Although proper manipulation of these experimental protocols has permitted assessment of tubular sites of action of several diuretics [32], such techniques have not been utilized to a large extent with toxicity testing.

Whole animal screening procedures have been used, however. For example, conscious rats can be housed in metabolism cages and timed urine samples collected. These urines can be assessed for osmolality with a simple freezing point depression apparatus. The animals can be monitored at defined time intervals for the duration of the experiment and can even be tested for maximal urinary concentrating ability by administration of a challenge dose of antidiuretic hormone. This screening procedure will not yield the quantitative clearance data that can be obtained with the above clearance experiments, but is very useful in the acquisition of survey-type data pertaining to nephrotoxins.

Nephrotoxins do cause a prompt and effective change in tubular fluid solute concentration. This has been demonstrated to be true whether or not one is dealing with heavy metals, organic solvents, etc. It is also true when the renal failure is of the high output variety as well as with oliguric failure. In each situation the decreased urine osmolality is sustained for as long as renal function is impaired.

DISTAL TUBULE-COLLECTING DUCT (E, FIG. 1)

The functions of the distal tubular apparatus is almost as complex and as varied as that of the proximal tubule [33]. Recent studies suggest the existence of several anatomical segments between the end of the thin ascending limb and the first confluence of the distal segment with another tubule. This segment has a straight part (thick ascending limb) reaching the region of the *macula densa*, and a convoluted part thereafter. Traditionally, the distal segment has been thought to start at the *macula densa*. At least four cell types have been identified documenting the morphological heterogeneity of this nephron segment [34]. Although specific structure-function relationships have not been developed completely in the distal tubule, one would not be surprised to learn that this segment with its varied anatomical conformations would also have a variety of functional and biochemical activities. Sodium and chloride reabsorption occurs in the distal segment with such facility so as to reduce significantly the tubular fluid concentration of those electrolytes as the fluid traverses the distal segment. In addition, at one segment in the nephron sodium movement out of the tubular fluid occurs at the same site as potassium entry into the tubular fluid (potassium secretion). Studies by Giebisch and others [summarized in 33] demonstrated that it is the sodium reabsorptive process that was responsible for potassium entry into the nephron in those species where the potassium entry event was passive, i.e. potassium entered the distal tubule along its electrochemical gradient.

Various organic compounds also are removed from the tubular fluid in the distal segment. Apparently active reabsorptive processes do not exist in the distal segment for organic compounds, but extensive passive reabsorption does. The extent of passive reabsorption varies depending upon the lipid solubility of the compound in question, its pKa, the volume flow of tubular fluid, and the pH of that fluid. That is to say, nonionic diffusion of organic compounds is a predominant event in the distal segment to a large extent because it is in this segment that the most drastic changes in tubular fluid pH occur. How important these passive mechanisms are in the ultimate disposition of compounds with nephrotoxic potential has not been clearly defined. Unquestionably these events are important in the renal management of a variety of exogenous drug substances, for example, salicylate or amphetamine, and one might anticipate similar results with nephrotoxic compounds depending on their chemistry.

Standard clearance experiments have been used extensively to assess distal tubular function. For example, the nonionic diffusion process has been described with clearance techniques for many substances. This is most easily managed since it is possible to regulate both urine pH and urine volume flow over relatively wide ranges. For example pretreatment with ammonium chloride or infusion of bicarbonate can cause wide changes in urine pH ($\sim$ 5 to 8). Hence assessment of urinary excretion of a given organic substance under these extremes of pH will give insights into the importance of passive renal handling of the substance.

Micropuncture techniques have also been used, but, as indicated above, this is a highly sophisticated and demanding procedure and is not a common laboratory tool in renal physiology laboratories, let alone toxicology laboratories. Nonetheless, the application of perfused nephron procedures to study the specific renal management of certain organic compounds could be a powerful technique for the description of the nonionic diffusion process and the assessment of the renal handling of xenobiotics.

The above represents a brief view of renal tubular function. In particular, an effort has been made to emphasize those aspects of renal physiology which are most relevant to the description and understanding of nephrotoxic events. Other aspects of renal function are unquestionably important in the development of the normal homeostatic processes, but not necessarily so for renal function related to nephrotoxicity.

REFERENCES

1. Wearn JT and Richards AN, Amer. J. Physiol. 71:209-219, 1924.
2. Brenner BM, Ichikawa I and Deen WM, In The Kidney I (Brenner BM and Rector FC, eds.). W. B. Saunders Co., Philadelphia, 1981 pp. 291-295. ISBN 0-7216-1967-3.
3. Valtin H, In Renal Function: Mechanisms preserving fluid and electrolyte balance in health, Little Brown and Co., Boston, 1973, pp.40-42. ISBN 0-316-89556-3.
4. Chang RLS, Deen WM and Robertson CR, et al. Kid. Intern. 8:212-218, 1975.
5. Valtin H, In Renal Dysfunction: Mechanisms involved in fluid and solute imbalance, Little, Brown and Co., Boston, 1979, pp. 205-216. ISBN 0-316-89554-7.
6. Tune BM, Burgs MB and Patlak CS, Amer. J. Physiol. 207:1057-1063, 1969.

7. Roch-Ramel F and Weiner IM, Kidney Intern. 18:665-676, 1980.
8. Roch-Ramel F, White F, Vowles L, Simmonds HA and Cameron JS, Amer. J. Physiol. 239:F107-F112, 1980.
9. Windhager EE, In Membrane Transport in Biology, Vol. IV B (Giebisch G, Tosteson DC and Ussing HH, eds.) Springer-Verlag, NY, 1979. ISBN0-387-08895-4.
10. Reuss L, In Membrame Transport in Biology, Vol. IV A (Giebisch G, Tosteson DC and Ussing HH, eds.) Springer-Verlag, NY, 1979. ISBN 0-387-08895-4.
11. Segal S and Thier SO, In Handbook of Physiology: Renal Physiology, Section 8 (Orloff J and Berliner RW, eds) American Physiology Society, Washington, DC, 1973, pp 653-676.
12. Burg, MB, In The Kidney, Vol. I, (Brenner BM and Rector FC, eds.) Saunders, WB, Philadelphia, 1981, pp. 330-337. ISBN 0-7216-1967-3.
13. Barany EH, Acta Physiol. Scand. 88:412-429, 1973a
14. Barany EH, Acta Physiol. Scand. 86:12-27, 1972.
15. Barany EH, Acta Physiol. Scand. 88:491-504, 1973b.
16. Pappenheimer JR, Heisey SR and Jordan EF, Amer. J. Physiol. 200:1-10, 1961.
17. Cserr HF and van Dyke DH, Amer. J. Physiol. 220:718-723, 1971.
18. Hook JB and Hewitt WR, Amer. J. Med. 62:497-506, 1977.
19. Cohen JJ and Barac-Nieto M, In Handbook of Physiology: Renal Renal Physiology, section 8, (Orloff J and Berliner RW, eds.) American Physiological Society, Washington, DC, 1973, pp 922-923.
20. Barac-Nieto, M and Cohen JJ, Amer. J. Physiol. 215:98-107, 1968.
21. Taggart JV, Silverman L and Trayner EM, Amer. J. Physiol. 173: 345-350, 1953.
22. Chung, St, Park YS and Hong SK, Amer. J. Physiol. 219: 30-33, 1970.
23. Berndt WO and Beechwood EC, Amer. J. Physiol. 208:642-648, 1965.
24. Peters L, Pharmacol. Rev. 12:1-35, 1960.
25. Berndt WO, Pharmacology 22:251-263, 1981.
26. Ross CR, Pessah NI and Farah A, J. Pharmacol. Exp. Therp. 160:375-380, 1968.
27. Koschier FJ and Berndt WO, Biochem. Pharmacol. 26: 1709-1713, 1977.
28. Mudge GH, Berndt WO Valtin H, In Handbood of Physiology: Renal Physiology Section 8, (Orloff J and Berliner RW, eds.), American Physiology Society, Washington, DC, 1973, pp 594-605.
29. Berndt WO, Environ. Health Persp. 15:73-88, 1976.
30. Berndt, WO, In Toxicology of the Kidney (Hook J ed.) Raven Press, NY, 1981, pp 1-32 ISBN 0-89004-475-9.
31. Jamison RL, In The Kidney, Vol. I (Brenner BM and Rector FC eds.), W. B. Saunders, Co., Philadelphia, 1981, pp 495-550. ISBN0-7216-1967-3.
32. Mudge, GH, In The Pharmacological Basic of Therpeutics, (Gilman, AG, Goodman LS and Gilman AG, eds), Macmillan Publishing Co., Inc. NY, 1980, pp. 885-892. ISBN 0-02-344720-6.
33. Giebisch G, Malnic G and Berliner RW, In The Kidney, Vol. I (Brenner BM and Rector FC, eds.) In B. Saunders Co., Philadelphia, 1981, pp. 408-439. ISBN 0-7216-1967-3.
34. Wright FS and Giebisch G, Amer. J. Physiol. 235: F515-F527, 1978.

MICRO-, MIDDLE AND MACROMOLECULES IN BLOOD AND URINE

J. S. L. Fowler

Imperial Chemical Industries, Pharmaceutical Division, Mereside, Alderley Park, Nr Macclesfield, Cheshire SK10 4TG, UK

Abstract: Assessment of kidney function is probably one of the most difficult tasks in clinical diagnosis. Data available from present methods of blood or urine analysis are often imprecise and ambiguous with respect to detection and localisation of renal lesions. Techniques presently available for use in animals provide only poor estimates of kidney function, and in turn are limited because of the difficulties in obtaining good quality samples in routine studies.

The use of a profile of relevant blood tests is not entirely satisfactory, but is to be preferred to analysis of single parameters. Serum creatinine and albumin concentrations are an essential component of such a profile but the latter may be limited by current methods of quantitation.

Urine assays do not add substantially to the precision of routine diagnosis of nephrotoxicity although recognition of glycosuria may be a sensitive index of tubular dysfunction.

Chemically induced nephrotoxicity most often manifests as proximal tubular damage, therefore efforts to improve the methods for recognition and quantification of tubular lesions in animals seem worthwhile. The least ambiguous methods for use in preclinical studies are still based on histopathological or histochemical assessment. More emphasis should thus be placed on the sequential study of analytes in plasma and urine, and considerable effort devoted to develop methods which utilise changes in urinary macromolecules where emphasis should be placed on molecular weight determination, identification and quantitation. The use of urinary enzymes, particularly where methods for isoenzymes are available, offers an alternative route forward.

There are no immediate prospects of a resolution of the problem facing the toxicologist or the clinician.

Nephrotoxicity, Microproteins, Urinary Enzymes.

INTRODUCTION

Blood as a tissue.   Assessment of kidney function in health and disease presents one of the most challenging problems which face clinical diagnosis. Blood may be regarded as a unique circulating tissue which is in a service role for tissues such as the brain, gastrointestinal tract, muscle, skin and skeleton; whereas it itself is serviced by other major organs such as the heart, lungs, liver, spleen and kidneys. Organs whose task it is to circulate or maintain the blood also utilise a substantial blood supply in order to maintain their own metabolic functions.

This unique quality of circulating blood, to supply substrates and remove metabolites, has encouraged the growth of the diagnostic laboratory sciences in particular, clinical biochemistry and haematology. Clinical chemistry and haematology utilise samples of the blood in order to identify alterations in the tissues which it perfuses or arises from: it is paradoxical that simultaneously activities occur whose object is to return the blood as rapidly as possible to its original state thus evening out the effects of metabolic processes. This homeostatic feature creates severe constraints for the analyst since methods must be both sensitive and specific. Also the investigatory protocol must be most carefully timed if changes which manifest in blood are to be detected. The study of renal function may be approached from two directions: either the study of blood which will require quite sensitive methodology or, alternatively, by study of the urine which provides an ideal non-invasive method and has been the subject of centuries of attention from physicians and scientists.

Components of blood.   Blood plasma and cells transport nutrient and waste products. The haemoglobin binds large amounts of oxygen and in doing so, the buffering power of haemoglobin is utilised as an important factor in maintaining homeostasis. Plasma proteins exert an oncotic pressure which influences the exchange of fluid between the blood and tissues. In addition plasma proteins have an important and unique role in that they combine with many substances to form relatively inert complexes, which are broken down to yield their component parts as and when required.

Role of the kidney. In man each kidney weighs about 150 grams and is responsible for processing the blood and rejecting its waste products as urine. Every day over 1500 litres of blood are processed by the kidneys leading to a filtered volume in the glomerulus in excess of 150 litres. This is reduced by the kidney tubules until approximately 1.5 litres of hypertonic urine is voided during each day. The minimal volume of fluid which is required to cover waste solutes is of the order of half a litre per day since the maximum concentration of urine cannot exceed a 10-fold multiplication of the osmolal concentration of the plasma. The work that the kidney tubules must do in reducing the filtered load to the voided volume is very great and it is the study of this process or lack of it, which may form the basis for recognition of kidney dysfunction.

Interference with kidney function.   Two types of chemical interference can be envisaged: i) diuretic substances alter the fluid status of the body by direct action on the renal tubules. A diuretic increases urine and solute production (1), but to be therapeutically useful the output of sodium as well as of water must be increased. ii)

The most important nephrotoxic agents similarly interfere with the tubular concentration process: about 60% of adverse renal actions attributed to chemicals take the form of damage to the proximal tubule (2).

Study of kidney function. Although an enormous amount is known concerning the structure of the kidney at the microscopic and electron microscopic levels this is not necessarily helpful when it comes to evaluation of kidney function. Information would be required on its performance both at rest and under-load together with an estimate of its efficiency and some idea as to the likelihood of its continued reliability in the face of the work which it has to do. Total renal failure is not consistent with life and in reaching a conclusion concerning renal function, estimates must be made of the extent to which kidney function is impaired and if this situation is improving or declining. The study of micro-, middle and macro-molecules of blood and urine is central to this matter.

MICRO, MIDDLE AND MACRO-MOLECULES: A CLASSIFICATION

The various molecules of interest may be classified micro-, middle or macro-as shown in Table 1 .

TABLE 1. Micro-, middle and macro-molecules in blood or urine: a classification.

MOLECULE	EXAMPLES
Micro-(1-200 daltons)	H^+ NH_4^+ Na^+ K^+ HCO_3^- Cl^- inorganic phosphate blood urea nitrogen creatinine
Middle (50-5000 daltons)	methylquanidine guanidinosuccinate volatile phenols aminoacids ?
Macro-(microproteins (10-70,000 daltons)	beta-2-microglobulin retinol binding protein lysozyme ligandin
(macroproteins (70,000 + daltons)	albumin transferrin N-acetylglucosaminidase IgA, IgG, IgM Tamm-Horsfall

RECOGNITION AND LOCALISATION OF KIDNEY DEFECTS

The study of known nephrotoxic agents in animal models has led to an enormous literature relating to the kidney. Unfortunately the techniques for recognition, let alone localisation of kidney defects in the intact animal or human are somewhat less advanced. Safety evaluation requires methods for early detection of relatively insidious or low-grade nephrotoxins but this is particularly poorly served.

No panacea is at present available to the toxicologist or the nephrologist. No single method seems to offer particular promise: the best opportunities for recognition of agents with kidney damaging potential still seems to lie in the careful design of studies incorporating contributions from a multi-disciplinary team.

STUDY OF MICROMOLECULES IN BLOOD

Profiles. The measurement of several parameters on a sample of blood from a patient or animal may indicate kidney dysfunction. (Table 2).

TABLE 2.   Simple Profile for Recognition of Kidney Disorders
               by Analysis of Plasma or Serum

bicarbonate	chloride	creatinine
sodium	potassium	glucose
blood urea nitrogen		

Changes in plasma or serum profiles may, however, be blurred by other effects. For example the overuse of diuretics elevate bicarbonate, with a reciprocal depression of chloride, hypokalemia, hyponatremia, elevated blood urea nitrogen and slight hyperglycemia. In pre-renal conditions and in renal failure there is hyponatremia, hyperchloremia and general metabolic acidosis. Blood urea nitrogen is generally very high and slight hyperglycemia may also be present. In pre-renal as opposed to renal insufficiency the ratio of blood urea nitrogen to creatinine is usually high. In renal tubular acidosis there is conservation of chloride with an associated depression of bicarbonate: these changes may be seen in potassium loss syndromes or certain drug therapies such as amphotericin treatment.

Single parameters. Use of single parameters is considerably less effective than use of profiles. Chloride can be raised in renal failure or reduced in renal disease. Bicarbonate can be raised during diuretic treatment but low in renal failure. Potassium is high in renal failure in acidosis and low following certain diuretics. Sodium is high in dehydration and over administration of intra-venous fluids, but low in advanced renal failure. Blood urea nitrogen is high in renal conditions but may also be high in pre-renal conditions such as myocardial infarction (3).

Creatinine is probably the most useful single parameter in routine screening for renal damage. Creatinine clearance calculation may not be worthwhile since reliable information about glomerular filtration rate is not necessarily obtained. Plasma creatinine alone, if elevated, indicates abnormal glomerular filtration which is sufficient to confirm that more detailed investigations should be undertaken (4). A reduction in glomerular function can occur without plasma creatinine becoming abnormal, but this is more frequently the case for creatinine clearance, and deterioration in glomerular function is detected less frequently with creatinine clearance than with plasma creatinine alone. The reciprocal of plasma creatinine has the further advantages that it changes in the same direction as, and in proportion to, the changes in glomerular function.

TABLE 3.   Full Profile for Recognition of Kidney Disorders
            by Analysis of Plasma or Serum.

bicarbonate	aspartate aminotransferase	inorganic phosphate
sodium	total protein	creatinine
glucose	lactate dehydrogenase*	calcium
blood urea nitrogen	chloride	albumin
alkaline phosphatase	potassium	

*not suitable for routine use in animals due to interference from blood cell enzyme.

MACROMOLECULES IN BLOOD

Incorporation of information relating to protein or enzyme concentration and activities into profiles of micromolecular data leads to considerably greater precision in the diagnosis of the various types of renal condition. For example, in the overuse of thiazide diuretics, which tend to cause dehydration, there is elevated blood urea nitrogen, total protein and albumin with a consequent increase in total calcium since it is largely albumin bound. Circulating enzyme activities such as lactate dehydrogenase or aspartate aminotransferase are usually in the high normal range.

In pre-renal conditions such as congestive heart failure or dehydration, blood urea nitrogen is elevated although creatinine is normal. Plasma albumin is reduced due to a marked loss of protein in the urine and total protein in blood will be affected to a slightly lesser extent. Lactate dehydrogenase and aspartate aminotransferase activities will be slightly elevated outside the normal range. In advanced renal conditions albumin will be quite markedly decreased due to proteinuria, whereas total protein may be low, but still close to the normal range. A consequence of chronically low circulating albumin will be low total calcium which in turn gives rise to compensatory secondary hyperparathyroidism leading to an elevated alkaline phosphatase (bone isoenzyme) activitiy in blood. Lactate dehydrogenase will be slightly higher due to retention, but aspartate aminotransferase activity is likely to be low. Hyperglycemia is a frequent observation in nephrotic states and may well be associated with anti-insulin activity which has been ascribed to the presence of middle molecules due to the uraemic state.

In renal tubular disease there is an osteomalacia due to chronic wastage of phosphate with a consequently raised alkaline phosphatase activity and an elevated blood urea nitrogen. Low circulating protein levels (in particular albumin) are seen and the consequent secondary reduction in total calcium is again apparent. In uremia blood urea nitrogen and creatinine levels are very high. In addition, 'middle molecules', some of which may arise from breakdown of creatinine for example, methylguanidine and guanidinosuccinic acid, are detectable and may be responsible for the toxemia of the uraemic state. Low circulating aspartate aminotransferase activity is commonly encountered when renal insufficiency is treated by dialysis it is thought to be due to the loss of the cofactor pyridoxine during the treatment. In these cases total calcium may become elevated even though albumin is still in the low range, the reason for this is unknown.

Single parameters. Albumin is raised in dehydration, but is usually low in renal disease. This is a most reliable parameter but, unfortunately, the methods which are currently employed in the majority of clinical analysers are based on the binding of bromo-cresol green and this method is quite unreliable for accurately detecting lower concentrations of albumin. Total protein is slightly reduced in renal disease but in renal infarction any of the enzymes (for example, alkaline phosphatase, lactate dehydrogenase or aspartate aminotransferase) may be elevated, due to destruction of renal tissue.

MICRO- AND MACRO-MOLECULES IN URINE

Since the blood parameters, even when assembled into profiles, are generally relatively insensitive and ambiguous in differential diagnosis of renal disease, considerable attention has also been focussed on urine parameters. Clearance calculations may be used, but creatinine clearance does not offer any particular advantage over plasma creatinine. As explained earlier, it is less effective in detecting abnormal glomerular filtration (4).

Determination of urinary electrolytes, osmolality or specific gravity can provide valuable information allowing differentiation of diuretic actions from nephrotoxic damage. Proteins and even cells are found in small amounts in normal urine but may be grossly elevated in renal disease. The detailed study of various proteinurias would seem to offer a promising approach which should be pursued actively in the future.

Serum proteins. Serum proteins may be found in urine and can be used to classify different types of renal disease (Table 4), according to their molecular weight. The pattern of proteins in the voided urine results from the interaction of the two main processes of glomerular filtration and tubular reabsorption, therefore ranking proteins by molecular weight can be helpful. Quantification of a large number of proteins is tedious, but using two proteins of dissimilar molecular weight (such as transferrin and IgG), the relative permeability of the glomerulus can be established (5).

A prognosis based on the amount of protein excreted in unit time should be regarded with great caution, because a reduction in protein excretion will occur as numbers of funtional glomeruli decline and also as the serum albumin level falls. Thus the determination of serum creatinine and albumin should always accompany estimates of voided protein.

TABLE 4. Classification of Renal Disease according to
         type of Protein in Urine. [8]

TYPE	IMPLICATION	CHARACTERISED BY
I	Normal	Traces of most serum proteins
II	Proximal Tubular Defect	Presence of microproteins from serum (up to 70,000 daltons)
III	Specific Glomerular Defect	Presence of certain (only) of the larger proteins from serum (70,000 + daltons)
IV	General Glomerular Defect	Presence of most of the larger proteins from serum.
V	Mixed Glomerular and Tubular Damage.	Presence of micro- and macro-proteins from serum

TABLE 5. Some Urinary Proteins from Renal Sources.

PROTEIN	ORIGIN
alkaline phosphatase aminopeptidase	brush border
N-acetylglucosaminidase	lysosomes
beta-glucosidase	cytosol
ligandin	proximal tubule (pars recta)
Tamm-Horsfall	ascending limb distal tubule collecting duct
lactate dehydrogenase	distal tubule

TABLE 6.   Some Urinary Enzymes of Value in Diagnosis of
            Renal Disease   (6)

DISEASE	ENZYMES
Glomerular	
aminonucleoside of puromycin	kallikrein, NAG, beta-galactosidase
anti-GMB antibody	kallikrein, alkaline phosphatase
glomerulonephritis	NAG
Proximal Tubular	
mercuric chloride chromate uranyl nitrate cadmium	ligandin alanine aminopeptidase leucine aminopeptidase alkaline phosphatase gamma-glutamyltranspeptidase NAG, glucosidases
Distal Tubular	
folate	lactate dehydrogenase alkaline phosphatase
Papilla	
ethyleneimine	NAG glucosidases alkaline phosphatase

Renal origin proteins. Proteins in urine may be of renal origin (Table 5). Several proteins found in urine may be enzymic and some of the most useful of these are shown in Table 6.

Many reviews of those urinary enzyme determinations which are useful in the differential diagnosis of renal lesions have appeared in the literature. Two of the most recent are Price (6), and Vanderlinde (7).

SOME SPECULATIVE AREAS FOR RESEARCH

MIDDLE MOLECULES IN BLOOD

There has been increasing interest in the study of uraemic states and abnormal metabolites which can be detected in such states. Three will be considered, the volatile phenols, methylguanidine, and guanidosuccinic acid. A brief note is made regarding glycosuria and molecules in the range 200-10,000 daltons.

Although the concept of 'middle molecules' is not utilised in biochemistry circles, it is important in the clinical sense since most of the important 'dialysable' entities will occupy this molecular weight range. Also in the middle-molecule range are all xenobiotics, and their Phase I and Phase II metabolites. Finally, the concept of middle-molecule is convenient since it separates the true micromolecules (e.g. to 200 daltons) from the macromolecules as visualised by the protein biochemist (e.g. 10,000-60,000 daltons).

Guanidines as uraemic toxins. Guanidinosuccinic acid (GSA) is regarded as a prime candidate for a uraemic toxin (9) as is methylguanidine (MG) (10). There is evidence that guanidines are haemolytic in vivo or ex vitro (11) and also are markedly toxic to dogs (12).

It can be demonstrated that GSA is elevated in both blood and urine of uraemic patients (13) and MG is similarly elevated and is distributed preferentially into blood cells and other tissues (14). Arginine and creatinine which was traditionally thought to be inert, are now known to be precursors of MG (15) and low nitrogen diets which have been empirically used in uraemic situations are now known to decrease the metabolic production of both MG and GSA (16), presumably by reducing the deamination load.

Although there seems little doubt of the importance of MG and GSA in uraemic states, it is doubtful that they will be useful parameters for early detection of nephropathy since elevated levels will follow and seem unlikely to precede this damage. These parameters, however, could be quite important where the objective is to monitor damage and determine a prognosis.

Glycosuria. Presence of glucose in urine is due to incomplete recovery of the filtered load. Glycosuria is seen after administration of several nephrotoxins (17) and correlates well with excretion of renal ligandin in mercuric chloride damage and low dose chromate damage (18). We have found that seqential determination of urinary glucose concentrations offers a suitable means for screening of compounds with straight or convoluted proximal tubular damaging actions: for example as caused by maleic acid or heavy metals.

Volatile compounds in urine. Development of sensitive gas chromatographic methods has led to detection of volatile materials in urine from man and rat (19,20). Eighty compounds of which sixty were identified for the first time, were confirmed by GC-MS (21) to be in the molecular weight range 44-154 daltons.

The importance of such molecules is unknown; they may arise in intestinal obstruction (22). Endotoxin of intestinal origin (23) may also be implicated in certain nephropathies. In view of the common site of origin of endotoxin and volatile phenols it is tempting to speculate on a correlation between abnormal bacterial activity in the gastro-intestinal tract, concomitant volatiles in blood or urine with the presence of a nephropathy.

Regardless of speculation, volatile phenols are found in serum of uraemic patients and are reduced by renal dialysis: p-cresol is the dominant compound so far identified (24).

Molecules 200-10,000 daltons. Although a wide range of molecules is known to be excreted within this size range, including nearly all drug metabolites and their conjugates, as yet there is little in the literature to suggest that use has been made of them in routine toxicological or clinical assessment of kidney damage.

MACROMOLECULES IN URINE

Microproteins. The presence of beta$_2$-microglobulin, alpha$_2$-microglobulin and lysozyme is regarded as indicative of tubular disease (25,26). It has recently been shown that normal tubular reabsorption of filtered microproteins will occur even in the presence of elevated serum levels. Quite high serum levels of microproteins can arise in malignant disease such as myelomatosis, but these will not necessarily lead to elevated levels in urine as long as tubular function is unimpaired (27).

The consensus of published material suggests that determination of microproteinuria would offer a means of early detection of renal tubular disease: however, in a recent study designed to determine the effects of cadmium in rhesus monkeys, this was not the case since all changes were relatively late in onset (28). Further studies in animals with other reference compounds would seem desirable.

Renal ligandin. Renal ligandin is present in proximal tubular cells as a component of the renal organic anion transport system (29) and may be induced by pretreatment with tetrachloro-dibenzo-p-dioxin. Purified ligandin is a 46,000-dalton protein and probably consists of two sub-units (22,000 and 24,000-daltons) which are monomers of two distinct proteins (30). Liganduria is an early indicator of mercuric chloride damage (proximal tubule: pars recta) and to a lesser extent, potassium dichromate damage (proximal tubule: pars convoluta). Glycosuria is simultaneously seen with the liganduria (18).

Despite early optimism, ligandin has not received as much attention recently, but the other components of the anion transport system may be important in consideration of chemically induced nephrotoxicity.

Urinary Enzymes. Most urinary enzymes probably derive intrinsically from the kidneys, since serum enzymes having a molecular weight greater than 70,000 daltons will be excluded by the glomerulus (See Table 5). Even so, assays of urinary enzymes are not at present recommended as screening procedures, due to the influence of extra-renal diseases and difficulty of analysis due to interfering substances. There may, however, be a case for their use in evaluation of functional nephrotoxic damage attributed to new drugs. Measurement of isoenzyme patterns offers greater diagnostic specificity

N-Acetyl-beta-glucosaminidase (NAG) has been studied in detail (31) and seems to offer some promise. Urinary NAG is elevated in several acute nephropathies, including acute tubular necrosis, active glomerular nephritis and analgesic nephropathy. The B isoenzymic form of NAG is particularly increased in renal disease and is indicative of tubular dysfunction, whereas the A^S form is likely to be related to glomerular disease (A^S = Serum origin) (32).

A feasibility study for introduction of a newly synthesised substrate incorporated in a dip-stick urine test for NAG has also been undertaken by Price (6).

Mucoproteins - Tamm-Horsfall protein.   A high molecular weight protein was identified by Tamm and Horsfall (33) with reactivity towards various viruses.   Tamm-Horsfall Protein (THP) is secreted by distal tubular cells and is a glycoprotein composed of multiple sub-units.   It is produced by and associated with plasma cell membranes of cells of the ascending limb of the loop of Henle and the distal convoluted tubule. THP has recently been found to cross react with two serum proteins having apparent molecular weights of 125,000 and 84,000 daltons (34) THP has been said to have a general similarity of structure to human erythropoietin (35). The role of THP is incompletely understood. It is reported able to trap E.coli and may therefore, have importance in the non-immunological anti-infectious mechanism of mucosal surfaces (36); a role for THP in tubular lithiasis has been suggested (37) although this must presently be regarded as controversial (38).

THP has been shown to be useful as an early indicator of chromate damage (39) and further studies seem warranted in animals with respect to a potential role for THP in nephrocalcinosis. Certainly, in view of the large variety of functions assigned to THP, its unique structure and site of elaboration, further study of aspects of its role seem obligatory.

CONCLUSIONS

If there is to be one single parameter which could be recommended for routine assessment of renal function then it would have to be plasma creatinine.   The   creatinine   method   unfortunately   is   inherently inaccurate and subject to interference by chromogens in the blood.   It seems unnecessary to determine creatinine clearance and urea does not offer a genuine alternative since it is elevated in so many pre-renal conditions.

The ability to produce a concentrated urine is also a good functional test of renal integrity.   In the concentration test, osmolality of concentrated urine in a water deprived patient or animal gives a good indication of efficiency of tubular conservation mechanisms. The urine analysis techniques have a major advantage in that they are non-invasive.   However, the quality of urine which may be available in routine animal studies is usually unsatisfactory for sophisticated analysis.

Proteinuria, of which enzymuria is a special case, is a common manifestation of renal disease; the separation of albumin and the microproteins enable detection of tubule dysfunction, whereas glomerular dysfunction is indicated by presence of the large proteins.

Unfortunately, the methods for characterization of proteins in urine are not suitable for adaptation to routine toxicological investigations. For   example,   the   sodium   dodecyl   sulphate-polyacrylamide   gel electrophoresis technique has the disadvantage of requiring extensive pretreatment of urine including concentration and incubation and a long destaining procedure after electrophoresis.   It is not, therefore, applicable to the continuous monitoring of animals, although as an analytical tool it is very powerful.

The use of urinary enzymes is similarly not immediately adaptable to routine toxicity trials; but N-acetyl-glucosaminidase (particularly if isoenzyme determinations can be done), seems to offer a specific means for detecting tubular damage.

Histological and histochemical investigations still provide an essential backup to these biochemical determinations. At present the best approach will be achieved by a combination of plasma creatinine and urinary protein determination combined with histochemistry and histopathology at the appropriate times.

It is hoped that real advances can be made in the applicability of some of the newer techniques to routine investigation of nephrotoxic potential of therapeutic or environmental chemicals.

REFERENCES

1.   Laurence DR & Bennett PN, Clinical Pharmacology 5th Ed: Churchill Livingston, 1980.
2.   Muehrcke RC, Acute Renal Failure. Diagnosis Management. C V Mosby Co. pp. 167-261, 1969.
3.   Moseley MJ, et al. Arch Intern Med 141: 438-440, 1981.
4.   Morgan DB et al, Post Grad Med J 54: 302-310, 1978.
5.   Kerr DNS & Davison JM, Brit J Hospital Med 361, 1975
6.   Price RG,submitted for publication.
7.   Vanderlinde RE, Ann Clin Lab Sci 11: 189-201, 1981.
8.   Balant L & Fabre J Diagnostic Significance of Enzymes & Proteins in Urine (UC Dubach & Schmidt, eds.) p. 216-223, 1979.
9.   Cohen BD, Arch Intern Med 126: 846-850, 1970.
10. Barsotti G, Arch Intern Med 131: 709-713, 1973.
11. Giovannetti S, et al. Clin Sci 34: 141-148, 1968.
12. Giovannetti S, et al. Clin Sci 36: 445-452, 1969.
13. Kopple JD, et al. J Lab Clin Med 90: 303-311, 1977.
14. Orita Y, et al, Nephron 27: 35-39, 1981.
15. Orita Y, et al, Nephron 22: 328-336, 1978.
16. Ando A, et al. Nephron 24: 161-169, 1979.
17. Wright PJ & Plummer DT, Biochem Pharmacol 23: 65-73, 1974.
18. Bass NM et al. Clin Sc 56: 419-426, 1979.
19. Dirmikis SM & Darbre AJ, Chromatogr 94: 169-187, 1974.
20. Yoshihara I, Agric Biol Chem 44: 1185-1187, 1980.
21. Miyashita K & Robinson AB, Mech Aging Develop 13: 177-184, 1980.
22. Tamm A & Villako K, Scand J Gastroenterol 6: 5-8, 1971.
23. Jacob AI, et al. Gastroenterology 72: 1268-1270, 1977.
24. Wengle B & Hellstrom K, Clin Sci 43: 493-498, 1972.
25. Peterson PA, et al. J Clin Invest 48: 1189-1198, 1969.
26. Johansson BG & Ravnskov U, Scand J Urol Nephrol 6: 249-256, 1972.
27. Engstrom W, et al. Clin Chim Acta 108: 369-374, 1980.
28. Nomiyama K, et al. Arch Environm Contam Toxicol 10: 297-304, 1981.
29. Kirsch R, et al. J Clin Invest 55: 1009-1019, 1975.
30. Bass NM et al. Biochim Biophys Acta 492: 163-175, 1977.
31. Price RA, Curr Probl Clin Biochem 9: 150-163, 1979.
32. Tucker SM, et al. Clin Chim Acta 102: 29-40, 1980.
33. Tamm I & Horsfall FL, Proc Soc Exp Biol & Med 74: 108, 1950.
34. Lynn KL, et al. Kidney International 19: 619, 1981.
35. Grant AMS & Neuberger A, Biochem J 136: 659-668, 1973.
36. Orskov I, et al. Lancet 1: 887, 1980.
37. Hallson PC & Rose GA, Lancet 1000-1002, 1979.
38. Sophasan S, et al. J Urol 124: 522-524, 1980.
39. Schwartz RH, et al. Lab Invest 27: 214-217, 1972.

THE URINARY EXCRETION OF TAMM—HORSFALL GLYCOPROTEIN

Anne B. St. J. Dawnay, Carolyn Thornley and W. R. Cattell

Departments of Chemical Pathology and Nephrology, St Bartholomew's Hospital, London EC1, UK

INTRODUCTION

Tamm-Horsfall glycoprotein (THG) is produced only by the kidney. It is predominantly excreted in the urine as aggregates which has hampered progress in assessing the value of its measurement. Thus insensitive assays have necessitated the use of laborious techniques in attempts to achieve a uniform state of disaggregation and, by implication, a degree of immunoreactivity proportional only to concentration. Aggregation is promoted by high cationic strength, low pH and high concentrations of THG. Simply by using a sufficiently sensitive method to allow a 1:100 or greater dilution of sample in distilled water prior to analysis, we have developed an assay which is unaffected by these factors. We present here the validation of this method and the excretion rates in a healthy population and in patients with chronic renal impairment.

METHODOLOGY

Assay. Concentrations of THG were determined by a rapid (2h) radioimmunoassay with a sensitivity of 20ng/ml. Samples with lower values were re-assayed by a more sensitive procedure capable of detecting 1.6ng/ml [1] . Intra- and inter-assay coefficients of variation were less than 10% at all concentrations.

Urinary aggregation of THG. The degree of aggregation of THG was crudely ascertained by comparing the amount of THG precipitated by centrifugation of 1ml of fresh urine at 2000rpm for 10 min with the amount remaining in the supernatant. As expected, increasing values of the ratio precipitated THG: supernatant THG correlated positively and significantly with high osmolality (r_s = 0.74, $p < 0.001$, N=20), low pH (r_s = 0.58, p 0.01, N=20)

and high concentrations of THG in the urine (r_s = 0.71, p < 0.001,
N=20). THG could not be precipitated from samples after a 1:100
dilution in distilled water.

   Disaggregation. Samples were either diluted 1:100 in distilled
water or 1:100 in assay diluent (0.065M sodium phosphate buffer
containing 0.01M EDTA and 2% (w/v) bovine serum albumin, pH 7.4) or in
varying proportions of the two. The concentrations of THG increased
with increasing dilution in water and plateaued at 1:20. (Figure 1.)
This effect paralleled the reduction in ionic strength which presumably
led to greater disaggregation and therefore allowed the detection of
previously buried antibody binding sites. A dilution of 1:100 in water
was subsequently used and results were independent of incubation time
at this dilution.
   The measurement of THG was not affected by variation of urinary pH or
calcium concentration or incubation in the presence of SDS provided
that samples had been diluted 1:100 in water.

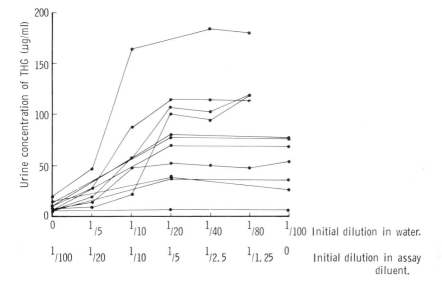

Figure 1. The effect of dilution in distilled water on the apparent
concentration of THG in urine.

   Storage. The freezing of urine either at -20°C or in a mixture of
methanol and carbon dioxide has been reported [2,3] to affect the
concentration of THG. We have found no such effect either before of
after dilution (1:100) in distilled water. Samples could be stored at
room temperature or at 4°C for at least 2 days without change in
concentration.

   Validation. Parallelism, and therefore immunological identity, was
demonstrated between the standard preparation and the samples at 4
dilutions (1:100, 1:200,1:400, 1:800). Occasionally, and especially in
concentrated urines, a deviation was seen at the lowest dilution but not
in the remaining three.
   THG in the range 94 to 1500 ng/ml was added to diluted (1:100) urines

containing 292 and 200 ng/ml. Recoveries of 96 to 114% (mean 106%) were
obtained.

APPLICATION OF THE ASSAY

   Normal range.   The excretion of THG in 15 females and 14 males with
normal renal function ranged from 22 to 56 mg/24h which is similar to
that found by others [2,4].   In the 22 individuals examined, a good
correlation was obtained between the THG/creatinine ratio in 24h
collections and in random samples from the same timed period   (Figure
2).
   The normal excretion ratio ranged from 16 to 52 mg THG/g creatinine
(median 31) in 45 healthy females and from 12 to 56 mg/g (median 23) in
44 males. This slightly lower median is due to the generally higher
creatinine excretion in males.   There was no correlation between the
THG/creatinine ratio and age (range 22-72 years).

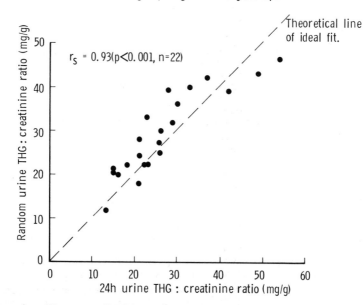

Figure 2.   The correlation of urine THG i.e. THG/creatinine or above
creatinine ratios in 24h collections and random samples from the same
timed period.

   Chronic renal failure.   24h urinary excretion of THG has been
correlated with simultaneous creatinine clearances in 29 healthy
individuals and in 18 patients with chronic, stable renal impairment
(Figure 3).   It can be seen that the correlation between the two is
tighter the greater the reduction in creatinine clearance.   Factors
determining variation in the urinary excretion of THG in relation to
creatinine clearance in normals remains to be defined but it is clear
that a valuable new tool for defining renal function in health and
disease has been developed.

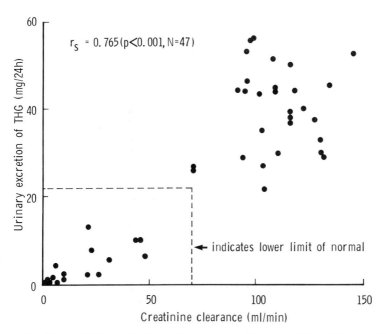

Figure 3. Correlation of the urinary excretion of THG with creatinine clearance in healthy individuals and in patients with chronic, stable renal impairment.

CONCLUSIONS

1. A urinary THG assay has been developed which is not interfered with by factors known to cause aggregation of this glycoprotein.
2. The urinary THG measured reacts in an immunologically identical manner to non-aggregated standard preparations and samples may be stored frozen.
3. THG excretion in health and disease shows a general relationship to creatinine clearance implying glomerulo-tubular balance. This is also shown in the THG/creatinine ratio in 24h and random urine samples. In normal subjects there is, however, a significant variation in THG excretion in relation to creatinine clearance which requires further study.

References

1.   Dawnay ABStJ, McLean C and Cattell WR.   Biochem J 185: 679-687, 1980.
2.   Grant AMS and Neuberger A. Clin Sci 44: 163-179, 1973.
3.   Goodall AA and Marshall RD.   Biochem J 189: 533-539, 1980.
4.   Samuell CT.   Clin Chim Acta 85: 285-293, 1978.

A PERSPECTIVE ON THE PATHOLOGY AND CYTOCHEMISTRY OF RENAL LESIONS

J. M. Faccini

Pfizer Central Research, Centre de Recherche, Laboratoires Pfizer, 37400 Amboise, France

ABSTRACT.   Despite common morphological features, it is difficult to extrapolate renal pathological findings from laboratory animals treated with potential nephrotoxic compounds to man. There is a high background of spontaneous nephropathies in laboratory animals especially rodents, the incidence and severity of which increases with age.
A full understanding of renal pathology in laboratory animals is best achieved by measuring as many parameters as possible including enzyme histochemistry coupled with quantitation of enzymes in urine, and electron as well as ligh microscopy. Studies carried out with gentamicin have shown a dose-related nephrotoxicity. When assessed by electron microscopy the lesion correlated better with the renal binding of the antibiotic than with light microscopic assessment.

KEYWORDS. Spontaneous renal disease, histochemistry, aminoglycosides, analgesics, histochemistry.

INTRODUCTION

The task of the pathologist in diagnosing human disease or evaluating toxicological pathology is to identify the aetiological agent that is responsible for the changes he observes. To do this, he must have a profound understanding of the physiology, normal anatomical variation and types of disease that affect the organ or tissue in question. No-where is this more important than in the study of the effects of chemicals on the kidneys of laboratory animals and in the subsequent extrapolation of these findings to assess the degree of hazard they represent for man.

Species differences in metabolism and physiology are sufficient to warrant caution when extrapolating the results of animal studies to man but, nevertheless, laboratory animals and the rat, in particular, have proved of immense value in predicting the potential toxicity of a wide range of chemicals including drugs.

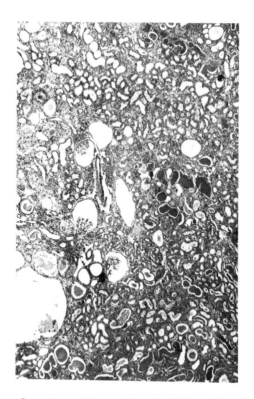

Figure 1. The renal cortex of an untreated 24-month old rat showing the fully developed form of progressive renal disease in this species - tubular dilatation, cysts, cast formation and fibrosis. H.E. x 40.

RENAL DISEASE IN LABORATORY ANIMALS

It is outside the scope of this article to give a comprehensive account of renal disease in laboratory animals ; a few of the more significant spontaneous diseases will serve as an illustration of their importance.

Progressive renal disease in rats (glomerulonephrosis). The single most important renal disease in adult and aged rats [1] which, in its established form in senile rats, is easily recognisable. The kidneys are enlarged and pale with cystic spaces, some of which are large enough to be visible to the naked eye. Microscopically, many tubules are dilated and frequently contain pink-staining proteinaceous material - "thyroid-isation" (Figure 1) ; tubular epithelium is both hyperplastic and atrophic with thickened basement membrane ; the glomeruli show a wide variety of changes - ranging from sequential to global glomeruloscle-rosis - the segmented form is reminiscent of the nodular lesions seen in the human glomerulus in diabetics.
Aged rats can have a 100% incidence of this disease, a situation which bedevils chronic studies with this species, especially if the test substance is suspected of producing nephrotoxicity. It is an interesting feature of this condition that the blood urea often remains within

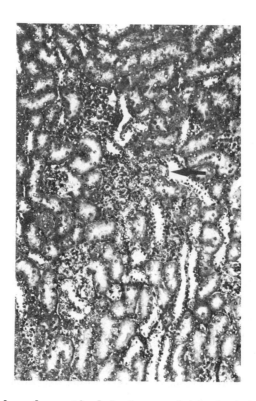

Figure 2. Minimal early cortical lesion, probably incipient glomerulonephrosis, in a 3-month old untreated rat (arrow), comprising tubular
dilatation, basophilia and a loss of tubular architecture. H.E. x 90.

normal limits despite the presence of dramatic histological changes. In
man too, the lack of sensitivity of blood urea measurements as an
indication of the severity of chronic renal disease is well known [2].
    Strain differences are important and in long term studies on un-
treated rats carried out at Amboise, we have found a higher incidence in
Long-Evans than Sprague-Dawley rats - males 74% against 56% ; females
44% against 13% respectively [3].
    The potential for this condition to cause confusion in toxicity
studies occurs with the initial phase of the disease. Although the
disease is age-related [4], [5], the onset may commence before six
months especially with such accelerating factors as high protein diets
[5] and transient potassium deficiency 6 . Such dietary and metabolic
disturbances are, incidentally, among the many aetiological agents that
have been suggested for this disease which, nonetheless, remains cryptogenic.
    Figure 2 illustrates a lesion that we recognise in the colony of rats
(Sprague-Dawley, Charles River France) that are used in Amboise and that
can occur as early as 3 months and increases in frequency and severity
with age. It corresponds to the description given in the literature and
the fact that it appears confined to tubules explains the popularity of
the hypothesis that glomerulonephrosis in rats is an incipiant tubular
lesion. A comparison of this lesion - tubular degeneration with an

adjacent round cell infiltrate - with the early lesion induced by aminoglycosides or heavy metals (Figure 5) illustrates the need for caution
in interpreting nephrotoxicity in this species. Nevertheless, the rat
remains in the author's view the species of choice for assessing nephrotoxicity because of its susceptibility to nephrotoxins.

   Renal amyloidosis. This is an important disease in some strains of
mice and syrian hamsters [1]. It occurs in approximately 5-30% of
untreated male and 2-5% of untreated female mice and 0-4% of untreated
male and 0-8% of untreated female hamsters used in our laboratory at
Amboise. In mice strains with a high incidence, the disease begins at
about 6 months of age and is important because it causes papillary
necrosis and is, therefore, a potential cause of confusion in assessing
analgesic and non-steroidal antiinflammatory agents in this species.

   Interstitial nephritis (focal). This condition occurs in all species
of laboratory animals [1]. In the rat, it may be a manifestation of
early glomerulonephrosis (see above). It produces distortion of tubules
accompanied by a focal mononuclear inflammatory cell infiltrate that has
to be distinguished from the subacute lesion seen with tubular toxins.
The focal nature of the spontaneous lesion with the lack of changes in
other parts of the kidney and the absence of biochemical changes help in
the differential diagnosis.

   Interstitial nephritis (diffuse). This condition is primarily of
importance in the dog. The acute form is rare and generally associated
with leptospira organisms [7]. The chronic form, which is much more
common, is cryptogenic although an infectious aetiology is suspected [8],
it only enters into the differential diagnosis with a possible nephrotoxic agent in the milder forms of the disease which produces multifocal
areas of fibrous tissue containing dilated and cystic tubules. This more
localised lesion resembles the hypercalcaemic nephropathy of hyperparathyroidism in man and can be produced experimentally by administration
of parathyroid hormone or large doses of vitamin D [9].

   Renal calcification (mineralisation). Focal mineral deposits in the
medulla are common to the laboratory rat and dog. They are unlikely to
cause confusion when it is recognised that they are a high incidence
phenomenon. Ultrastructural studies suggest that shed microvilli can
initiate intraluminal microliths [10]. They stain positively with the
Von Kossa technique for calcium. They are commoner in female rats and
this would appear to be a hormonal phenomenon as ovariectomy inhibits
the development of the lesion and oestrogens induce it in males [11].
Their presence correlates with the calcium/phosphorus ratio in the
diet [12].

RENAL TUBULAR ENZYMES AND NEPHROTOXICITY

   Given the high histochemical activity of a number of relatively
easily measured enzymes in the renal tubular epithelium and the fact
that some of these enzymes can be recovered from the urine, it is not
surprising that these techniques have gained a wide popularity as
indications of nephrotoxic potential. In addition, urinary enzyme assays
have the obvious attraction that they constitute a non-invasive technique that can be employed on human subjects and would, therefore,

appear to satisfy the ultimate goal of the toxicologist – a test that can be easily applied to both the experimental animal and man.

Attempts to correlate urinary enzyme activities with histology and histochemistry are hindered by the technical difficulties of obtaining uncontaminated 24-hour urine samples from rats, together with the fact that there are considerable variations in urinary enzyme activity in normal rats. Following a detailed study comparing histochemical activity in the renal cortex of the same enzymes measured in urine, Cottrell and his co-workers [13] concluded that the value of urinary enzyme measurements in the rat was limited.

In a series of experiments carried out by Pfizer Central Research [14], the same problems were encountered but it was concluded that under certain conditions urinary enzymes could be of value. It was found that the type of metabolism cage was important, collecting the urine in vessels surrounded by ice reduced the contamination of microorganisms which interfered with the assays and dialysis of urine samples increased the enzyme values. A period of acclimatisation before treatment is also especially important : high values of enzyme activity are obtained after transferring rats to metabolism cages and changing them from nightly to daily feeding, for example, requiring an optimum period of acclimatisation of six days before any treatment is started. The range for 80 consecutive 24-hour urine samples collected from 40 untreated rats after a period of acclimatisation is given in Table 1.

Table 1. Normal ranges for values for cell counts and enzyme levels obtained from 80 rat urine samples.
ULN : Upper limits of normal, LLN : Lower limits of normal, and SD : Standard deviation.
GOT = glutamate-oxalacetate transaminase, GPT = glutamate-pyruvate transaminase, LDH = lactate dehydrogenase, ALP = alkaline phosphatase, ICDH = isocitrate dehydrogenase, and γ-GT = gamma-glutamyl transpeptidase.

	Cell counts	Enzyme levels (IU/L)					
		GOT	GPT	LDH	ALP	ICDH	γ-GT
ULN	400	10.0	8.4	16.0	148	3.9	2541
LLN .	100	2.5	1.3	2.4	18	1.1	495
Mean	136	5.5	3.7	7.2	54	2.6	660
± SD	60	1.5	1.4	2.8	25	0.7	232

It can be seen that there is still considerable variation between the high and low values obtained. The choice of enzymes at the time of these experiments was fairly arbitrary but, for example, treatment with variable doses of intraperitoneal mercuric chloride and collecting the urine over the subsequent 24 hours showed a dose-related correlation in groups of 3 rats per dose level (Table 2).

A similar correlation with time is seen after consecutive doses over 3 days (0.2 mg/kg i.p.) in Table 3.

After a single high dose (2.7 mg/kg s.c.) and then continued 24 hours monitoring over 13 days is given in Table 4.

Table 2. A comparison of parameters used to assess kidney damage in rats treated with mercuric chloride. ULN = upper limit of normal.

Dose (mg/kg i.p.)	GOT	Enzyme levels (IU/L)					Blood urea (mg %)	Cell counts (x10^2)
		GPT	LDH	ICDH	ALP	γ-GT		
0	5.4	2.6	7.3	2.1	64	1091	44	2.0
0.1	7.0	2.3	12.1	2.2	50	692	41	1.7
0.3	9.2	3.7	21.9	15.8	58	815	43	5.3
0.6	98.0	6.2	197	312	78	1575	68	15.6
1.0	310	17.3	806	437	199	2901	76	44.6
2.7	365	27.2	1025	942	1968	5364	160	250
ULN	10.0	8.4	16.0	3.9	148	2541	56	4.0

Table 3. The effect of daily injections of mercuric chloride (0.2 mg/kg i.p.) on parameters used to assess kidney damage in rats. Values in brackets are from 3 rats treated with saline.

Day of treatment	GOT	Enzyme levels (IU/L)			Blood urea (mg %)	Cell counts (x10^2)
		LDH	ICDH	ALP		
1	9.3	22.5	12.5	72	–	4.7
	(5.7)	(8.6)	(2.1)	(41)		(2.0)
2	140	170	133	348	–	37
	(5.9)	(10.6)	(1.9)	(52)		(1.7)
3	206	508	254	854	95	123
	(5.7)	(9.6)	(1.7)	(48)	(48)	(2.0)

Table 4. Urinary changes following 2.7 mg/kg single injection s.c. mercuric chloride-induced kidney damage in rats and during the subsequent healing period.

Days post treatment	GOT	GPT	Enzyme levels (IU/L)				Cell counts (x 10^2)
			LDH	ICDH	ALP	γ-GT	
1	370	17.2	1157	942	1969	5634	260
2	60	5.5	265	138	140	1650	80
3	25.0	3.6	47.0	6.7	49	758	53
4	18.0	4.3	25.0	2.3	38	711	28
5	14.3	3.8	26.3	2.0	41	721	44
6	12.8	4.4	20.0	1.8	34	700	33
7	14.4	2.4	28.0	2.0	74	967	55
8	13.9	4.0	21.0	2.0	58	897	21
9	9.9	3.3	16.2	1.8	40	662	28
10	10.5	4.6	15.0	1.7	60	1010	22
11	7.4	3.7	13.6	2.3	56	660	33
12	6.1	4.0	11.3	3.2	50	670	23
13	6.3	3.8	8.8	1.9	40	500	13

Mean blood urea level was 59.5 mg % at day 13.

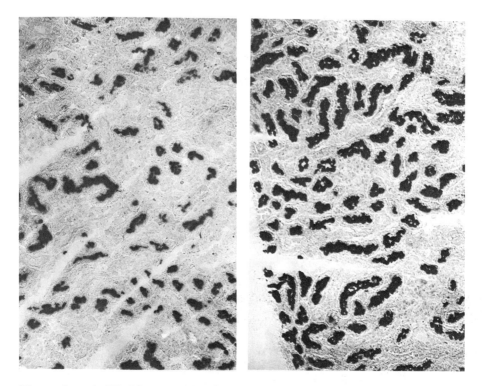

Figure 3. a) Alkaline phosphatase activity in the renal cortex of a rat
treated for 3 days with 100 mg/kg gentamicin s.c. There is a loss of
activity in comparison with a control rat (b) injected with distilled
water. Gomori technique x 90.

It can be seen that only LDH and GOT remain raised and in other
similar experiments with neomycin the only consistant enzyme to be
raised was LDH, this led to the subsequent use of LDH assays of urine
samples as a convenient method of assessing nephrotoxic potential of
aminoglycosides. The fall off in enzyme activity with time despite
persistent, histochemical and histological evidence of continued cellular damage has been noticed by several workers [13], [15] but it does
not diminish the value of these and other enzymes, for example β-galactosidase,N-acetyl-β-D-glucosaminidase [16] and maltase [17], as indicators
of initial nephrotoxicity. The value of certain enzymes in man may be
even greater. Mondorf measuring the urinary activity of the human brush-
border enzyme, alanine aminopeptidase, in healthy volunteers showed it
to be a sensitive index of minimal nephrotoxicity with a variety of
aminoglycoside antibiotics at therapeutic dose levels [18].
    In the experimental animal, enzyme histochemistry affords an oppor-
tunity with electron microscopy of identifiying the cellular component
that is damaged by nephrotoxins. Its value, in this respect, nevertheless, is limited.

Alkaline phosphatase. One of the earliest targets of nephrotoxic
agents e.g. heavy metals or aminoglycoside antibiotics is the brush

border of the proximal convoluted tubule [17], [18]. As alkaline phosphatase is a brush border enzyme, a reduction in its activity can be shown histochemically [13], [16]. Figure 3 shows the alkaline phosphatase activity demonstrated by the Gomori technique [19] in the kidney of a rat treated with 100 mg/kg body weight of gentamicin given subcutaneously for 3 days and then killed on the fourth day. A partial loss of staining is apparent when compared to a control rat. Following the same protocol but killing the rats 48 hours after cessation of treatment rather than 24 hours, however, would reveal a much greater reduction in enzyme activity [16]. Measurement of alkaline phosphatase activity in the urine of rats treated with nephrotoxins has shown that increases in the activity of this enzyme are adequate indices of nephrotoxicity but according to Stroo et al. [12] it is no more sensitive than other methods and, to Cottrell et al. of limited value in the rat [13]. From the various studies carried out at Pfizer Central Research and those of Wellwood et al. [16] among others, it is apparent that, in rats given aminoglycoside antibiotics, raised levels of alkaline phosphatase appear in the urine soon after the initiation of treatment. A subsequent loss of this enzyme activity in cortical proximal convoluted tubules is only evident later on when, as would be expected, the urine enzyme

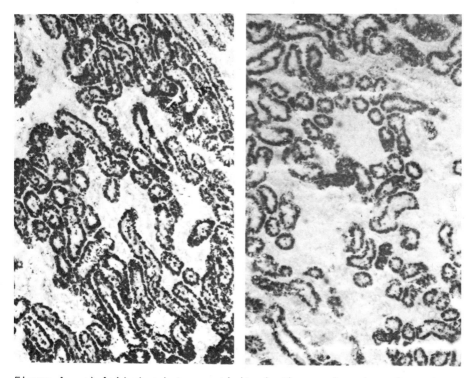

Figure 4.   a) Acid phosphatase activity in the renal cortex of a rat treated for 3 days with 100 mg/kg gentamicin s.c. The reaction product is more diffusely distributed than in the control rat (b) indicating increased lysosomal activity. Technique of Baker and Anderson [24] x 90.

activity has fallen. Therefore, although of limited value as indices of nephrotoxicity, these techniques do throw some light on the mechanism involved.

Lactic dehydrogenase. A number of investigations have shown that this enzyme when measured in the urine is a sensitive index of renal tubular damage [13], [14], [20], [21]. With stain histochemistry, rats treated with 100 mg/kg b.w. of gentamicin for 3 days (as above) did not show any modification of enzyme activity in tissue sections, whereas much lower dosage of this antibiotic and neomycin have been found to produce significant rises in urinary activity [14], [22].

Acid phosphatase. The proximal convoluted tubule is rich in lyso-somal acid phosphatase [23] and just as electron microscopy demonstrates increased numbers of lysosomes with nephrotoxins so enzyme histochem-istry reveals modifications in activity. The changes observed depend to some extent on the method employed and are best understood by the concomitant demonstration of other lysosomal enzymes such as leucyl-aminopeptidase. Using the technique of Barker and Anderson [24] on renal cortical tissue from rats given gentamicin (as above) an initial in-crease in activity with a diffuse "staining" is apparent when compared to controls (Figure 4). With the ensuing necrosis a total loss of this enzyme from the cortex is found [16].

Glucose-6-phosphatase. This enzyme has a rich distribution in proximal convoluted tubules [24] and although in the liver it is esta-blished as a good indicator of tissue damage, we did not found it of great value as such in the kidneys of rats treated with gentamicin.

Succinic dehydrogenase. As a mitochondrial component, this enzyme is found in all parts of the renal tubule especially the thin ascending limb [25]. It is apparent from electron microscopic studies that changes in membranes and cytosegregosomes occur before any modifications in mitochondria which diminishes the importance of this enzyme as a histo-chemical indicator of the initial effects of most of the common nephro-toxins.

THE NEPHROTOXICITY OF AMINOGLYCOSIDE ANTIBIOTICS

The histochemical changes produced by gentamicin described above are a reflection on the susceptility of the rat proximal tubular cell to the effects of aminoglycoside antibiotics. Lesions can also be demonstrated by both light and electron microscopy ; they are highly reproducible and give a good indication of potential toxicity.

The acute changes or those induced by mildly toxic doses can only be detected by electron microscopy but with chronic administration or moderately toxic doses, lesions are evident by light microscopy. The established lesion, which is one of acute proximal tubular necrosis, comprises epithelial flattening with cytoplasmic basophilia and nuclear pyknosis with evidence of regeneration manifested by mitoses (Figure 5) ; amorphous deposits are present in the lumina and there is some tubular dilatation. With chronic dosing, foci of fibroblastic proliferation and lymphocytic infiltration of the interstitium appear. These changes are illustrated in Figure 6 taken from a male rat given 40 mg/kg b.w./day of gentamicin for 4 weeks.

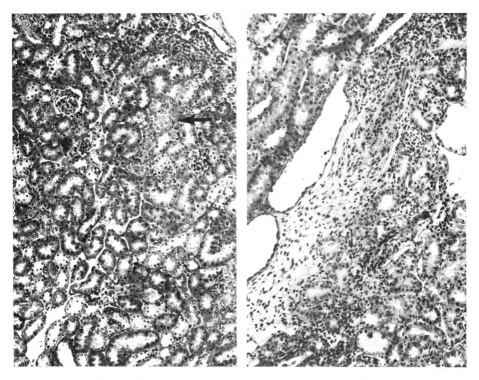

Fig. 5   Fig. 6

Figure 5. Early changes of acute tubular necrosis in a rat given
20 mg/kg b.w. of gentamicin subcutaneously for 7 days. There is a focus
of tubular basophilia only (arrow). H.E. x 90.

Figure 6. Renal cortical changes in a rat given 40 mg/kg b.w. of
gentamicin for 4 weeks. There is tubular dilatation and focal adjacent
fibrosis with round cell infiltration. H.E. x 90.

   The severity and extent of such lesions lend themselves to a form of
grading which can be useful in assessing new antibiotics and comparing
them in a semi-quantitative manner with marketed compounds. Figure 7
shows the results of a study in which 10 rats/sex/dose group were given
10, 20 and 40 mg/kg body weight of gentamicin intramuscularly per day
for four weeks. Scoring the resultant tubular necrosis minimal 1,
moderate 2 and marked 3, a histogram can be constructed which shows that
the pattern of severity is dose-related, especially in males. This
correlated with clinical chemistry parameters and renal weights.
   In a subsequent series of experiments, we attempted to correlate
these changes and those seen by electron microscopy with plasma and
renal levels of gentamicin. In one study, three rats per sex were given
gentamicin at 5 and 20 mg/kg subcutaneously in one group once, and
another, consecutively for 7 days ; the animals were killed 24 hours
after the last dose. Light microscopic evidence of nephrotoxicity was
seen in some but not all of the rats, but this did not correlate with

GENTAMICIN DOSE GIVEN INTRAMUSCULARLY FOR 1 MONTH

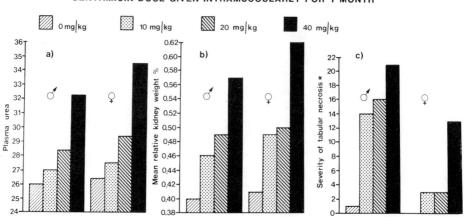

Figure 7. The effect of gentamicin treatment (0, 10, 20 and 30 mg/kg, intramuscularly for 4 weeks) on (a) plasma urea (b) relative kidney weight (c) severity of tubular necrosis* in male and female rats.

* derived from number of animals x degree of necrosis, where minimal = 1, moderate = 2, marked = 3.

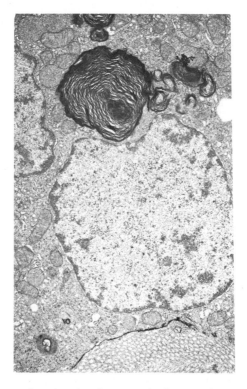

Figure 8. Electron micrograph of a proximal convoluted tubular cell of female rat given 40 mg/kg b.w. of gentamicin for 2 weeks. The characteristic cytosegrosomes are seen adjacent to the nucleus.   x 7056.

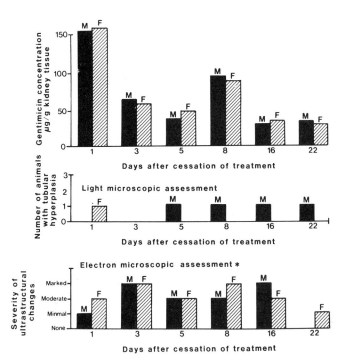

Figure 9. Renal concentrations of gentamicin compared with light and electron microscopic assessment of nephrotoxicity in male and female rats following gentamicin treatment 5 mg/kg/day subcutaneously for 7 days (3 animals / sex sampled at days 1,3,5,8,16 and 22 following cessation of treatment).

* The severity of nephrotoxicity is related to the concentration of intracellular myelin figures and cytosegrosomes. (M = male, F = female)

the plasma or renal concentrations of drug. Electron microscopy, on the other hand, even after a single dose correlated well. Cytosegregosomes and myelin figures were observed in the cytoplasm of proximal convoluted tubular cells from both males and females. Their distribution was more extensive and their size greater in animals of both sexes receiving the higher dosage (Figure 8).

In a separate study, 18 male and 18 female rats received 5 mg/kg gentamicin for 7 days and were then killed in groups of 3/sex 1, 3, 5, 8, 16 and 22 days after the last dose. Gentamicin kidney concentrations declined from about 150 µg/g of fresh kidney tissue one day after the last dose to about 25 µg/g at day 22. A striking rebound in kidney concentrations was noted on day 8 (Figure 9). Acute tubular necrosis and resultant hyperplasia were only seen sporadically by light microscopy but electron microscopy showed evidence of marked renal damage even 16 days after the last dose.

In general, the degree of nephrotoxicity of gentamicin, as with other aminoglycoside antibiotics, is dependant upon the amount administered and the species or even strain of animal being studied 26 . As plasma

levels and the extent of renal binding are dependant upon dose and
length of administration [27], a close correlation between binding and
nephrotoxicity would be anticipated.

However, as 75% of gentamicin is taken up by the luminal surface of
the proximal convoluted cells [28], the extensive renal damage that
occurs with high dosage limits the amount of aminoglycoside taken up by
the kidney and, consequently, no correlation between dose and tissue
damage is observed with such high doses [29]. With lower doses or
shorter periods of administration, conventional light microscopy does
not detect nephrotoxicity [16]. This has led to the assumption that
there is no good correlation between renal binding and nephrotoxicity [30].
The use of electron rather than light microscopy, however, shows that
this is not the case, particularly with moderate doses of aminoglycosides.

THE NEPHROTOXICITY OF NON-STEROIDAL ANTIINFLAMMATORY (NSAI) AGENTS AND ANALGESICS

Whereas the kidneys of rats and indeed other laboratory animals
including the dog, are adequate models for the toxic effects of amino-

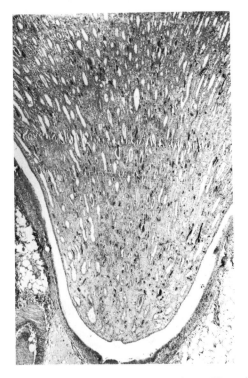

Figure 10. The renal papilla of a male rat given 50 mg/kg b.w. phenylbutazone for 24 months showing diffuse necrosis. H.E. x 40.

glycoside antibiotics, this is not the case with NSAI agents and analgesics. The characteristic and limiting renal toxicity of NSAI agents in
chronic animal toxicity studies is papillary necrosis. All compounds of
this class appear to cause this lesion in all animal species to which
they have been administered in adequate doses over long periods of
time [31]. Figure 10 illustrates the renal papilla of a male rat given
50 mg/kg body weight of phenylbutazone orally for 2 years : the tissue
is necrotic with merely the outline of the collecting tubules apparent
and a few remaining vesicular nuclei. A clear demarcation between the
necrotic papilla and the surviving medullary tissue is usually seen. An
associated cortical interstitial nephritis is induced by this phenomenon
and can be prevented by prior surgical removal of the papilla [32].

The rat is especially sensitive to the effects of NSAI agents and the
sensitivity has been shown to vary with different strains [33]. The
ratio of the dose causing renal papillary necrosis in animals – especially rats and mice – to the usual clinical dose administered to man is
consequently comparatively low. This has stimulated a universal critical
evaluation of renal function tests in clinical trials and a search for
renal papillary necrosis in man. Whereas patients show altered renal
function during therapy with NSAI agents, they do not have the same
susceptibility to papillary necrosis. In contrast, in man, this lesion
is associated with analgesic agents, especially those containing phenacetin 34 . When these analgesic compounds are given to animals, however, they do not produce papillary necrosis unless administered in
exceptionally high (lethal or sublethal) doses [35] or accompanied by
such draconian measures as dehydration [36]. A rat model does exist but
this is the Gunn strain bred from mutant Wistar rats which has a profound deficiency of glucuronyl transferase which results in the progressive accumulation of unconjugated bilirubin in the renal papilla [37]. To
further add to the differences between animals and man, the usual lesion
induced in animals is tubular necrosis and this again necessitates high
dosage [35] unless such precipitating factors as dietary manipulation
are employed [38].

The lack of correlation between the animal experiments and man in
this respect led Rosner in his comprehensive review of the subject [35]
to the pessimistic view that "had the histopathologists and the clini-
cians not drawn attention to the problem of nephropathy induced by
analgesic abuse, the toxicologist would never have suspected, foreseen
or predicted the existence of such a syndrome". In the five years that
have ensued since the appearance of that review, however, it has been
established that prostaglandins are exceptionally important to the renal
circulation [39] and that profound differences exist between experimental animals and man and even between sexes within the same species in
the relative importance of the different prostaglandins [40], [41]. This
helps to explain the different reactions between species to NSAI agents
which inhibit prostaglandins, and it can be hoped that further dis-
coveries of that nature and a better understanding of mechanisms will
help in the extrapolation of animals studies in general to man.

I should like to acknowledge the collaborative work of my colleagues
in Pfizer Central Research and particularly that of C. Charuel, M.J.
Gallimore, E. Irisarri and J. Martin.

REFERENCES

1. Casey HW, Ayers KM and Robinson FR, in Pathology of Laboratory
    Animals, Vol. 1 (K Benirschke, FM Garner and TC Jones, eds.).
    Springer-Verlag, New York, 1978, pp. 115-166. ISBN 0-387-90292-9.
2. Dossetor JB, Ann Intern Med 65:1287-1299, 1966.
3. Greaves P and Rabemampianina Y, Arch Toxicol in press.
4. Bras G and Toss MH, Tox appl Pharm 6:247-264, 1964.
5. Durand A, Allen M, Fisher M and Adams M, Arch Pathol 77:435-450,
    1964.
6. Kennedy GC, Glear CTG and Parker RA, Quart J Exptl Physiol 45:82-87,
    1960.
7. Taylor PL, Hanson LE and Simon J, Am J Vet Res 31:1033-1049, 1970.
8. Krohn K, Mero M, Oksanen A and Sandholm M, Am J Pathol 65:157-170,
    1971.
9. Epstein FM, J chron Dis 11:255-277, 1960.
10. Nguyen HT and Woodward JC, Am J Pathol 100:39-56, 1980.
11. Armstrong WG and Horsly HJ, Nature 21:980-981, 1966.
12. Clapp MJL, Lab Animals 14:253-261, 1980.
13. Cottrell RC, Agrelo CE, Gangolli SD and Grasso P, Fd Cosmet Toxicol
    14:593-598, 1976.
14. Gallimore MJ, Pfizer Internal Report 19/12/75.
15. Spangler WL, Adelman RD, Gonzelman GM and Ishizaki O, Vet Pathol
    17:206-217, 1980.
16. Wellwood JM, Lovell D, Thompson AE and Tighe JR, J Path 118:171-182,
    1976.
17. Stroo WE and Hook JB, Toxicol appl Pharmacol 39:423-434, 1977.
18. Mondorf AW, Breier J, Hendus J et al., Eur J clin Pharmacol 13:133-
    142, 1978.
19. Chayen J, Bitensky L and Butcher R, Practical Histochemistry.
    John Wiley, London, 1973, p. 111. ISBN 0-471-14950-0.
20. Wright PJ and Plummer DT, Biochem Pharmacol 23:65-73, 1974.
21. Leathwood PD, Gilford MK and Plummer DT, Enzymologia 42:285-301,
    1971.
22. Gregory MH, M.Sc. Thesis, University of Surrey, 1977.
23. Ericson JLE and Trump BF, Histochemie 4:470-479, 1965.
24. Barka T and Anderson PJ, J Histochem Cytochem 10:741-753, 1962.
25. Heptinstall RH, In Pathology of the Kidney, Vol. 1, 2nd edit.
    Little Brown & Co., Boston, 1974, p. 1. ISBN 0-316-35795-2.
26. Cuppage FE, Setter K, Sullivan LP, Reitzes EJ and Melnykovych AO,
    Virchows Arch B Cell Path 24:121-138, 1977.
27. Reiner NE, Bloxham DD and Thompson WL, Clin Res 25: 460A, 1977.
28. Collier VU, Mitch WE and Lietman PS, Clin Res 26: 288A, 1978.
29. Nieminen L, Kasanen A, Kangas L, Sairo E and Anttila M, Experientia
    34:1335-1336, 10, 1978.
30. Gilbert DN, Plamp P, Starr P, Bennett WM, Houghton DC and Porter G,
    Agents Chemother 13:34-40, 1978.
31. Wiseman EH and Reinert H, Agents Actions 5:322-325, 1975.
32. Hardy TL, Brit J exp Pathol 1:591-600, 1970.
33. Bokelman DL, et al Tox appl Pharmacol 19:111-124, 1971.
34. Dubach UC, Levy PS, Rosner B, Baumeler HR, Muller A, Peier A and
    Ehrensperger T, Lancet 1:539-545, 1975.
35. Rosner I, CRC Crit rev Toxicol 4:331-352, 1976.
36. Goldberg M, Myers CL, Peshel W, McCarron D and Morrison AB, J clin
    Invest 50:37-44, 1971.

37. Axelsen RA, J Path 120:145-150, 1976.
38. Maclean A, Chenery R, Nuttall L and Fisher C, J int Med Res 4:79-82, Suppl 4, 1976.
39. Editorial, Lancet 11:287-289, 1981.
40. Ubaidi F and Bakhle YS, J Physiol 291:41-42, 1979.
41. Gecse A, Ottlecz A, Schaeffer I, Bujdoso A and Telegdy G, Biochem Biophys Res Commun 86:643-647, 1979.

THE USE OF HISTOCHEMICAL TECHNIQUES ON 1 MICRON METHACRYLATE SECTIONS OF KIDNEY IN THE STUDY OF CEPHALORIDINE NEPHROTOXICITY IN RATS

Roger Burnett

The Boots Co. Ltd, Pathology Department, Biological Research R3, Pennyfoot Street, Nottingham NG2 3AA, UK

INTRODUCTION

Early nephrotoxic changes have been detected by enzyme histochemical methods, using frozen sections. There are however technical problems involved in handling sufficient sections, at any one time, to allow for valid comparisons.

With the advent of commercially available water soluble methacrylates it is possible to produce 1 micron sections with excellent definition and negligible shrinkage of the tissue. In addition, the retention of enzyme activity in methacrylate embedded tissues has been reported [1].

Cephaloridine has been reported to cause acute damage to the proximal tubules in rodents [2] and has been used to investigate urinary enzymes in the rat [3].

MATERIALS AND METHODS

Groups of 15 female Charles River CD rats (100–120 g bodyweight) were given a single subcutaneous injection of 0.5, 1, 2 or 4 g/kg of Cephaloridine ('Ceporin' Glaxo Laboratories) as a 20% (w/v) aqueous solution. A control group was given a subcutaneous injection of saline. Three rats from each dosage group were killed on days 1, 2, 3, 4 and 10.

The kidneys were quickly removed, weighed, and cut into 4–5 mm slices which were fixed at 4°C in buffered formalin on a roller mixer for 24 hours. The tissues were then dehydrated in 70, 85, 90 and 100% ethanol for 20 min each stage, and infiltrated overnight on the roller mixer at 4°C, in non polymerised JB–4 plastic (solution A) with a catalyst (Windsor Laboratories UK). The tissues were then transferred to fresh plastic, containing the catalyst, according to the manufacturer's instructions. The polymeriser (solution B) was mixed 1 : 40 with the plastic. This was placed into Sorval moulds, with aluminium holders and allowed to cure in a vacuum. The blocks were taken from the moulds, wiped and allowed to dry, and sectioned at 1 μm on a

Reichert Autocut motor driven rotary microtome using glass knives. The
sections were taken up onto numbered slides, air dried, and stored until
required.

Kidney sections were stained with haematoxylin and eosin, and
toluidine blue. A variety of enzyme histochemical techniques were
applied; only those found to be consistently reproducible are reported
here, others are under investigation.

On each occasion sufficient media was made to incubate 75 slides
plus controls, in Coplin jars. The following methods were used (no
rehydration is required):-

Alkaline phosphatase (AP):- The Gomori method [4], with incubation
for 21 h at pH 9.4 at 37°C. After treatment, sections were counter
stained with methyl green, dried on a hot plate and mounted in
Ralmount (R A Lamb Ltd) mounting media.

Adenosine Triphosphatase (ATPase):- The calcium-cobalt method
of Padykula and Herman [5] with pre-incubation at pH 4.6 in veronal
buffer at room temperature for 15 min and incubation for 20 h at pH
9.4 at 37°C. Sections were finally dried and mounted.

Non-specific Esterase (NSE):- The α naphthyl acetate method
of Davis and Ornstein [4], with incubation for 18 h at pH 6 at 37°C,
sections were then dried and mounted.

Controls:- Media without the substrate was used in each case.

RESULTS

Enzyme methods:- No specific staining was seen in the negative
controls. The three methods worked repeatedly giving precise enzyme
localisation with excellent structural detail. The AP and ATPase
activity was similar in distribution and confined mainly to the brush
borders (fig. 1). The NSE activity was largely confined to the
lysosomes, with some cytoplasmic staining in the cells of the proximal
tubules (fig. 3).

The calcium method for AP was more reproducible than the azo dye or
substituted naphthol methods, giving a stronger reaction and less
deposit. The calcium method for ATPase gave better results than
the Wachstein lead method as this procedure produced much more deposit.
Pre-incubation at pH 4.6 for 15 min gave a better demonstration of
brush borders in the proximal tubules than with no pre-incubation or
with 15 min pre-incubation at pH 4.2, 5, 9 or 9.4. The NSE α naphthyl
acetate method using pararosanilin produced a better localiation
than other techniques and this was further enhanced by reducing the
pH to 6.

Amongst the other enzymes investigated was acid phosphatase; the
standard method gave no reaction with these sections.

Cephaloridine nephrotoxicity study:- 4 g/kg produced severe proximal
tubular necrosis on the first day and killed 8/15 rats. All rats had
died or were killed by day 4.

2 g/kg caused degenerative changes by day 1, the earliest changes
were in the brush borders and these were readily detected by the
marked reduction in AP/ATPase activity (fig. 2). There was also
a marked loss of lysosomal NSE activity in the proximal tubules
(fig. 4). These changes progressed to necrosis of the proximal tubules
(particularly the first segment) on day 2, reaching a maximum by day 3.

1 g/kg and 0.5 g/kg caused hydropic change and some loss of indiv-

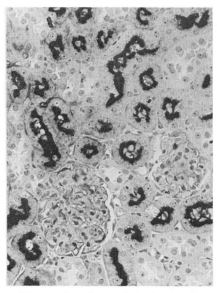
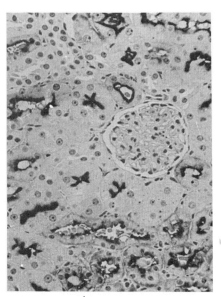

Figure 1 : Control rat kidney
Normal ATPase activity (X160)

Figure 2 : 2 g/kg Cephaloridine Day 1
disrupted brush borders (ATPase X160)

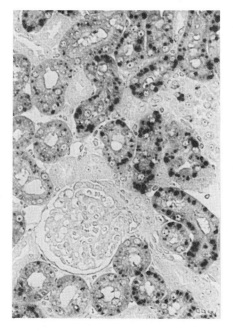
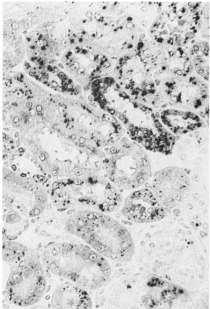

Figure 3 : Control rat kidney
Normal NSE activity (X160)

Figure 4 : 2 g/kg Cephaloridine Day 1
reduced NSE activity (X160)

idual cells in the proximal tubules, these were accompanied by slight changes of the marker enzymes, which was most noticeable on day 3.

Even in the most severely affected animals given 2 g/kg the basement membranes appeared to be intact. Regenerative changes occurred from day 4, with a gradual re-epithelialisation of the tubules. In the less damaged tubules resolution occurred by division of adjacent cells but in the severely denuded tubules mitotic activity was seen in the distal portion of the proximal tubules and cells appeared to spread up the nephron. The low cuboidal epithelium of the regenerated tubules was lined by a narrow band of AP/ATPase activity.

Animals killed on day 10 showed virtual complete resolution of the architecture and the enzyme distribution was similar to that of the controls. The brush borders appeared lower than in the controls.

DISCUSSION

Demonstrable amounts of AP, ATPase and NSE are retained in methacrylate embedded tissue which has been fixed in formalin for 24 h at 4°C, but a prolonged incubation of up to 24 h is required. The level of activity is low when compared with that in fresh frozen tissue, but because of the good localisation and fine preservation of tissue structure, the technique has much to commend it. The ability to cut, store and bulk stain a large number of slides makes direct comparison between sections from several blocks all stained together possible. Histochemical and light microscopy methods can be used on serial sections. Shorter fixation times gave only a marginal increase in activity. Washing of the tissue after fixation had a similar effect, but also increased the background staining. The use of different fixatives and fixation times may enable different enzyme systems to be demonstrated, eg others [1] used Karnovsky's fixative and achieved staining for acid phosphatase but not alkaline phosphatase. This pattern was reversed after fixation in formalin. The incubation times required have been seen to vary greatly with the pre-treatment and can only be determined empirically.

In this study, at a time when the toluidine blue stained sections were equivocal, the marker enzymes, particularly those of the brush border, gave a clear demonstration of the cellular damage.

The application of enzyme techniques to 1 μm methacrylate embedded tissue can be recommended for investigations where the detection of early changes is required without recourse to electron microscopy.

REFERENCES

1. Higuchi S, et al. Stain Technol 54 (1) 5-12, 1979
2. Atkinson R M, et al. Toxicol Appl Pharmacol 8, 398-406, 1966.
3. Ngaha E O and Plummer D T. Biochem Med 18, 71-79, 1977.
4. Bancroft J D and Stevens A, Theory and Practice of Histological Techniques. Churchill Livingstone, Edinburgh and London, 1977 Chapter 18. ISBN 0-443-01534-1.
5. Bancroft J D and Stevens A, Histopathological stains and their diagnostic uses. Churchill Livingstone, Edinburgh and London, 1975, p. 131. ISBN 0-443-01226-1.

THE CHOICE OF ANIMALS FOR NEPHROTOXIC INVESTIGATIONS

Hilmar Stolte and Jeanette M. Alt

Hannover Medical School, Department of Internal Medicine and Department of Physiology, Laboratory of Experimental Nephrology, Hannover, FRG

ABSTRACT

In studies concerned with nephrotoxicity there is no general preference for any single species or strain of research animal. The selection depends on the aim of the study as well as particular functional or anatomical features of the animal's kidney plus availability, ease of handling etc.

In many investigations in experimental nephrology the animal of choice is the rat due to the development of micropuncture techniques and micro-analytical methods which may yield more insight into kidney function in health and disease at the single nephron level. The rat kidney is also used for isolated organ perfusion and for biochemical studies of cellular or subcellular fractions. However, the utility of the rat in the investigation of proteinuria as a symptom of the diseased kidneys is limited. In contrast to man there is a pronounced proteinuria in rats, which is age related and depends on strain and sex. Other animal species used for specific experimental studies include the rabbit (isolated perfused tubules), the hamster (renal papilla), or necturus (electrophysiology).

In experimental medicine the results of animal studies are often extrapolated to man. These interspecies comparison may be complicated by many factors such as the selection of an adequate reference e.g. body surface, body weight or kidney weight. Moreover, nephrotoxic drugs may cause species and strain dependent effects that differ quantitively, even though there are well documented similarities in both functional and morphological lesions.

Keywords: Nephrotoxicity, laboratory animals, renal physiology, proteinuria

INTRODUCTION AND GENERAL ASPECTS

The choice of animal models in medical and particularly in experimental nephrotoxicity studies depends on the aim of the study and the applicability of the results to man or clinical medicine.

Table 1 summarises the more general aspects of the selection of research animals used in science or industry. Industry is mainly concerned with different species for screening tests and less with questions about pathomechanisms. Scientific studies require a smaller number of animals and the application of more sophisticated techniques.

Table 1.   General aspects

- Science or industry
- Availability (costs)
- Handling (size, sensitivity to stress)
- Standardization (inbred, outbred, food, sex, age)
- Background information

The costs of handling and standardization are equally important for both science and industry. In the USA "The Animal Welfare Act", which became law in 1966, has influenced the choice of animals by protecting dogs, cats, hamsters, rabbits and all wild warmblooded animals, but not rats or mice.

In order to reduce the number of test animals when searching for small effects standardization is essential. Matching for age and sex of reference and test animals is obligatory. Moreover, maintenance and diet have to be standardized. Differences to diet alone can provoke functional changes such as increased or decreased albumin excretion (Hackbarth, personal communication). A reduced uptake of electrolytes and other food components can also influence the response of the test animals to experimental conditions. An important advantage of barrier maintained specific pathogen free animals is that infectious diseases may greatly increase the inter-animal variability. The question of whether inbred or outbred strains are to be preferred depends on the type of investigation. When looking for small differences between test and control, inbred strains should be used, but whenever the range of possible reactions is broad (i.e. for the detection of rare side effects of drugs) outbred strains with great genetic variability may be preferred.

To compare different species the allometric function for interspecies relation can be used. This function has been determined for different parameters such as glomerular filtration rate or organ weights (for further detail see: "Research animals and concepts of applicability to clinical medicine", Exp.Biol.Med., Vol.7, editors: K.Gaertner, H.J. Hackbarth, H. Stolte, Karger, Basel, 1982, in press). The susceptibility of some animal species deviates from the rule which complicates the prediction of how they might react to the experiment.

There are no general preferences of research animals in nephrotoxicity studies. To exclude nephrotoxicity of certain substances at least three different species should be used with only one rodent species. The rat is the animal choice in nephrology, due to the development of micropuncture techniques and microanalytical methods, which were an important step forward, yielding more insight into kidney function in health and disease at the single nephron level [1-5]. Therefore most animal models for investigation of renal physiology and pathophysiology are now based on the rat.

This presentation will be focussed on the advantages, disadvantages and special choices of research animals presently used in nephrology with particular emphasis on nephrotoxicity studies.

RESEARCH ANIMALS USED IN EXPERIMENTAL MEDICINE AND NEPHROLOGY

In 1961 Schmidt-Nielsen [6] surveyed the physiological abstracts submitted to the Federation Proceedings on research animals used including man.   Dogs, rats, primates and cats were used in 88% of 700 studies. Twenty years later a similar survey [7] has showed that rats, men and mice have gained the lead.   Dogs are still used, but in a much smaller percentage.   In experimental medicine this change is certainly influenced by the general aspects discussed above including the "Animal Welfare Act" in the USA.

It is also of interest that mice are only used extensively in immunology, but rats are used in 6 out of 8 categories of disciplines. In a survey by ourselves from data published in Index Medicus 1978 the rat was found to be used in most disciplines (Table 2).

Table 2.   Comparison of the percentage of studies undertaken on man and the rat in experimental medicine.

	Percentage	
	Man	rat
- Circulation	31	23
- Respiration	16	9
- Kidney	10	15
- Intestine	14	13
- Hormones	14	24
- Nutrition Metabolism	15	16

AIM OF STUDY AND CHOICE OF ANIMALS

Before it is possible to discuss the choice of animal the different aims of a study have to be considered.   Table 3 summarizes different topics which are often combined, for example: site of action and vascular or tubular effects.   Last, but not least, the aim of the study should always be relevant to man or clinical medicine.

Table 3.   Possible criteria to be evaluated in the study of nephrotoxins.

- Changes in renal excretory function
- Renal excretory mechanisms or metabolic pathways for nephrotoxins
- Intra-renal distribution of nephrotoxins
- Site of action within the kidney
- Vascular and/or tubular effects
- Pathomechanisms at cellular or subcellular level
- Acute or long term toxicity
- Dosage dependence
- Early functional and/or late morphological changes by nephrotoxins
- Nephrotoxicity and gestation
- Relevance to clinical medicine

In addition general aspects (see above) have to be discussed such as the use of animals in science or industry. Most important, however, is the selection of research animals by the planned technical approach and by anatomical and functional features (see Table 4). One well known example for functional disorder is the Brattleboro rat, first described by Valtin [8], which lacks anti-diuretic hormone and therefore cannot regulate its urinary osmolality.

Table 4. Factors effecting the choice of animal in the study of nephrology

Rat	- free flow micropuncture, microperfusion, collecting duct catherization, microcinematography
	- isolated perfused kidney
	- cellular and subcellular fractions
Dog	- clearance and stop-flow techniques
	- blood flow measurements
	- isolated kidney
Rabbit	- in vitro microperfusion
Golden hamster, gerbil, psammomys	- micropuncture in renal papilla
Chicken	- use of portal circulation
Necturus, frog, toad, amphiuma, lizard	- electrophysiological recordings
	- micropuncture of distal tubule
	- intra- and extra-cellular measurements
Goosefish, dogfish, flounder, hagfish	- clearance techniques
	- in vitro microperfusion
	- cellular and subcellular fractions

Modified from Hierholzer [3]

Progress in the understanding of kidney function has mainly been increased by defining the basic mechanisms underlying renal transport processes at the cellular or subcellular level. This understanding has been greatly improved in the last 15 years by the use of new techniques and analytical methods in suitable experimental animals. The application of different in vivo and in vitro micropuncture techniques for comparative studies has evolved using species such as the fish, especially, for questions involving cellular mechanisms of tubular transport [9-11].

When applying these techniques, differences in anatomy, physiology and development of the nephron should be considered. The drawing (Fig. 1) from Long and Giebisch [12] compares the common features of the nephron of different species, the particular arrangement within the kidney and the presence or lack of a counter current system.

An example of different tubular functions is the significant acidification of proximal tubular fluid in most mammalian kidneys and its absence in necturus and the frog [5]. The distal nephron with the distal tubule, collecting tubule and collecting duct has a much tighter epithelium than the proximal tubule. Whereas in the proximal tubule the

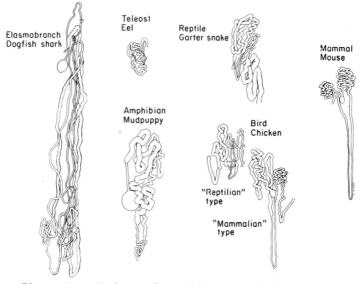

Figure 1.   Nephrons from different animals species.
From Long and Giebisch [12].

bulk of fluid and solutes is reabsorbed, in the distal nephron higher
transepithelial concentration differences are achieved to form a hypotonic
urine, unless there is a counter current concentration mechanisms as in
the mammalian kidney [5, 12].   Para-aminohippurate (PAH) transport seems
to be more powerful in later potions of proximal tubules of mammals and
snakes than in earlier portions [13].   Fluid, sodium, glucose or amino
acid reabsorption is significantly less in the straight segments than in
convoluted tubules [5, 14-16].

This subdivision into nephron portions and subportions on the basis of
functional and structural criteria has been described by the term
heterogeneity.   However, this term is used in several senses.   It has
been used to the distinguish the glomeruli into those of superficial,
midcortical and juxtamedullary localisation within the kidney [17].
There are great species differences in the distribution of various nephron
segments, their vascular supply (e.g. chicken kidney with portal
circulation) and, in the case of the mammalian kidney, the course of
Henle's loop and its histological relationships [17].

The rat is most often used in nephrology research because micropuncture
techniques are well developed, as are isolated organ perfusion and
cellular or subcellular fractionation techniques.   This enables a good
comparison of the overall kidney function with that at the single nephron
level.   Thus, during the last few years a large amount of information has
been gathered on kidney function in one mammalian species.

However, for specific studies such as blood flow measurements, the dog
is species of choice and studies on the mammalian concentration mechanism
make use of the hamster [7] because of the high urinary concentrating
capacity where the counter current system in the elongated renal papilla
is easily accessed by micropuncture techniques.   Microdissection is
easily performed in the rabbit kidney, thus this species is used for the
in vitro microperfusion of isolated tubular segments [18-20], a technique
which has recently also been applied to human collecting ducts [21].

Tubular secretory processes are best studied in the chicken because the
portal circulation supplies primarily the renal tubular apparatus, but
this approach has largely been confined to pharmacology [27].   Necturus
has been used for electrophysiological recordings and for the study of
local mechanisms in renal physiology and the aglomerular goosefish ·has
been used to study special tubular secretory transport processes.   [5,23]
The elasmobranch fish *Squalus acanthius*   lacks the enzyme carbonic
anhydrase, thus comparing its renal function to mammals reveals more
insight into the action of inhibitors on this enzyme.   It has been of
special   interest   to   compare   the   bicarbonate   reabsorption   in
S. acanthius   with that of mammals after the application of large doses
of acetazolamide [24].

Using different techniques (see Table 4) at the single nephron level
some nephrotoxic substances and their effects on the kidney are selected
(see Diezi and Roch-Ramel, this volume).   One well known example is the
action of mercuric chloride on the single nephron which has been studied
by Biber et al. [25].   As revealed by microdissection in these
experiments mercuric chloride treatment is followed by destruction of the
proximal tubule including the pars recta.   Free-flow micropuncture
technique, however, showed an almost normal fractional fluid uptake in the
diluting segment with a tubular fluid:plasma ratio for inulin of 5.7 and a
ratio for osmolality of 0.65 (see figure 2 in ref. 25).

Table 5 summarizes data on the effect of gentamicin on glomerular
function [26, 27].   This study is also a good example of the application
of a specific rat strain with superficial glomeruli which are directly
accessible for micropuncture [28].   A decrease of the single nephron
filtration rate from 36 to 22 nl/min is followed by a decreased total
kidney glomerular filtration rate (GFR) and accompanied by a lowered mean
value of the ultrafiltration coefficient from 0.072 to 0.034 nl/s.mmHg.

The ultrafiltration coefficient K_F, which is the product of hydraulic
conductivity and total glomerular surface area, is restored when captopril
- the antagonist of angiotensin II - is administered in addition to
gentamicin.   Morphologically the glomerular were normal but tubular
lesions could be seen.   From which it was concluded that angiotensin II
mediated the defect of glomerular ultrafiltration.   Gentamicin caused a
significantly greater reduction of SNGFR than tobramycin when given in an
identical dose [26].

Although the rat is the most frequently used research animal in
nephrology and nephrotoxicity studies other animals are of value [29,30].

Table   5.   Study   in   superficial   glomeruli-filtration   rats   in
          Munich-Wistar rats treated with Gentamicin

	GFR	SNGFR*	K_F
	µ l/min	nl/min	nl/s.mm Hg
Controls	1.00	36	0.072
Gentamicin	0.58	22	0.034
G + Captopril	0.84	32	0.062

Data from Schor et al [27].   Gentamicin dose: 40 mg/kg/day i.p. for 10
days.   Captopril dose: 20 mg/kg p.o.   *SNGFR=single nephron GFR.

Table 6.   Species differences in glomerular filtration rate and total
           number of glomeruli

	GFR $(ml/min/m^2)$	Number of glomeruli in both kidneys
- Man	75	2.0×10^6
- Horse	57	5.5×10^6
- Pig	72	2.0×10^6
- Dog	104	8.8×10^5
- Guinea Pig	40	1.5×10^5
- Rat	35	6.0×10^4
- Mouse	50	2.2×10^4

Experiments by Miller [31] illustrates how the flounder kidney can be used
to study secretory processes in isolated tubules.   In these experiments
the uptake of PAH was decreased by the application of two different dose
of mercuric chloride.   In the ouabain treated tubules reductions of PAH
uptake correlated with total tissue Na and K.   Plasma membrane vesicles,
which were prepared from flounder kidneys, provide a good example of the
vital role which a comparative approach has played in the development of
renal physiology and pharmacology [32].
     In addition to the monkey [33], the pig is a good choice of animal for
experimental nephrology because of its gross anatomical similarity to man
(the kidneys are multipapillate) and a close functional relationship.
Table 6 compares the total kidney glomerular filtration rate and the
number of glomeruli in different mammalian species.
     The closest correlation to man is found in the pig.   One example of
the use of the pig in nephrotoxicity studies is the effect of mycotoxins
on the kidney [34].   These experiments have shown that the pig is
sensitive to Ochratoxin A fed in the diet. Ochratoxin A fed at low levels
for long periods of time reduces both GFR and renal blood flow.   Another
good example of the choice of the pig are studies of foetal renal function
[35,36].   It is important to note, that such experiments could be
undertaken chronically for several days, for example between the 100 and
110 day of gestation.
     Another factor which requires consideration is the use of anaesthetized
and unaesthetized animals.   A model has been described with a special
training, unrestrained and with catheters inserted in blood vessels such
as the aorta or with cuffs around the renal artery [37].   Thus longterm
studies of the effects of different drugs on blood pressure and on renal
blood flow could be performed.

APPLICABILITY TO CLINICAL MEDICINE

     There are marked interspecies variations in sensitivity to
nephrotoxins, such as urographic radiocontrast drugs [38], in animals and
man.   Whereas rabbits, guinea pigs, monkeys and humans are sensitive to
cephalosporins, rats are unusually resistant [39-41].   Rabbits are more
resistant to aminoglycosides than rats and humans (see also Table 7).
From this it follows that the rat is not always the animal of choice for
the study of dose related changes in humans.

Table 7.   Species differences in drug sensitivity

Species	Ethacrynic acid	Ouabain	Aminoglycosides	Cephalosporins
Man	+	+	+	+
Monkey	+	+		+
Dog	+	+	(+)	+
Rabbit	(+)		(+)	+
Guinea Pig	(+)		(+)	+
Rat	(+)	-	+	(+)

   + = sensitive   - = resistant to nephrotoxic effects

   It is important that the threshold for drug action might be different between species although these seem to be well documented similarities in functional and morphological lesions [39,41].
   In addition to different species' sensitivity to drugs, there are functional disorders which are difficult to assess and to compare with man.   The following discussion will be focussed on the symptom of proteinuria, which is most used to diagnose renal disease in man.
   The rat has a marked normal proteinuria which shows strain and sex differences, as well as functional changes related to puberty and ageing. The strain differences in albumin excretion can be quite great (see Table 8).   A subline of the Munich Wistar rats (MWF/Ztm) with surface glomeruli has a sieving coefficient for Albumin of 0.0004, which is 20 fold higher than in all other rat strains studied in our laboratory (42 and unpublished observation).

Table 8.   Albuminuria in different sublines of Wistar rats.

Wistar sublines	Albumin Excretion (µg/h/animal)
WC/Ztm	43.0 ± 16.0
MWF/Ztm	1,610.0 ± 1,150.0
Han:W	9.4 ± 0.8
ACI/Ztm	95.0 ± 66.0
Han: SPRD	35.0 ± 53.0

In contrast to man there is a sex dependent excretion of low molecular weight,(LMW-) proteins which are more pronounced in the male rat than in the female (Fig. 2).   These sex dependent LMW-proteins in the male rat increase dramatically after puberty and vanish with age.   Castration abolishes this LMW-protein excretion.   This has to be considered in experimental studies with increased proteinuria.   Therefore, for studies of tubular dysfunction, which in man is congruent with the increased excretion of LMW-proteins because of a decreased tubular uptake, only female rats should be chosen.
   Proteinuria caused by nephrotoxins in man should, therefore, be studied by analysing the qualitative and quantitative distribution of urinary proteins.   This will also allow conclusions to be made in respect to the

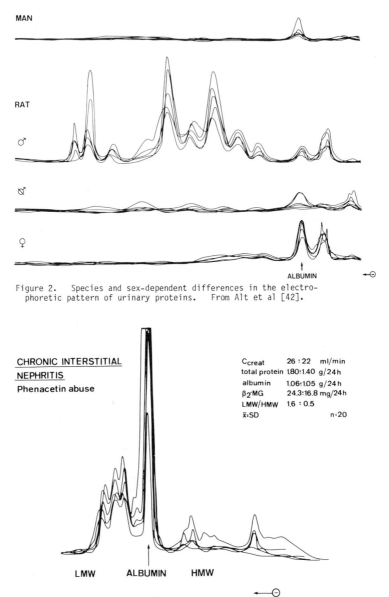

MAN

RAT

♂

♂

♀

ALBUMIN ⟶⊖

Figure 2.   Species and sex-dependent differences in the electrophoretic pattern of urinary proteins.   From Alt et al [42].

CHRONIC INTERSTITIAL
NEPHRITIS
Phenacetin abuse

C_{creat}	26 : 22	ml/min
total protein	1,80 : 1,40	g/24h
albumin	1,06 : 1,05	g/24h
$\beta_2\text{-MG}$	24,3 : 16,8	mg/24h
LMW/HMW	1,6 : 0,5	
$\bar{x} \pm SD$		n = 20

LMW   ALBUMIN   HMW

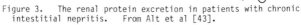

⟵⊖

Figure 3.   The renal protein excretion in patients with chronic
intestitial nepritis.   From Alt et al [43].

pathomechanism.   Figure 3 shows the electrophoretic pattern of protein excretion as determined by gradient electrophoresis in patients with analgesic nephropathy [43].   There is an increased excretion of LMW-protein confirming the involvement of the proximal tubule segment.   This tubular involvement is demonstrated by an increased albumin and β_2-microglobulin (1180 dalton) excretion, as well as by a low ratio of low molecular weight over high molecular weight proteins.   This ratio excludes albumin, the excretion of which is determined by the restriction at the glomerular site as well as by the tubular uptake [44].

FUTURE ASPECTS

As has been mentioned, for clinical medicine, the applicability of results from studies with research animals is of importance.   Due to the fact that the application of new techniques at the single nephron level are not easily performed in man, isolated and in vitro cultured kidney cells are a step nearer to learning more about human kidney function in health and disease.   This technique is especially useful in the investigation of metabolic pathways or immunological mechanisms [45,46]. However, even if it leads to a better understanding of toxicology in man and reduces the number of research animals that have to be used, we will still need animals to study the complexity of the drug action.

Supported by Deutsche Forschungsgemeinschaft

Dedicated to Jan Brod, M.D., F.R.C.P., Professor of Internal Medicine, on the occasion of his 70th birthday.

REFERENCES

1. Andreucci VE(ed.), Manual of Renal Micropuncture, Idelson, Naples, 1978.
2. Giebisch GH (ed.),Yale J Biol Med 45:187-456,1972.
3. Hierbolzer K, Exp Biol Med 7: in press, 1982.
4. Stolte H and Alt J (eds.), Contr Nephrol 19:1-249,1980.
5. Windhager EE, Micropuncture Techniques and Nephron Function. Butterworth, London, 1968.
6. Schmidt-Nielsen B, Fed Proc 20:902-912, 1961.
7. Schmidt-Nielsen B, Exp Biol Med 7:in press, 1982.
8. Valtin H, J Clin Invest 45:337-345, 1966.
9. Goldstein L and Schmidt-Nielsen B (eds.),J Exp Zoology 199:296-457, 1977.
10. Goldstein L (ed.),Yale J Biol Med 52:495-568,1979.
11. Hodler J et al, Am J Physiol 183:155-162, 1955.
12. Long S and Giebisch G, Yale J Biol Med 52: 525-544, 1979.
13. Roch-Ramel F and Weiner IM, Kidney Int 18:665-676, 1980.
14. Eisenbach GM et al, Pfluegers Arch 357:63-76, 1975.
15. Mudge GH et al, In: Handbook of Physiology.   Renal Physiology (J Orloff and RM Berliner eds.) American Physiological Society, Washington, pp. 587-652, 1973.
16. Tune BM et al, Am J Physiol 217:1057-1063, 1973.

17. Kriz W and Kaislling B, in Proc. VII, Int Congr Nephrol, Montreal, Karger, 1978, pp. 217-233. ISBN 38055-2915-5.
18. Burg MB et al, Am J Physiol 210:1293-1298, 1966.
19. Burg MB et al, Am J Physiol 215:788-794, 1968.
20. Burg MB, Yale J Biol Med 45:321-326, 1972.
21. Grantham JJ and Chonko AM, in Contemporary Issues in Nephrology (BM Brenner and JH Stein, eds.) Churchill Livingstone, New York, 1978.
22. Rennick BR, Am J Physiol 217:247-250, 1969.
23. Forster RP and Berglund F, J Gen Physiol 39:349-359, 1956.
24. Maren TH, J Pharmacol Exp Ther 139:140, 1963.
25. Biber TU et al, Am J Med 44:664-705, 1968.
26. Baylis C et al, Kidney Int 12:344-353, 1977.
27. Schor N et al, in: Tel Aviv Satellite Symposium on Acute Renal Failure (Abstracts), Tel Aviv, Israel, 1981.
28. Martin JB et al, Endocrinology 94:1359-1364,1974.
29. Guarino AM et al, Cancer Treat Rep 63:1475-1483,1979.
30. Pritchard JB and Miller DS, Fed Proc 39:3207-3212,1980.
31. Miller DS, J Pharmacol Exp Ther: in press.
32. Eveloff J et al, Am J Physiol 237:F291-F298,1979.
33. May DG and Weiner JM, J Pharmacol Exp Ther 176:407-417,1971.
34. Krog P et al, Acta Pathol Microbiol Scand 81:689-695,1973.
35. Alt JM et al, Quart J Exp Physiol:in press, 1982.
36. Macdonald AA and Colenbrander B, Adv Physiol Sci 8:319-325,1980.
37. Gellai M and Valtin H, Exp Biol Med 7, in press,1982.
38. Mudge GH, Kidney Int 18:540-552,1980.
39. Falco FG et al, J Infect Dis 119:406-409,1969.
40. Kaloyanides GJ and Pastoriza-Munoz E, Kidney Int 18:571-582,1980.
41. Kosek JC et al, Lab Invest 30:48-57,1974.
42. Alt JM et al, Lab Animals 14:95-101,1980.
43. Alt JM et al, Contr Nephrol 19:79-87,1980.
44. Alt JM et al, Contr Nephrol 24:115-121,1981.
45. Atkins RC et al, Kidney Int 17:515-527,1980.
46. Horster M, Klin Wochenschr 58:965-973,1980.

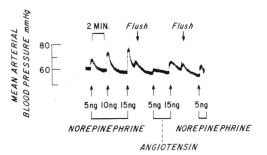

study the tubular effects of known nephrotoxic agent such as
aminoglycoside antibiotics, maleic acid, lithium, vanadate, etc.
Some aspects of the tubular transport of several of these compounds
and of other drugs such as salicylic acid or paracetamol (acetaminophen) have been investigated by micropuncture studies.

The purpose of the present short review is 1. to discuss briefly
the technical approaches which have been used in this type of
experimental studies, and 2. to describe the various toxic compounds
which have been investigated at the single nephron level.

EXPERIMENTAL METHODS

The uses and limitations of the main techniques used in toxicity
studies at the single nephron level are summarized below. A more
detailed discussion of these methods may be found in references [1-3].

Free-flow micropuncture : the collection of tubular fluid flowing
freely into a micropipet, inserted at a known point along the nephron,
permits an estimate of fluid and solute net transport from the
glomeruli to the point of puncture. Measurement of the inulin
concentration in tubular fluid (TF) and plasma (P) (ratio inulin TF/P)
provides an evaluation of net water transport, and permits the
calculation of fractional delivery of any solute at (or fractional
reabsorption down to) the puncture site. Single nephron filtration
rate (SGFR) is usually calculated by multiplying the TF/P inulin
ratio by the tubular flow rate. The tubular segments accessible to
micropuncture include the convoluted portion of the superficial
proximal tubule, part of the descending and ascending limbs of
Henle's loop, parts of the superficial distal and collecting tubules
and the medullary collecting ducts. Glomerular and peritubular blood
capillaries are also accessible to micropuncture. Blood from efferent
arterioles can be collected and analysed for plasma protein concentration. Micropipets inserted into capillary and tubular structures
may also be used for measuring hydrostatic pressure, which may be
continuously recorded by a micro-pressure transducer system.
Tubular pressure has often been measured in experimental models of
acute renal failure, in order to delineate the role of tubular
obstruction as a mechanism of renal shut down : tubular obstruction
is expected to entail an upstream increase of intraluminal pressure
and a sharp decrease of filtration rate. On the other hand, pressure
measurements in glomerular capillaries and Bowman's space, and
analysis of efferent arteriolar plasma permit a direct assessment of
ultrafiltration dynamics in vivo, and have contributed to our
understanding of the mechanisms responsible for the decrease of SGFR
induced by toxic agents such as aminoglycoside antibiotics.

Stationary tubular micro-perfusion ("split-drop") : the capacity
of a particular nephron segment accessible to micropuncture to
carry out net fluid and solute transport may be evaluated by inserting
into a tubule a droplet of known chemical composition, isolated at
both ends by two oil columns. The rate of fluid reabsorption, measured
by volume changes of the "shrinking droplet" in serial microphoto-

graphs, permits an estimate of the rate of absorption. When impermeant
molecules (e.g. raffinose) are added to the droplet, samples of the
droplet fluid may be analysed after different time intervals in order
to determine the transepithelial concentration gradients built up
by tubular cells.

Continuous tubular microperfusion : defined tubular segments
may be perfused through micropipets, one of which is connected to
a pump delivering known amounts of artificial tubular fluid. The
difference between the composition of the fluid flowing into the
collecting pipet and that of the perfusion fluid reflects the
transport activity of the nephron segment under study. Peritubular
capillaries may be microperfused simultaneously in order to control
the composition of the peritubular fluid. This technique has been
used to determine the rate of net transport of various solutes
across the tubular epithelium, and to understand some aspects of the
transport mechanisms. Other applications include investigations
on the role of changes in fluid composition on nephron function,
as for instance in studies on the regulation of SGFR by early
distal fluid flow rate and/or composition ("tubulo-glomerular
feed-back" mechanism; recently reviewed in ref. [4]). The function
and role of this feed-back system has been looked at after
administration of various nephrotoxic compounds; its activation may
be causally related to the fall of GFR associated with acute renal
failure.

Tubular microinjection : serial collection of ureteral urine
immediately after microinjection of a radioactively labelled compound,
together with inulin, into a tubule permits to evaluate the overall
reabsorptive activity, related to the investigated compound, of
tubular segments located beyond the injection site. The fraction of
the radioactivity recovered in the final urine is compared to that of
inulin. Fractional recovery of inulin, in standard conditions, must
be equal or close to 100 % to validate the microinjection. Reduced
levels of recovery of normally impermeant molecules such as inulin
after toxic injury have been considered as evidence for the presence
of tubular lesions and transepithelial leaks. Microinjection at
different tubular levels may be used to localize more precisely the
site of epithelial injury.

Microperfusion of isolated tubules "in vitro" : nearly all
tubular segments have been investigated by this technique, mostly in
physiological studies. Briefly, the technique consists in a microdissection of single tubular segments from kidney slices. The
tubule is then mounted, in a thermostatically controlled bath,
between a perfusion and a collection pipet. Fluid transport across
the epithelia wall is evaluated by measuring the changes in luminal
concentration of an impermeant molecule. This technique has not yet
been used often in pharmacological or toxicological studies. Obvious
advantages of this approach include complete control of luminal and
peritubular fluid composition, a clear-cut definition of the nephron
segment under study, the absence of systemic effects of applied
drugs or other chemicals, etc.

Study of non-perfused single tubules : in vitro measurements of
uptake of organic ions into isolated nephrons has provided informa-
tions about the tubular heterogeneity, and interspecific variations,
of peritubular transport of such molecules [5].   The distribution
of intracellular accumulation of gentamicin in various nephron
segments has been investigated by such technique.

HEAVY-METAL INDUCED NEPHROTOXICITY

Inorganic salts of various heavy metals have been used as tools in
micropuncture studies investigating the pathophysiology of acute
renal failure (ARF). Such studies were usually aimed at recognizing
the contribution of various mechanisms of toxicity to the fall of
GFR associated with ARF. Such mechanisms include tubular obstruction,
back-leak of tubular fluid through damaged epithelia, activation of
the "feed-back" mechanism of control of GFR, afferent arteriole
vasoconstriction and a decrease of renal blood flow.

Heavy metals which have been used in such experiments include
mercuric, uranyl and chromate ions. In addition, subacute effects of
lead acetate in young animals have been reported recently.

Mercuric chloride [ref. 6-18]: Doses of 4 to 15 mg $HgCl_2$/kg were
injected into rats; micropuncture was carried out in the first hours
or days after injection.   Though the results reported in the different
studies are partly conflicting, there is evidence that the time course
of appearance of toxic ARF depends on the dose of $HgCl_2$, and may vary
between strains of rats. Marked functional differences between similar
nephrons at the cortical surface develop during the establishment of
ARF [6,8,9,11,12,14,16].   The experimental observations, thus, may
depend on the choice of the punctured tubules.

Three days after 5-10 mg $HgCl_2$/kg, s.c., kidney surface nephrons
appeared normal on microscopic examination, but intratubular
injection of nigrosin revealed that a variable number of tubules had
no or low flow [8], probably as a consequence of tubular obstruction.
SGFR in apparently normal nephrons of intoxicated rats was not
different from that measured in antidiuretic control rats. Isotonic
fluid reabsorption occured at a normal rate in proximal convoluted
tubules, whereas fluid reabsorption between late proximal and early
distal segments was markedly reduced, as indicated by a smaller
increase in the TF/P inulin ratio than in controls. Mason et al
confirmed, by in vivo microperfusion, that the ability of
"Henle's loop" to reabsorb sodium was decreased after $HgCl_2$ [18].
The distal nephron, in contrast, did not exhibit an abnormal
behaviour [8].   Intraluminal secretion of an organic ion
(p-amino-hippurate, PAH) in $HgCl_2$ poisoned rats, was found to be
normal in most of the convoluted proximal tubules, but severely
impaired in the final portion of these tubules. This observation
again points to a late-proximal site of the toxic effect of inorganic
mercury, a finding which agrees well with morphological data
which show tubular necrosis to occur predominantly in the pars recta
[8].   Biber et al proposed that, under the influence of $HgCl_2$, a
variable proportion of nephrons is obstructed, particularly at the

end of the proximal tubule, and that this fact results in a major decrease of whole kidney GFR, despite a near-normal filtration rate in the un-obstructed nephrons (8).

After 12 mg $HgCl_2$/kg, Flanigan et al observed significant decreases of tubular pressure 8-26 hours following the toxic injury, while tubular pressure was normal in the first hours [6]. On the other hand, Flamenbaum et al reported that, 24 hours after 5mg $HgCl_2$/kg despite evidence for intraluminal presence of cell debris and partial tubular obstruction, the pressure in the proximal tubules was normal [11]. This observation was interpreted as indicating a decrease of effective filtration pressure in these nephrons, which, when the obstruction to fluid flow was removed, showed only a slight decrease of SGFR. Intratubular hydrostatic pressure was also found to be normal by Mason et al 5 - 12 hours hours after 4.5 mg $HgCl_2$/kg while a small increase was found after 6 mg $HgCl_2$/kg [14]. This increase, however, appeared too small to explain the drop of SGFR. In another study carried out in the first hours following a very large dose of mercuric chloride (15 mg/kg), a 50 % decrease of SGFR was measured, a drop of a magnitude similar to that observed in whole kidney GFR [9]. In the same study, there was no evidence for abnormal tubular permeability (i.e. transepithelial diffusion of inulin). In contrast, Bank et al (7), as well as Steinhausen et al (10) reported that after 4 mg $HgCl_2$/kg the tubules of poisoned rats were permeable to inulin, as shown by the finding of an apparent decrease of SGFR when measured at different sites along the nephron (7), or by a near 90 % loss of radioactive inulin after intratubular injection into proximal tubules (10). Abnormal tubular permeability, however, was not confirmed by Olbricht et al, who used microinjections of labelled inulin 3-12 hours after 6 mg $HgCl_2$/kg (15).

These apparent discrepancies may be explained in part by the marked nephron heterogeneity following poisoning with mercuric ions, as supported by the findings of Huguenin et al (16). These authors reported that 48 hours after 4 mg $HgCl_2$/kg, more than half of the superficial tubules appeared opaque and collapsed, whereas the remaining tubules had a normal appearance. The ability to reabsorb isotonic saline, studied by the "split drop" technique, was reduced in the normal-looking tubules, while the more rapid reabsorption observed in the collapsed tubules was considered a consequence of abnormal tubular leakiness of the damaged epithelium. Tubular collapse following $HgCl_2$ could be prevented by chronic salt loading; under these conditions the reabsorptive capacity of punctured tubules was uniformly decreased [16].

Taken together, these studies suggest that, reabsorption of fluid and Na decreases first in "Henle's loops", but later or after larger doses of Hg^{++}, also in the convoluted proximal tubules which, besides, may become abnormally leaky.

The tubulo-glomerular feed-back mechanism does not appear to be impaired in $HgCl_2$ induced ARF [17]. The decrease of SGFR generally observed under these conditions could, therefore be due to an increase of the fluid and salt load to the early distal tubules, which would activate the "feed-back" mechanism [12,13]. A similar hypothesis was also proposed by McDowell et al [19]. Activation of the feed-back mechanism in mercury poisoned rats, appears to be independent of the renin-angiotensin system [20].

The fate of mercuric ions within the kidney has also been investigated by micropuncture techniques. In these experiments $^{203}HgCl_2$ was microinjected into tubules or peritubular capillaries of the dog kidney. The absence of specific effects of various, known metabolic inhibitors of active transport led the authors to conclude that there is no active transport mechanism either reabsorptive or secretory of inorganic mercury. The low recovery rate of Hg after intraluminal (8 %) or peritubular (1 %) injection indicates that the metallic ion is rapidly taken up and stored by tubular cells [21].

Uranyl nitrate (U.N.)(ref. 14,15,20,22-26) : parenteral injection of 10 or 15 mg/kg to rats rapidly induced ARF. Six hours after 10 mg/ kg, GFR in whole kidney and superficial tubules decreased by 30-35 % while intratubular pressure did not increase [14,22]. There was no evidence for either tubular obstruction or tubular "leakage" (investigated by inulin microinjections)[15,22] in these rat studies, after up to 15 mg U.N./kg,whereas in dogs, 48 hours after 10 mg/kg of U.N., only 14 % of the inulin injected into tubules was recovered [23]. In dogs the data suggested a significant "leak" from the straight portion of the proximal tubules. The difference between rats and dogs, however, is quantitative rather than fundamental : in rats injected with 25 mg/kg U.N. there was some evidence for an epithelial "leak" [24]. Free-flow micropuncture studies indicate that Na delivery to the distal tubule increases after uranyl nitrate [25], a finding compatible with the involvement of a "feed-back" mechanism in the decrease of GFR. Renin activity was found to increase in the juxtaglomerular apparatus of superficial and deep nephrons [26]. If this were so, the feed-back mechanism involved could be mediated by an intrarenal renin-angiotensin system. Evidence to the contrary, however, was published by Mason et al, who reported that the depression of SGFR due to toxic injury is independent of the renin activity in the juxtaglomerular apparatus [20], and concluded that the depression of SGFR is not due to an activation of the renin-angiotensin system.

Direct measurement of the effective filtration pressure in single glomeruli "in vivo" showed that, 25 mg/kg U.A. induce a primary decrease of glomerular permeability which contributes to the decrease of GFR [24].

The studies discussed, thus, indicate that uranyl ions entail a significant decrease of GFR and may inhibit Na reabsorption at sites between the late proximal and the distal tubule. Depression of GFR appears to result from abnormal epithelial leakiness and from glomerular alterations. The role of the "feed-back mechanisms" under these conditions is equivocal.

Dichromate (ref. 8, 27,28) : acute and chronic renal lesions were induced in rats by 7-15 mg/kg potassium dichromate. Twenty-four hours after 15 mg/kg, SGFR decreased by 80% in animals given a salt-restricted diet which stimulates the renin-angiotensin system, while the decrease was much less marked (35 %) in salt-loaded, "renin-depleted", animals [27]. Tubular transport mechanisms also were impaired : the proximal reabsorptive half-time ("split-drop") was consistently increased in poisoned rats. Glomerular capillary pressure was moderatly reduced [27]. These observations were made in selected superficial nephrons, since many tubules were collapsed. Though intratubular hydrostatic pressure was not clearly elevated, dichromate was suspected to induce tubular obstruction, because many tubules were seen to contain cellular debris [8]. Three days after dichromate (7-15 mg/kg) a persistent inhibition of isotonic fluid reabsorption ("split-drop") was reported [8]; functional and morphological lesions appeared to predominate in the convoluted portions of the proximal tubule. Thus, PAH secretion was strongly inhibited in early segments of the proximal tubule, but appeared much less affected in the straight portion [8].

Though whole kidney GFR was clearly depressed 3 days after dichromate, SGFR in non-collapsed surface nephrons was not decreased, and these tubules were not abnormally leaky to inulin, in contrast to nephrons visibly obstructed by cell debris. Biber et al therefore conclude that dichromate injury induces a marked morphological and functional tubular heterogeinity, with maintenance of normal filtration in part of the nephrons [8]. A similar study was carried out 3-4 weeks after injecting 15 mg/kg dichromate [28]. Again, pronounced morphological and functional heterogeneity was recorded. The range of SGFR was large, but measurements of proximal fluid reabsorption in this highly heterogenous nephron population indicated that glomerulo-tubular balance (i.e. the relationship between rate of filtration and of tubular fluid reabsorption) was well maintained in these tubules.

Inorganic lead : mean term exposure to lead acetate (1 % solution in drinking fluid during 6 weeks) appears to affect renal functions in young rats (exposure starting at weaning) [29]. Renal functions were measured 3 and 16 weeks after cessation of exposure. Micropuncture of proximal tubules showed a significant depression of SGFR in rats exposed to lead between 12 and 25 weeks of age. The decrease was of similar magnitude for the whole kidney GFR and the renal blood flow.

MYOHEMOGLOBINURIC NEPHROPATHY

Several micropuncture investigations have been carried out during early stages of renal failure associated with myohemoglobinuria, induced by intra-muscular injection of glycerol [30-33] or by direct administration of methemoglobin [14,15,17,18,34-35]

In the first hours following injection of glycerol (10 ml/kg of a 50 % solution), tubular flow rate was markedly reduced and low levels of intratubular pressure were measured, but there was no evidence for intratubular obstruction or abnormal tubular leakiness. SGFR was reduced by 50-60 % when compared to controls, but, as in other models of chemically-induced acute renal failure, a profound heterogeneity in macroscopic appearance and function between different superficial nephrons was noted [30]. Estimates of SGFR based on fluid samples obtained from the least abnormal nephrons, therefore, tend to underrate the decrease of ultrafiltrate formation in the damaged kidneys [30]. This decrease entailed a drop of absolute fluid reabsorption from proximal tubules. An observed depression of the rate of fluid reabsorption from "split drops" [30], on the other hand, suggests that this type of poisoning also directly impairs the reabsorptive salt and water transport in proximal tubules. Since the fall of SGFR after injections of glycerol could not be explained by tubular obstruction, by a fall of blood pressure, or by tubular leakiness, it was suggested that reduction of net filtration pressure accounts for the drop in filtration rate [30].

Additional investigations, intended at elucidating the mechanisms of glycerol toxicity, were performed in animals infused with mannitol and/or saline before injecting glycerol [31]. These types of pretreatment afforded some protection against the effects of glycerol, apparently by reducing the proportion of severely damaged tubules. SGFR, however, remained abnormally low in individual tubules. Chronic saline loading did not inhibit the toxic effects of glycerol, but resulted in a more rapid rate of functional recovery, when compared to non-expanded control animals [35]. Involvement of vasopressin in the development of acute renal failure was considered unlikely, following the observation that toxic alterations after glycerol were similar in tubules from Brattleboro rats 34 .

Another micropuncture study, carried out at later times, provides an insight into the functional disturbances still present up to the 6th day after injecting glycerol. While return of tubular flow in damaged tubules appeared to follow the recovery of adequate effective glomerular filtration pressure the inhibition of fluid reabsorption from proximal tubules was observed to persist for longer times [36].

Investigations on the renal toxic effects of exogenous methemo-globin provided results reasonably similar to those obtained by the use of glycerol. Reduced glomerular filtration pressure [32,33], rather than tubular obstruction or large back-diffusion of filtrate [14,15], appeared to be responsible for the low rates of SGFR.

ANTIBIOTICS

Aminoglycosides : both the renal transport and the renal toxicity of gentamicin and of tobramycin have been investigated by micro-puncture studies [37-40].

Tubular transport of gentamicin was evaluated in rats by tubular and capillary microinjections [38], or by free flow micropunctures [39]. After microinjection into early proximal tubules of a droplet containing a low or a high concentration of gentamicin, the fraction of gentamicin absorbed by tubular cells down to the final urine was found to range between 14 % (high concentration) to 30 % (low concentration) [38]. The recovery was greater after late proximal microinjection and the injected drug was nearly completely recovered after distal microinjections. These observations indicate tubular absorption of gentamicin along the convoluted part of the proximal

tubule and "Henle's loop", presumably in the straight portion of the
proximal tubule. There was no evidence for transtubular secretion
of gentamicin following capillary microinjection [38]. Additional
evidence for net reabsorption of gentamicin along the proximal
tubule was provided by the free-flow micropuncture studies of
Senekjian et al [39] which indicate that the fractional reabsorption
of the drug along the convoluted part of the superficial proximal
tubule approximated 30-40 % of the amount filtered, depending on
the experimental condition. Further net reabsorption occurred along
"Henle's loop", since except after furosemide or bicarbonate
administration, only 25-30 % of the filtered amount of gentamicin
reached the superficial distal tubules.

   In all experimental conditions, fractional delivery of gentamicin
into final urine was higher than that measured in distal superficial
tubules, a finding suggesting different tubular handling of
gentamicin in superficial and deep nephrons, or, alternatively,
secretion of gentamicin in the collecting tubule system [39].

   The mechanisms involved in the uptake of gentamicin by tubular
cells are still unclear. Studies with separated renal tubules
suggested that gentamicin uptake requires metabolic energy and
reaches saturation at high concentration of the drug in the medium
[41]. Uptake of gentamicin, however, appears to be heterogeneous along
the nephron and to reach the highest levels in the distal segments
of the proximal tubule [42].

   The nephrotoxic effect of aminoglycoside antibiotics, particularly
the influence of these drugs on the dynamics of glomerular ultrafiltration, have been investigated by micropuncture experiments in
vivo in a strain of rats having accessible glomeruli at the surface
of the kidney. Baylis et al [37] found that the dose-related drop of
SGFR following gentamicin injection (4 or 40 mg/kg during 10 days)
resulted predominantly from a decrease of the glomerular capillary
ultrafiltration coefficient. In a later study by the same group [40],
tobramycin (40 mg/kg during 10 days) was found to impair
glomerular filtration much less than gentamicin (40 mg/kg during 10
days). The depression of the ultrafiltration coefficient and nephron
plasma flow, induced by gentamicin, were nearly completely prevented
when captopril, a converting enzyme inhibitor, was given before and
during exposure to gentamicin. Angiotensin II, thus, may be involved
in the impairment of glomerular functions by gentamicin. Captopril,
however, did not prevent the occurrence of gentamicin-induced
morphological damage in the proximal tubule epithelium.

   Benzylpenicillin and carbenicillin : a free flow micropuncture
study [43], aimed at characterizing the sites of tubular transport of
these 2 penicillins, confirmed and extended earlier conclusions
derived from clearance experiments. Benzylpenicillin and carbenicillin
were secreted into the lumen of the proximal tubule only, the former
more rapidly than the latter. A small but significant proportion of
the intratubular benzylpenicillin was reabsorbed along the
collecting duct at very low urine flow rates [43].

   Puromycin aminonucleoside : this compound has been frequently used
to produce a model of "glomerular proteinuria" in experimental animals.

Micropuncture investigations showed that the decrease of SGFR induced by puromycin is due to a depression of the glomerular capillary ultrafiltration coefficient [44]. Four days after puromycin injection, quantitation of albumin concentration in proximal tubular fluid and in final urine suggested that only a small fraction of the filtered albumin was absorbed by the tubular epithelium [45].

URATE NEPHROPATHY

Acute renal failure may follow any sudden and major increase of the urate concentration in blood or in the urine. Clinically, such situations occur during treatment of leukemia by cytostatic drugs or by irradiation, or at the beginning of courses of uricosuric drugs. Experimentally, urate nephropathy may be reproduced by loading rats with uric acid and oxonate (an inhibitor of uricase) either parenterally [46], or with the diet during 2 to 7 days [47,48].   Such treatment induces a six - fold [47,48] to 17-fold [46] increase of the plasma urate concentration.   In the loaded animals the superficial tubules appeared distended, and occasionally contained crystalline material [46]. The SGFR of these nephrons was reduced by nearly 70 %, while whole kidney GFR decreased by 86 % [46]. Intratubular pressure in proximal and distal tubules was increased to 2-3 times its normal value [46,48]. There were, however, large differences between identical superficial nephrons : part of the tubules showed normal flow and pressure, while others had high tubular pressure and no flow [47]. Microinjection studies with inulin did not indicate abnormal tubular leakiness [47]. Morphological examination of tubules suggested that tubular obstruction was secondary to deposition of crystalline material in the collecting ducts. The decrease of GFR might be related in part to the tubular obstruction and the resulting increase of intratubular pressure [46,47,48].

Increased hydrostatic pressure was also measured in efferent arterioles and peritubular capillaries [46,49], as a likely consequence of deposition of crystals in the latter. In another study, however, decreased rather than increased pressure was measured in peritubular and glomerular capillaries [47].

The experimental studies, thus, suggest, that urate nephropathy is due to an obstruction of collecting tubules and ducts [46-49], an impairment of renal capillary blow flow [46], and/or to a decrease of glomerular filtration pressure [47]. High tubular flow rate and urinary dilution prevent the appearance of acute urate nephropathy, despite a high plasma concentration of uric acid [49]. This observation suggests that tubular obstruction may be the predominant pathogenetic mechanism [49]. Incidentally, the same mechanism appears to be involved, on the other hand, in the acute renal failure induced by large doses of *folic acid* [50].

Micropuncture, microperfusion and microinjections techniques have been extensively used to investigate the *tubular transport of uric acid*. Bidirectional (i.e. secretory and reabsorptive) transport of urate occurs across the proximal tubular epithelium [see 51]. In the rat, at endogenous plasma urate levels the reabsorptive transport predominates along the whole length of the proximal tubule. When plasma urate concentration increased by injection of oxonate and uric acid, net secretion of urate occurs in very early proximal convolutions, whereas net reabsorption persists in the second half of the proximal convoluted tubule [52]. When plasma urate concentration is increased, higher loads of urate reach the distal tubule. Under these conditions, the distal tubular urate concentration approximates 15 to 25 mg %, a concentration well below the solubility of urate in buffer at pH 7. A concentration of urate well above the solubility of urate, however, is reached in the ureteral urine of hyperuricemic rats (200-250 mg %) [52]. In these experiments GFR was not depressed, presumably because the high urine flow rate (obtained by infusion of mannitol) prevented the precipitation of urate and the occurrence of tubular obstruction.

Free-flow micropuncture has been used to investigate the tubular transport of urate in a few other mammalian species. Species in which urate reabsorption overwhelmingly predominates over secretion across the whole kidney include man, the Cebus monkey and the mongrel dog [see 51]. In the two latter species micropunture experiments showed a predominance of urate reabsorption both in the convoluted and in the straight parts of the superficial proximal tubules. In other species, such as the Dalmatian coach hound, the rabbit and the pig, tubular secretion of urate prevails over reabsorption at normal or at slightly elevated plasma urate concentration. Micropuncture experiments showed that the main site of tubular urate secretion in the rabbit and the Dalmatian coach hound is the straight portion (pars recta) of the proximal tubules [see 51], while in the pig [53] urate is mainly secreted by the convoluted part of the proximal tubules.

Tubular urate transport albeit under physiological conditions and not in urate nephropathy, has also been studied in the isolated perfused rabbit proximal tubule in vitro. Net urate secretion occurred across the epithelium of the pars recta, but not in the convoluted part of the proximal tubule [54]. Finally, the uptake of radiolabelled urate by various segments of the proximal tubule has been measured by in vitro incubation of non-perfused nephrons [55]. The intracellular accumulation of urate in such experiments reflects the transport across the peritubular membrane, i.e. the first step of transepithelial secretory movement. In the rabbit, the first parts of the straight portions of the proximal tubules were able to concentrate urate against a greater gradient than the convoluted portions [55]. The opposite observation was made in pig próximal tubules [5]. These findings confirm the conclusions of the in vivo micropuncture investigations concerning the tubular sites of net urate secretion. The segmental localization of tubular accumulation or secretion of p-amino-hippurate studied, respectively, by in vitro incubation or by in vivo micropuncture, showed that the secretion of urate and PAH occurred at the same sites in both species, i.e. in the convoluted segment in the pig [5], and in the pars recta in the rabbit [55]. Such observations validate the use of the in vitro incubation technique for predicting the tubular topography of secretory sites for drugs and other chemicals along renal tubules.

ANALGESICS

The pathogeny of human analgesic nephropathy, characterized by chronic interstitial nephritis and papillary necrosis, is still unclear. Despite many attempts to induce similar lesions in experimental animals by repeated administration of large doses of various analgesics, no functional studies at the single nephron level appear to have been carried out in these conditions. More experimental emphasis has been placed on the search for possible biochemical mechanisms of nephrotoxicity [see 56].

By contrast, the renal fate of salicylate and of paracetamol has been investigated in some detail by free-flow micropuncture techniques. In rats with a low urine flow rate, infused with salicylate to obtain a plasma concentration averaging 0.6 mM, net secretion of salicylate occurred across the epithelium of the early proximal tubule (the fractional delivery reaching 125 % of the ultrafiltered amount); salicylate was reabsorbed along the remaining part of the convoluted proximal tubule (fractional delivery at end-proximal convoluted tubule : 100 %)[57]. Much more effective reabsorptive occurred between the end of the superficial proximal and the distal tubule "Henle's loop" (85 % of the amount filtered) since the early distal delivery of salicylate amounted to only 15 % of the ultrafiltered load. Additional reabsorption continued along the distal tubule (fractional delivery at late distal sites : 7 %), and the collecting duct system (fractional excretion into the final urine : 0.5 %)[57]

Similar studies on the tubular fate of paracetamol(unpublished observations)showed no evidence for tubular secretion of the drug. Net reabsorption occurred along the proximal tubule, approximating 45 % of the amount filtered. The fractional reabsorption over "Henle's loops" was much smaller than that measured for salicylate, and averaged 15 % of the amount filtered. Since fractional delivery at the end of the distal tubule was about 25 % and the fractional excretion in the final urine was 5 %, it appears that a rather large amount of the drug (about 20 % of the amount filtered) may be absorbed along the collecting duct system, i.e. a much larger fraction than for salicylate. This difference may explain the fact that paracetamol is accumulated in the inner medullary tissue to a larger extent that salicylate [58]. This conclusion, however, remains conjectural since the role of juxtamedullary nephrons under these conditions has not been yet investigated.

MISCELLANEOUS NEPHROTOXIC CHEMICALS

Lithium : Renal functional lesions which have occurred after acute or short-term lithium administration include a decrease of maximal concentrating ability, consecutive to interference of lithium with the action of vasopressin [59] and/or to a decrease of the corticopapillary solute gradient [60]; a fall in proximal tubular Na and phosphate reabsorption [61,62]; an impairment of urinary acidification and potassium excretion (63), and a decrease of GFR and of renal plasma flow [64]. Chronic administration of lithium to patients has been suspected to entail renal interstitial damage [65].

Free-flow micropuncture was used to investigate the effect of lithium administered to rats either acutely [61] or for 10-12 days [62]. Plasma lithium concentrations averaged 2-3 mM and 0.6 mM, respectively. Both studies indicate that lithium depressed fluid and Na reabsorption along the proximal tubule by 8-12 %. Sodium reabsorption was increased in the "Henle's loop" and decreased in the distal tubule after acute administration of lithium [61], while fluid reabsorption was decreased in "Henle's loop" and increased distally after more prolonged exposure [62]. Both studies however point to the fact that lithium alters fluid and electrolyte transport at multiple nephron sites. A discussion on the possible mechanisms of interference between lithium and electrolyte transport systems in various tissues may be found in reference [66]. A free-flow micropuncture study investigating the renal handling of lithium indicates that reabsorption occurs along the proximal tubule, including the pars recta, while no net transepithelial movement of lithium occurs in the distal part of the nephron [67].

Orthovanadate : This compound induces diuresis and natriuresis, probably as a consequence of an inhibition of tubular Na-K-ATPase activity [68]. The tubular effects of 0.5 or 1.0 μmole of vanadate injected into rats were investigated by free-flow micropuncture [69]. Either dose of vanadate entailed a significant decrease of approximately 30 % of fluid reabsorption along the proximal tubule, but no change of SGFR. The enhanced sodium excretion in the final urine, which occurred after both doses, therefore, appeared to be due to an inhibition of Na reabsorption from the proximal tubule, in the absence of a compensatory increase of Na reabsorption at more distal sites of the nephron. The mechanism of this transport inhibition has not been investigated.

Maleic acid : Parenteral maleic acid (100-200 mg/kg) increases the urinary excretion of water, electrolytes, amino acids and glucose 70,71 . Some characteristics of this experimental nephropathy have been investigated by in vivo micropuncture techniques in the rat [70-72]. While one study [72] suggests that the functional alteration due to maleic acid results from an increased permeability of tubular cells to amino acids and to glucose, which are released into the urine by increased efflux from distal epithelial cells, another study [71], by contrast, concludes that the abnormality of urine composition is the consequence of an inhibition of the saturable reabsorptive mechanism of amino acids along the proximal tubule by maleic acid. No clear-cut explanation for this contradiction is apparent at this time.

CONCLUSION

This present brief survey pertains to review the most important functional studies at the single nephron level in the field of renal toxicology. Many of the contributions reviewed were designed to elucidate the mechanisms of acute renal failure (ARF), particularly the cause of the decrease of GFR in ARF : micropuncture studies permit a critical evaluation of the role of tubular back-flow of filtrate as an explanation for the drop of GFR [73]. Other important contributions include a detailed analysis of the "tubulo-glomerular feed-back" in ARF [13], an investigation on the nature of glomerular functional alterations produced by aminoglycoside antibiotics and the delineation of the tubular topography of several transport systems for urates, antibiotics, analgesics or lithium.

With only few exceptions, micropuncture studies on nephrotoxicity have been carried out shortly after the administration of the toxic compound. Investigations on tubular functions in chronic poisoning or in chronic states induced by acute poisoning have been exceptional, and should be given more attention in future studies. Similarly, practically no micropuncture experiments on toxic interactions in the kidney have been carried out.

While several problems could be solved by further investigations using micropuncture techniques, it should be borne in mind that these methods have technical limitations. Thus, cortical tubular micropuncture gives access to only a very restricted nephron population situated in the outermost cortex, while morphological and functional heterogeneity among nephrons of various cortical layers has often been described [74]. Furthermore, as repeatedly stressed in this survey, even the most superficial nephron population may become markedly heterogenous after toxic injury, a fact which severely limits the possibility of extrapolating from measurements made in selected nephrons to the whole population.

The use of in vitro tubular microperfusion techniques may obviate some of the shortcomings of in vivo micropuncture. This method, however, has only exceptionally been used in studies on renal toxicology.

Finally, in vitro studies of defined non-perfused segments of tubules have been used more extensively in recent times in order to characterize enzyme activities (75,76), organic ion uptake (55) or specific "receptors" (42). In the future, such studies will probably contribute to a better understanding of the mechanisms involved in toxic injuries to the renal tubule.

REFERENCES

1. Andreucci VE, ed., Manual of Renal Micropuncture. Idelson, Naples, 1978.
2. Blantz RC and Tucker BJ, in Methods in Pharmacology, vol. 4B: Renal Pharmacology (M Martinez-Maldonado, ed.). Plenum Press, New York and London, 1978, chap. 6, pp. 141-163. ISBN 0-306-35265-6.
3. Chonko AM, Irish JM III and Welling DJ, in Methods in Pharmacology, vol. 4B: Renal Pharmacology (M Martinez-Maldonado, ed.). Plenum Press, New York and London, 1978, chap. 9, pp. 221-258. ISBN 0-306-35265-6.
4. Wright FS and Briggs JP. Physiol Rev 59:958-1006, 1979.
5. Schäli C and Roch-Ramel F. Am J Physiol, in press (accepted June 1981).

6. Flanigan WJ and Oken DE. J Clin Invest 44:449-457, 1965.
7. Bank N, Mutz BF and Aynedjian HS. J. Clin Invest 46:695-704, 1967.
8. Biber TUL, Mylle M, Baines AD, Gottschalk CW, Oliver JR and
   MacDowell MC. Am J Med 44: 664-705, 1968.
9. Barenberg RL, Solomon S, Papper S and Anderson R. J Lab Clin Med
   72:473-484, 1968.
10. Steinhausen M, Eisenbach GM and Helmstädter V. Pfluegers Arch
   311:1-15, 1969.
11. Flamenbaum W, McDonald FD, DiBona GF and Oken DE. Nephron
   8:221-234, 1971.
12. Thiel G, Hugenin M, Brunner F, Peters L, Peters G, Eckert H,
   Torhorst J and Rohr HP. J Urol Nephrol 79:967-977, 1973.
13. Mason J. Kidney Int 10:S106-S114, 1976.
14. Mason J, Olbricht C, Takabatake T and Thurau K. Pfluegers Arch
   370:155-163, 1977.
15. Olbricht C, Mason J, Takabatake T, Hohlbrugger G and Thurau K.
   Pfluegers Arch 372:251-258, 1977.
16. Huguenin M, Thiel G and Brunner FP. Nephron 20:147-156, 1978.
17. Mason J, Takabatake T, Olbricht C and Thurau K. Pfluegers Arch
   373:69-76, 1978.
18. Mason J, Gutsche HU, Moore L and Müller-Suur R. Pfluegers Arch
   379:11-18, 1979.
19. McDowell EM, Nagle RB, Zalme RC, McNeil JS, Flamenbaum W and
   Trump BF. Virchows Arch B 22:173-196, 1976.
20. Mason J, Kain H, Shiigai T and Welsch J. Pfluegers Arch 380:
   233-243, 1979.
21. Cikrt M and Heller J. Environ Res 21:308-313, 1980.
22. Flamenbaum W, Huddleston ML, McNeil JS and Hamburger RJ.
   Kidney Int 6:408-418, 1974.
23. Stein JH, Gottschall J, Osgood RW and Ferris TF. Kidney Int
   8:27-41, 1975.
24. Blantz RC. J Clin Invest 55:621-635, 1975.
25. Flamenbaum W, Hamburger R and Kaufman J. Pfluegers Arch
   364:209-215, 1976.
26. Flamenbaum W, Hamburger RJ, Huddleston ML, Kaufman J, McNeil JS,
   Schwartz JH and Nagle R. Kidney Int 10:S115-S122, 1976.
27. Henry LN, Lane CE and Kashgarian M. Lab Invest 19:309-314, 1968.
28. Kramp RA, MacDowell M, Gottschalk CW and Oliver JR. Kidney Int
   5:147-176, 1974.
29. Aviv A, John E, Bernstein J, Goldsmith DI and Spitzer A.
   Kidney Int 17:430-437, 1980.
30. Oken DE, Arce ML and Wilson DR. J Clin Invest 45:724-735, 1966.
31. Wilson DR, Thiel G, Arce ML and Oken DE. Nephron 4:337-355, 1967.
32. Wilson DR, Thiel G, Arce ML and Oken DE. Nephron 6:128-139, 1969
33. Thiel G, McDonald FD and Oken DE. Nephron 7:67-79, 1970.
34. Ruiz-Guinazu A, Coelho JB and Paz RA. Nephron 4:257-275, 1967.
35. Jaenike JR. J Lab Clin Med 73:459-468, 1969.
36. Oken DE, DiBona GF and McDonald FD. J Clin Invest 49:730-737,
   1970.
37. Baylis C, Rennke HR and Brenner BM. Kidney Int 12:344-353, 1977.
38. Pastoriza-Munoz E, Bowman RL and Kaloyanides GJ. Kidney Int
   16:440-450, 1979.
39. Senekjian HO, Knight TF and Weinman EJ. Kidney Int 19:416-423,
   1981.

40. Schor N, Ichikawa I, Rennke HG, Troy JL and Brenner BM. Kidney Int 19:288-296, 1981.
41. Barza M, Murray T and Hamburger RJ. J Infect Dis 141:510-517, 1980.
42. Vandewalle A, Farman N, Morin JP, Fillastre JP, Hatt PY and Bonvalet JP. Kidney Int 19:529-539, 1981.
43. Bergeron MG, Gennari FJ, Barza M, Weinstein L and Cortell S. J Infect Dis 132:374-383, 1975.
44. Brenner BM, Bohrer MP, Baylis C and Deen WM. Kidney Int 12:229-237, 1977.
45. Oken DE, Cotes SC and Mende CW. Kidney Int 1:3-11, 1972.
46. Conger JD, Falk SA, Guggenheim SJ and Burke TJ. J Clin Invest 58:681-689, 1976.
47. Cook MA, Adkinson JT. Proc Soc Exp Biol Med 163:187-192, 1980.
48. Spencer HW, Yarger WE and Robinson RR. Kidney Int 9:489-500, 1976.
49. Conger JD and Falk SA. J Clin Invest 59:786-798, 1977.
50. Huguenin ME, Birbaumer A, Brunner FP, Thorhorst J, Schmidt U, Dubach UC and Thiel G. Nephron 22:41-54, 1978.
51. Weiner IM. Am J Physiol 237:F85-F92, 1979.
52. Rougemont D de, Henchoz M and Roch-Ramel F. Am J Physiol 231:387-392, 1976.
53. Roch-Ramel F, White F, Vowles L, Simmonds HA and Cameron JS. Am J Physiol 239:F107-F112, 1980.
54. Chonko AM. Am J Physiol 239:F545-F551, 1980.
55. Schäli C and Roch-Ramel F. Am J Physiol 239:F222-F227, 1980.
56. Duggin GG. Kidney Int 18:553-561, 1980.
57. Roch-Ramel F, Roth L, Arnow J and Weiner IM. J Pharmacol Exp Ther 207:737-747, 1978.
58. Bluemle A and Goldberg M. J Clin Invest 47:2507-2514, 1968.
59. Singer I and Forrest JN Jr. Kidney Int 10:82-95, 1976.
60. Carney S, Rayson B and Morgan T. Pfluegers Arch 366:19-23, 1976.
61. Hecht B, Kashgarian M, Forrest JN Jr and Hayslett JP. Pfluegers Arch 377:69-74, 1978.
62. Carney SL, Wong NLM and Dirks JH. Nephron 25:293-298, 1980.
63. Galla JN, Forrest JN Jr, Hecht B, Kashgarian M and Hayslett JP. Yale J Biol Med 48:305-314, 1975.
64. Thomsen K and Olesen OV. Toxicol Appl Pharmacol 45:155-161, 1978.
65. Hestbech J, Hansen HE, Amdisen A and Olsen S. Kidney Int 12:205-213, 1977.
66. Ehrlich BE and Diamond JM. J Membr Biol 52:187-200, 1980.
67. Hayslett JP and Kashgarian M. Pfluegers Arch 380:159-163, 1979.
68. Balfour WE, Grantham JJ and Glynn IM. Nature 275:768, 1978.
69. Higashi Y and Bello-Reuss E. Kidney Int 18:302-308, 1980.
70. Bergeron M and Vadeboncoeur M. Nephron 8:367-374, 1971.
71. Günther R, Silbernagl S and Deetjen P. Pfluegers Arch 382:109-114, 1979.
72. Bergeron M, Dubord L and Hausser C. J Clin Invest 57:1181-1189, 1976.
73. Oken DE. Am J Med 58:77-82, 1975.
74. Valtin H. Am J Physiol 233:F491-F501, 1977.

75. Schmidt U and Horster M, in Methods in Pharmacology, vol. 4B: Renal Pharmacology (M Martinez-Maldonado, ed.). Plenum Press, New York and London, 1978, chap. 10, pp. 259-296. ISBN 0-306-35265-6.
76. Morel F, Chabardès D and Imbert-Teboul M, in Methods in Pharmacology, vol. 4B: Renal Pharmacology (M Martinez-Maldonado, ed.). Plenum Press, New York and London, 1978, chap. 11, pp. 297-323. ISBN 0-306-35265-6.

THE USE OF ISOLATED KIDNEY CELLS, GLOMERULI AND SUBCELLULAR FRACTIONS FOR ASSESSING RENAL FUNCTION

Kari Ormstad

Department of Forensic Medicine, Karolinska Institutet, S-104 01 Stockholm 60, Sweden

ABSTRACT

The complex functions and the highly organized structure of the kidney render certain limitations to *in vivo*-systems and isolated perfused kidney for the investigation of separate functions at a cellular and subcellular level. For such purposes techniques have been developed for the isolation of intact glomeruli, various cell populations and subcellular organelles.

A technique for obtaining viable tubular epithelial cells by collagenase perfusion of isolated kidneys has recently been developed and used for studies of glutathione turnover, drug metabolism and amino acid uptake. The cells are viable and actively metabolizing for 2-3 h, they exhibit an active uptake of amino acids and a rapid turnover of their glutathione content. The capacity for drug (paracetamol) conjugation is lower than in the liver, but qualitatively, the same conjugates are formed. Glutathione-S-conjugates undergo a stepwise breakdown similar to that involved in the catabolism of extracellular glutathione. In contrast to hepatocytes, kidney cells oxidize GSH to GSSG, and they take up low-molecular disulfides which subsequently undergo an intracellular reduction.

These processes have been further studied in subcellular fractions. The GSH oxidase activity is found exclusively in the plasma membrane fraction - most probably in the basolateral part - and is due to a metal-containing enzyme distinctly separable from γ-GT. Disulfide reduction takes place in the cytosolic fraction, and a 3-step reaction involving thiol transferase and glutathione reductase is suggested.

Key words: Glomeruli, isolated kidney cells, glutathione, drug metabolism.

INTRODUCTION

The complex and highly organized structure of the kidney makes it difficult to study the various specialized functions separately in the intact organ. For this purpose isolated tissue and cell fractions constitute valuable model systems, and various techniques have been developed for the preparation of isolated glomeruli, tubular fragments, single cells and subcellular organelles.

The function of lower parts of the nephron can be studied by microperfusion after puncture in situ or after dissection of single tubular units in vitro. However, these techniques are presented elsewhere in this issue and a further description is therefore outside the scope of the present paper.

ISOLATED GLOMERULI

The most common technique employed for the isolation of intact glomeruli consists of a sequential passing of anemized and homogenized renal cortical tissue through a series of stainless steel or nylon sieves with varying mesh size [1,2] whereby a preparation consisting of >90%-95% intact glomeruli without Bowman's capsule is obtained. The isolation procedure takes about 50-60 min, and the yield amounts to 80-90% of the estimated number of glomeruli present in the kidney. After isolation, the viability of the preparation is assessed in terms of lactate dehydrogenase (LD) leakage and trypan blue exclusion, and the integrity of the glomeruli seems to be maintained for many hours under favorable conditions. The glomeruli have been studied morphologically, used for purification of basal membranes, used as a cell source for primary culture and employed in incubation experiments to study their O_2 uptake, metabolism and response to hormones and xenobiotics, as well as the synthesis of basal membrane matrix [3] and prostaglandins [4]. Mostly, rats have been used as experimental animals for these studies, but in a recent paper Peterson et al. [5] reported results from chickens, where the mixed function oxidase catalyzing the 1α- and the 24-R-hydroxylation of 25-hydroxycholecalciferol was demonstrated in nuclei from isolated glomeruli.

ISOLATED CELLS

Isolation procedure. In our laboratory a technique has been developed for the isolation of a single tublular epithelial cells [6,7]. The isolation procedure involves collagenase perfusion, gentle dispersal of the tissue and filtering through a nylon mesh sieve which retains glomeruli, connective tissue and undigested tissue fragments. The procedure takes about 60 min and the cell yield is $10-15 \times 10^6$ cells per kidney. The cell population is somewhat heterogeneous, but according to morphological criteria, ca. 75% consists of uniformly spherical cells with a well-developed fur coat of microvilli. From enzymatic and functional studies we assume that this major fraction represents tubular epithelial cells. We have not further separated the various cell types and we use the total cell yield as it is. Heidrich and Dew [8] however reported that structurally and functionally homogenous cell preparations have been obtained from rabbit kidney cortex by free flow electrophoresis, and this possibility further refines the system.

The viability and integrity of isolated kidney cells prepared according to our technique is established by testing trypan blue exclusion, NADH penetration, glutathione (GSH) status and respiration rate (Table 1). Under control conditions, the cells are intact and actively metabolizing for at least 3 hours, which makes this system a convenient and versatile tool in studies of tubular functions at a cellular level. Routinely, we perform cell experiments as short time incubations in a carbogen-gassed, thermostatted system of round-bottom siliconized glass flasks and remove samples from the incubate at pre-set time points. Cell viability is checked every half hour.

Table 1. Characteristics of isolated kidney cells

Yield	$\approx 10^7$ cells/kidney
Trypan blue exclusion	85-95%
NADH penetration	10-15%
Packed cell volume	14-15 $\mu l/10^6$ cells
GSH content	28-32 nmol/10^6 cells
Protein content	≈ 2 mg/10^6 cells
Respiration rate	22-26 nmol $O_2/10^6$ cells per min

Transport functions. Among the functions tested in isolated kidney cells is amino acid uptake [9]. We have found that the cells rapidly accumulate all amino acids tested at rates compared to that observed in isolated hepatocytes i.e. 1.5-6 nmol/10^6 cells/min. Certain differences have been observed though, since in contrast to hepatocytes kidney cells are able to take up cystine as well as other low molecular disulfides. For more than 10 years it has been discussed whether the brush-border enzyme γ-glutamyltransferase (γ-GT) is involved in renal tubular amino acid absorption [10,11] and so far no conclusive answer has been reached. In vivo it has been observed that patients congenitally deficient in γ-GT activity exhibit no abnormal aminoaciduria [12] whereas in various cellular systems a coupling between γ-GT activity and amino acid transport has been described [13,14]. We have earlier reported [9] that in the presence of serine·borate (20mM) uptake of Glu, Cys, Met and Cys-S-Cys is inhibited whereas Gly uptake is unaffected. However, with a newly described γ-GT inhibitor, Anthglutin [15], no effect on absorption is observed (Table 2). This is taken to indicate that the effect of serine·borate was a more unspecific one and not related to γ-GT inhibition, and a quantitatively important involvement of γ-GT in renal tubular amino acid transport thus seems to be quite a posibility.

Table 2. Amino acid uptake in isolated kidney cells
Results given as a mean $\pm$ SD of at least 3 experiments

		nmol taken up/10^6 cells per min	
		+ serine·borate	+ Anthglutin
	Control	20mM	1 mM
Cysteine	5.2 ± 0.9	3.9 ± 1.0	5.3 ± 1.1
Cystine	1.9 ± 0.5	1.0 ± 0.3	2.1 ± 0.5
Methionine	2.8 ± 0.6	1.5 ± 0.5	2.6 ± 0.7
Glutamate	3.3 ± 0.7	1.9 ± 0.4	3.4 ± 0.7
Glycine	5.6 ± 1.1	5.4 ± 1.2	5.8 ± 1.3
Leucine	4.9 ± 1.0	3.8 ± 0.9	4.5 ± 1.2

Turnover of cellular glutathione. The turnover of renal tissue glutathione has been extensively studied by Meister et al. [10] and under in vivo conditions, a half-life of 30 mins has been observed, which apart from plasma glutathione turnover ($t_{1/2}$= 1-2 min [16]) is the most rapid rate found in any tissue.

We have studied the glutathione status in isolated kidney cells and could confirm the observation that it is rapidly turning over under control conditions and even more so in the presence of certain amino acids [9]. This supports the operation under certain conditions of the so-called γ-glutamyl cycle, with intracellular glutathione acting as a γ-Glu group donor and amino acids as acceptors. However, with amino acid concentrations and pH in the more in vivo-like range, glutathione hydrolysis and not transpeptidation in the preferred γ-GT-mediated reaction [17], so in accordance with studies of renal amino acid uptake in the absence of γ-GT activity, a quantitatively important involvement of the γ-glutamyl cycle seems difficult to visualize.

Under control conditions, renal cells were able to maintain a normal level of glutathione for hours [6]. In cells isolated from kidneys pre-perfused with diethylmaleate, which depletes cellular glutathione to ca. 30% of control values, replenishment occurred within 30 min in the presence of the proper precursor amino acids in the medium (resynthesis rate 0.6-1.0 nmol/10^6 cells per min) [9]. Like in hepatocytes [18], intracellular access to cysteine moieties appeared to be the rate-limiting step for glutathione synthesis, but kidney cells showed a somewhat different preference for the source of cysteine [9]: In hepatocytes, extracellular methionine can substitute for cysteine since after uptake it is rapidly converted to cysteine via the cystathionine pathway [19]. This was not the case in kidney cells, apparently because of a lack of activity of the enzyme cystathionase [20]. Cystine, on the other hand, is not taken up in hepatocytes, but quite rapidly in kidney cells, and here it appears to be the preferred sulfur source for glutathione synthesis.

In addition to de novo synthesis, kidney cells also seem to have another mechanism to keep cellular glutathione at an optimal level, i.e. direct uptake across the plasma membrane (cf. [21]). The main route of transport in the intact kidney is from the peritubular capillaries to the interior of tubular cells and probably further to the urine, and it has been reported that up to 90% of plasma or perfusate glutathione is extracted during one passage through the renal vascular bed [22]. The exact nature and the possible physiological role of this transport remains however to be stated.

STUDIES INVOLVING CELLS AND SUBCELLULAR FRACTIONS

Disulfide reduction. As mentioned, low molecular disulfides are taken up into isolated renal cells. However, the disulfides are never seen to accumulate within the cells, they undergo a rapid reduction and are either stored intracellularly in thiol form, processed further or re-excreted to the surrounding medium. This was first observed with cystine [9], and in order to determine the localization and nature of the reduction mechansim we incubated cystine with various subcellular fractions and possible cofactors. A measurable reduction to cysteine could only be observed with the cytosolic fraction (i.e. post-105,000 x g supernatant) and in the presence of NADPH and reduced glutathione (GSH)(Fig.1) which led us to suggest the following reaction mechanism:

I.   Cys-S-Cys + GSH $\longleftrightarrow$ GS-Cys + CysH
II. GS-Cys + GSH $\longleftrightarrow$ GSSG + CysH
III. GSSG + NADPH $\longleftrightarrow$ 2GSH + NADP$^+$

where reactions I and II are catalyzed by thiol transferase and reaction III by glutathione reductase.

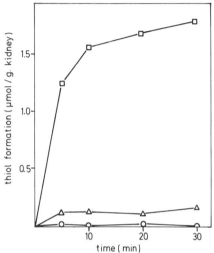

Fig. 1. Thiol formation in rat kidney cytosolic fraction incubated with cystine, 0.2 mM under N$_2$-atmosphere. Additions as indicated: O–O no additions; △–△ GSH, 0.5 mM; □–□ GSH, 0.5 mM + NADPH, 1.0mM.

This sequence of reactions has later been further substantiated by results obtained with purified thiol transferase (a generous gift from Dr Mannervik's laboratory, University of Stockholm) and glutathione reductase (Boehringer Mannheim GmbH, W. Germany).

Drug metabolism. A variety of endogenous and xenobiotic substrates undergo oxidative, conjugative and degradative reactions in the kidney (cf. [7]). We have exposed isolated kidney cells to the analgesic drug paracetamol via the incubation medium and followed the effect on cell viability as well as the pattern of metabolites formed [23]. During 2 hours' incubation, paracetamol concentrations up to 5 mM did not exert any toxic effect on the cells as judged from routine viability criteria. Like in hepatocytes, glucuronide and sulfate conjugates of paracetamol were formed, but although the cellular concentration of glutathione is high and glutathione S-transferase is present, glutathione-S-paracetamol could only be detected in trace amounts. Instead, cysteine and N-acetylcysteine conjugates appeared in the medium. Under conditions where the glutathione-degrading enzyme γ-glutamyltransferase was inhibited (20 mM serine·borate added to the incubate), however, glutathione-S-glutathione (synthetized by isolated hepatocytes) was incubated with kidney cells (Fig.2). Thus, we concluded that in addition to forming glutathione-S-conjugates, the kidney is also metabolizing those by a reaction sequence initiated by the γ-GT-mediated splitting of the γ-Gly-Cys peptide bond, followed by a cleavage of the Cys-Gly peptide bond catalyzed by a particular peptidase (amino-peptidase M) also present in renal tissue [24] and finally an N-acetylation of the residual cysteine conjugate.

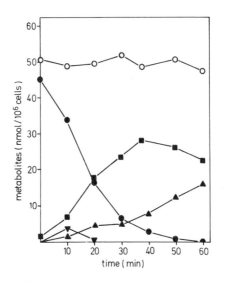

Fig. 2. Metabolites formed during incubation of isolated kidney cells with 25 μM paracetamol-S-glutathione. Filled symbols denote the absence, open symbols the presence of the γ-glutamyltransferase inhibitor Anthglutin, 1 mM. ○–○ paracetamol-S-glutathione; ▽–▽ paracetamol-S-cysteinylglycine; □–□ paracetamol-S-cysteine; △–△ paracetamol-S-N-acetylcysteine.

This pathway has also been suggested by others [24,25] for the degradation of glutathione-S-conjugates and unsubstituted glutathione in vivo, which was even more firmly supported by our observation that addition of glutathione to the incubate in a competitive fashion inhibited metabolism of glutathione-S-paracetamol.

The final N-acetylation appeared to be the rate-limiting step in the suggested reaction sequence. This may partly be due to a limited cellular capacity for uptake of the cysteine conjugate. Incubations with purified subcellular fractions have demonstrated that both γ-GT [26] and aminopeptidase M [27] are located in the brush border of tubular epithelial cells whereas all known N-acetyltransferases are intracellular (cf. [28]) and uptake thus is a prerequisite for acetylation to take place. Furthermore, the availability of AcCoA and the capacity for transporting the N-acetylcysteine conjugate out of the cell may limit the excretion of N-acetylcysteine conjugates in the kidney.

Glutathione oxidation. During incubations of isolated kidney cells with unsubstituted glutathione it was observed that irrespective of whether GSH or GSSG was added to the incubate, the metabolites appearing were the same, i.e. they all contained a cystine moiety, which suggested that the initial step in the handling of GSH was an oxidation to GSSG [23]. Addition of GSH to a kidney cell suspension led to a very rapid disappearance of the tripeptide, and this phenomenon was not affected by inhibition of γ-GT. On the other hand, when γ-GT activity was blocked (by serine·borate or Anthglutin) GSSG accumulated in the medium in stoichiometric proportion to GSH loss. Further studies with purified subcellular fractions have demonstrated the existence of a GSH-oxidizing enzyme clearly distinct from γ-GT and strictly confined to the plasma membrane fraction [29], and recent observations by Lash and Jones [26] have supported results obtained in our laboratory with isolated perfused kidney, that the enzyme is restricted to the basolateral part of the tubular epithelial plasma membrane [30].   The enzyme has now been purified [31, 32] and has proven not to be strictly specific for GSH but also to accept some other low molecular thiols as substrates.   This inhibition is reversible upon addition of copper ions, but not iron or zinc, which suggests an involvement of copper in the active form of the enzyme.   Preliminary results of electron paramagnetic resonance (EPR) and atomic absorption spectrometry (Kroneck & Ormstad, unpublished results) also suggest that the renal thiol oxidase is a metalloenzyme.

The reaction with GSH requires molecular O_2, and H_2O_2 is formed in stoichiometric proportion to GSH disappearance and GSSG formation. However, it seems likely that O_2^- is formed as an intermediate during GSH oxidation and subsequently is dismutated spontaneously or catalyzed by superoxide dismutase to H_2O_2.   Thus, we suggest the following reaction:

$$2GSH + O_2 \longleftrightarrow GSSG + 2\ O_2^- \xrightarrow{2H^+} GSSG + H_2O_2 + O_2$$

Although the existence of renal GSH oxidation has been known for more than 35 years [33] the exact nature of the reaction and its possible physiological significance are still incompletely known.

In view of the basolateral localization of the enzyme [26,30,] the high apparent K_m (-0.5 mM) for GSH and the very low GSH concentration in peripheral plasma (<3-5 μM [16,34]) it seems unlikely that the physiological function of the enzyme is to oxidize extracellular GSH. Another possibility is that the enzyme in vivo functions to modify the activity of thiol containing locally-acting peptide hormones or to facilitate binding to receptor sites on the tubular epithelial cells.

REFERENCES

1.   Cook WF and Pickering GW, Nature 182: 1103-1104, 1958
2.   Misra RP, Am J Clin Pathol 58: 135-139, 1972
3.   Hjelle JT, Carlsson EC, Brendel K and Meezan E, Kidney
         International 15: 20-32, 1979
4.   Schlondorff D, Rocznialk S, Satriano JA and Flokert Vw, Am J
         Physiol 239: 486-495, 1980
5.   Peterson EW, Ghazarian JG and Garancis JC, Calcif Tissue Internat
         33: 19-25, 1981
6.   Jones DP, Sundby GB, Ormstad K and Orrenius S, Biochem Pharmacol
         28: 929-935, 1979
7.   Ormstad K, Jones DP and Orrenius S, Meth Enzymol 77: 137-146, 1981
8.   Heidrich HG and Dew ME, J Cell Biol 74: 780-788, 1977
9.   Ormstad K, Jones DP and Orrenius S, J Biol chem 255: 175-181, 1980
10. Meister A, In Metabolism of Sulfur Compounds (DM Greenberg, ed.)
         Acad press, New York, 1975, pp. 101-188
11. Curthoys NP and Hughey R, Enzyme 24: 383-403, 1979
12. Schulman JD, et al. Biochim Biophys Res Commun 65: 68-74, 1975
13. Osuji GO, FEBS Lett 105: 283-286, 1979
14. Mooz ED, Biochem Biophys Res Commun 90: 1221-1228, 1979

15. Minato S, Arch Biochem Biophys 192: 235-240, 1979
16. Wendel A and Cikryt P, FEBS Lett 120: 209-211, 1980
17. Elce JS and Broxmeyer B, Biochem J 153: 223-232, 1976
18. Reed DJ and Orrenius S, Biochem Biophys Res commun 77: 1257-1264, 1977
19. Beatty PW and Reed DJ, Eur J Biochem 116: 13-16, 1981
20. Moldeus P, Ormstad K and Redd DJ, Eur J Biochem 116: 13-16, 1981
21. Ormstad K, Lastbom T and Orrenius S, FEBS Lett 112: 55-59, 1980
22. Haberle D, Wahllander A and Sies H, FEBS Lett 108: 335-340
23. Jones DP, et al. J Biol Chem 254: 2787-2792, 1979
24. Hughey RP, et al. Arch Biochem Biophys 186: 211-217, 1978
25. Wendel A, Heinle H and Silbernagl S, Hoppe-Seyler's Z Physiol Chem 358: 1413-1414, 1977
26. Lash LH and Jones DP, Personal communication
27. Okajima K, Inoue M and Morino Y, Biochim Biophys Acta 675: 379-385, 1981
28. Tate SS, In Enzymatic Basis of Detoxication (W Jakoby, ed.) Acad Press, New York. 1980, pp. 95-120, ISBN 0-12-380002-1 (V.2)
29. Ormstad K, Moldeus P and Orrenius S, Biochem Biophys Res Commun 89: 497-503, 1979
30. Ormstad K, Lastbom T and Orrenius S, Biochim Biophys Acta, in press
31. Ashkar S, Binkley F and Jones DP, FEBS Lett 124: 166-168, 1981
32. Ormstad K, Lastbom T and Orrenius S, FEBS Lett 139: 239-243, 1981
33. Ames SR and Elvehjem CA, J Biol Chem 159: 549-562, 1945
34. Tietze F, Anal Biochem 27: 502-522, 1969

THE HEMODYNAMIC BASIS FOR EXPERIMENTAL ACUTE RENAL FAILURE

Donald E. Oken, Douglas M. Landwehr and Barry B. Kirschbaum

Departments of Medicine, Medical College of Virginia and the Veterans Administration Hospital, Richmond, Virginia, USA

Various lines of evidence point toward, and others away from, a pathogenetic role of the renin angiotensin axis, the prostaglandins, and kinins in acute renal failure (ARF). A neurogenic cause for impaired filtration seems rather less likely since classical ARF occurs in totally denervated, transplanted kidneys. However mediated, filtration failure must relate to a reduction in net filtration pressure or glomerular capillary hydraulic conductivity (Kf). In the presence of normal blood pressure and serum protein concentration, we thus must envision significantly altered renovascular resistances and/or, high proximal tubule pressure as the cause if altered hydraulic conductivity is not responsible. These three factors might operate in concert and to a varying extend in different models. Since markedly suppressed filtration in several murine and canine ARF models coexists with essentially normal renocortical blood flow, simple preglomerular vascular constriction (such as seen in human ARF) is precluded as the cause. Tubule pressures in most ARF models are not greatly elevated, ruling out tubule obstruction as the essential factor. Analysis shows that the glomerular capillary membrane must become virtually impermeable before hydraulic conductivity alone can cause filtration failure. A relatively modest relaxation of the postglomerular vasculature will greatly depress glomerular filtration, an effect augmented by any elevation in tubule pressure or fall in Kf that might coexist in any given model. It seems likely that no single determinant of glomerular dynamics is responsible for all models of ARF in the rat. Although great progress has been made in understanding the pathophysiology of experimental ARF, considerable work is needed to identify the mediator(s) and the glomerular mechanisms involved.

Acute renal failure; glomerular dynamics; hemodynamics.

Glomerular filtration and tubular transport processes must be precisely matched to maintain normal fluid, electrolyte, and hydrion balance. In man, some 180 liters of filtrate containing 25,000mEq of sodium, 800mEq of potassium, 4,600mEq of bicarbonate and 180g of glucose, together with large amounts of divalent ions, amino acids and other vital materials, are presented to the tubules for absorption each day. Urea, creatinine and other wastes in the filtrate are excreted to differing degrees. Well maintained filtration in the face of tubular injury would put the organism at risk of life threatening volume depletion, electrolyte disorders and malnutrition. There is, therefore, significant survival value to curtailing glomerular filtration (GFR) whenever the tubule's absorptive capacity is seriously impaired [1] -- for a short period of time, at least. Pathologic retention of toxic metabolites with impaired ability to excrete excesses of ingested water and electrolyte ultimately must outweigh any earlier benefits obtained by the cessation of filtration, but the fortunate victim might have the opportunity to repair tubular epithelial integrity before that point is reached. At present, we know of no mechanism for "cross-talk" between an injured renal tubular epithelium and the glomerulus. Normal "glomerulo-tubular balance" with which tubular absorption is regulated according to GFR nowadays is attributed to hydrostatic and colloid oncotic pressure differences between the tubule lumen, interstitium and peritubular capillaries rather than a chemical mediator, but one could easily envision a messenger substance released by injured tubular epithelium which is capable of shutting off glomerular filtration. Osswald [2] has presented evidence suggesting that adenosine might serve as this mediator between tubular injury and failed filtration in the rat, a very attractive theory which has yet to be confirmed. Unfortunately, we have been unable to find any salutory effect of prolonged intravenous infusions of imidazole on the filtration failure of rats with glycerol induced myohemoglobinuric acute renal failure (unpublished observation) although this substance is a very potent antagonist of the known vascular effects of adenosine [3].

There is presently little doubt that glomerular filtration is truly maximally impaired and tubular function significantly depressed in both experimental and human acute renal failure [4-7]. In past years, however, several investigators have suggested that filtrate actually is formed at a normal or near normal rate but is then nearly totally absorbed across defects in the tubular epithelial barrier [8-10]. Some degree of tubular "leakiness" can, indeed be demonstrated by direct renal micropuncture in certain models of ARF [8-10], but that does not negate a mass of evidence which shows that the filtration process is maximally suppressed in all the acute renal failure models studied to date. Intravenously injected lissamine green can be seen to be filtered and to fill the tubular system of normal rats and dogs whose kidneys are under direct microscopic visualization during micropuncture experiments. In most experimental models of acute renal failure, by contrast, lissamine green appears promptly in the peritubular capillary circulation but fails to appear in any surface glomeruli or proximal tubules [11]. Tubules in most models are totally collapsed and fail to yield any significant volume of fluid on insertion of a micropipet. Isotonic fluid injected into such tubules in retrograde

fashion to the glomerulus remains unabsorbed for several minutes,
an indication that fluid absorption in proximal segments of the
nephron is very depressed rather than augmented by tubular leakage.
Thus, the inability to collect filtrate by proximal tubular
micropuncture is a direct reflection of failed filtration.

The depression of glomerular filtration in human acute renal
failure is readily explained on the basis of hemodynamic phenomena.
Although one cannot fruitfully employ classical PAH clearance
techniques for studies of renal blood flow in the presence of gross
tubular transport dysfunction, inert gas washout techniques have
proven very satisfactory as indicators of renal blood flow independent
of and unaffected by tubular defects. Several investigators [12-14]
have found renocortical blood flow in human acute renal failure to be
depressed to some 20-30 percent of normal. On angiography, preglomerular
vascular constriction and virtual disappearance of the outer cortical
arteriolar pattern are clearly demonstrable [15]. Renovascular
resistance must increase three to five-fold before renocortical
ischemia of this degree is obtained and, with the degree of preglomerular
vasoconstriction evident on angiography, glomerular filtration must
inevitably be massively reduced regardless of any other abnormality
present.

The situation in experimental acute renal failure of the rat is
very different and rather more puzzling. Very few studies have found
renocortical ischemia of a degree approaching that reported for man,
and most recent studies have shown nearly normal or even supernormal

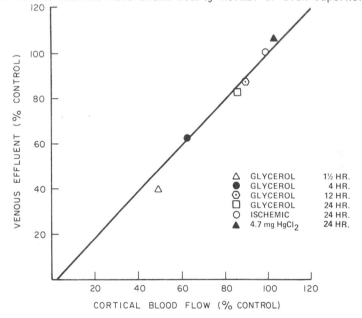

Figure 1.   Renocortical blood flow measured with implanted
              platinum electrodes in rats with acute renal failure
              due to 1 hour of total renal arterial occlusion
              (ischemia), 4.7 mg/Kg body weight HgCl$_2$ or 10 ml/Kg
              body weight 50 percent glycerol (Reproduced from
              reference 17 with permission of Nephron).

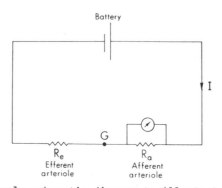

Figure 2.   A simple schematic diagram to illustrate the
                 relationship between renovascular resistances, blood
                 flow and "filtration pressure" in the glomerular
                 capillary (G). Blood flow (I) is determined by the
                 sum of the two resistances in series (RA and RE). The
                 filtration pressure at point G (glomerulus) is set by
                 the pressure drop across RA and is determined by the
                 ratio RA/RE. Blood flow and glomerular filtration are
                 thus regulated quite independently.

renocortical blood flow values [16, 17]. Studies from our laboratory
[17] illustrating the time course of cortical blood flow change in
rats subjected to mercury poisoning, total renal ischemia for 1 hour,
or glycerol induced myohemoglobinuria are shown in (Figure 1). It
may be seen that blood flow was within + 20 percent of control in all
three models, a finding which has been interpreted by some to
indicate that glomerular blood flow is adequate to sustain filtration
and that tubular factors therefore must be the root cause of acute
renal failure. In fact, they prove nothing of the kind.

Reduced to its simplest form the renocortical circulation may be
compared to an electrical circuit in which a battery provides the
blood pressure (Figure 2). Two resistors in series, one placed
before and the other after the glomerulus, serve to regulate current
(i.e. blood) flow and set the voltage (i.e. hydrostatic filtration
pressure) in a glomerulus placed between those two resistors. Flow
through this circuit may be controlled by manipulating the
preglomerular resistance, or both. Decreasing the value of either
lowers total resistance and thus increases flow if the voltage (or
blood pressure) remains constant; increasing one or both resistances
has the inverse effect. An individual resistance thus might increase
markedly without affecting flow through the circuit in any fashion
if a reciprocal decrease in its companion keeps the total resistance
of the circuit unchanged. In short, normal renocortical blood flow
does not necessarily imply either a normal preglomerular resistance
or a normal glomerular filtration pressure, and in no way rules out
the possibility that impaired filtration in experimental models of
renal failure reflect a primary vasomotor phenomenon.

Glomerular capillary pressure is only one of the determinants of
glomerular filtration, the single nephron filtration rate being
determined according to the equation: $SNGFR = Kf [(Pg - (COP + Pt)]$
where Kf is glomerular capillary hydraulic conductivity (nl/min
mmHg), and Pg, Pt, and COP are glomerular capillary, proximal tubule

and mean colloid oncotic pressures (mmHg), respectively. Thus, filtration is regulated by the hydraulic conductivity (permeability) of the filtration barrier and the algebraic difference between the filtration pressure promoting filtration, on the one hand, and the tubular and oncotic pressures which oppose the process on the other. There is ample evidence that, early in the course of post-ischemic acute renal failure produced by either renal artery clamping or prolonged norepinephrine infusions, proximal tubule pressure is so massively elevated as to inevitably to cause filtration to stop [18, 19]. In various other models, however, proximal tubule pressure is either normal or variably depressed [20, 21], so that such a mechanism cannot be impuned as the usual cause of filtration failure. Mean glomerular capillary colloid oncotic pressure is a function of the serum protein concentration and of the degree of glomerular filtration occurring within the glomerulus. Serum protein concentrations are not generally elevated in either human or experimental acute renal failure, and mean colloid oncotic pressure at any given serum protein concentration is at its absolute minimum in the absence or near absence of ongoing filtration. An abnormality in glomerular capillary hydraulic conductivity (Kf) is the remaining determinant that could produce filtration failure, in theory at least. Blantz [22] has incriminated decreased Kf as a major contributor to the reduced filtration found in uranium poisoned rats. Daugharty et al [23], on the other hand, could find no alteration in Kf during studies of rats with mild, post-ischemic renal failure. Further studies of the role of altered hydraulic conductivity in the pathogenesis of acute renal failure clearly are needed but, until they appear, a more precise idea of the practical importance can be gleaned with network modelling [24].

As discussed earlier, glomerular capillary pressure is determined by the dividual resistances before (RA) and after (RE) the glomerulus and the mean arterial blood pressure. The resistance of the glomerular capillary itself (Rcap) is assumed to be very small [25] although it, too, contributes to the overall vascular resistance. We have determined the degree of change in RA, RE, Pt and Kf needed to lower glomerular filtration to a level consistent with ARF by using a network thermodynamic model and the SPICE computer simulator program. Filtration failure is arbitrarily defined here as a single nephron GFR < 7 percent of control. It is found that RA must rise from its reported normal value of 3.8×10^{10} dyne sec cm $^{-5}$ in the rat to some 7.8×10^{10} dyne sec cm $^{-5}$ or RE must fall from 1.9×10^{10} dyne sec cm $^{-5}$ to 0.5×10^{10} dyne sec cm $^{-5}$ to produce effective filtration failure when proximal tubule pressure is held at its putative normal value of 11 mmHg. Even more marked changes in these resistances must occur in the presence of a reduced proximal tubule pressure such as found in various murine models [20, 21]. On the other hand, the degree of resistance change required to produce renal failure is rather less in the presence of an elevated proximal tubule pressure. Recalling that tubule pressure and glomerular blood flow have been found to be near normal in most ARF models, however, and noting that an increase in RA to 7.8×10^{10} dyne sec cm $^{-5}$ is associated with a 48 percent fall in GBF, it seems inconsistent to suggest that increased preglomerular resistance alone can be the usual cause of experimental acute renal failure in the rat. A decrease in postglomerular resistance to a degree that, in and of itself, reduces the filtration rate to less than 10 percent of normal necessarily raises GBF by some 20 percent above its normal value, but again the degree of change required to produce filtration failure is rather less in the presence of increased proximal tubule pressure. Raising RA and decreasing RE reciprocally maintains both total vascular resistance and glomerular blood flow at essentially normal levels. Following such a maneuver and holding proximal tubule pressure normal, we find from our model that filtration almost stops when RA is assigned a value of 4.9×10^{10} dyne sec cm^{-5} (a 29 percent rise), while RE is reduced to 0.8×10^{10} dyne sec cm^{-5} (approximately one-half of control). At a tubule pressure of 19 mmHg (normal = 11 mmHg), moreover, an increase in RA of only 16 percent with a fall in RE of 32 percent is sufficient to produce filtration failure.

Glomerular filtration in the rat is remarkably insensitive to proximal tubule pressure change when all other determinants are held constant at control values. There is an almost linear decrease in SNGFR as tubule pressure is raised from its normal value of 11 mmHg to 32 mmHg, but filtration remains at some 15 percent of normal after increasing this pressure to 30 mmHg. Changes up to this magnitude, therefore, cannot of themselves produce the near cessation of glomerular filtration found in acute renal failure. Only in those models where proximal tubule pressure may rise to a value above some 30 mmHg [18] can tubular obstruction be incriminated as the sole or major cause of failed filtration.

While intuition might argue to the contrary, change in hydraulic conductivity produces an important decrease in SNGFR only when extreme (Figure 3). Thus, reducing Kf in the rat from its reported

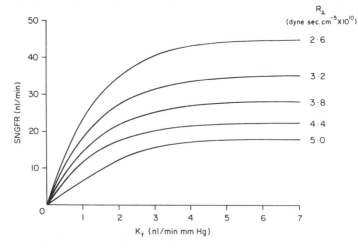

Figure 3.   The relationship of single nephron filtration rate (SNGFR) to glomerular capillary hydraulic conductivity in the rat at various values for afferent arteriolar resistance (RA), (normal RA = 3.8×10^{10} dyne sec cm^{-5}). Note that the effect of Kf change on SNGFR is very small at all assumed values of RA until Kf falls below 2 nl/min mmHg (normal 5 nl/min mmHg). A GFR < 2 nl/min as in ARF requires a Kf < 0.5 nl/min mmHg. Adapted from reference 24).

normal value of 5 nl/min mmHg [25] to 1.5 nl/min mmHg will cause SNGFR to fall by only one-third, full filtration failure requiring a reduction in Kf to approximately 5 percent of its control value. Although superimposing a decrease in hydraulic conductivity upon changes in RA and RE inevitably lowers SNGFR below the value obtained with a normal Kf, its potential contribution to filtration failure remains quite small until the Kf is very markedly reduced. Our model thus shows that the 70 percent reduction in Kf found by Blantz [22] in uranium poisoned rats would contribute in only a modest way to the reduction in SNGFR that he observed.

The "failed reflow" hypothesis suggests that the low SNGFR which typifies acute renal failure is brought about by increased glomerular capillary resistance and that this, in turn, is brought about by glomerular capillary endothelial cell swelling [26]. Wardle [27] has proposed an alternate explanation: increased capillary resistance due to intracapillary fibrin deposition. It is generally accepted that the resistance of the normal glomerular

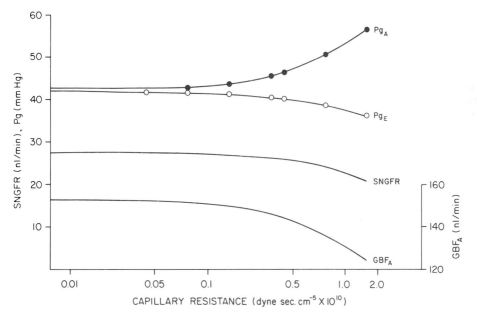

Figure 4.   The effect of glomerular capillary resistance on single nephron filtration rate (SNGFR) glomerular blood flow (GBFA), and glomerular capillary pressure at the beginning (PgA) and end (PgE) of the glomerular of the rat. Normal resistance is believed to be $< 10^9$ dyne sec cm $^{-5}$. SNGFR is almost unaffected until capillary resistance exceeds 2×10^{10} dyne sec cm $^{-5}$, a value comparable to that of the total postglomerular resistance of the rat. This high capillary resistance value produces a significant axial pressure drop along the capillary and causes a 20 percent fall in blood flow. (Reproduced from reference 24, with permission of Kidney International).

capillary is extremely low [25]. We find from our analysis that a solitary increase in glomerular capillary resistance of whatever cause has remarkably little effect on SNGFR of the rat until a resistance is reached that must also cause renocortical blood flow to fall drastically (Figure 4). With renocortical blood flow so well maintained in rat models of acute renal failure, it would seem that neither the failed reflow phenomenon nor capillary occlusion with fibrin products plays a significant pathogenetic role.

In sum, acute renal failure in the rat seems unlikely to be due to a solitary change in preglomerular or glomerular capillary resistance unless present estimates of blood flow are wrong. Only extreme changes in hydraulic conductivity can cause filtration failure, and tubular obstruction in most models can play only a contributory role by reducing the degree of vascular resistance change otherwise needed. With well maintained blood flow, then, we are left with efferent arteriolar relaxation (with or without some degree of change in afferent arteriolar resistance Kf and/or Pt) as the likely essential cause of filtration failure in various rat models of acute renal failure. The glomerular dynamic abnormalities in murine models thus seem to contrast sharply with those in man where preglomerular vascular constriction, in and of itself, is sufficient to explain the development of filtration failure. Although the rat has served as the prime experimental subject for studies of toxicologic renal injury, it might be wise to employ caution in extrapolating between the two species.

For reasons outlined elsewhere [28], acute renal failure is more apt to represent intrinsic abnormalities within the kidney than to be the product of some presently unidentified circulating factor. Indeed, we have found that animals with either glycerol induced myohemoglobinuric renal failure or mercury poisoning shown no improvement in their filtration rate when cross circulated with normal rats for several hours, and their normal cross-circulated partners experience no significant deterioration of renal function (Jackson B, Kornetsky K, and Oken DE, unpublished observation). A role of renal nerves seems unlikely since acute renal failure occurs in both man and the rat whose kidneys have been totally denervated by renal transplantation [29]. Several experimental findings tend to incriminate the renin-angiotensin system in the pathogenesis of acute renal failure, as first suggested some 35 years ago [30]. Plasma volume depletion markedly predisposes to the development of this syndrome, and the relationship between plasma volume depletion and renin release is well established. Long-term salt loading in the rat predictably prevents the development of several models of acute renal failure [31, 32] while greatly depressing both the renal and the plasma renin titres [33]. In addition, plasma renin and angiotensin levels are elevated in patients [34] and rats [35] with this syndrome, although filtration remains depressed in the rat long after the plasma renin activity has normalized [35]. It has been reported that passively transferred rabbit antiangiotensin antibody prevents the expected reduction in filtration rate of rats put at risk of myohemoglobinuric acute renal failure [36], and such a finding would strongly support an essential pathogenetic role for the renin system. We, on the other hand, have not been able to confirm that result [37]. Nor

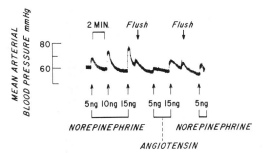

Figure 5.   Blood pressure response to graded doses of
               norepinephrine and angiotensin 2 of pentolium treated
               rats to be challenged with myohemoglobinuric acute
               renal failure. The response to angiotensin is
               normally several-fold greater than to norepinephrine,
               but here the animals were relatively refractory to
               angiotensin. They nonetheless showed no protection
               from renal insufficiency. (Reproduced from reference
               49 with permission of the American Journal of
               Physiology).

have we had any greater success with active immunization of the
rat against angiotensin despite the fact that extreme resistence
to the systemic effects of exogenous angiotensin was documented
(Figure 5). Such experiments and the evident failure of various
angiotensin antagonists to reverse glomerular insufficiency [36]
do not support the renin hypothesis and argue against the importance
of circulating renin or angiotensin in this process. A local
action of the renin-angiotensin system in the pathogenesis of
acute renal failure still is by no means disproven by such experiments
since the large antibody molecule might not be able to penetrate
to the intrarenal angiotensin effector and the concentration of
angiotensin inhibitors reaching this site may be too small to
negate angiotensin's effects. Nevertheless, unilateral renal
artery banding in the rat, a maneuver which greatly increases
ipsilateral renal renin content while depressing that of the
contralateral kidney, reportedly provides no detectable difference
in the susceptibility to, and severity of, renal failure produced
in the two kidneys [38]. Kidneys of rats recovering from prior
renal failure have an entirely normal renal renin content [39],
and release renin normally after either hemorrhage or isoproterenol
injections (Figure 6), yet they are highly refractory to a
second renal failure challenge [39]. Their renocortical blood
flow response to angiotensin, furthermore, is not depressed,
and, with all facts taken together, it seems that resistance
afforded by prior renal failure is not necessarily attributable
to impairment of renin-angiotensin axis function.
    Osswald et al [2] have found a sharp increase in renal tissue
levels of adenosine as well as the related compounds, inosine and
hypoxanthine in rats subjected to renal artery clamping. Levels
of these compounds fell promptly to normal after restoration of
the renal circulation, however. Adenosine is an interesting
compound. As already mentioned, it has been incriminated as a
possible mediator linking tubular injury and abnormalities of

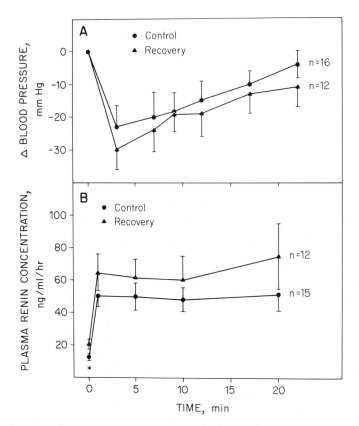

Figure 6.   Plasma renin release in response to acute
                 hemorrhage of normal control rats and animals recently
                 recovered from prior myohemoglobinuric acute renal
                 failure (Panel B). The blood pressure change is shown
                 in Panel A. Refractoriness of "recovery" animals to
                 ARF cannot be attributed to abnormality in their
                 capacity to normally release renin. (Reproduced from
                 reference 50 with permission of Nephron).

glomerular function in acute renal failure. While adenosine
produces vasodilation in most tissues, it appears to be a potent
constrictor of the renal circulation. Houck and coworkers [40]
have reported that the compound causes glomerular filtration to
decrease more than renal blood flow and, therefore, postulated
that it causes afferent arteriolar constriction with dilation of
the postglomerular circulation - the very effect that would seem
most likely to be compatible with the production of acute renal
failure in the rat. The effect of adenosine on the renovascular
tree has been found to closely parallel plasma renin activity,
however; even its constrictor activity, like that of angiotensin,
can be markedly decreased by long term salt loading. (It may be
recalled that long term salt loading also is an effective means
of preventing experimental acute renal failure in rats). Any
relationship between tubular injury and depressed glomerular

filtration in acute renal failure attributable to adenosine
release thus might well be produced by way of the renin-angiotensin
axis.

The apparent relationship between adenosine and angiotensin is
not unique. In fact, it is now well established that there is a
complex interrelationship between the prostaglandins, kinins,
dopamine, catecholamines, and angiotensins. In general, maneuvers
that produce renovascular constriction promote the release of
prostaglandins and kinins. The latter, powerful vasodilators,
modulate the degree of vasoconstriction that normally follows the
administration of angiotensin 2 [41], norepinephrine [42] and
renal nerve stimulation. Conversely, renin release in rabbit
renocortical slices has been shown to be significantly augmented
by the addition of either prostaglandin I2 or arachidonic acid,
an effect which clearly is independent of alterations in hemodynamics,
neural influences, and angiotensin [43]. Stimulation of renin
release has also been demonstrated in vivo after intraarterial
infusions of prostaglandins [44]. It is well established that a
variety of stimuli for renin release also induce prostaglandin
release by normal kidneys [45]. In turn, the prostaglandins as a
class modulate neurotransmission [42], regulate intrarenal
distribution of blood flow [46], and induce other effects which
might influence the development of acute renal failure. Within
the family of prostaglandins, PGE2 and PGI2 generally serve as
vascular dilators and produce a preferential increase in renocortical
blood flow [47]. Curiously, PGE2 in the rat acts as a vasoconstrictor
[47], rather than a dilator. Thromboxane A2 appears to be a
renovascular constrictor in all species and thus is particularly
suspect as a potential contributor to the vasomotor abnormalities
of ARF [48]. With this complex interaction between hormones
produced in the kidney, however, some potentiating and others
negating the effect of others, we are in no position at the
present to determine whether any of the known hormones directly
produces the vasomotor abnormalities of acute renal failure, and
it is entirely conceivable that a mediator or mediators yet to be
discovered is the prime determinant of this syndrome.

The past fifteen years have seen significant advances in our
understanding of the pathophysiologic events attendant upon acute
renal failure. Much more needs to be learned, however. In human
acute renal failure, the profound preglomerular vasoconstriction
that has been found universally offers a very adequate explanation
for the near cessation of glomerular filtration. The immediate
cause of this vasoconstriction unfortunately remains entirely
unknown. In the rat, whose renal failure is attended by essentially
normal renocortical blood flow, it appears that postglomerular
vascular relaxation is an essential component of failed filtration.
The contributory role of concomitant preglomerular vascular
constriction, change in capillary hydraulic conductivity and
proximal tubule pressure demand elucidation. Establishment of
the pathogenetic basis for such abnormalities as might be present
must await further clarification of the dynamic aberrations at
play.

REFERENCES

1. Oken, D.E. In: Pathogenesis and Clinical Findings with Renal Failure. (U. Gessler, K. Schroder, and H. Weidinger, eds.). Georg Thieme Verlag, Stuttgart, 1971 p 118-124.
2. Osswald, H., Schmitz, H.-J., and Kemper, R. In: Europ. J. Physiol. Pflugers Arch., 1977, 371:45-49.
3. Martinez, J.R., and A.M. Martinez. In: European Journal of Pharmacology 18, 1972, p 386-391.
4. Brun, C. and Munck, O. In: Lancet i: 1957, 603-607.
5. Meroney, W.H., and Rubini, M.E. In: Metabolism 8, 1959, 1.
6. Wilson, D.R., Thiel, G., Arce, M.L., and Oken, D.E. In: Nephron 6, 1969, 128-139.
7. Thiel, G., McDonald, F.D., and Oken, D.E. In: Nephron 7, 1970, 67-79.
8. Bank, N., Mutz, B.F., Aynedjian, H.S. In: J. Clin. Invest., 1967, 46:695-704.
9. Steinhausen, M., Eisenbach, G.M., Helmstadter, V. In: PflugersArch., 1969, 311:1.
10. Tanner, G.A., Sloan, K.L., Sophoson, S. In: Kidney Int., 1974, 1:406.
11. Henry, L.N., Lane, C.E., Kashgarian, M. In: Lab Invest., 1968, 19:309.
12. Brun, C., Crone, C., Davidsen, H.G., Fabricius, J., Hansen, A.Lassen, N.A., Munck, O. In: Proc. Soc. Exp. Biol. Med., 1955, 89:687-690.
13. Hollenberg, N.K., Adams, D.F. In: Proc. Conf. on Acute Renal Failure. Friedman, E.A. and Eliahou, H.E. Eds. DHEW Publication, 74-608, 1973, pp 209-229.
14. Reubi, F.C., Grossweiler, N., Furtler, R. In: Circulation, 1966, 33:426-442.
15. Hollenberg, N.K., Adams, D.F., Oken, D.E., Abrams, H.L., Merrill J.P. In: N. Engl. J. Med, 1970, 282:1329-1334.
16. Steinhausen, M., Eisenbach, G.M., Bottcher, W. In: Pflugers Arch., 1975, 339:273-288.
17. Churchill, S., Zarlengo, M.D., Carvalho, J.S., Gottlieb, M.N., and Oken, D.E. In: Kidney Int., 1977, 11:246-255.
18. Tanner, G.A., Sloan, K.L., and Sophasan, S. In: Kidney Int., 1973, 4:377-389.
19. Arendshorst, W.J., Finn, W.F., and Gottschalk, C.W. In: Circ. Res., 1975, 37:558-568.
20. Flanigan, W.J., and Oken, D.E. In: J. Clin. Invest., 1965, 44:449.
21. Oken, D.E., Arce, M.L., and Wilson, D.R. In: J. Clin. Invest., 1966, 45:724.
22. Blantz, R.C. In: J. Clin. Invest., 1975, 55:621.
23. Daugharty, T.M., Ueki, I.F., Mercer, P.F., and Brenner, B.M. In: J. Clin. Invest., 1974, 53:105-116.
24. Oken, D.E., Thomas, S.R., Mikulecky, D.C. In: Kidney Int., 1981, 19:359-373.
25. Brenner, B.M., Troy, J.L., and Daugharty, T.M. In: J. Clin. Invest., 1971, 50:1776-1780.
26. Flores, J., DiBona, D.R., Beck, C.H., and Leaf, A. In: J. Clin. Invest., 1972, 51:118.
27. Wardle, E.N. In: Nephron, 1975, 14:321.
28. Oken, D.E. In: Kidney Int., 1976, 10:S-94-S-99.

29. Silber, S.J. In: Surgery, 1974, 75:573-577.
30. Goormaghtigh, N. In: Proc. Soc. Exp. Biol. Med., 1945, 59:303.
31. Thiel, G., McDonald, F.D., Oken, D.E. In: Nephron, 1970,
     7:67-79.
32. McDonald, F.D., Thiel, G., Wilson, D.R., DiBona, G.F., Oken,
     D.E. In: Proc. Soc. Exp. Biol. Med., 1969, 131:610-614.
33. Flamenbaum, W., Kotchen, T.A., and Oken, D.E. In: Kidney
     Int., 1972, 1:406.
34. Kokot, F., and Kuska, J. In: Nephron, 1969, 6:115.
35. DiBona, G.F., and Sawin, L.L. In: Lab. Invest., 1971, 25:528.
36. Powell-Jackson, J.D., MacGregor, J., Brown, J.J., Lever, A.F.,
     and Robertson, J.I.S. In: Proc. Conf. Acute Renal Failure.
     Friedman, E.A. and Eliahou, H.E. Eds. DHEW Publication, 74-608,
     1973, pp. 74-608.
37. Oken, D.E., Cotes, S.C., Flamenbaum, W., Powell-Jackson,
     J.D., and Lever, A.F. In: Kidney Int., 1975, 7:12-18.
38. Churchill, P.C., Bidani, A., Fleischmann, L., and Becker-
     McKenna, B. In: Nephron, 1978, 22:529-537.
39. Oken, D.E., Mende, C.W., Taraba, I., and Flamenbaum, W. In:
     Nephron, 1975, 15:131-142.
40. Houck, C.R., Bing, R.J., Craig, F.N., and Visscher, F.E. In:
     Amer. J. Physiol, 1948, 153:159-168.
41. Bergstrom, S., Farnebo, L.O., and Fuxe, K. In: Europ. J.
     Pharmacol., 1973, 21:362-368.
42. Lonigro, A.J., Terragno, N.A., Malik, K.U., and McGiff, J.C.
     In: Prostaglandins, 1973, 3:595-606.
43. Horton, A.R., Misono, K., Hollifield, J., Frolich, J.C.,
     Inagami, T., Oates, J.A. In: Prostaglandins, 1977, 14:1095-
     1104.
44. Gerber, J.G., Branch, R.A., Nies, A.S., Gerkins, J.F., Shand,
     D.G., Hollifield, J., Oates, J.A. In: Prostaglandins, 1978,
     15:81-88.
45. Tannenbaum, J., Splawinski, J.A., Oates, J.A., Nies, A.S.
     In: Circ. Res., 1975, 36:197-203.
46. Herbaczynska-Cedro, K., Vane, J.R. In: Circ. Res., 1973, 33:
     428-436.
47. Malik, K.U., McGiff, J.C. In: Circ. Res., 1975, 36:599-609.
48. Feigen, L.P., Chapnick, B.M., Flemming, J.E., Flemming, J.M.,
     Kadowitz, P.J. In: Am. J. Physiol., 1977, 233:H573-H579.
49. Oken, D.E., Biber, T.U.L. In: Amer. J. Physiol., 1968,
     214:791-795.
50. Carvalho, J.S., Landwehr, D.M., and Oken, D.E. In: Nephron,
     1978, 22:107-112.

THE EFFECTS OF NUTRITIONAL FACTORS ON RENAL RESPONSE TO TOXINS

James W. Bridges, Peter H. Bach, Frank W. Bonner and Eleanor M. Beaton

Robens Institute of Industrial and Environmental Health and Safety, and the Department of Biochemistry, University of Surrey, Guildford, Surrey GU2 5XH, UK

ABSTRACT

The composition of animal diets varies both between sources, and between batches form the same source. Similarly, the composition of tap water varies both seasonally and between sources. In addition both food and water may contain trace amounts of an array of established toxicants, some of which are known to accumulate. Thus nutrition can play a decisive and uncontrolable role in the development of nephrotoxic lesions in experimental animals.

Gross dietary inadequacies (such as fat-free diet,choline- and vitamin-deficiency, and protein-calorie malnutrition) may cause renal changes comparable with toxic insult. Equally, however, it is now becoming clear that unlimited quanties of food and/or excesses of certain types of food constituents may also have deleterious effects over long term studies, and the type of protein may also affect the kidney (e.g. diets high in gelatin cause both renal hypertrophy and hyperplasia).

Relatively little is known about the altered sensitivity of the kidney to toxic substances when dietary factors are sub-optimal, nor how subtle changes in individual food constituents could alter the development and the course of nephrotoxicity.

A clear appreciation of how these many nutritional factors affect renal function and renal functional reserve may serve to:-

i) define those spontaneous age relate lesions which are nutritionally induced,

ii) characterise the dietary factors which exacerbate chemically induced renal lesions,

iii) establish the criteria by which to assess the validity of extrapolating data from experimentally induced renal lesion to risk analysis in humans,

iv) explain the variability in the response of both animals and man to nephrotoxic substances, and

v) identify those nutritional factors which will provide the maximum protection against toxic insults, and promote the most favourable recovery of renal function after toxic damage in both the experimental and the clinical situations.

KEY WORDS: Dietary variablity, Food contaminants, Myctoxins, Lipids, Vitamins, Protein.

INTRODUCTION

The importance of nutrition, in its fullest context, has become increasingly apparent in human health and disease, but its relevance to the scientific assessment of experimental toxicity data still needs to be carefully evaluated.

The level of our scientific understanding of nutritional needs and excesses is still inadequate and it is frequently difficult to separate fact from heresay.   Whereas the vitamin requirements for normal development and function have been recognized for some considerable time, it is only recently that a relationship between diet and drug metabolising activity has received attention.   However, there remains a paucity of reliable information on the effects of nutritional factors on the response to toxic insult, especially with regard to the kidney. The little information that is available is derived mainly from experimental animals.   This paper will, therefore, concentrate mainly on data obtained from laboratory animals, particularly the rat, but will try to indicate the possible relevance of such findings to man.

NUTRITIONAL FACTORS IN THE DESIGN OF TOXICITY STUDIES

Diet is one of a large number of variables (e.g. species, strain, sex,   age, health of animal, caging density, temperature, humidity, lighting intensity etc.) which must be considered when designing, conducting and interpreting experiments which involve the use of live animals (1). The very wide availability of "standardised" commercial animal diets has had many benefits, but an unfortunate consequence has been the widespread neglect of the possible contribution of subtle dietary factors to research findings.   The toxicologist is concerned with the relationship between the dose of chemical and its biological effect(s) in animals.   It is   therefore salutary to be reminded that the great majority of "new" molecules, with which the cells of the body come into contact, arise from ingested foodstuffs.   Moreover, the amount of food consumed per day may be a significant proportion of the body weight (e.g. man 1 to 4%, rat 4 to 7.5%; hamster 10 to 12% and mouse 10 to 15%).

Dietary factors may contribute to changes observed in animals during a toxicological study in a number of ways.

Direct changes due to:-

i)   a general dietary deficiency or excess e.g. carbohydrate, protein or
     lipid, the best known of which is protein-calorie malnutrition,

ii) a deficiency or excess of specific micro-nutrient(s) e.g. an amino
     acid, essential fatty acids, vitamin etc.,

iii) an imbalance of dietary constituents e.g. high protein, fat-free
     etc.

iv) the presence of toxic non-nutritive constituents or contaminants
     e.g. cadmium, lead , nitrosamines or mycotoxins,

Indirect Changes due to :-

i)   alteration in xenobiotic metabolising activity may modify the
     course or formation of toxic metabolites and/or detoxication
     products e.g. many vegetables of the brassica family induce mixed
     functional oxidase metabolism,

ii) modification in the uptake, transport, excretion and/or tissue
     retention and concentration of the toxin and/or its metabolites e.g.
     phytates and metals, phosphate may precipitate calcium,

iii) changes in cellular response to the chemical and its metabolites or
     to antigens, and

iv) a markedly changed cellular or organ requirement for specific
     nutrient(s) as a direct consequence of the toxic insult.

     It is, therefore, important to consider the nutritive and non-
nutritive composition of the diet, the amount of food likely to be
consumed and the efficiency of its utilization in both the generation
and interpretation of toxicological data.
     There are, however, several important constraints in selecting the
most appropriate diet.   For example, there is very little reliable
information on the nutritional requirements of laboratory rats over
their entire lifespan, and data on other animal species is even more
limited.   Moreover, the contributions of food-food interactions and
trace levels of dietary toxic constituents and contaminants to long term
health have been largely neglected.   A major problem is to identify the
most appropriate parameters by which to define "dietary adequacy".
Should we aim for a diet that maximises the growth rates, that which
provides an adequate storage and excretion of important individual
nutrients (and if so which) or should the diet be provided ad lib?   In
their natural environment animals are rarely in this "nutritional
cocoon", instead they are forced to be mobile and under "hunting
stress";   all factors which may make an important contribution to the
health of the animal.   An interesting pointer to the importance of the
quantity of diet that is consumed has been the demonstration (2) that
the incidence of tumours, in various tissues of the mouse, could be
dramatically reduced from 80% to 10% by changing from ad lib feeding
to a mild dietary restriction (about 86% of the ad lib animal intake).
     The problem of selection of an appropriate diet is exacerbated by the
fact that both tap water and apparently similar diets from various
manufacturers show very large differences (often 10 fold and on occasion
200 fold) in the content of particular nutrients (see Tables 1, 2 and
3). Moreover, different batches of a specified diet from the same
manufacturer may also vary considerably in composition (3-5).

     Water as a nutritional variable.   The addition of fluoride to
drinking water has now been widely accepted as the most suitable means
of circumventing the geographical and the seasonal variability in the
normal concentrations of this ion.   Recently, a possible relationship
between the hardness of water and the incidence of cardiovascular
disease   has   been   suggested   (3)   and   there   have   been   several
epidemiological   studies   on   the   possible   role   of   drinking   water
contaminants in carcinogenesis (7)

Table 1. Variability in the composition of commercially available rat diets.

Nutrient Substance	Concentration Range minimum-maximum	Estimated Requirement	Fold Variation
Minerals			
Phosphorous(%)	0.20-1.90	0.44	> 9
Magnesium(%)	0.01-1.2	0.04	120
Calcium (%)	0.27-1.67	0.56	6
Selenium (ppm)	0.001-0.21	0.04	210
Zinc (ppm)	5.0-43	13.3	> 8
Copper (ppm)	38-90	5.6	> 20
Iodine (ppm)	0.08-2.00	0.17	25
Amino Acids			
Methionine (%)	0.13-1.21	0.67	9
Tryptophan (%)	0.08-0.39	0.17	4
Vitamins			
Vit A (mg/kg)	0.23-3.75	0.67	16
Vit D (IU/kg)	650-5100	1108.0	> 7
Riboflavin (mg/kg)	3.0-63.4	2.8	> 20
Vit B12 (mg/kg)	0.0010-0.024	0.0056	> 20
Choline (mg/kg)	1000-6000	800.0	6
Protein (%)	21.7-44.4	-	2
Fat (%)	4.0-6.6	-	1.5

Data from Newberne (5).

Table 2. Variability in the composition of tap water, showing the maximum range both within and between sources of samples over 3 years*.

Substance	Minimum	Maximum	Units	Fold variation
Nitrate	0.3	13.8		> 40
Fluoride	<0.2	1.08		> 5
Sulphate	8	206		> 25
Orthophosphate	0.03	3.09	mg/L	>100
Sodium	31	53		± 2
Potassium	4.5	9.2		± 2
Iron	<0.01	0.53		> 50
Manganese	<0.01	0.04		> 4
Chromium	<10	<20		± 2
Zinc	<10	210		> 20
Copper	<10	<100		± 10
Cadmium	<1	2		> 2
Lead	<10	20	µg/L	> 2
Mercury	<0.2	<1		± 5
Selenium	<1	<5		± 5
Arsenic	<10	10		-

*Data from UK Water Statistics 1976/77, 1977/78 and 1978/79.

Table 3. Non-nutrients and contaminants in commercially available rat diets.

Substance	Concentration Range (ppm)	Toxic Level	Pathophysiological response
Mercury	0.007-0.16	2-5	Nephrotoxicity
Arsenic	0.010-0.92	5-10	-
Cadmium	0.005-0.168	0.2	Nephrotoxicity, Hypertension
Aflatoxin B_1	0-0.2	0.01-1	Tumours
Heptachlor	0.0002-0.012	1-5	DM* Induction or inhibited
Malathion	0.005-2.4	380	Cholinesterase depression
Nitrates	0-90	-	Nitrosamine tumours
Lead	0-9.0	10	Lead nephropathy
DDT	0-5.0	1	DM induction

*DM - Drug metabolism   Data from Greenman et al (4) and Newberne(5).

     The role of drinking water as an uncontrolled variable in experimental research remains uncharted, although it is likely to profoundly affect the kidney and possibly other organs.   The normal water intake of experimental animals depends on an array of factors such as species, strain, age; extra-renal factors such as anti-diuretic hormone synthesis, environmental humidity, stress and possibly the amount and type of food consumed.   Any attempt to define water balance obviously becomes more difficult when animals are to be treated experimentally.   Here stress may affect them and a variety of chemicals may cause either direct nephrogenic or extra-renal changes in water intake and excretion.
     In common with commercially prepared diets (Table 1) the different constitutents in tap water may vary markedly between any two sources and the composition of water from a single source may also change from day to day (Table 2).   Water is easily contaminated from air borne material and especially from those surfaces in which it is stored or carried. The uncertain composition of tap water may be exacerbated by the recycling of waste water, irregular and unpredictable environmental contaminations, and the fact that tap water from a single outlet may, in fact, be supplied from more than one source, depending on circumstances such as demand, purification plant and water pipe repairs, etc.
     The real significance of these variables is uncertain.   Chemically they may represent only a small change, but the kidney handles vast quantities of water and over the duration of a long term toxicity study trace constituents may cause an accumulative effect.   These unknowns could account, in part, for failure to induce lesions reproducibly.
     One possible approach to avoiding this problem is the use of distilled water in place of tap water.   Distilled water is, however, most prone to contamination from storage containers and gaseous dissolution.

THE KIDNEY AS A TARGET FOR DIETARY INDUCED DISEASES

The kidney is a common focus for both direct and indirect dietary induced diseases. There are a number of contributing reasons. The kidney :-

(a) Represents 0.4% of the total body mass, but as the major excretory organ it receives 20-25% of the resting cardiac output. Consequently, the kidney is exposed to a very wide range of endogenous substances, food constituents and contaminants, together with deliberately administered chemicals and their metabolites. Some of these may reach abnormally high concentrations because of the active renal transport processes which underly homeostasis.

(b) Has a high metabolic rate and consequently requires a considerable and regular supply of nutrients.

(c) Is concerned with the uptake and storage of many nutrients particularly, carbohydrates, amino acids, electrolytes and trace constituents such as vitamins and metal ions.

(d) Produces a tubular filtrate which, with the exception of the mature male rat, is free of protein. Protein binding plays an important role in limiting the toxicity of many natural and synthetic chemicals in other regions of the body (8) and its absence may enhance tubular toxicity. Moreover, the tubular filtrate is acidic and may cause the precipitation of certain acidic dietary constituents (e.g. oxalate).

(e) Possesses an active drug metabolising capability and may, therefore generate chemically reactive metabolites (9).

EXAMPLES OF DIRECT EFFECTS OF DIETARY FACTORS ON RENAL DISEASE

The direct effect of dietary factors on human disease is an important subject in its own right. The increasingly widespread availability of high potency, low bulk nutritional preparations means that direct toxic effects may be more likely to occur now than in the past (10). Dietary factors also contribute directly to the background incidence of disease in animals and they are therefore of concern to the animal toxicologist. In addition it is known that certain chemicals produce a nutritional deficiency through directly antagonising the effects of vitamins or minerals, or damage to tissue may result in its failure to retain essential nutrients. For example, chemicals which produce interstitial nephritis may cause a systemic nutrient deficiency resulting in osteodystrophia fibrosa (5)   Thus it is important for the toxicologist to be able to identify nutritional diseases. It should be pointed out, however, that with our present state of knowledge, it is difficult to differentiate between those changes which reflect a direct deleterious effect of malnutrition of the kidney, and those produced by the kidney as an adaptation to a nutritional "insult".

PROTEIN DEFICIENCY OR EXCESS

It is well established, both in experimental animals and man, that modification of the protein content of diets affects renal function. Glomerular filtration rate (GFR) and renal plasma flow (RPF) decreased in normal adults fed low protein diets and increased when the dietary protein content was replaced. A high protein diet was also associated with an increased p-aminohippurate (PAH) transport maxima (11). Others have reported a consistent decrease in GFR (as measured by creatinine clearance) in normal human subjects fed on calorie-deficient diet, irrespective of the contribution of calories from protein, fat or carbohydrate (12). Similar findings have been reported in malnourished children (13). Experimental animals fed protein deficient diets tend to exhibit smaller glomeruli and consequently have a diminished capillary surface available for filtration. Klahr and Alleyne (14) have reviewed the effects of chronic, protein-calorie malnutrition on the kidney. In addition to the above effects on GFR and RPF, the following observations were made :-

i)   urea clearance was decreased in protein deficient humans,

ii)   plasma levels of creatinine and urea nitrogen tended to be low in protein-deficient humans, despite decreased GFR, and

iii) polyuria and nocturia were common features of malnourished patients.

There may be decreased acid excretion during malnutrition, but few histological changes have been desribed in protein-calorie malnourished humans though swelling of the capsule epithelium and hyalinization of the glomerulus have been reported in malnourished children who had died (15).
Diets which are rich in certain proteins tend to cause kidney hypertrophy in rats. Halliburton (16) has shown that a high protein, isocalorific diet (containing 30% zein protein or 45% casein, compared to 15% in control diets, produced roughly similar increases of 20 percent in kidney weight, but had no effect on the DNA content. In contrast, a diet containing 30% gelatin caused both a marked hypertrophy (kidney weight increased by about 60%) and a hyperplasia. This effect of gelatin could not be ascribed solely to its unusual high glycine content because a normal diet supplemented with high levels of this amino acid produced no hyperplasia and only a 20% hypertrophic change. The practice of using gelatin to make up special diets may, therefore, need to be reconsidered, especially if the renal effects of a toxicant or a constituent in this special diet are of interest. Clapp (3) has observed a reversible renal pelvic dilatation in rats which correlated with the total amount of protein in the diet. Although the cause is unknown, it is unlikely to be due to the blockage of the ureter or bladder. Interestingly, no correlation with kidney weight was noted in these experiments which would seem to lend support to the contention that the nature of the protein is a crucial determinant of the hypertrophic effect. The previous dietary history of the individual may also influence the severity of renal lesions arising from high protein diets, for example obese rats are more vulnerable than are normal or underfed ones.

The feeding of high protein diets to rats causes, in itself, a pronounced chronic nephritis and proteinuria (17, 18) and has, therefore, generally been considered to be a factor which predisposes to renal disease.   Recently Neuhaus et al (19) have used an hepatically synthetized low molecular weight protein, α2u-globulin, as a means of assessing the efficiency of the uptake of filtered protein by the nephron.   They found that a protein free diet markedly reduced both urinary α2u and albumin, but a high protein diet (50% casein) decreased α2u reabsorption, although it had no effect on urinary albumin.   This observation highlights some of the misleading data that may be derived from measuring only on quantitative "proteinuria" and not establishing the distribution of protein molecular weight, from which it may be possible to differentiate between "high molecular weight" glomerular leakage,"tubular proteins" and failure to reabsorb polypeptide molecules.   Neuhaus et al (19) concluded that dietary protein levels may affect the renal homeostasis where amino acids could be conserved when protein intake was low, or protein molecules were selectively not reabsorbed when the protein uptake was high.

Both excessive calorific intake (carbohydrate and/or lipid) and starvation (20) have been demonstrated to induce certain intermediary metabolism enzymes [e.g. fatty acids induced peroxisome proliferation and, ω and ω -1 laurate hydroxylase(21)].   In addition, the over-consumption of food due to experimental hypothalamic lesions in rats (22) has been associated with the development of senile kidney lesions. There is good evidence that prolonged administration of high energy diets to rats does reduce longevity and increases the general incidence of tumours (2, 23).   In relation to the findings of Roe (2), it is interesting to note that Bras and Ross (24) have observed a high incidence of progressive glomerularnephrosis in rats fed a standard commercial diet ad libitum, but a restricted intake of protein, and/or carbohydrate decreased the incidence of the renal lesion.

Deficiency or excess of specific nutrients.   The normal distribution, tissue concentrations and likely biochemical roles of the vitamins in the kidney have been reviewed by Weber and Wiss (25).   The morphological zones that undergo pathophysiological changes due to a specific deficiency or excess of a vitamin or mineral often occurs in those areas in which the particular nutrient is normally stored.

Some of the vitamin deficiency-induced effects may, however, be secondary, particularly due to hormonal changes, rather than as a primary result of the vitamin deficiency.   The renal hypertrophy observed in thiamine deficient rats, for example, is probably due to prolonged negative nitrogen balance caused by insuficient calorie intake (26), and the pyridoxine deficiency associated renal changes may be related to haematuria (27).   Occasionally the offspring of vitamin-deficient animals develop renal changes rather than the parent. Vitamin B12 depletion of female rats from before mating to the end of gestation results in degenerative changes of the kidneys of the newborn pups which includes poorly differentiated glomeruli and tubules (28). Hypervitaminosis may also be associated with renal changes.   Excess vitamin A-induced glomerulonephritis and necrotising nephrosis has been described in laboratory animals (29).

Normally the kidney requires high concentrations of flavoproteins which reflects its high metabolic activity.   As a consequence the kidney (along with the liver) is very vulnerable to riboflavin deficiency.   Dietary riboflavin deficiency produces a number of ultrastructural changes in the mouse kidney which are largely confined to the pars recta of the proximal tubule (30).   These changes include both peroxisome and lysosomal proliferation and the formation of giant mitochondria, which may be due to mitochondrial fusion.   These ultrastructural changes generally parallel those that have been observed following the hyperlipidaemic agents e.g. diethyl-hexyl-phthalate and clofibrate. This may indicate that there is a common initiating stage, perhaps the inhibition of fatty acid oxidation in the mitochondria which would lead to a concomitant build up of fatty acids within the cell (31).

Moderate choline deficiency in weanling rats has been demonstrated to cause haemorrhagic lesions with subsequent hypertension, while severe deficiency causes a rapid onset of anaemia, frequently with deaths. Costa and coworkers (32) have ascribed these effects to an increase in renal catecholamines and a posible decrease in acetylcholine within the renal circulation, producing a marked vasoconstriction and increased blood pressure. The most important initial factor appears to be the reduction in renal adrenaline levels.   Other significant changes which may contribute to the observed nephrotoxic effect of choline deficient diets include a considerable disturbance in the pattern of phospholipid synthesis and probably also its degradation by the kidney (33).

Potassium deficiency affects both the heart and the kidney in many animal species and in man.   The main effects are typically vacuolation of the epithelium of the cortex, dilation of the tubules at the corticomedullary junction and some shedding of the epithelium (5). Potassium deficiency also causes marked changes in the number and size of the lipid droplets in the medullary interstital cells (34).   The exact functional consequences of these changes are uncertain, but there is evidence to suggest that these intra-cellular structures are related to either medullary prostaglandin synthesis, the state of diuresis and/or to hypertension (35). The topic is, however, most controversial.

Recently Brinker et al (36) have shown that potassium deficient dogs were much more sensitive to the nephrotoxic effects of gentamicin, although the possible mechanism(s) remain uncertain.   By contrast sodium chloride loading is known to ameliorate the nephrotoxic effects of chemicals (37).   High sodium diets may also induce hypertension in newborn rats (5), and may contribute to secondary hypertensive changes (see Thurston this volume).

High doses of fluoride have been shown to produce polyuria, albuminuria, haematuria, hyperphosphaturia, tubular degeneration and necrosis (38,39).   Within a few hours after fluoride infusion, urine osmolality, GFR and excretion rates of sodium, chloride and potassium were decreased in a dose-related manner (38).   Recovery of urinary osmolality took several days, probably due to the rather prolonged effects of fluoride on the permeability of the glomueruli and/or the redistribution of renal blood flow (see also Mazze this volume).   The marked renal damage associated with an excessive inorganic phosphate intake has been well documented (40), but the mechanism which underlies these pathophysiological changes is not yet understood.

An Imbalance of Dietary Constituents.   One of the major difficulties in identifying dietary requirements is that levels of one component may influence the dietary needs for another.   Thus the dietary requirements for choline (and the magnitude of the lesions produced by choline deficient diets) may be reduced by the presence of other lipotrophic factors such as methionine, vitamin E, and selenium.

Conversely vitamin E is subject to oxidation when dietary levels of unsaturated fats are high, and rats fed on diets low in vitamin E may show increased lipid peroxidation in the kidneys. These peroxidative changes may be most marked at autopsy, unless appropriate steps are taken to prevent them.

Renal disease may also be exacerbated by an imbalance of inorganic dietary constituents. The ratio of calcium to phosphate, for example, has a major influence on the development of nephrolithiases in female rats (3, 40). The available evidence indicates that the development of nephrocalcinosis is favoured by a bioavailable calcium:phosphate ratio of less than one. (This bioavailability will be affected by both the dietary levels of the ions and the presence of binding agents such as phytate). The presence in the glomerular filtrate of other ions such as magnesium and citrate, as well as urinary pH, also affect the development of the lesion, presumably by influencing the precipitability of calcium phosphate in the tubular lumen (42). Magnesium ions appear to reduce precipitation by stabilising supersaturated solutions of calcium phosphate within the tubule. Circulating oestrogens probably also contribute directly to nephrocalcinosis. This may explain the sex specificity of the lesion and the relative immunity of immature female rats to it.

Van Reen (43) has recently shown that pregnant rats fed a diet that was sub-optimal for the duration of the gestation period produced pups which (after weaning), when challenged with a diet known to promote urolithiases, were found to be much more suceptible to both urinary tract and bladder stone formation. This suggests that the response to toxic insults may yet be shown, in some instances, to be affected by the maternal nutritional while in utero or during lactation.

Exposure to various toxic metals such as cadmium may alter the homeostasis of essential metals, for example zinc, copper and iron (44). This may be brought about by several means:

i.   By competition for binding and uptake in the gut.

ii. By increased biological demand for zinc/copper since these
     metals are bound by the cadmium-induced metallothionein.

iii. Cadmium-induced renal damage leads to an excessive loss of
     essential metals in the urine and increases the nutritional
     requirements for these metals. Both zinc and copper are
     essential for normal bichemical functions in the kidney. Thus
     the loss of either as a result of exposure to toxic heavy metals
     may have significant deleterious effects.

The presence of toxic constituents and contaminants. Standard laboratory diets may vary considerably in their content of toxic contaminants (4). In most cases the levels of individual substances are well below the level known to produce toxicity (see Table 3), but this is not invariably the case, for example cadmium levels of 0.17 ppm have been reported in a commercially available rat diet, a level very close to that of 0.2ppm which has been recorded to cause adverse effects. Furthermore, an additive effect of the various individual dietary toxins may occur. The possible nephrotoxicity of non-nutritive food constituents has not been investigated extensively. α-Solanine, a glycoalkaloid present in damaged potatoes, has been shown to produce

severe congestion and hyperaemia in the kidneys of mice given an acute
dose of this compound (45).   It is likely that related glycoalkaloids,
which are commonly present in food, also have nephrotoxic effects.
     The kidney lesions induced by mycotoxins are well known (Table 4) and
have been associated with the use of mouldy foodstuff.   A more detailed
account of mycotoxin-associated nephropathy can be found elsewhere.
(Berndt, this volume).

Table 4. Mycotoxins and the various species in which they are known to
cause nephrotoxic effects.

MYCOTOXIN	SPECIES AFFECTED
Aflatoxin B1	monkey
Aflatoxin G1	rat
Sterigmatocystin	rat, monkey
Cyclopiazonic acid	rat
Penitrem A	chicken, rat, rabbit, guinea-pig, mouse
Rubratoxin B	dog, chicken, rat, mouse, guinea-pig, cat
Ochratoxin A	rat, dog
Sporidesmin	sheep
Lupinosis toxin	sheep, horse
Patulin	mouse
Citrinin	mouse, rat, rabbit, guinea-pig
12,13-Epoxytrichothecenes	dog

Data from Terao and Ueno (46)

EXAMPLES OF INDIRECT EFFECTS OF DIETARY FACTORS ON RENAL DISEASE

     Alteration of drug metabolising activity.   Drug metabolising
activity in a number of tissues may be modified by dietary factors.   As
a consequence the rate of formation of active metabolites and/or
detoxication products, delivery to the kidney (or produced within it)
may be reduced or diminished considerably.   Dietary factors may have a
selective effect on the drug metabolising enzymes of a particular
tissue.   For example, kidney cortex arylhydrocarbon hydroxylase
(benzpyrene hydroxylase) is induced by a 20% protein diet supplemented
with either 5-10% coconut or herring oil, whereas no induction occurred
in either the liver or lung (48, 49).   The induction effect in the
kidney appears to be independent of the extent of saturation of the
fatty acid (see below).   It differed from the induction of this enzyme
by polycyclic hydrocarbons in that the rate of induction is much slower.
This selective induction effect may provide a partial explanation of the
observation (50), that dimethylnitrosamine, which is known to produce
its toxic effect through the aegis of a reactive metabolite(s), induces
considerably more tumours in the kidneys of rats fed a low protein, high
lipid, high carbohydrate diet than in those on a standard diet.
     Recent work from Zenser (51) and Duggin (52) have highlighted the
previously unappreciated role of medullary cyclo-oxygenase in the cooxidative generation of biologicially reactive intermediates, which have
been speculatively linked to the pathogenesis of bladder carcinoma (51)
and renal papillary necrosis (52).   There is increasing evidence to
suggest that nutritional essential fatty acid (EFA) deficiencies affects

not only malnourished children, but also particularly patients who are receiving total parenteral nutrition (53). Limited EFA may, in itself, alter the effective co-oxygenation of xenobiotics. EFA deficiency has been shown to increase the potential of the papilla to oxidise more arachidonic acid, when the concentration of this molecule was no longer limiting (54). In addition to the possible interactive effects caused by other lipid related molecules in the diet (see above), dietary iron has also been shown to affect the relative tissue levels of unsaturated fatty acids in EFA deficient rats (55). This area of nutrition is obviously most complex and warrants further investigations, especially because it may be relevant to hospitialised patients who may be given a wide variety of medications as part of a chronic or intensive care programme.

Various naturally occurring xenobiotics are present in some foods and may reduce mixed function oxidase activity. For instance, safrole, flavones, xanthines and indoles, and the effect of such compounds upon the kidney should be assessed. In addition diet may be contaminated with substances containing enzyme-inducing activity. Dietary exposure of rats to polybrominated biphenyls stimulates microsomal enzyme activity. Similarly, 2,3,7,8-Tetrachlorodibenzo-p-dioxin (TCDD), one of the most persistent of all the environmental contaminants, is a most potent mixed functional oxidase inducer in the kidney (57). The significance of such observations in relation to the possible sensitisation of the kidney to toxicity produced by other drugs, environmental and industrial chemicals needs to be considered (see Rush and Hook, this volume).

MODIFICATION IN THE DISTRIBUTION OF CHEMICAL AND/OR ITS METABOLITES

i) Uptake. Hyper-absorption of dietary oxalate has been shown to occur in vitamin B6 deficient rats (58). The absorption of oxalate from the intestine appears to be at least partially a carrier mediated mechanism; it has been postulated that the increased oxalate absorption may arise from enhanced synthesis of the transport protein in response to the vitamin B6 deficiency. This mechanism may explain the great frequency of urinary calcium oxalate stones that occur in the Northern latitudes of India where vitamin B6 deficiency is very common (58). High carbohydrate diets e.g. xylitol have also been shown to cause hyperabsorption of dietary oxalate in laboratory rats (59) which may explain the high incidence of oxalate stones and bladder hyperplasia in rats maintained chronically on high carbohydrate diets.

The uptake, tissue deposition and subsequent development of toxicity of metals is also greatly modified by dietary factors; this is reported in more detail by Bremner (this volume). Compounds with chelating-properties such as phytate may impede the absorption of some metals e.g. zinc. Other factors known to influence metal absorption include protein, milk, vitamins C and D and calcium (60).

ii) Tissue Binding. Many chemicals are transported in the bloodstream bound to proteins, notably serum albumin. In low protein states such as kwashiorkor there is a very significant decrease in serum albumin (61) and as a consequence there may be significantly higher circulating levels of unbound chemical which may lead to enhanced toxicity (8). Low protein diets, particularly those deficient in sulphur containing amino acids might be expected to reduce the levels of cellular binding proteins and peptides e.g. metallothioniens and glutathione with a possible increased nephrotoxicity of chemicals such as cadmium and paracetamol.

iii) Excretion   Reduced urinary and biliary excretion may arise through dietary deficiency or excess of various nutrients.   The various nutritional factors which alter GFR and other renal functional factors have been described above.

CHANGES IN CELLULAR RESPONSE

i)   To chemical and/or metabolites.   The altered cellular responses to nephrotoxic insult in potassium depleted (36) and salt loaded animals has already been described (37).   Vitamin deficiencies have also been noted to modify the toxicity of some drugs.   Deficiencies of Vitamin A, biotin and pyridoxine have been shown to enhance the nephrotoxicity of benzylpenicillin in the rat (62).   Protein deficiency enhances the toxicity (nephritis) of the herbicide Diuron [3-(3,4-dichlorophenyl)-1,1-dimethylurea] (63).   The mechanism of these effects is not known but may be mediated by modification of the cellular response to those chemicals.

ii)   To antigenic materials.   Newberne and colleagues (5) have observed that rats littered to dams that had been made marginally deficient in the lipotrophic substances choline and methionine, were significantly less resistant to salmonella infection than control animals.   The effect appears to be direct one on the thymo-lymphatic system, resulting in a significant reduction of cell mediated immunity.   Interestingly a number of highly lipophilic compounds e.g. TCDD and polyhalogenated biphenyls have been reported to produce a similar effect.   It remains to be established whether increased infection of the kidneys may arise through this mechanism.

iii)   Through initial damage to other organs.   Dietary factors may, of course, also cause toxicity to the kidney as a secondary consequence of tissues changes in other organs (see Table 5).   For example, pyridoxine deficiency may provoke adrenal insufficiency and haematuria, which may in turn lead to calcium deposition in the corticomedullary zone. Thiamine deficiency may cause kidney hypertrophy through the initiation of a general negative nitrogen balance (7).

CONCLUSIONS

The implications for the effects of nutritional factors on nephrotoxicity are far reaching and deserve significantly more attention:

1. Diet is an important component in the spontaneous occurrence of long term renal lesions in experimental animals. .Spontaneous pathology can only serve to complicate and hinder the assessment of long term toxicity data and attempts to minimise this possibility will therefore promote more sensitive detection of chemically-induced lesions and may help to reduce the number of animals required for toxicity assessment.

Table 5. Effect of Dietary Nutrient excess and/or deficiency on the kidney.

NUTRIENT	LESION	POSSIBLE CAUSES
Vitamins		
Thiamine (d)	Hypertrophy	Indirect due to negative nitrogen balance
Riboflavin (d)	Hypertrophy, Lipid degeneration of proximal tubules	Adrenal insufficiency
Pyridoxine (d)	Calcium deposits in cortico-medullary zone, destruction of renal papilla	Haematuria, adrenal insufficiency
Nicotinic acid (d)	Tubular degeneration	Reduced cofactor levels
Pantothenic acid (d)	Degenerated tubule cells Proximal and distal cells very distended	Adrenal insufficiency
Choline (d)	Haemorrhagic necrosis of proximal tubule and subsequent hypertension	Lipid peroxidation, reduction in catecholamines, phospholipid disturbances
Vitamin A (d)	Desquamation of tubular epithelium and enlargement of distal convoluted tubules and collecting ducts	
Vitamin A (e)	Renal calcification	
Vitamin E (d)	Granulation of tubular epithelium and separation of basement membrane	Lipid peroxidation
Essential fatty acids (d)	Renal papillary necrosis	Disturbance in prostaglandin levels or in lipid synthesis.
Essential fatty acid (e)	Proximal tubule damage	Lipid peroxidation

Table 5 - cont.

Minerals

Chloride (d)	Renal fibrosis	
Magnesium (d)	Calcification	Precipitation of calcuim phosphate
Calcium:Phosphate ratio low	Calcification	Precipitation of calcium phosphate
Potassium (d)	Tubular epithelium degeneration	
Sodium (d)	Juxtaglumerular index increased	
Sodium (e)	Hypertension in newborn rats	

    d = deficiency in the diet and e = excess in the diet.

From data of Newberne (5).

2.   A fuller appreciation of the various dietary factors known to influence nephrotoxicity may help to explain species variability in the response to toxic insult and facilitate the extrapolation of data from experimental situations to man.

3.   Cultural and dietary habits vary tremendously among the human population e.g. trace element deficiencies are common in some Middle Eastern countries.   Such factors may contribute towards the incidence of kidney disease (e.g.Itai-itai disease, Balkan nephropathy) or increase the susceptibility to the other nephrotoxic chemicals.

4.   Chronic disease state in man may influence nutritional status and this should be considered when long term drug therapy is prescribed, since the response to the drug and/or susceptibility to its side effects may be modified.

5.   Modification of dietary constituents may help to protect the kidney against chemically-induced insult, an approach that has far reaching therapeutic implications in preventing iatrogenic renal damage.

REFERENCES

1.   Baker HJ et al, in The Laboratory Rat (HJ Baker, JR Lindsey and SH Weisbroth eds.), Vol 1, Academic Press, New York, 1979,pp. 169-192. ISBN 0-120-74901-7.
2.   Roe FJC, Proc Nutr Soc 40:37-65,1981.
3.   Clapp MJL, Lab Animals 14:253-261,1981.
4.   Greenman DL et al, J Toxol Env Health 6:235-246,1980.

5. Newberne PM in Pathology of Laboratory Animals (K Bernirsche, FM
    Garner and TC Jones eds.) Vol 2, Springer Verlag,Berlin, 1978, pp.
    2065-2171. ISBN 3-540-90292-9.
6   Crawford MD et al, Lancet 2:327-329,1971.
7. Wilkins JR et al, Amer J Epidemiol 110:420-448,1979.
8. Wilson AGE and Bridges JW Prog Drug Metab 1:193-247,1976.
9. Bridges JW and Fry JR, in The Induction of Drug Metabolism (R
    Estabrook and E Lindelaub eds.) Schattauer Verlag, Stuttgart, 1978,
    pp.343-354, 1978.
10. Campbell TC et al, Nutr Rev 39:249-256,1981.
11. Pullman TN et al, J Lab Clin Med 44:320-332,1954.
12. Sargent F and Johnson RE, Amer J Clin Nutr 4:466-481,1956.
13. Alleyne GAO, Pediatrics 39:400-411,1967.
14. Klahr S and Alleyne GAO, Kidney Int 3:129-141,1973.
15. Bras G et al, West Ind Med J 6:33-42,1957.
16. Halliburton IN, in Compensatory Renal Hypertrophy (WW Newinski and
    RJ Cross eds.), Academic Press, New York, 1969, pp. 101-128.
17. Saxton JA and Kimball GC, Arch Pathol 32:951-965,1941.
18 Newburgh LH and Curtis AC, Arch Intern Med 42:801-821,1928.
19. Newhaus OW et al, Nephron 28:133-140,1981.
20. Jakobsson SV et al, Biochem Biophys Res Commun 39:1073-1079,1970.
21. Ellin A and Orrenius S, Chem-Biol Interac 3:256-261,1971.
22. Kennedy GC, Brit Med Bull 13:67-70,1957.
23. Gallatly M, in Mouse Hepatic Neoplasia (WH Butler and P Newberne
    eds.) Elsevier, N-Holland, Amsterdam, 1975.
24. Bras G and Ross MH, Toxicol Appl Pharmacol 6:247-262,1964.
25. Weber W and Wiss O, in The Kidney, Morphology Biochemistry and
    Physiology, Vol 4 (C Rouiller and AF Muller eds.) Academic Press,
    New York, 1971, pp 271-295.
26. Skelton FR, Proc Soc Exp Biol Med 73:516-519,1950.
27. Agnew LRC, J Pathol Bacteriol 63:699-705,1951.
28. Newberne PM and O'Dell BL, J Nutr 68:343-357,1959.
29. Nieman C and Obbink HJK, Vitamins Hormones 12:69-99,1954.
30. Kobayashi K et al, Virchows Arch B Cell Pathol 34:99-109,1980.
31. Hinton RH et al, unpublished observation.
32. Costa RS, Brit J Exp Pathol 60:613-619,1979.
33. Monserrat AJ et al, Arch Pathol 85:419-432,1968.
34. Nissen HM, Z Zellforsch 85:483-491,1968.
35. Bohman S-O, in The Renal Papilla and Hypertension (AK Mandal and S-O
    Bohman eds.), Plenum Medical Books, New York, pp. 7-33, 1980, ISBN
    0-306-40506-7.
36. Brinker KR et al, J Lab Clin Med 98,292-301,1981.
37. Haley DP, Lab Invest 46:196-208,1982.
38. Kessabi M etal, Toxicol Letters 5:169-174,1980.
39. Whitford GM and Stringer GJ, Proc Soc Exp Biol Med 157:44-49,1978.
40. Mackay EM and Olivier J, J Exp Med 61:319-333,1935.
41. Moore T and Sharman IM, Wld Rev Nutr Diet 31:173-177,1978.
42. Bunce GE et al, J Exp Med Pathol 33:203-210,1980.
43. Van Reen R, Nutr Rep Int 24:295-303,1981.
44. Bonner FW, PhD Thesis, University of Surrey,1980.
45. Jadhau SJ et al, CRC Crit Rev Tox 9:21-104,1981.
46. Terao K and Ueno Y, in Toxicology, Biochemistry and Pathology of
    Mycotoxins (K Uraguchi and M Yamazaki, eds.) Wiley, New York, 1978,
    pp. 189-238. ISBN 0-470-26423-3.
47. Ford SM et al, Fd Cosmet Toxicol 18:15-20,1980.

48. Angeli-Greaves M and McLean AEM, in Drug Toxicity (J Gorrod ed.)
    Taylor and Francis, London, 1980, pp 91-100.
49. Swann P and McLean AEM, Biochem J 124:283-288,1971.

RENAL PAPILLARY NECROSIS PRODUCED BY LONG-TERM FAT-FREE DIET

Elizabeth A. Molland

Robens Institute of Industrial and Environmental Health and Safety, University of Surrey, Guildford, Surrey GU2 5XH, UK

INTRODUCTION

Burr and Burr (1,2) reported that rats reared on a fat-free diet lost weight and died after 32 weeks; many had developed haematuria and had abnormal kidneys which were thought to be the immediate cause of death. Borland and Jackson (3) described the morphological changes: of 21 animals on a totally fat-free diet, there were 7 cases of total necrosis of the renal papilla. Other changes, seen by light microscopy, included fine particulate fat in the medullary and cortical tubular epithelium, focal calcification at the cortico-medullary junction, and hyperplasia of pelvic epithelium.

The experiment was repeated to confirm the above observations, and to make a more detailed examination of the medulla by light and electron micoscopy.

MATERIALS AND METHODS

Ten female Black-hooded Lister rats, 6 weeks old, were put on a vitamin-supplemented fat-free diet (ICN Pharmaceuticals Inc.), and 10 controls received Heygate's modified Thompson pellet diet. Both groups had unlimited drinking water. Animals were weighed throughout the experiment.

After 46 weeks the kidneys were perfused in vivo with 2.5% glutaraldehyde, the papilla of one being divided transversely into 3 blocks, post-fixed in Palade's 1% osmium tetroxide, and embedded in Araldite. Areas for ultrastructural examination were selected from $1 \mu m$ Toluidine-blue stained sections, and ultra-thin sections stained by uranyl acetate and lead citrate

The other kidney was sectioned horizontally through the papilla tip, and paraffin-embedded sections examined in the light microscope after staining by haematoxylin and eosin, periodic-acid Schiff (PAS), von Kossa's technique for calcium, Perl's stain for iron, Alcian blue pH 2.5 for mucopolysaccharides, Sudan Black B, and frozen sections by Sudan III for lipids.

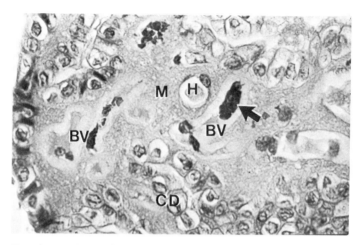

Fig 1. Fat-free diet 46 weeks. Intermediate necrosis of papilla
showing fibrillar matrix (M) with loss of interstitial cells. Walls
of blood vessels (BV)are thickened with sludged red cells in the lumen
(arrowed). Partly necrotic loop of Henle (H) contains granular cast.
Collecting duct (CD) is intact.
    H and E X 560

RESULTS

One test animal died at 10 weeks (no histology performed). There was
a significant difference between the mean weight of the test group (198g)
and the control group (244g) at 46 weeks. All test animals had
generalized loss of body fat,and three had generalized hair loss, with
heavy scaling of their tails. Test kidneys were all enlarged, and one
pair were diffusely scarred.

Light microscopic findings. The cortex of test kidneys showed no
glomerular changes, but there was marked increase of fat, and a smaller
increase in finely granular iron in the proximal tubular epithelium.
Clumps of haematoxyphilic material, containing calcium and iron, were
present within degenerating tubules at the cortico-medullary junctions.
The kidneys with macroscopic scarring showed segmental scarring of the
cortex.
    There was intermediate necrosis of the papilla in 6 pairs of kidneys,
although none were totally necrotic. The matrix was fibrillar, with loss
of acid mucopolysaccharides and of interstitial cells (Fig. 1). Blood
vessels were lined by a thick, indistinct layer of material (Fig. 1)
which appeared blue in H & E stained sections, and showed purple
metachromasia in toluidine-blue stained sections. Loops of Henle were
necrotic,containing granular casts; collecting ducts were preserved.
One specimen showed hyperplasia of surface epithelium.   There was a
marked increase of lipid in interstitial cells in the outer medulla, and
non-necrotic papilla, and in the interstitium of the vascular bundles.
Lipid was usually absent from areas of intermediate necrosis.

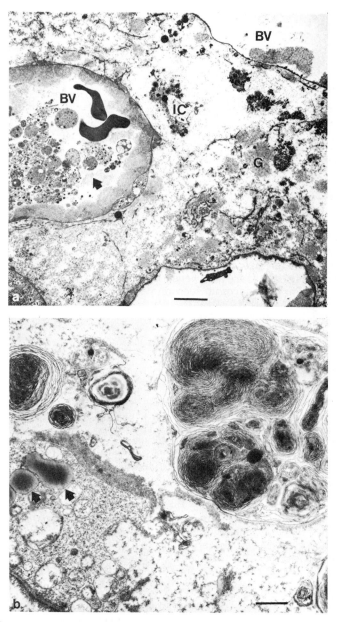

Fig. 2 Fat-free diet 46 weeks. Papilla,
(a)Matrix contains remnants of interstitial cells (IC) and granular
material (G) with strands of basement-membrane-like material. Blood
vessels (BV) are lined by granular material with a rim of basement
membrane. Red cells, platelets and cell fragments (arrowed) lie in
the lumen of one vessel.Bar 5 microns
(b)Fat-free diet 46 weeks. Large lipid body with myelin degeneration
lies free in the matrix. Adjacent smaller bodies (arrowed) have
translucent borders.Bar 1 micron

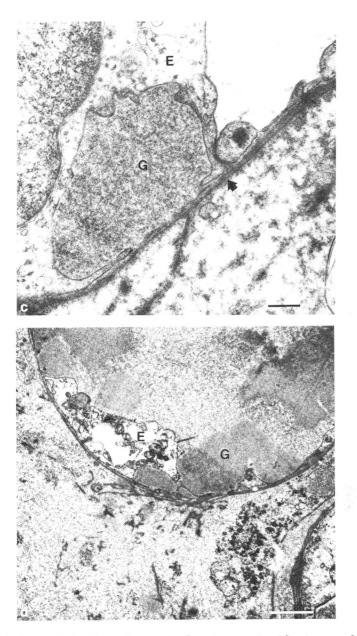

(c) Fat-free diet 46 weeks.   Early change in blood vessel wall.
Granular material (G) distends the overlying endothelial cell (E) and
is continuous with the basement membrane which has a dense outer rim
(arrowed). Bar 1 micron
(d) Fat-free diet 46 weeks.   Later change in blood vessel wall.
Degenerating endothelial cell (E) is partly detached from basement
membrane.
Granular material (G) extrudes into the blood vessel lumen. Bar 2
micron.

       Lead citrate and uranyl acetate.

Electron microscopic findings. In the inner medulla the disintegration of interstitial cells in areas of intermediate necrosis was confirmed. The matrix containing collections of cell remnants, including granular material, vesicles and membrane-bound bodies, and there was also a diffuse increase of granular material, with strands of basement membrane like material in the matrix (Fig 2a). In the outer medulla, intact interstitial cells showed dilated cisternae and granular cytoplasm which suggested degenerative change. Lipid bodies were abundant, within interstitial cells or lying free: many showed myelin degeneration and some had translucent borders (Fig. 2b).

The basement membrane of blood vessels showed focal granular material bulging inwards, distending the overlying endothelial cell (Fig 2c). The material appeared to extrude into the lumen, with degeneration of the endothelial cell, (Fig 2d) and it finally lined the entire circumference of the vessel (Fig 2a). Collections of platelets and cell debris were seen in the lumens (Fig.2a).

The epithelium of Henle's loop contained autophagocytic vesicles with electron-dense droplets and myelin bodies, and in many tubules had disintegrated, the lumen being filled by degenerating cell organelles. Collecting duct epithelium contained numerous electron-dense droplets, and showed generalized shrinkage.

DISCUSSION.

These results confirm that renal papillary necrosis may be induced by a fat-free diet, although the present lesions were at a less advanced stage than those reported by Burr and Burr (1,2). Insufficient diet was available to continue the experiment beyond 46 weeks).

It has been shown that the lesion may be corrected by the administration of unsaturated long-chain fatty acids, particularly linoleic acid (2). Since these may be the precursors of renal medullary prostaglandins (4), it is possible that deficiency of the latter may be involved in the pathogenesis of the lesion. Rabbits on a diet deficient in essential fatty acids have been shown to have a reduced prostaglandin content in the medulla (5). However, the only morphological change described in the latter model was a fall in the quantity of medullary lipid droplets. There is, therefore, insufficient evidence at present to relate the necrosis specifically to prostaglandin deficiency. The increase of lipid in the outer medulla may indicate a utilization block or a shift of lipogenic metabolism from the damaged inner medulla.

The pathogenesis of the vessel changes is also uncertain. Possibly a specific lipid factor is necessary for the integrity of the basement membrane, although this would imply a unique structure, since the changes were not seen in vessels in other organs. The morphological evidence of stasis in affected vessels, suggests that local ischaemia may contribute to the necrosis of the papilla, but its aetological role is uncertain.

It is hoped to extend the studies on this model, maintaining animals on the diet for longer periods, and undertaking more detailed morphological and biochemical investigations.

REFERENCES.

1. Burr GO and Burr MM, J Biol Chem 82:345-367, 1929.
2. Burr GO and Burr MM, J Biol Chem 86:587-621, 1930.
3. Borland VG and Jackson CM, Arch Path 11:687-708, 1931.
4. Hamberg M FEBS Letters 5:127-130, 1969.
5. Van Dorp DA, Ann NY Acad Sci 180:181-199, 1971.

NEPHROTOXIN-INDUCED CHANGES IN KIDNEY IMMUNOBIOLOGY WITH SPECIAL REFERENCE TO MERCURY-INDUCED GLOMERULONEPHRITIS

P. Druet, B. Bellon, C. Sapin, E. Druet, F. Hirsch and G. Fournié*

Hôpital Broussais, 96 rue Didot, 75674 Paris Cedex 14, France, and
*Hôpital Purpan, 31052 Toulouse Cedex, France

ABSTRACT.   A number of toxic agents are thought to be responsible for immunologically mediated nephritides in human and in experimental animal models. Glomerulonephritis and acute tubulo-interstitial nephritis are both encountered. Heavy metals and drugs are most often concerned. The same agent is able to induce, in different patients, various types of immunologically mediated glomerulonephritis, suggesting that the immune reactivity of individuals is a major determinant in the clinicopathological presentation of drug toxicity. The mechanism of action of toxic agents is poorly understood, toxins are thought to act either as haptens or by modifying normal constituents and rendering them antigenic. Recent experiments also suggest that some drugs may directly act on immunoregulation. We have developed an experimental model of immunologically mediated glomerulonephritis in rats chronically intoxicated with mercury. Results can be summarized as follows: a) Brown-Norway (BN) rats develop a biphasic disease with first anti-glomerular basement membrane antibodies and then an immune complex type disease; b) immunological and serological studies have clearly shown that this disease is self-limited, suggesting the occurrence of an efficient auto-regulation process; c) there is evidence that in the BN rat model mercury acts directly on immuno-competent cells inducing a T dependent polyclonal activation; d) genetic control of susceptibility to the disease observed in BN rats mainly depends on major histocompatibility linked genes; e) the study of other inbred rat strains clearly established that susceptibility depends on the strain tested and that, under similar experimental procedure, the phenotypic expression of the disease also depends on genetic factors.

KEY WORDS.   Immunologically mediated nephritis - Toxic - Mercury - Rat Genetic control - Immune complexes.

BASIC MECHANISMS RESPONSIBLE FOR IMMUNOLOGICALLY MEDIATED EXPERIMENTAL NEPHRITIS.

The responsibility of antibodies reactive with various renal structures and of immune complexes in the induction of immunologically mediated experimental nephritis, has been well established since the pioneering work of Dixon [1,2] and Germuth [3]. However the respective role of antibodies and immune complexes either formed in situ or circulating is now a matter of discussion [4]. In contrast, the role of cell mediated immunity has rarely been investigated in experimental models while it is suggested to play a major role in some kinds of drug induced tubulo-interstitial nephritis in human [5].

Humoral immunity. The earliest work was based on immunomorphological data. Most of our knowledge was, and is still, based on the rather simple immunofluorescent technique. It was first considered that a linear smooth pattern of fixation of the anti-Ig conjugate along basement membranes (glomerular or tubular) was suggestive of an antibody mediated nephritis while a granular pattern of fixation along the glomerular basement membrane (GBM) or tubular basement membrane (TBM) or vessels from the interstitial tissue was the hallmark of an immune complex (IC) mediated disease [6]. Although this concept is still valid in most cases, it is now clear, from experimental data, that it may be misleading to draw definite conclusions from immunomorphology alone (Table 1).

Antibody mediated nephritis.

Anti-basement membrane antibodies. Anti-GBM antibodies, either heterologous or autologous, have been induced in experimental animals immunized with either heterologous or autologous GBM 1. It has been well demonstrated that anti-GBM antibodies are responsible for glomerular injury through various complement dependent or complement independent processes [7,8]. The role of cells such as polymorphs or macrophages attracted to the glomeruli as a consequence of antibody fixation on GBM also seems of relative importance [7,9]. Anti-TBM antibodies can also be induced in experimental animals either immunized with heterologous [10] or allogeneic combination of TBM [10]. Here again, tubulo-interstitial damage is mediated by antibodies. In addition, recent results suggest that the mononuclear cells found in the interstitium are probably present as a consequence of cell mediated immunity and responsible for tubulo-interstitial injury.

Non-anti-basement membrane antibodies. In the past few years, it has become more and more evident that circulating antibodies directed against a non classical BM antigen can also induce glomerular or tubular disease. Some of the involved antigens (Heymann's antigen, Tamm-Horsfall's protein) belong to kidney structure. Others, so-called "planted" antigens, are non renal products which bind to renal structures and stimulate the production of antibodies which in turn react with those products (Concanavalin A, DNA, cationic ferritin).

Renal antigens. Heymann's antigen is present on glomerular epithelial cells. Rats immunized with this antigen develop an IC type glomerulonephritis (GN) with granular IgG deposits along the GBM [11,

TABLE 1 :   ANTIBODY AND IMMUNE COMPLEX MEDIATED NEPHRITIS.

Basement membrane antigen (ag) [6,10]
   Glomerular   anti-GBM or anti-TBM anti-
   Tubular   bodies fixed in a linear
                                       pattern along the BM.

Non basement membrane ag
  Renal ag :
    Heymann's nephritis [13,14]
    Tamm-Horsfall protein [15]

    Planted ag :   Antibodies elicited bind
           (Concanavalin A [16]   in a linear or granular
    Non immune (DNA   18   pattern in the glomerular
           (Cationized ferritin [17]   capillary wall or TBM
                                  depending on the antigen
    Immune reactants [19]   distribution.
    (Heterologous or autologous anti-
     body fixed on kidney structure)

Endogenous or exogenous ag without   Circulating IC deposited
  affinity for kidney structures [6]   in a granular pattern.

12]. It has recently been demonstrated that this GN is due to the fixation of free circulating antibodies on the glomerular antigen which is irregularly distributed along the glomerular capillary wall and is therefore responsible for the irregular, granular, fixation observed [13, 14].

An IC type tubulo-interstitial nephritis has also been induced in rats immunized with Tamm-Horsfall's protein. This protein is synthetized by cells from the ascending thick limb of the loop of Henle. The protein is expressed at the level of cell membranes but does not circulate. Circulating antibodies will bind to the antigen in an irregular granular pattern [15].

Planted antigens. A number of products can bind for physico-chemical reasons to various renal structures. These products, called "planted" antigens, can elicit antibody formation. Examples of planted antigens are concanavalin A which binds to BM sugars, cationised ferritin and cationic DNA which will bind to oppositely charged glomerular capillary walls. Antibodies against these products will then bind to the "planted" antigen responsible for a linear or granular pattern of fixation of the conjugates depending on the antigen distribution [16, 17, 18] (Table 1).

Immune complex disease. This concept arose from experimental findings in acute and chronic serum sickness [2]. It was clearly shown that, after injection of a foreign protein such as bovine serum albumin (BSA), circulating immune complexes appear, preceeding the deposition of IC in various renal and extra-renal structures in a typical granular pattern as observed by immunofluorescence [1].

Many endogenous or exogenous antigens in human and in experimental conditions have been considered to be responsible for the occurrence of an IC type disease on the finding of a granular pattern of fixation of adequate conjugates [6]. It is however difficult to differentiate in most cases the respective role of free antibodies and that of IC, either formed in situ or circulating. Characterization of IC, of circulating antibodies and direct analysis of the immune reactants found in the kidney may help differentiate these mechanisms. This distinction is not only academic and could have important therapeutic implications.

Cellular immunity. While the role of cells (monocytes, polymorphs) in the efferent limb of immunologically mediated nephritis is well known, the role of cell mediated immunity as initiating kidney lesions is poorly understood today. There is no clear demonstration that cell mediated immunity plays any role in experimental glomerular disease [20]. In contrast, recent data suggests that cell mediated immunity is most important in tubulo-interstitial lesions induced in mice and guinea-pigs immunized with TBM. These animals develop anti-TBM antibodies but it has been shown in mice that these antibodies do not play a major role in tubulo-interstitial injury while mononuclear cells are most important [21]. It has also been demonstrated in guinea-pigs with anti-TBM nephritis that these animals do develop lymphocytes which are cytotoxic for kidney cells 22 . There is also some evidence that cell mediated immunity is responsible for drug induced acute tubulo-interstitial nephritis in man (see below).

IMMUNOLOGICALLY MEDIATED NEPHRITIDES INDUCED BY TOXIC AGENTS.

We will first consider the features which suggest an immunological reaction after toxic exposure and then the various mechanisms which can induce such a reaction. Lastly, we will describe the different drug-induced nephritides which are probably immunologically mediated.

Features suggesting an immunological reaction. Drug hypersensitivity is usually an acute, unforeseeable reaction which occurs in a small proportion of people. There is some indication that susceptibility to some drugs is genetically controlled. Such adverse effects are not dose related, they improve after withdrawal of the toxin and recur, sometimes dramatically, after re-exposure. Clinical symptoms (fever, skin rash, liver involvement, arthralgia, eosinophilia) are often associated. The histological findings will be described further but some of them e.g. presence of anti-GBM or anti-TBM deposits,of an IC type nephritis or of cells (mononuclear cells, eosinophils) infiltrating interstitium lend support to the hypothesis of an immune process. The demonstration of an immune response (humoral or/and cellular) against the offending agent or induced by it would provide an additional argument which, in fact, is often lacking. It is therefore often difficult to differentiate direct toxic effect from hypersensitivity.

Mechanisms of drug hypersensitivity. Most of the classical hypersensitivity reactions can be induced by drugs. a) Anaphylactic reactions mediated by reaginic antibodies are probably important in acute interstitital nephritis in humans but there is only indirect evidence for it (the presence of eosinophils in the interstitium and high serum IgE level). Positive passive anaphylaxis cutaneous reactions have occasionally been reported. b) Drugs can induce a variety of antibodies: anti-GBM and anti-TBM antibodies have been observed after D-Penicillamine [23], mercury [24] or methicillin exposure [25].

Antibodies to drugs have been detected in rifampicin treated patients
[26]. Antinuclear antibodies have been described in patients treated
with a number of drugs [27] and mainly after hydralazine or procainamide
treatment [27]. c) Immune complex type disease is one of the best
delineated immune reactions in drug induced nephropathies as will be
described below. d) Although there is indirect evidence suggesting that
cell mediated immunity is implied, namely during drug induced acute
interstitial nephritides, it remains difficult, especially for
methodological reasons, to ascribe a definite role for cell mediated
immunity in such situations.

The precise mechanism of action of drugs in inducing such reactions is
only poorly understood. It has been known for a long time that drugs
behave like haptens and become immunogenic when linked to proteins [28].
This is thought to explain the appearance of anti-rifampicin antibodies
[26] for example. Drugs may also modify or enhance the antigenicity of
components to which they are bound rendering them antigenic. Such a
mechanism has been postulated for methyl dopa induced anti-erythrocyte
antibodies [29] and for hydralazine or procainamide induced anti-
nuclear antibodies [27]. Other experiments with procainamide [30]and

TABLE 2 : NEPHROTOXIN INDUCED IMMUNOLOGICALLY MEDIATED NEPHRITIS.

AGENT RESPONSIBLE	IMMUNO-MORPHOLOGY	
	HUMAN	ANIMAL
Heavy metals		
Mercury	Lin,Gra,	Lin, Gra,
Gold salts	Gra, MGC	Gra,
Lead, silver, bismuth	Gra?	/
Hydrocarbon solvents	Lin?Gra?	none
Drugs		
D-Penicillamine (and related)	Lin,Gra,MGC,	Gra,
Captopril	Gra,	/
Para and Trimethadione	Gra,MGC,	?
Non-steroidal anti-inflammatory		
drugs	Gra,MGC	/
Levamisole,		
Tolbutamide, Carbutamide,	Gra,	/
Ethosuccimide,		
Phenindione, Probenecid, Lithium	MGC,	/
Alcohol	Gra,	/
Vaccine	Gra?MGC	/

Lin : linear, Gra : granular Ig deposits,
MGC : minimal glomerular changes

methyl dopa [29] in man suggest that these drugs may act by triggering immune cells and therefore by modifying immunoregulation [29,30]. Experimental results which will be discussed below indicate that mercurials can also modify immune regulation.

Drug induced immunologically mediated nephritides.   We will now describe the various immunologically mediated nephritides probably induced by drugs (Table 2). Most of the known examples come from human pathology except for the mercury induced auto-immune disease which has been extensively studied in rat and rabbit and will be described separately.

Anti-glomerular basement membrane glomerulonephritis.   This severe form of GN, characterized by linear IgG deposits along the GBM, is sometimes associated with lung involvement (Goodpasture's syndrome) because anti-GBM antibodies also react with alveolo-capillary BM. Definite diagnosis needs the demonstration of circulating anti-GBM antibodies and/or of the anti-BM activity of eluted Igs from the diseased kidney. In most situations the etiology is unknown. There is indirect evidence, from epidemiological data, that anti-GBM GN would be more frequent among subjects exposed to hydrocarbon solvents [31]. Anti-GBM antibodies have not been induced in experimental animals submitted to gazoline vapors [32]. Some patients treated with D-Penicillamine have been reported to develop Goodpasture's syndrome or GN with linear IgG deposits, but anti-GBM antibodies were not further characterized [23,33]. Mercury is also able to induce GN with linear IgG deposits in human [24] and anti-GBM antibodies have been experimentally induced in BN rat [34] and rabbits [35].

Immune complex type glomerulonephritis.   This group of GN mainly includes in man : a) membranous glomerulopathy (MGP) characterizd by granular IgG deposits along the glomerular capillary wall corresponding to subepithelial electron dense deposits, b) membrano-proliferative GN (MPGN) characterized by the presence of Ig and C3 deposits along the glomerular capillary wall and mesangium, and c) Berger's disease characterized by IgA mesangial deposits. Numerous toxic agents have been described associated with the occurrence of IC type GN in human [36], but most of our knowledge relies on epidemiological data.

Heavy metals.   Since the first reports of Becker et al., [37] and Mandema et al., [38], numerous cases of MGP with IgG and C3 granular deposits have been described in patients treated with mercury containing drugs or as a consequence of occupational or environmental exposure (reviewed in [39]). Although mercury is no longer used as a therapeutic agent, it may play an unsuspected role because it is still present in many preservatives, in the environment, and some workers may also be at risk. The prognosis of this GN is usually good and most patients recovered after removal from exposure. Very little is known concerning the mechanisms of action of mercury in human, It was tempting to speculate that mercury could act as a hapten or by modifying a serum or structural proteins rendering them antigenic because of the well known affinity of mercury for SH groups. There is no proof for it. The only available studies in humans suggest that mercury probably acts on lymphocytes [40, 41]. Recent studies with our experimental model are in accordance with this suggestion.

An IC type GN occurs in rheumatoid arthritis (RA) patients treated with gold salts. The percentage of patients with proteinuria varies from 1 to 10%. A typical MGP is usually encountered and often in patients with seronegative RA [42]. It usually appears after a few weeks or months and proteinuria disappears after withdrawal of the drug while immune deposits may persist for a long time. The mechanism of action of gold salts is unknown. An hypersensitivity reaction is suspected from the finding of skin rash,eosinophilia and increase in serum IgE level in these patients. Microanalytical studies failed to detect gold within deposits [43]. An IC type GN has also been induced in Wistar rats receiving sodium aurothiomalate [44].

Few cases concerning patients intoxicated with lead, or silver and presenting with nephrotic syndrome (NS) have been described [45], but renal biopsies were not studied by immunofluorescence. In a recent case (J.F. Bernaudin : personnal communication), spontaneous silver deposits were observed in the GBM suggesting that non-immune deposits containing silver might be responsible for glomerular damage. Immunofluorescent studies were negative.

D-Penicillamine and related drugs. Nephrotic syndrome frequently occurs in patients treated with drugs with sulfhydryl groups. Among them D-Penicillamine is the best known. Proteinuria with or without NS frequently occurs in patients with RA [46], chronic hepatitis, biliary cirrhosis, Wilson's disease or cystinuria and receiving D-Penicillamine [47]. Nephrotic syndrome which occurs in about 7% of RA patients treated with D-Penicillamine, usually occurs during the first year of treatment and disappears after withdrawal of the drug. Most of the patients studied exhibited a MGP. Immune deposits usually persist even after proteinuria has disappeared [48]. Similar IC type deposits were induced in Sprague-Dawley rats intoxicated with high doses (2g/kg/day) of D-Penicillamine [49]. Immune deposits appeared progressively and a typical MGP developed after two months of treatment. Interestingly, deposits always disappeared after intoxication was discontinued [49]. No data was reported concerning the mechanism of action of D-Penicillamine.

Several other drugs with sulfhydryl groups (thiopronin, pyrithioxine, methimazole) have also been reported to induce NS in man [36,50].

Recent reports have described the occurrence of proteinuria with eventually NS in hypertensive patients treated with captopril [51]. A typical MGP was observed. Moreover it was found that patients treated with captopril, but not showing proteinuria, which underwent a renal biopsy, often had granular IgG deposits suggesting that IC type GN may be quite frequent [51]. Anti-nuclear antibodies were detected in some patients but their role in the pathogenesis of the disease was not demonstrated [51].

Other drugs. About 40 patients have been reported which presented NS and/or proteinuria after trimethadione or paramethadione treatment [52]. A typical MGP was found in one case [53] but complete immunomorphological studies were not performed in the other cases. It was first reported that Sprague-Dawley rats receiving trimethadione developed a NS 54 but this could not be confirmed [52].Membranous glomerulopathy has been described in patients treated with levamisole [55], diclofenac [56], or ethosuccimide [57].

Systemic lupus erythematosus like-syndrome. Many drugs are known to be inducers of anti-nuclear antibodies with occasionally a lupus like-syndrome. These syndromes are characterized by the absence of renal involvement. However, some patients with drug induced systemic lupus erythematosus had renal involvement. Procainamide is usually responsible for it [58]. Another case of NS with anti-nuclear antibodies has been described after practolol treatment [59]another drug known to induce lupus a like syndrome.

Alcohol. Several reports have clearly shown that GN with mesangial IgA deposits or MPGN with IgA deposits were frequently encountered in alcoholic patients [60,61]. It is likely that, as in Berger's disease or Henoch-Schonlein purpura, IC containing IgA are responsible for this disease but they have not been identified. It is suspected that liver injury may be responsible for modifications in occurrence and clearance of IC containing IgA.

Minimal glomerular changes. This entity is characterized by a NS without detectable immuno-morphological abnormalities by light or electron microscopy and with negative immunofluorescent findings. Although there is no immunomorphological evidence suggesting an immune process, several data suggest that cell mediated immunity could be involved. Abnormalities of T cell function have been reported [62], lymphocytes from these patients release a factor which enhances permeability [63] and NS with minimal glomerular changes (MGC) has been described in patients with lymphoma [64] and in allergic patients [65].
    It is of interest to note that NS with MGC has been reported in a number of well studied patients receiving various drugs such as D-Penicillamine [66], gold salts (J.F. Girard, unpublished observations), trimethadione and fenoprofen [67,68]. In these cases, the NS disappears when treatment is discontinued. It is remarkable that several toxins are able to induce either a NS with MGC or an anti-GBM GN or an IC type GN. Although there is no proof that the NS with MGC is immunologically mediated, it is quite likely that the same toxic agent may induce immunologically mediated glomerulonephritides in different ways.
    A number of other drugs were found associated with NS: phenindione, probenecid, phenylbutazone, tolbutamide, carbutamide (reviewed in: 36) and lithium carbonate [69]. It is often difficult to incriminate the drug in these individual cases and, moreover, renal histology does not always allow for differentiation between MGC and MGP. In addition, there is no way to differentiate a direct toxic effect of the drug, as demonstrated in rats for aminonucleoside [70] from a NS with minimal glomerular changes. A direct toxic effect is probably responsible for the NS encountered in patients treated with mitomycin-C [23] or in heroin addict subjects [71].
    Lastly, NS with MGC has also been described after vaccination possibly
as a consequence of immunological imbalance induced by reaction to the vaccine. These NS resolve spontaneously. They must be differentiated, in our opinion, from the few cases of NS with IC type GN observed in patients after hyperimmunisation and which are not a consequence of vaccine itself [72-75].

Acute tubulo-interstitial nephritis. In contrast, with the above immunologically mediated GN, features of hypersensitivity reaction are often present in cases of drug induced acute tubulo-interstitial nephritis (ATIN). Suggestive features remain the immunomorphological characteristics such as: infiltration with mononuclear cells and eosinophils, presence of IgE containing plasma cells or of antibodies reactive with a kidney structure.

Many drugs have been incriminated [5, 36]. The more frequently encountered are: methicillin, rifampicin, phenindione and glafenine. Some of these are now rarely used. In all these cases renal biopsy shows mononuclear cells infiltration of interstitium with few eosinophils. IgG linear deposits have been found along the TBM together with a derivative of methicillin : dimethoxi-phenyl-penicilloyl (DPO). Two hypothesis were raised : a) DPO binds to normal TBM and induces anti-TBM formation [25]; b) DPO binds to TBM only in patients with interstitial nephritis [76,77]. In that latter hypothesis anti-TBM hypothesis would be a secondary event.

Anti-TBM antibodies have not been found in other forms of ATIN. Antibodies to rifampicin together with cell mediated immunity have been found [26] in most patients with ATIN induced by rifampicin. However the immune nature of this disease is debatable and its mechanism is unknown.

Phenindione induces a severe ATIN which is probably an hypersensitivity reaction because it is associated with skin rash and liver involvement. There is an important infiltration of interstitium with mononuclear cells [78].

Vasculitis. Necrotizing vasculitis is occasionally induced by drugs. Skin and kidney are often affected. Penicillin was one of the drugs most often implicated but other drugs (sulfamides, phenylbutazone, thiazidic and, more recently, allopurinol [36]) have also been incriminated.

MERCURY INDUCED IMMUNE GLOMERULONEPHRITIS.

In order to clarify the mechanism of immunologically mediated GN induced by toxic agents, we described several years ago a model of GN induced by $HgCl_2$ in outbred Wistar rats [79]. A percentage of rats injected with doses of $HgCl_2$ ranging from 0.1 to 0.4 µg per 100g bodyweight three times a week developed after several weeks a typical MGP. The role of the strain used was then suspected to be most important and we have tested the susceptibility of 18 inbred rat strains characterized by their haplotype (RT1) at the major histocompatibility complex (MHC). The Brown-Norway rat strain was extensively studied and results obtained in studying this strain will be first summarized. Then we will briefly present results obtained using other inbred strains.

Auto-immune disease induced by $HgCl_2$ in the BN rat.

Immuno-morphological findings. Brown-Norway rats injected with various doses of $HgCl_2$ (from 0.2 to 0.05 g per 100 bodyweight) develop a biphasic disease. Eight days after the first injection of mercury, linear IgG deposits are seen along the glomerular capillary wall [34]. The presence of anti-GBM antibodies has been confirmed in two ways: a) Igs eluted from diseased kidneys were shown to have an anti-GBM activity both in vivo and in vitro [34] ; b) circulating anti-GBM antibodies were detected using two assays from day 11 following the first injection [80]. Linear IgG deposits are still more intense on day 15, and are associated with C3 deposits [34]. Renal histology shows a monocytic afflux within the glomerular capillary lumen with focal endothelial detachment

[81] . Moreover, classical tubular toxic lesions are seen. Linear IgG deposits are also observed in most organs [82].

Proteinuria and NS appear in most of the rats during the second or third week [83] even when rats were previously decomplemented [84]. Several rats die during this period probably as a consequence of intra-vascular coagulation evidenced by heavy intra-luminal fibrin deposits associated with biological evidence of intra-vascular coagulation [85]. This is probably a consequence of immune glomerular injury. Interestingly, those rats which survive this phase will remain alive until the end of the experiment while proteinuria disappears in spite of the fact that $HgCl_2$ injections are pursued.

The second phase appears earlier than previously suspected. It is characterized by granular IgG and C3 deposits which progressively appear from about day 15 [80] and are prominent on days 30 and 60 [83]. These deposits are found in the glomerular capillary wall (in a subepithelial position), in the mesangium and in the wall of renal vessels [83]. Similar deposits were found in the vessels of most of the organs tested [82] : spleed, liver, intestine, lung, heart, choroid plexus, ciliary processes. In several rats, linear deposits were no longer observed at time of sacrifice which, together with the fact that proteinuria disappears, suggests that the disease is self-limited. The antigen responsible for the second phase has not been characterized. However, when diseased kidneys with granular IgG deposits, but without detectable linear IgG deposits were eluted, IgG with anti-GBM activity was recovered which suggests that a BM antigen might be involved [83].

Serological findings. Anti-GBM antibodies and circulating immune complexes (CIC) were sequentially searched for in BN rats injected with HgCl . The Raji cell assay and the fluid phase Clq binding assay were used to detect CIC like material. Two sensitive assays were used to characterize anti-GBM antibodies. Anti-GBM antibodies were detected from day 11 with a peak from days 16-20. They progressively disappeared from day 30 and were no longer found on day 60. This confirms the transient character of the anti-GBM antibody response. Circulating immune complexes were also transiently detected between days 11 and 31.

Several immuno-morphological and serological data therefore show that most of the abnormalities encountered are transient. This means that the disease induced by HgCl is self-limited and that auto-regulation processes of immune response (suppressor cells?, anti-idiotypic antibodies? and/or immune complexes ?) are efficient. This is an interesting feature of this drug induced disease which contrasts with the regulation defect(s) of mice with spontaneous lupus syndrome [86].

Influence of the chemical form of mercury and of its route of administration. A quite similar disease was obtained when organic mercurial (CH_3HgCl) was injected or when various mercury containing drugs were tested: mercuresceine applied on the skin, ointment containing ammoniated mercury, mercurobutol in the form of pessaries or applied on the skin [87]. $HgCl_2$ and CH_3HgCl were also efficient in inducing the disease whatever the route of administration: digestive or respiratory route, subcutaneous or intravenous injections [88].

Mechanism of action of mercury. As said above, mercury could act as a hapten or by modifying a self-component rendering it antigenic or by triggering immunocompetent cells. The latter possibility was first

tested because we observed a polyclonal increase in total serum IgE in BN
rats injected with HgCl [89].

Serum IgE in Brown-Norway rats injected with $HgCl_2$. Non-specific
total serum IgE was sequentially measured in BN rats injected with $HgCl_2$.
IgE levels increased from day 5 to reach a maximum value by day 15. The
maximum value could reach 2,000 μg/ml (normal value : 2 g/ml). Then, IgE
level decreased. No specificity could be found for IgE induced by $HgCl_2$
[89]. This was reminiscent of findings in rats infected with parasites
which induce a polyclonal increase of serum IgE [90]. We suspect that
$HgCl_2$ also enhances the IgE response to various environmental antigens.
Indeed, we could demonstrate that $HgCl_2$ potentiates the IgE response to
an unrelated antigen such as ovalbumin [89].

Evidence for in vivo and in vitro polyclonal activation induced by
$HgCl_2$ in Brown-Norway rats. Spleen and lymph nodes from $HcCl_2$ injected BN
rats were enlarged on day 12. This was also suggestive of an in vivo
polyclonal activation (PA). We measured the anti-DNA and anti-TNP
response since these antibody specificities are considered as good
markers of PA. Anti-DNA antibodies transiently increased on day 7 and
there was also a transient increase in both IgM and IgG anti-TNP plaque
forming cells (PFC) on day 12 in the spleen of BN rats injected with
$HgCl_2$ (Table 3) [91].
$HgCl_2$ also induced a significant increase of IgM and IgG anti-TNP PFC on
day 4 of culture of normal BN rat spleen cells [91]. This demonstrates
that $HgCl_2$ acts on immunocompetent cells to induce PA.   Recent
experiments suggest that $HgCl_2$ does not act directly on B cells because T
cells are required to obtain in vitro PA. Other experiments in PVG/c
rats by Weening et al., [92] demonstrated that $HgCl_2$ reduced the
generation of supressor cells.

Genetic control of susceptibility to auto-immune disease induced by
$HgCl_2$ in Brown-Norway rats. Brown-Norway rats bear the RTI^n haplotype
and Lewis (LEW) rats the RT haplotype. While BN rats are highly

TABLE 3 : IN VIVO ANTI-TNP RESPONSE INDUCED BY $HgCl_2$ ON DAY 12 AFTER
THE FIRST INJECTION OF $HgCl_2$.

STRAIN	$HgCl_2$	PFC PER 10^6 SPLEEN CELLS $\pm$ SEM		PFC PER SPLEEN $\pm$ SEM (10^3)	
		DIRECT PLAQUES	INDIRECT PLAQUES	DIRECT PLAQUES	INDIRECT PLAQUES
BN	+	17 $\pm$ 8	2 $\pm$ 0.6	9.34 $\pm$ 5.27	1.27 $\pm$ 0.39
BN	–	40.2● $\pm$ 3.7	27 ○ $\pm$ 8.7	44.13■ $\pm$ 5.18	32.45■ $\pm$ 5.9
LEW	+	27.4 $\pm$ 0.5	4.7 $\pm$ 1.8	18.02 $\pm$ 0.32	3.09 $\pm$ 1.18
LEW	–	23.1 $\pm$ 4.7	5.1 $\pm$ 1.5	14.18 $\pm$ 2.88	3.13 $\pm$ 0.92

●$p < 0.05$, ○$p < 0.02$, ■$p < 0.01$ compared to the control rats.

TABLE 4 : IMMUNOFLUORESCENCE FINDINGS IN BN AND LEW RATS AND IN SEGRE-
GANTS OBTAINED BETWEEN BN AND LEW RATS INJECTED WITH $HgCl_2$.

RATS	RT1 HAPLOTYPE	$HgCl_2$ DOSE (μg)	LINEAR IgG DEPOSITS (n pos/n tested)	GRANULAR IgG DEPOSITS (n pos/n tested)
BN	n	100	20/20	20/20
LEW	l	100	0/11	0/11
	n	400	0/15	0/15
(LEW x BN) F_1	l/n	100	14/14	11/11
	l/n	100	31/42	37/38
(LEW x BN) F_2	n/n	100	15/17	15/16
	l/l	100	0/16	0/16
(LEW x BN) F_1 x LEW	l/n	100	9/38	30/30
	l/l	100	0/40	0/33
(LEW x BN) F_1 x BN	l/n	100	40/40	34/34
	n/n	100	30/30	25/25

susceptible, LEW rats were found consistently resistant: none of the manifestations described in the BN strain were seen in the LEW strain.

We therefore tested the susceptibility of segregants obtained between the BN and the LEW strains, F and F hybrids (LEW x BN) F x BN and (LEW x BN) F x LEW backcrosses were tested for their ability to develop both phases of the disease. All the rats were injected with HgCl and their RT haplotype was determined. Results obtained clearly demonstrated that genetic control of susceptibility to the induction of both phases of the disease is inherited as an autosomal, dominant trait and depends on MHC linked gene(s) (Table 4). Data also suggest that few non MHC linked genes are involved [93,94].

Other experiments have shown that the resistance of LEW rats can be overcome provided they receive immuno-competent cells from a susceptible strain. Lewis rats were sublethally irradiated and reconstituted with spleen or bone marrow cells from F hybrids. These chimaeric rats then developed both phases of the disease [95]. This suggests that gene products which control susceptibility are expressed on immuno-competent cells.

Mercury induced glomerulonephritis in other inbred rat strains [96]. Seventeen in bred rat strains were tested as described for BN rats (Table 5). a) None of these strains developed anti-GBM antibodies. b) All the strains tested bearing the RT haplotype (LEW, F.344, BS and AS) were found to be resistant, even when receiving very high $HgCl_2$ doses (0.4 μg for two of them). c) LOU, Wistar AG and LEW.1U ($RT1^u$) were also found to be resistant even when injected with high $HgCl_2$ doses, while Wistar Furth ($RT1^u$) rats developed a typical MGP when injected with high HgCl doses (0.4 g). This suggests either intra-MHC differences between these strains or/and that the genetic control of susceptibility does not depend on MHC linked genes in Wistar-Furth rats. The MGP we obtained in these rats is reminiscent of the GN initially found in some outbred Wistar rats. The antigen responsible is unknown. d) PVG/c and AUG (RT1) DA and AVN (RT1),BDV and LEW.1D (RT1), OKA (RT1), BUF (RT1)and AS

TABLE 5 :   IMMUNOFLUORESCENCE FINDINGS IN RATS INJECTED WITH $HgCl_2$.

STRAIN	RT1 HAPLOTYPE	$HgCl_2$ DOSE	GRANULAR IgG DEPOSITS ON DAY 60
F.344	1	0	0/7
		400	0/5
BS	1	0	0/2
		100	0/5
AS	1	0	0/6
		100	0/8
WAG	u	0	0/7
		400	0/15
LOU	u	0	0/4
		100	0/5
W.Furth	u	0	0/9
		400	5/5
LEW.1U	u	0	0/5
		400	0/6
PVG/c	c	0	0/15
		100	30/30
AUG	c	0	0/3
		100	4/4
DA	a	0	0/10
		100	16/16
AVN	a	0	0/10
		100	3/6
BDV	d	0	0/8
		100	9/9
LEW.BDV	d	0	0/5
		100	6/6
AS_2	f	0	0/6
		100	8/8
OKA	k	0	0/5
		100	5/5
BUF	b	0	0/6
		100	13/15

(RT1) rats developed only an IC type GN. Anti-nuclear antibodies with anti-SS DNA specificity were found in several of these strains and anti-SS DNA antibodies were eluted from diseased kidneys from PVG/c rats. This suggests that these antibodies may play a pathogenic role. Similar findings were previously reported by Weening et al., in PVG/c rats [97].

CONCLUSION.

From our studies we can conclude that mercurials induce in the rat a well defined auto-immune disease, the phenotypic expression of which greatly depends on the strain tested. Brown-Norway rats developed a biphasic disease with anti-GBM antibodies and then an IC type GN. No anti-GBM antibodies were found in the other rat strains tested nor in seven inbred mice strains (unpublished data). The other rat strains tested were found to be resistant or to develop an IC type GN. Interestingly rabbits do develop a disease quite similar to that we have described in BN rats [35].

Three major points emerge from our experiments in BN rats. a) Susceptibility to the induction of the disease is genetically controlled and MHC linked gene(s) are involved. That susceptibility to induction of immunologically mediated GN induced by gold salts is also genetically controlled in human has been suggested by Wooley et al., [98]. Patients bearing the DRW3 haplotype develop MGP more frequently than patients bearing other DRW haplotypes. b) The auto-immune disease induced by $HgCl_2$ is self-limited. This fact points to the importance of auto-regulation processes in this model. c) Several experimental data indicate that mercurials act, at least in part, as polyclonal activator and modify immunoregulation.

This work was supported by DGRST (78/7/2625) and INSERM (CRL 805023 and 805037).

REFERENCES

1. Unanue ER and Dixon FJ, in Adv Immunol 6:1-90, 1967.
2. Dixon FJ, Amer J Med 94: 493-498, 1968.
3. Germuth FG and Rodriguez E, in Immunopathology of the renal glomerulus: immune complex deposit and anti-basement membrane disease. Little Brown and Company, Boston, 1973.
4. Couser WG and Salant DJ, Kidney Int 17:1-13, 1980.
5. Mery JP and Morel-Maronger L, in Proceedings 6th International Congress of Nephrology, Florence, Karger, Basel, 1976, pp. 524-529.
6. Wilson CB and Dixon FJ, in the Kidney (BM Brenner and FC Rector eds.), WB Saunders Company, Philadelphia, 1976, pp. 838-940.
7. Cochrane CG and Koffler D, in Adv Immunol 16: 185-264, 1973.
8. Couser WG et al. Kidney Int 11:170-180, 1977.
9. Schreiner GF et al. J Exp Med 147:369-384, 1978.
10. Andres GA and McCluskey RT, Kidney Int 7:271-289, 1975.
11. Heymann W et al. Prc Soc EXp Biol Med 100:660-666, 1959.
12. Edgington TS et al. Science 155:1432-1434, 1967.
13. Vandamme BJC et al. Lab Invest 38:502-510, 1978.
14. Couser WG et al. J Clin Invest 62:1275-1287, 1978.

15. Hoyer JR, Kidney Int 17:284-292, 1980.
16. Golbus S and Wilson CB, Kidney Int 16:148-157, 1979.
17. Batsford SR et al. Clin Nephrol 14:211-216, 1980.
18. Izui S et al. J Exp Med 144:428-443, 1976.
19. Mauer SM et al. J Exp Med 137:553-570, 1973.
20. Dixon FJ, New Engl J Med 283:536-537, 1970.
21. Rudofsky UH et al. Lab Invest 43:463-470, 1980.
22. Neilson EG and Philips SM, J Immunol 123:2381-2385, 1979.
23. Fillastre JP et al. Proceedings 8th International Congress
    of Nephrology, Athens, Karger, Basel, 1981, pp. 745-752.
24. Lindqvist KJ et al. E Afr Med J 51:168-169, 1974.
25. Border WA et al. New Engl J Med 291:381-384, 1974.
26. Pujet JC et al. Brit Med J 2:415-418, 1974.
27. Tan EM, Fed Proc 33:1894-1897, 1974.
28. Landsteiner K, The specificity of serological reactions,
    Harvard University Press, Cambridge, 1945.
29. Kirtland HH et al. New Engl J Med 302:825-832, 1980.
30. Bluestein HG et al. Lancet 2:816-819, 1979.
31. Zimmerman SW et al. Lancet 2:199-201, 1975.
32. Wilson CB, Immunological Rev 55:257-297, 1981.
33. Gibson T et al. Ann Intern Med 84:100, 1976.
34. Sapin C et al. Clin Exp Immunol 28:173-179, 1977.
35. Roman Franco AA et al. Clin Immunol Immunopathol 9:464-481, 1978.
36. Mery JP and Fillastre JP, in Nephrology (J Hamburger,
    J Crosnier and JP Grunfled eds.), J Willey, New York, 1979,
    pp. 1169-1187.
37. Becker et al. Ann Int Med 110:178-186, 1962.
38. Mandema E et al. Lancet 1:1266, 1963.
39. Kazantzis G, Environ Health Perspect 27:111-118, 1978.
40. Caron GA et al. Int Arch Appl Immunol 37:76-87, 1970.
41. Charpentier B et al. Nephrologie, in press, 1981.
42. Tornroth T and Skrifvars V, Amer J Pathol 75:573-590, 1974.
43. Watanabe I et al. Arch Path Lab Med 100:632-635, 1976.
44. Nagi AH et al. Exp Molec Path 15:354-362, 1971.
45. Blanc-Brunat N et al, in Rein et Toxique,Masson, Paris, 1975,
    pp. 31-52.
46. Bacon PA et al. Quart J Med 45:661-684, 1976.
47. Jaffe IA et al. Ann Int Med 69:549-554, 1968.
48. Matthes KJ, Contr Nephrol 24:109-114, 1981.
49. Seelig JP et al. Res Exp Med 170:35-55, 1977.
50. Amor B et al. Nouv Presse Med 8:2023-2024, 1979.
51. Hoorntje SJ et al. Lancet 1:1212-1215, 1980.
52. Heymann W, Pediatrics 22:614-615, 1958.
53. Drummond KN et al. J Clin Invest 45:620-630, 1966.
54. Heymann W, JAMA 202:127-128, 1967.
55. Menkes CJ et al. Nouv Presse Med 7:2654-2655, 1978.
56. Ducret F et al. Nephrologie 1:143-144, 1980.
57. Silverman SH et al. Amer D Dis Child 132:99,1978.
58. Zech P et al. Clin Nephrol 11:218-221, 1979.
59. Farr MJ et al. Brit Med J 2:68-69, 1975.
60. Callard P et al. Amer J Pathol 80:329-1979.
61. Nochy D et al. Clin Nephrol 6:422-427, 1976.
62. Shalboub RJ, Lancet 2:556-559, 1974.
63. Lagrue G et al. Lancet 1:271-272, 1975.
64. Sherman RL et al. Amer J Med 52:699-706, 1972.

65. Wittig HJ and Goldman AS, Lancet 1:542-543, 1970.
66. Herve JR et al. Nouv Presse Med 9:2847, 1980.
67. Bar-Khayim Y et al. Amer J Med 54:272-280, 1973.
68. Brezin JH et al. New Engl J Med 301:1271-1273, 1979.
69. Richman AV et al. Ann Intern Med 92:70-72, 1980.
70. Ryan GB et al. Lab Invest 33:461-468, 1975.
71. Cunningham EE et al. Amer J Med 68:47-53, 1980.
72. Kuzemko JA, Brit Med J 4:665-666, 1972.
73. Rohwedder HJ and Volzke E, Arch Kinderheilk 168:53-56, 1963.
74. Bishop WB et al. New Engl J Med 2:616-619, 1966.
75. Boulton-Jones JM et al. Brit Med J 3:373-426, 1974.
76. Baldwin DS et al. New Engl J Med 279:1245-1252, 1968.
77. Colvin RB et al. Ann Intern Med 81:404-405, 1974.
78. Michielsen P and DE Schepper PJ, in Drug induced diseases
      (L Meyler and HM Peck eds.), Excerpta Medica, Amsterdam,
      1972, pp. 261-324.
79. Bariety J et al. Amer J Pathol 65:293-302, 1971.
80. Bellon B et al. Eur J Clin Invest 11:3, 1981.
81. Hinglais N et al. Lab Invest 41:150-159,1979.
82. Bernaudin JF et al. Clin Exp Immunol 38:265-273, 1979.
83. Druet P et al. Ann Immunol 129C:777-792, 1978.
84. Capron M et al. submitted for publication.
85. Michaud A et al. Eur J Clin Invest 9:25, 1980.
86. Theofilopoulos AN and Dixon FJ, Immunological Rev
      55:179-216, 1981.
87. Druet P et al. Nephron, in press, 1981.
88. Bernaudin JF et al. Clin Immunol and Immunopathol 20:
      129-135, 1981.
89. Prouvost-Danon A et al. J Immunol 126:699-702, 1981.
90. Urban JF et al. J Immunol 119:583-590, 1977.
91. Hirsch F et al. 8th International Congress of Nephrology,
      Athens, 1981, 138.
92. Weening J et al. Clin Exp Immunol 45:64-71, 1981.
93. Druet E et al. Eur J Immunol 7:348-351, 1977.
94. Sapin C et al. Transplant Proc 13:1404-1406, 1981.
95. Sapin C et al. Eur J Immunol 10:371-374, 1980.
96. Druet E et al. Transplant Proc 11:1600-1603, 1979.
97. Weening JJ et al. Lab Invest 39:405-411, 1978.
98. Wooley PH et al. New Engl J Med 303:300-302, 1980.

RENAL ENDOCRINE AND EXOCRINE FUNCTION, BLOOD PRESSURE AND NEPHROTOXICITY

H. Thurston

Department of Medicine, Clinical Sciences Building, Leicester Royal Infirmary, P.O. Box 65, Leicester LE2 7LX, UK

ABSTRACT

The kidney functions as a major homeostatic regulator of body fluids and blood pressure and this complex role involves both excretory and endocrine mechanisms. Until recently the majority of studies have been concerned with a 'prohypertensive' role for the kidney which involves sodium and water retention and increased activity of the vasoconstrictor renin angiotensin system. However, over the past decade there has been increasing evidence for a renal antihypertensive function. Currently there are three renal vasodilator systems, prostaglandins, kinins and antihypertensive renomedullary lipids which may mediate this blood pressure lowering effect. These vasodilator substances may serve to counterbalance the vasoconstrictor action of the renin angiotensin system and maintain normal blood pressure. It follows therefore that a deficiency of the renomedullary vasodepressor system could lead to the development of hypertension. There is little information about the effects of renal damage on these systems, but since blood pressure may depend upon a delicate balance between renal vasodilator and vasopressor mechanisms nephrotoxic agents may disturb this balance and cause hypertension.

Key Words   Blood pressure; Renin; Prostaglandins; Kallikrein; Nephrotoxicity; Renomedullary lipids.

INTRODUCTION

The association between renal disease and blood pressure was postulated by Richard Bright (1) in 1836. At the turn of the nineteenth century the renal pressor substance renin was discovered(2) and a reciprocal relationship between blood pressure and salt intake in hypertensive patients was demonstrated(3) although this phenomenon was wrongly attributed to changes in chloride balance. An unproductive period followed because of repeated unsuccessful attempts to confirm

the presence of renin and the failure to develop a reproducible
experimental model of renal hypertension. The latter problem was
resolved by Goldblatt (4) with the production of sustained hypertension
in the dog by bilateral renal artery construction. This stimulated an
immediate search for a humoral pressor agent and attention was again .
drawn to renin. A stable renin extract was prepared (5,6) and in 1938
renin was detected in the renal venous blood of Goldblatt hypertensive
dogs (7). That renin was an enzyme discovered by chance in 1940 when it
was demonstrated that renin itself had no pressor activity but acted
upon plasma to produce a short-acting vasoconstrictor hormone (8,9).
This was the first indication that renin was only the initiating step
of the renin-angiotensin system.

Despite a long period of research the renin-angiotensin system
remains the only known pressor system in the kidney for which there is
any evidence for involvement in the pathogenesis of hypertension.
However, sodium retention is an important factor in the development of
hypertension in patients with chronic renal insufficiency. Thus,
patients with terminal renal failure or bilaterally nephrectomised
patients only become hypertensive when sodium loaded (10,11). The
concept of a prohypertensive function for the kidney by these two
mechanisms is now firmly established. However, there is evidence that
the kidney may exert a blood pressure lowering action by a non-excretory
endocrine function (12). Furthermore the antihypertensive effect may
be mediated by vasodepressor substances secreted from the interstitial
cells of the renal medulla (13). In addition Muirhead (14) has proposed
that the prohypertensive and antihypertensive renal actions counterbalance each other to maintain blood pressure homostasis.

The purpose of this review is to examine the evidence for this
hypothesis and discuss the effects of nephrotoxicity induced renal
damage on the endocrine functions of the kidney with particular reference
to blood pressure control.

THE RENIN ANGIOTENSIN SYSTEM

The release of renin, by the kidney, initiates a sequence of enzymic
reactions which lead to the formation of an active polypeptide hormone
(15). Renin acts upon its substrate, a glycoprotein alpha globulin
synthesised by the liver, to produce the largely inactive decapeptide
angiotensin I. Converting enzyme, a depeptidyl carboxypeptidase which
is found mainly in lung (16) and also in plasma and blood vessel wall
(17) removes the carboxyterminal amino acids Histidine-Leucine from
angiotensin 1 to generate the octapeptide angiotensin 11 (Fig 1). This

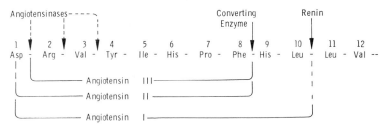

Figure 1   The terminal amino acid sequence of renin substrate
                  (angiotensinogen) and the points of cleavage by renin,
                  converting enzyme and angiotensinases.

peptide which is the most potent naturally occurring vasoconstrictor substance known, functions as the effector hormone of the renin angiotensin system (15) although the heptapeptide des-Asp-angiotensin II (Angiotensin III) may have important actions in some sites (18). Both of these hormones are rapidly degraded to peptide fragments in the peripheral capillary beds by a group of enzymes collectively called angiotensinases (19).

Synthesis and storage of renin   Renin is a glycoprotein enzyme of molecular weight 39,400 - 43,000. It is synthesised and stored in the juxtaglomerular apparatus which lies at the vascular pole of the glomerulus (20). This structure consists of modified granulated smooth cells of both the afferent and efferent arterioles which lie in close association with a group of specialised cells of the distal convoluted tubule, the macula densa (21).

Renin release by the kidney   Renin secretion is controlled by two receptor mechanisms (22):   (1) The juxtaglomerular baroreceptor which responds to a fall in pressure by stimulating renin release. The sympathetic nervous system also acts at this site. Renal beta adreno-ceptors stimulate renin release whereas alpha adrenoceptors inhibit renin secretion. (2) The chemoreceptor macula densa responds to changes in fluid composition in the distal tubule. The nature of this mechanism is controversial, however changes in the rate of delivery of sodium and chloride appear to be involved. Angiotensin II inhibits renin release by a negative feedback loop. Renin secretion is also depressed by potassium or antidiuretic hormone. Recent evidence from in vitro and in vivo studies, suggests a role for prostaglandins in the control of renin release. Thus prostaglandin PGI_2 and prostaglandin PGE_2 stimulate renin secretion in both renal slices and intact kidney preparations (23).

Extra renal renin   Renin-like enzymes, which split the substrate leucyl-leucine bond to form angiotensin, have been found in many tissues (24). These include uterus, placenta, fetal membranes, amniotic fluid, brain, adrenal glands, lung, liver, spleen, submaxillary glands and blood vessel walls. However, one of these enzymes 'pseudo-renin' can only form angiotensin I from the synthetic tetradecapeptide substrate but not from homologous substrate (25). Moreover, although a variety of proteolytic enzymes such as cathepsin D and pepsin are capable of generat-ing angiotensin I from homologous substrate at low pH (26), it is unlikely that significant generation would occur at physiological pH. Some workers however, have attributed a local function to renin-like activity found in the brain, uterus and blood vessel walls (27) but in all except the latter case the evidence is conflicting. Furthermore, there is increasing evidence to suggest that renin activity in blood vessel walls is ultimately derived from the kidney and the physiological actions of the renin-angiotensin system may be more closely associated with vascular rather than plasma renin levels (28).

Inactive renin   The activity of renin in plasma or renal extracts can be increased substantially in vitro by acidification to pH 3.3, trypsin, kallikrein treatment, or incubation at $-5^{\circ}C$ (29). Renin activation may represent the removal of an inhibitor, or the splitting of a higher molecular weight precursor. Whether activation occurs in vivo is not

known and its significance remains unclear. However, since inactive
renin persists in the circulation after bilateral nephrectomy it
may be synthesised at an extra renal site. At the present time the
only clinical significance of inactive renins lies in its effect
upon some assay procedures which activate renin during an acidification
pretreatment stage (30).

Inhibition of the renin-angiotensin system   Measurements of circulating
levels of renin-angiotensin 11 may neither reflect the concentration
of the receptor site or the degree of vasoconstriction produced in the
peripheral arterioles. Recently, several agents have been developed for
the pharmacological blockade of the renin angiotensin system at two
sites: conversion of angiotensin I into angiotensin II (inhibition of
converting enzyme) and angiotensin II receptor binding (blockade by
competitive angiotensin II antagonists). Three agents have been used
in this context, teprotide (31) (Sq 20881) the nonapeptide and captopril
(32) (Sq 14225) which are converting enzyme inhibitors and the octapeptide
angiotensin II antagonist, sarcosine I alanine 8 angiotensin II,
saralasin (33) (P113). These agents have been used to define the role of
the angiotensin system in various physiological and pathological states.
However, saralasin has intrinsic agonist actions (33) and converting
enzyme inhibition prevents the degradation of bradykinin which has
vasodepressor action (33,34). Thus changes in blood pressure observed
with administration of converting enzyme inhibitors cannot be confidently
attributed to angiotensin II blockade alone (35).

Renin-angiotensin system and blood pressure control   Renin has no
intrinsic pressor activity of its own but raises blood pressure by the
generation of angiotensin II which is the major active vasoconstrictor
hormone of the renin-angiotensin system (15). Although angiotensin II is
by weight the most potent vasoconstrictor substance known in nature (36)
it can raise blood pressure in several ways:
(i)   A direct action on vascular smooth muscle causing widespread
      vasoconstriction.
(ii) An indirect effect via the sympathetic nerve system acting both at
      a central level, increasing sympathetic outflow (37), and peripherally
      by enhancing noradrenaline release from sympathetic nerves (38).
(iii) Stimulation of adrenal aldosterone secretion, promoting renal
      absorption of sodium.
(iv) A direct action upon the kidney at low doses which promotes salt
      and water retention.
   The renin-angiotensin system has an important role in regulating
arterial blood pressure and aldosterone secretion in both homeostasis and
disease (39,40). However, the role of renin in hypertension is much more
controversial. It is, however, important in the rare form of hypertension
caused by renin secreting tumours (41) and in patients with advanced
renal failure and hypertension which is resistant to fluid removal by
renal dialysis (42,43). Renin is probably important also in surgically
correctable renovascular hypertension (44) although such patients
occasionally have normal renin levels (45). The role of renin in essential
hypertension is most controversial and is found to be elevated in only
a minority of patients (46).

OTHER RENAL PRESSOR SYSTEMS

The failure to implicate the renin angiotensin system in the pathogenesis of many forms of hypertension has stimulated a search for additional pressor agents. Even experimental hypertension and renovascular hypertension caused by renal ischaemia cannot be accounted for by the renin angiotensin system alone. Thus, sodium depletion in combination with renin angiotensin blockade (47) does not restore blood pressure to normal in hypertension produced by unilateral renal artery constriction (Goldblatt 2 kidney 1 clip hypertension). However, removal of the constricting clip produces an immediate fall in blood pressure with normal blood pressure levels achieved at 24 hours (48). Moreover, haemodynamic studies indicate that the reversal of hypertension is caused by a fall in total peripheral resistance which cannot be explained by structural changes or reduction of plasma renin (49). In addition sodium balance studies demonstrated sodium retention in association with the fall in blood pressure (50). Several alternative humoral pressor factors have been suggested and the best characterised of these include:
1) Nephrotensin - renal pressor substance found in plasma of dogs with renal hypertension (51).
2) Renopressin - found in the renal cortex and produces a slow sustained pressor response which can be blocked by specific antibodies (52).
3) Tonin - an enzyme which hydrolyses renin substrate and angiotensin I to generate angiotensin II and has been claimed to be present in increased amounts in human and experimental hypertension (53).

SODIUM RETENTION AND BLOOD PRESSURE

Some forms of experimental and clinical hypertension depend upon sodium retention and salt restriction has been used to treat hypertensive patients with renal failure (54). Moreover, the majority of patients with terminal renal failure or bilaterally nephrectomised patients only develop hypertension when salt loaded (11) and the same phenomenon can be observed in bilaterally (55) or partially nephrectomised dogs (56).
The mechanism by which sodium retention causes hypertension is the subject of much debate. Sodium loading produces an increase in venous return to the heart and consequently cardiac output rises. Early studies confirmed this sequence of events and it was proposed that the increase in cardiac output induced an autoregulating rise in peripheral resistance to protect the tissues from overperfusion (57). However, there is evidence, from experimental models of hypertension (58) and salt loaded renal dialysis patients (59), that a primary rise in peripheral resistance may occur without the necessity of initial increase in cardiac output. Since the protective autoregulatory mechanism cannot be invoked sodium must operate through another mechanism. The three alternative mechanisms which have been postulated are: (i) changes in serum sodium concentration, (ii) water logging of vascular walls, and, (iii) a raised intracellular sodium content of vascular smooth muscles (30).

RENAL VASODEPRESSOR SYSTEMS

Although the kidney was suspected of having an antihypertensive role over a century ago the basic observations were not made until 1932 when a rise in blood pressure following subtotal nephrectomy was noted (60).

These findings were confirmed in 1933 (61) and shortly afterwards a
more marked rise in blood pressure was demonstrated in the dog
following bilateral nephrectomy(62,63). This form of hypertension was
called 'renoprival hypertension' and it was maintained that sodium
retention could not account for the raised blood pressure (64). On the
other hand, whilst confirming these observations Tobian (64) also
observed a striking reduction in hypertension by salt restriction.

The controversy which ensued centred around whether the rise in
blood pressure resulted from sodium retention alone or the removal of
a renal vasodepressor system. Thus, in dogs hypertension could be
prevented if a single kidney was left 'in situ' with the ureter
implanted into the intestine or vena cava (63). Furthermore, renal
transplantation ameliorated renoprival hypertension despite the continued
maintenance of the salt and water overload (65). In contrast however,
bilaterally nephrectomised patients maintained on regular dialysis
only become hypertensive when allowed to become sodium loaded (66).

Renoprival hypertension therefore depends upon two components:
(1) sodium and water retention as a result of renal excretory failure
(2) a non-excretory endocrine vasodepressor system. The ability of the
kidney to excrete a salt and water overload is now accepted by most
workers to be a major antihypertensive function but the role of an
endocrine vasodepressor system remains in doubt. However, in the past
decade further evidence has gathered in support of a non excretory
antihypertensive action by the kidney. Thus uterocaval anastomosis
but not ureter ligation prevents renoprival hypertension in the rat(67).
Implantation of fragments of renal medulla prevents the development of
hypertension or lowers the blood pressure in hypertensive rats (13).
Histological studies of the transplants showed complete reabsorption
of the tubular elements with the persistence of lipid laden renomedullary interstitial cell (13). Muirhead (14) has continued his studies
and has now extracted a number of lipid substances which possess
significant vasodepressor properties.

Currently, there are three renal vasodilator systems which may
mediate the antihypertensive function of the kidney and thus play an
important role in blood pressure control: (i) the kallikrein kinin system,
(ii) renal prostaglandins and (iii) the antihypertensive renomedullary
lipids.

i) Kallikrein-kinin system   Kallikreins are serine proteases which
generate potent vasodilator peptides (kinins) from plasma substrates
called kininogens (68). There are two classes of kallikrein, plasma and
glandular. Both act on the same substrate but plasma kallikrein generates
bradykinin whereas glandular kallikrein forms an intermediate peptide
kallikrein (Lys-bradykinin) which must be converted to bradykinin by the
enzyme aminopeptidase (Fig 2). Renal kallikrein is found bound to the
plasma membranes of the cells of the distal convoluted tubule (69)
and part of the enzyme is in an active form (70). Kallikrein is
released into the renal tubules and kinins may be generated within
the tubules and lower urinary tract (71).

There is some evidence which suggests that kallikrein released by
the distal tubule reaches the interstitial and vascular spaces of
the kidney (Fig 3). Thus, it is possible that kinins may be found in
these spaces and so influence local blood flow. However, whether
kallikrein enters the circulation is uncertain but in any case it
would be rapidly inactivated by plasma inhibitors. The cells of
proximal tubule are rich in kininase which is identical to angiotensin

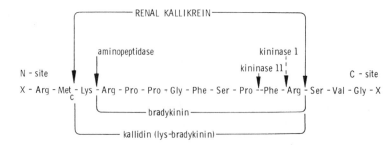

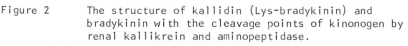

Figure 2   The structure of kallidin (Lys-bradykinin) and
              bradykinin with the cleavage points of kinonogen by
              renal kallikrein and aminopeptidase.

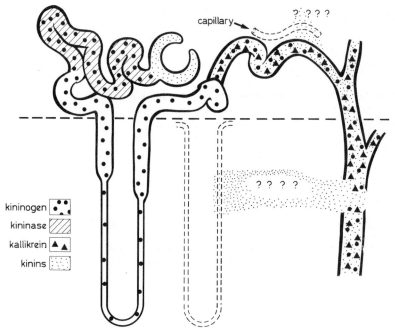

Figure 3   Localisation of renal kallikrein-kinin system in the
              renal tubule.

converting enzyme and present an effective barrier to filtered
bradykinin reaching the distal tubule (Fig 3). Thus even injections
of pharmacological amounts of bradykinin into the renal artery fail
to appear in the urine (72). It is likely therefore that the
considerable quantities of kallikrein and bradykinin found in urine
must be formed by, and within, the kidney. Furthermore, when urine
remains in the bladder for a long period kinin levels fall despite
continued generation suggesting that urine not only contains
kallikrein and kininogen but also kininase.

    Our current knowledge indicates that kinins are unlikely to serve
as the circulating antihypertensive hormone from the kidney since

a very large portion of bradykinin is inactivated during its
passage through the pulmonary circulation by angiotensin converting
enzyme (73). It is more reasonable to consider the system as acting
as a local intrarenal hormonal system (68). The following intrarenal
effects may be of importance.
(1) Renal prostaglandins may be controlled by the kallikrein-kinin
system. Thus kinins infused into the kidney stimulate the synthesis
of PGE$_2$ in the medulla and PGI$_2$ in the arterioles (74).
(2) Kinins stimulate renal renin release and moreover urinary
kallikrein in vitro converts inactive renin to active renin and it
has been suggested that kallikreins may perform this function in vivo(29).
(3) The renal kallikrein-kinin system may regulate renal salt and water
excretion. However, the capacity of bradykinin to produce a water
diuresis may depend upon its ability to induce the synthesis of PGE$_2$.
In addition, kinins may determine the principle produce of
prostaglandin synthesis in the medulla by regulating the enzyme
PGE-9-ketoreductase (75). Thus, in the presence of sodium depletion,
kinins may stimulate the production of PGF$_{2\alpha}$ and promote sodium and
water retention by blocking the intrarenal effects of kinins.
    In addition to interactions with prostaglandins there is evidence
that angiotensin II and aldosterone both stimulate kallikrein
release (76). One major advantage of such a response would be in
the maintenance of renal vasodilation during the renin-angiotensin
induced systemic vasoconstriction. In recent years it has been
suggested that renal kallikrein deficiency may play a role in the
pathogenesis of hypertension in man and experimental animals (68).
However, how locally generated kinins may regulate blood pressure is
unclear but it has been suggested that the prostaglandin PGE$_2$ could
mediate an important part of this antihypertensive function (75).

ii)   Prostaglandins   Prostaglandin biosynthesis and metabolism in
the kidney has been extensively reviewed (77). The arachidonic acid
precursor released by phospholipase from phospholipid stores is
converted by prostaglandin cyclo-oxygenase to produce a series of
prostaglandins which include PGE$_2$, PGF$_{2\alpha}$ and possibly PGI$_2$ and
thromboxinine A (Fig 4). PGE$_2$ and PGF$_{2\alpha}$ are predominantly synthesised

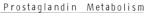

Prostaglandin Metabolism

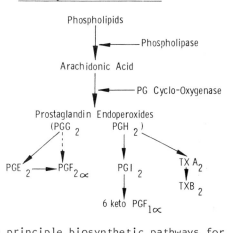

Figure 4   The principle biosynthetic pathways for prostaglandins.

by the interstitial and tubular cells of the renal medulla and papilla
(78). Prostacyclin (PGI_2), which is synthesised by microsomal enzymes
in arterial walls (79), however is mainly produced by the renal
cortex (78). The prostaglandins formed by the kidney may enter the
renal tubule or pass into the vascular compartment. Thus, the
prostaglandin levels in renal venous blood and probably urinary
prostaglandin excretion are thought to reflect renal biosynthesis.

Prostaglandins PGE_2 and PGI_2 are potent vasodilator compounds and
have been demonstrated to lower blood pressure in man and animals.
There is considerable evidence that prostaglandins act together with
the kallikrein-kinin system to comprise a major vasodilator system
in the kidney (75). Moreover, some of the diuretic and natriuretic
actions of bradykinin may depend upon prostaglandin PGE_2. Renal
prostaglandin synthesis is stimulated by a variety of stimuli which
include increased activity of the renin-angiotensin system, the
adrenergic nervous system, bradykinin and renal ischaemia (78). On
the other hand, prostaglandin PGE_2 and PGI_2 both stimulate renin
release in vitro and in vivo (80). The interaction between
prostaglandins and the renin-angiotensin system in the vascular and
interstitial compartments of the kidney is of great importance for
the control of the renal circulation, particularly during stress such
as hypertension or the administration of nephrotoxic substances.
Therefore together with the kinin system renal prostaglandin may
defend the kidney when the renal circulation is threatened. Thus,
indomethacin a potent cyclo-oxygenase inhibitor causes renal vasoconstriction and renders the renal microcirculation more sensitive to
vasoconstrictor substances (81). Whether renal prostaglandins produce
systemic vasodilatation is still debatable. Prostaglandin PGE_2 is
rapidly degraded by a single passage through the pulmonary circulation
and although PGI_2 is not cleared by the kidney it is not known whether
it is released in sufficient amounts to exert a blood pressure
lowering effect.

iii)   Antihypertensive renomedullary lipids   Muirhead and his
associates have isolated two antihypertensive renomedullary lipids
from the renal medulla which are distinct from prostaglandins (14).
Moreover, they propose that the vasodepressor action of transplanted
renal medulla or cultured renomedullary interstitial cells may be
mediated by one of these substances, the antihypertensive neutral
renomedullary lipid (ANRL). Unlike prostaglandins the intravenous
injection of ANRL is accompanied by a slow decline in blood pressure
in Goldblatt 1 kidney 1 clip hypertensive rats with recovery taking
60 minutes or more. The antihypertensive polar renomedullary lipid (APRL)
induces an immediate fall in blood pressure which is of a shorter
duration. However, multiple intravenous injections or infusions of
APRL produce a prolonged depressor response lasting from 24 to >60
hours (82). The antihypertensive response was not associated with an
increase in salt and water excretion even in sodium volume expanded
hypertensive rats and since cardiac output was unchanged the vasodepressor response is dependent upon a potent vasodilator action (83).

Unfortunately, purification and characterisation of the active
principle of ANRL has not been achieved but even so the secretion
of antihypertensive renomedullary lipids by the renomedullary
interstitial cells is probably the most attractive mechanism by which
the kidney can mediate an antihypertensive action. At the present
time the mechanism which signals the medulla to release antihypertensive

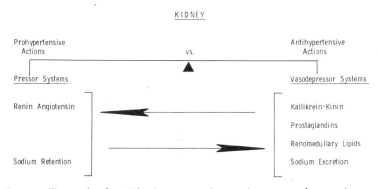

Figure 5   The relationship between the prohypertensive and
                antihypertensive actions of the kidney as related to
                renal hormones and sodium excretion by the kidney.

substances is not known but sodium overload may stimulate secretion
whereas renal artery constriction appears to depress the function of
the renomedullary interstitial cells (84).

Muirhead has proposed a mirror image relationship between
prohypertensive and antihypertensive renal systems (Fig 5). The
prohypertensive actions include the activation of the renin angiotensin
system and sodium retention. The antihypertensive actions include
renal excretion of sodium and the activity of the three renal
vasodepressor systems. When arterial blood pressure is controlled
these systems should be in balance.

VASODEPRESSOR FUNCTIONS OF THE RENAL MEDULLA IN EXPERIMENTAL HYPERTENSION

Complete reversal of 2 kidney 1 clip hypertension in the rat
cannot be achieved by either blockade of the renin-angiotensin
system alone or in combination with salt depletion (47). However,
removal of the renal artery constriction restores blood pressure
to normal levels even after several months of hypertension (48).
The fall in blood pressure is not associated with a natriuresis
or dependent upon renin or the reversal of structural vascular
changes (50). A search for an alternative mechanism has focussed
attention upon the vasodepressor properties of the renal medulla.
Chemical medullectomy has little effect on the blood pressure of
normal rats (85) but slightly higher blood pressures have been
observed in medullectomised Goldblatt hypertensive rats (86). However,
removal of the renal artery clip was associated with only a partial
reversal of hypertension when compared to animals with intact
medullae (87). Further studies using indomethacin and trasylol to
inhibit prostaglandins and the kallikrein kinin system failed to
modify the blood pressure response to unclipping of hypertensive
rats(88). This indirect evidence suggests that fall in blood pressure
which follows removal of the constricting clip may depend on the
secretion of antihypertensive lipids from the renomedullary
interstitial cells.

TOXIC NEPHROPATHY, RENAL HORMONES AND BLOOD PRESSURE

There are a host of diverse physical and chemical substances which
have been shown to damage the kidney. Moreover, the majority of
studies of nephrotoxicity have been concerned mainly with the
disruption of renal excretory function, the extent of damage to the
renal architecture and biochemical mechanisms which produce cellular
injury. As a consequence much less is known about the effect of renal
toxins upon blood pressure or vasoactive renal hormones. However,
changes in both renal hormones and blood pressure have been recorded
in three forms of toxic nephropathy: (i) heavy metal toxicity (ii) acute
renal failure (iii) analgesic nephropathy.

i)   Heavy metal toxicity   A number of heavy metals cause renal damage
but only cadmium and lead have been associated with arterial hypertension.
The role of cadmium in hypertension is still controversial and dosage
may be a critical factor. Thus, chronic low dose administration of
cadmium to rats (89) and rabbits (90) produces a rise in blood pressure.
High dosage however causes more severe renal damage and blood pressure
decreases (91). Similarly, in man industrial exposure is usually
associated with evidence of renal tubular damage (92) with glycosuria,
aminoaciduria, phosphaturia and proteinuria. On the other hand it is
claimed that low dose environmental exposure may be an important cause
of hypertension (93). The mechanism for cadmium-induced blood pressure
elevation is not clear. Cadmium has been shown to cause hyper-
reninaemia (94) and to decrease urinary sodium excretion (95). In
addition several studies have demonstrated a reduction of urinary
kallikrein in rats (89), rabbits and man (96) chronically exposed to
cadmium. Thus, if subnormal levels of urinary kallikrein reflect
a decrease in renal kallikrein the consequent reduction of kinins
may lead to salt and water retention and be a possible explanation
for cadmium-induced hypertension.
      Severe lead intoxication has also been linked with hypertension
(97) but lesser degrees of lead ingestion are not (98). In contrast
however, one epidemiological study showed raised plasma lead
levels in hypertensive patients (99). Plasma renin activity was
found to be suppressed in subjects suffering from chronic plumbism
due to drinking 'moonshine whisky' (100) and renin suppression could
be reversed by long term treatment with chelating agents (101).
However, in a more recent study plasma renin concentration levels in
patients with occupational lead exposure were normal and rose in
response to frusemide administration (102). Finally, urinary
kallikrein has been found to be reduced in lead exposed workers (103)
and it has been suggested that screening for changes in urinary
kallikrein excretion could provide a means of detecting early evidence
of renal toxicity from lead or cadmium (96).

ii)   Acute renal failure   Plasma renin and angiotensin II levels
are usually, but not invariably elevated in acute tubular necrosis
in both man and experimental animals (104 - 106). The renin angiotensin
system has been implicated in the pathogenesis of acute renal failure
and the evidence for and against such a role has been reviewed
extensively elsewhere (107,108). However, it is entirely possible that
increased activity of the renin-angiotensin axis is the result,
rather than the cause, of acute tubular necrosis. What is more neither
specific angiotensin II antibodies (109) or inhibition of the renin

angiotensin system (110) appear to significantly protect rats from acute renal failure. Thus, there is no evidence that circulating renin and angiotensin have an important role in causing renal dysfunction.

However, intrarenal generation of angiotensin II may still play a part in the regulation of renal blood flow and glomerular filtration rate. Moreover, chronic saline loading prevents the development in several models of acute renal failure (108) and this effect has been attributed to renin depletion in the kidney. On the other hand others have argued that saline diuresis per se confers considerable protection irrespective of the renin concentration in the kidney (111). These apparent contradictions may depend on differences between renal renin and intrarenal angiotensin II concentrations since there is evidence that intrarenal angiotensin II concentration may not necessarily parallel renal renin in some models of acute renal failure (112).

Sodium overload commonly occurs in acute renal failure but unlike sodium overload in chronic renal failure, hypertension is rarely observed (113). This is all the more surprising in view of the high circulating levels of renin and angiotensin II found in acute tubular necrosis. However, the pressor response to infused angiotensin II is depressed in acute renal failure and it has been suggested that the effect may depend upon a circulating inhibitor (114). Moreover, vasodepressor substances have been found in renal venous blood from ischaemic dog kidneys (113). Thus, hypertension may be prevented in acute renal failure by one or more of the vasodepressor systems which are thought to mediate the endocrine antihypertensive function of the kidney.

iii)   Analgesic nephropathy   The reported incidence of hypertension in analgesic nephropathy varies from 15 to 70% and malignant hypertension has been observed in about 7% of patients (115). Renal papillary necrosis is the primary and predominant pathological lesion of analgesic nephropathy and most workers now regard the changes of renal cortical 'interstitial nephritis' as a secondary phenomenon (116). Thus, the depletion of renomedullary vasodilator systems is the most likely mechanism to produce hypertension in analgesic nephropathy. However, rats with experimental papillary necrosis are usually normotensive (85,86) although sodium loading may cause an elevation of blood pressure in these animals (85). Similarly, surgical papillectomy in salt resistant rats only raised blood pressure on a high salt diet (84). These observations suggest that loss of the renomedullary vasodilator mechanisms does not directly cause hypertension. Therefore, it is more than likely that hypertension associated with papillary necrosis produced by long term analgesic abuse may depend on the extent of renal cortical interstitial nephritis.

References

1. Bright R, Guy's Hospital Rep 1: 380-400, 1836.
2. Tigerstedt R and Bergman PG, Skand Arch Physiol 7-8: 223-271, 1898.
3. Ambard L and Beaujard E, Arch Gen Med SH 1: 520-533, 1904.
4. Goldblatt H,et al. J Exp Med 59: 247-379, 1934.
5. Pickering GW and Prinzmetal M, Clin Sci 3: 211-227, 1938.
6. Landis EM et al. J Clin Invest 17: 189-206, 1938.
7. Fasciolo JC et al. J Physiol, Lond 94: 281-292, 1938.

8. Page IH and Helmer OM, J Exp Med 71: 29-42, 1940.
9. Braun-Menendez E et al, J Physiol, Lond 98: 283-298, 1940.
10. Kolff WJ et al, Circ Res 30: Suppl II, 23-28, 1964.
11. Vertes V et al, N Engl J Med 280: 978-981, 1969.
12. Fasciolo JC, Soc Argent de Biol Rev 14: 15-24, 1938.
13. Muirhead EE, Adv Intern Med 19: 81-107, 1974.
14. Muirhead EE, Hypertension 2: 444-464, 1980.
15. Peart WS, Pharmacol Rev 17: 143-182, 1965.
16. Ng KKF and Vane JR, Nature 216: 762-766, 1967.
17. Aiken JW and Vane JR, Circ Res 30: 263-273, 1972.
18. Freeman RH et al, Fed Proc 36: 1766-1770, 1977.
19. Peach MJ, Physiol Rev 57:313-330, 1977.
20. Swales JD, Pharmac Ther 7: 173-201, 1979.
21. Heptinstall RH, in Pathology of the Kidney, Little Brown and Co.,
     Boston 1974, pp 26-30. ISBN 0-316-35795.
22. Davis JO and Freeman RH, Physiol Rev 56: 1-56, 1976.
23. Weber PC et al, Klin Wochenshr 57: 1021-1029, 1979.
24. Ganten D et al, AM J Med 60: 760-772, 1976.
25. Skeggs LT et al, Fed Proc 36: 1755-1759, 1977.
26. Reid IA, Circ Res 41: 147-153, 1977.
27. Swales JD, Cardiovascular Rev and Reports 1: 309-315, 1980.
28. Thurston H et al, Hypertension 1: 643-649, 1979.
29. Sealey JE, in Frontiers in Hypertension Research (JH Laragh
     et al, eds) Springer Verlag, New York, 1981, pp 246-257
     ISBN 0-387-90557.
30. Swales JD, in Recent advances in clinical chemistry (K.G.M.M.
     Alberti and C.P.Price, eds) Churchill Livingstone,Edinburgh
     London 1981, pp 170-195.
31. Ondetti MA et al, Science 196: 441-444, 1977.
32. Engel SL et al, Proc Soc Exp Biol Med 140: 240-244, 1972.
33. Pals DT et al, Circ Res 29: 673-681, 1971.
34. Murthy et al, Circ Res 43: Suppl 1: 41-45, 1978.
35. Thurston H, in Angiotensin Converting enzyme inhibitors
     (ZP Horovitz ed) Urban and Schwarzenberg, Baltimore-Munich,
     1981, pp 141-159. ISBN 0-8067-0821-2.
36. Bohr DF, in Angiotensin (IH Page and FM Bumpus eds) Springer
     Verlag, Berlin, Heidelberg New York, 1974, pp 424-440
     ISBN 3-540-06276-9.
37. Buckley JP and Jandhyala BS, Life Sciences 20: 1485-1494, 1977.
38. Malik KU and Nasjletti A, Circ Res 38: 26-30, 1976.
39. Laragh JH and Sealey JE, in Handbook of Physiology: Renal
     Physiology (J Orloff and RW Berliner eds)American Physiological
     Society, Washington DC, 1973, pp 831-908.
40. Davis JO et al, Circ Res 34: 279-285, 1974.
41. Robertson PW et al, Am J Med 43: 963-976, 1967.
42. Williamson R et al, Quart J Med 39: 377-394, 1970.
43. Weidman P et al, Kidney Int 9: 294-301, 1976.
44. Vaughan ED et al, in Hypertension Manual (JH Laragh ed) Yorke
     Medical Books, New York 1974, pp 559-582. ISBN 0-914316-00-1.
45. Marks LS et al, Lancet 615-617, 1977.
46. Brunner HR, N Engl J Med 286: 441-449, 1972.
47. Swales JD and Thurston H, Clin Sci 52: 371-375, 1977.
48. Thurston H et al, Clin Sci 58: 15-20, 1980.
49. Russell GI, Clin Sci, in press, 1981.
50. Thurston H et al, Hypertension 2: 256-265, 1980.
51. Grollman A and Krishnamurty VSR, Am J Physiol 221: 1499-1506,
     1971.

52. Skeggs LT et al, Circ Res 40: 143-149, 1977.
53. Boucher R et al, Clin Sci 55: Suppl 4, 183s-186s, 1978.
54. Ulvila JM et al, JAMA 220: 233-238, 1972.
55. Houck CR, Am J Physiol 176: 183-189, 1954.
56. Guyton AC et al, Circ Res 26: Suppl II, 135-147, 1970.
57. Guyton AC et al, in Hypertension Manual (JH Laragh ed) Yorke
      Medical Books, New York, 1974, pp 111-134. ISBN 0-914316-00-1.
58. Conway J and Hatton R, Circ Res 43: Suppl 1, 82-86, 1978.
59. Kim KE et al, Clin Sci Mol Med 51: Suppl 3, 223s-225s.
60. Chanutin A and Ferris E, Arch Intern Med 49: 767-787, 1932.
61. Wood JE and Ethridge C, Proc Soc Exp Biol Med 30: 1039-1041,
      1933.
62. Braun-Menendez E and Von Euler VS, Nature (Lond) 160: 905, 1947.
63. Grollman A et al, Am J Physiol 157: 21-30, 1949.
64. Tobian L, J Clin Invest 29: 849 (abstract), 1950.
65. Kolff WJ and Page IH, Am J Physiol 178: 75-81, 1954.
66. Merrill JP et al, Am J Med 31: 931-940, 1961.
67. Floyer MA, Clin Sci 14: 163-181, 1955.
68. Carretero O and Scicli AG, Am J Physiol 238: F247-F255, 1980.
69. Ørstavik TB et al, J Histochem Cytochem 24: 1037-1039, 1976.
70. Carretero O et al, in Mechanism of hypertension (M Sambhi ed)
      Excerpta Medica, New York, 1973, pp 290-299.
71. Hial V et al, Biochem Pharmacol 25: 2499-2503, 1976.
72. Nasjletti A et al, Circ Res 37: 59-65, 1975.
73. Erdos EG, Am J Med 60: 749-759, 1976.
74. Nasjletti A and Malik KU, Life Sci 25: 99-110, 1979.
75. McGiff JC, Clin Sci 59: 105s-116s, 1980.
76. Mills IH, Nephron 23: 61-71, 1979.
77. Dunn MJ and Hood VL, Am J Physiol 233: F169-F184, 1977.
78. Weber PC, et al, Klin Wochenschr 57: 1021-1029, 1979.
79. Moncada SR, et al, Nature 263: 663-665, 1975.
80. Gerber JG, Kidney Int 19: 816-821, 1981.
81. Dunn MJ and Zambraski EJ, Kidney Int 18: 609-622, 1980.
82. Muirhead EE and Pitcock JA, in The Renal Papilla and Hypertension
      (AK Mandal and SV Bohman eds) Plenum Medical Book Company,
      New York and London, 1980, pp 35-61. ISBN 0-306-4506-7.
83. Prewitt RL et al, Hypertension 1: 299-308, 1979.
84. Sušić D, in The renal papilla and hypertension (AK Mandal and
      SV Bohman eds) Plenum Medical Book Company, New York and
      London, 1980, pp 63-76. ISBN 0-306-4506-7.
85. Shimamura T, Exp Mol Pathol 25: 1-8, 1976.
86. Heptinstall RH et al, Am J Pathol 78: 279-308, 1975.
87. Bing RF et al, Clin Sci (in press).
88. Russell GI et al, Clin Sci (in press).
89. Boscolo P et al, Toxicol Lett 7: 189-194, 1981.
90. Thind CS et al, J Lab Clin Med 76: 560-568, 1970.
91. Perry HM et al, J Lab Clin Med 76: 541-547, 1970.
92. Kazantzis G et al, Quart J Med 32: 165-192, 1963.
93. Bousquet WF, in Cadmium Toxicity (JH Mennear ed) Marcel
      Dekker, New York, 1979, pp 133-157.
94. Perry HM and Erlanger MW, J Lab Clin Med 76: 852 (abstract)
      1970.
95. Lener J and Musil J, Experientia 27: 902, 1970.
96. Iannaccone A et al, Adv Exp Med Biol 120:683-684, 1979.
97. Lane RE, Br J Mol Med 6: 125-143, 1949.
98. Cramér K and Dahlberg L, ibid 23: 101-104, 1966.

 99. Beevers DG et al, Lancet ii: 1-3, 1976.
100. Sanstead HH et al, Arch Environ Health 20: 356-363, 1970.
101. McAllister RC et al, Arch Intern Med 172: 919-923, 1971.
102. Campbell BC, Arch Environ Health 34: 439-443, 1979.
103. Boscolo G et al, Br J Ind Med 35: 226-229, 1978.
104. Massani ZM et al, Clin Sci 30: 473-483, 1966.
105. Brown JJ et al, Br Med J 1: 253-258, 1970.
106. Dibona GF and Swain LL, Lab Invest 25: 528-532, 1971.
107. Flamenbaum W, Arch Intern Med 131: 911-928, 1973.
108. Oken DE, Kidney Int 10: 594-599, 1976.
109. Oken DE, Kidney Int 7: 12-18, 1975.
110. Powell-Jackson JD et al, in Proc Conf on Acute Renal Failure
        (Friedman EA and Eliahou HE eds) US Government Printing
        Office, Washington DC, 1973, pp 281-289.
111. Bidani AK and Churchill PC, Am J Physiol 241: F34-F38, 1981.
112. Mendelsohn FAO and Smith EA, Kidney Int 17: 465-472, 1980.
        1980.
113. Swales JD, in Sodium in Metabolic Disease, Lloyd-Luke, London,
        1975, pp 174-175. ISBN 0-85324-116-3.
114. Agrest A and Finkielman S, Am J Cardiol 19: 213-220, 1967.
115. Murray TG and Goldberg M, Kidney Int 13: 64-71, 1978.
116. Gloor FJ, Kidney Int 13: 27-33, 1978.

RENAL DRUG METABOLISM AND NEPHROTOXICITY

G. F. Rush and J. B. Hook

Department of Pharmacology and Toxicology, Center for Environmental Toxicology, Michigan State University, East Lansing, Michigan 48824, USA

ABSTRACT

Xenobiotic metabolism in the liver may result in both inactivation and activation of a variety of chemicals. Metabolic activation of a chemical may result in the production of electrophiles or free radicals which may covalently bind to cellular proteins and disrupt normal cell function. The kidney appears to have at least two independent systems for bioactivating chemicals. Renal cytochrome P_{450} mediated drug metabolism is restricted to the kidney cortex and has been suggested to mediate the metabolic activation of chloroform, carbon tetrachloride and paracetamol (acetaminophen). In contrast, prostaglandin endoperoxide synthetase is localized to the inner medulla and papilla and is capable of cooxygenating a variety of substrates with arachidonic acid. Cooxygenation can result in the production of reactive metabolites capable of binding covalently to cellular protein. In addition, cooxidation of compounds like benzidine or N-[4-(5-nitro-2-furyl)-2-thiazolyl]formamide (FANFT) may be involved in their carcinogenic actions.

KEY WORDS: Metabolic activation; cytochrome P_{450}; prostaglandin endoperoxide synthetase; xenobiotic metabolism; cooxidation; acetaminophen; chloroform; carcinogen

INTRODUCTION

Metabolism of xenobiotics, although traditionally considered a detoxifying process, may result in the formation of toxic reactive metabolites, generally electrophiles or free radicals, which may covalently bind to cellular macromolecules and disrupt normal cell function [1,2]. In addition to the extensively studied hepatic systems, drug metabolizing enzymes are also present in many extrahepatic organs including the kidney [3]. Intrarenal drug metabolism is quantitatively much less than hepatic metabolism and appears to make only a minor contribution to total body metabolism of most chemicals (Table 1). However, in specific cases, intrarenal metabolism may play a crucial role in nephrotoxicity. We became interested in the role of renal drug metabolism in nephrotoxicity following the contamination of the food chain in Michigan by a complex mixture of polybrominated biphenyls (PBBs) [4]. PBBs, by themselves, appear to produce no functional or morphological toxicity in laboratory animals. However, they increase markedly the activities of both hepatic and renal mixed function oxidases (MFOs) [5]. PBBs are considered to be mixed inducers, that is, they induce rat liver MFOs in a fashion similar to a mixture of phenobarbital and 3-methylcholanthrene (3MC) [6]. PBBs, by virtue of their ability to induce renal MFOs have also been shown to potentiate the nephrotoxicity of chemicals such as chloroform and carbon tetrachloride [7].

Recently, another mechanism for the metabolic activation of nephrotoxic chemicals has been proposed to proceed via cooxidation with arachidonic acid by prostaglandin endoperoxide synthetase [8,9]. The purpose of this report is to provide a review of the mechanisms involved in renal drug metabolism and their role in chemically induced renal damage.

TABLE 1.   Rat liver and kidney mixed function oxidases

Tissue	Cytochrome P_{450}[a]	Ethoxyresorufin O-deethylase[b]	Benzphetamine N-demethylase[b]
Liver	0.50	2.10	1.8
Kidney	0.07	0.02	N.D.

[a] nmoles/mg protein.   [b] nmoles product/min/mg protein.
N.D. = not detected.

TARGET ORGAN TOXICITY

The kidney, unlike the liver, contains marked structural, biochemical, histochemical and functional heterogeneity. Likewise, enzymes capable of transforming endogenous and exogenous chemicals are not uniformly distributed within the kidney but have a limited distribution among cell types [10,11]. Zenser et al. [10] have shown that cytochrome P_{450} and monooxygenase activity exhibit a cortico-papillary gradient, being greatest in the cortex and least in the inner medulla and papilla (Table 2). NADPH cytochrome P_{450} reductase, an essential electron transport component of the cytochrome P_{450} MFO system, has been localized to a discrete nephron segment (late proximal tubule) by immunohistochemical techniques [12]. Fowler et al. administered 2,3,7,8- tetrachlorodibenzo-p-dioxin (TCDD) to rats and observed a proliferation of the endoplasmic reticulum in the S_3 cells of the proximal tubule while the anatomically adjacent S_2 cells were unaffected [11]. Recently, using an antibody prepared against cytochrome P_{450} from pig kidneys, Masters et al. have demonstrated that the morphological localization of cytochrome P_{450} to the proximal tubule is similar to NADPH cytochrome P_{450} reductase [13]. Thus, it is not surprising that administration of nephrotoxic chemicals that undergo bioactivation by renal mixed function oxidases may result in renal cortical damage that is confined to the late proximal tubule (e.g., chloroform).

Another characteristic of the mammalian kidney is that it contains two independent mechanisms for bioactivation of chemicals, each with distinct

anatomical locations [14]. When examining the nephrotoxic effects of acetaminophen, Joshi et al. observed that the inner medulla covalently bound more
radiolabeled acetaminophen than the cortex [15]. Since MFOs were virtually
absent in this section of the kidney, there must have been an alternative pathway
for metabolic activation [16]. This pathway may involve a prostaglandin
endoperoxide synthetase, requiring arachidonic acid and O_2 [17]. Many
compounds are known to be cooxidized with arachidonic acid by prostaglandin
endoperoxide synthetase to a chemically reactive species capable of covalently
binding to cellular proteins. Counter to the MFO system, renal prostaglandin
endoperoxide synthetase exhibits a papillary to cortical gradient (highest in the
papilla) (Table 2) [14]. By employing histological, immunofluorescence techniques, Smith et al. have shown that prostaglandin endoperoxide synthetase is
located primarily in the epithelial cells of the cortical and medullary collecting
ducts, arterial vascular endothelial cells and medullary interstitial cells [18].
Recently, Zenser et al. have suggested that prostaglandin endoperoxide synthetase may be involved in the activation of FANFT and other known bladder
carcinogens [9,19].

TABLE 2. Oxidation of 1,3-diphenylisobenzofuran by
NADPH and arachidonic acid dependent pathways in different segments of the kidney

Tissue	Cooxidation (nmol/mg/min)
Cortex	
Arachidonic acid	0.5 ± 0.2
NADPH	10.0 ± 1.1
Outer Medulla	
Arachidonic acid	1.0 ± 0.4
NADPH	3.0 ± 0.6
Inner Medulla	
Arachidonic acid	10.2 ± 1.4
NADPH	0.7 ± 0.2

Modified from Zenser et al. [9].

RENAL DRUG METABOLISM

Mixed function oxidases. Cytochrome P_{450} is the terminal component of an
electron transport chain responsible for the oxidation of many xenobiotics and
endogenous compounds. When this cytochrome is reduced with dithionite and
saturated with CO it has an absorption maxium at 450 nm. Like the liver, the
kidney contains a system involving NADPH and cytochrome P_{450} for metabolizing both endogenous and exogenous substrates. In many respects, this system is
very similar to that in the liver. For example, many of the different substrates
metabolized by hepatic enzyme systems are also metabolized by renal enzymes.
Oxidative drug metabolism in the renal cortex is thought to involve the same
electron transport systems (NADPH and NADH) as the liver. In fact, renal
NADPH cytochrome P_{450} reductase is immunologically identical to that found
in the liver. Like the liver, the kidney also appears to contain multiple forms of
cytochrome P_{450} some of which may be identical to the hepatic forms [20,21].

Renal MFOs also have important differences from the hepatic system. The absorption maximum of the reduced hemoprotein CO complex is at 452 to 454 nm in the kidney rather than 450 nm as in the liver [22]. While ω and $\omega-1$ hydroxylation occurs in both liver and kidney, the liver system appears to involve multiple forms of cytochrome P_{450} while the kidney system involves only one form [23]. Like the liver, renal arylhydrocarbon hydroxylase and other enzymes have an absolute requirement for NADPH; however, renal laurate hydroxylation can be supported by NADH alone ($\approx$50% of the NADPH dependent rate) [24]. In addition, antibodies to cytochrome b5 will inhibit both the NADPH and NADH dependent renal drug metabolism suggesting a more definitive role of NADH in renal drug metabolism [23]. Recently, Masters et al. have successfully isolated and purified a form of porcine renal P_{450} with a molecular weight of approximately 56,000 daltons [13]. In a reconstituted system, this P_{450} supported the hydroxylation of lauric acid. The addition of NADH and cytochrome b5 stimulated lauric acid hydroxylation by 4-fold and antibodies prepared against this P_{450} inhibited both the ω and $\omega-1$ hydroxylation of lauric acid in a reconstituted system [25,26].

Some of the agents known to induce hepatic MFOs will also induce renal MFOs. This induction is, however, species specific (Table 3). While it is well known that phenobarbital and β-naphthoflavone will induce rat and mouse hepatic MFOs in distinctive fashions, only β-naphthoflavone will induce the rat kidney; phenobarbital has no effect. In contrast, rabbit renal MFOs are inducible with phenobarbital [27,28] (Table 3). Data on renal MFOs in the hamster are not yet available but preliminary results in the guinea pig indicate that like the rat, the guinea pig kidney responds only to β-naphthoflavone (J. Smith, G. Rush and J.B. Hook, unpublished observations).

Prostaglandin Cooxidation.   Prostaglandin endoperoxide synthetase (PES) is an enzyme found in highest concentrations in seminal vesicle, platelets and kidney medulla [29]. This enzyme catalyzes the oxygenation of polyunsaturated fatty acids (primarily arachidonic acid) to hydroxy endoperoxides called PGHs

TABLE 3.   The effects of inducers on renal MFOs in the rat and rabbit

	Cytochrome P_{450}[a]	Ethoxyresorufin O-deethylase[b]	Benzphetamine N-demethylase[b]
Rat			
Control	0.06	0.02	N.D.
Phenobarbital	0.06	0.02	N.D.
β-Naphthoflavone	0.21[c]	16.07[c]	N.D.
Polybrominated Biphenyls	0.09[c]	4.13[c]	N.D.
Rabbit			
Control	0.10	0.01	0.19
Phenobarbital	0.40[c]	0.01	1.08[c]
β-Naphthoflavone	0.20[c]	1.13[c]	0.20
Polybrominated Biphenyls	0.40[c]	1.66[c]	0.52[c]

[a]nmoles/mg protein.   [b]nmoles product/mg protein/min.   [c]Significantly different from control.   N.D. = not detected.

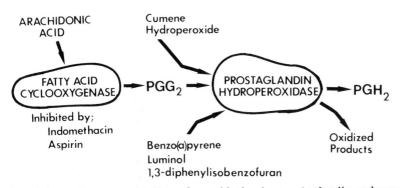

Fig. 1. Schematic representation of cooxidation by prostaglandin endoperoxide synthetase.

[30,31]. Free fatty acid concentrations are normally very low in most cells and a lipase catalyzed release of substrate from intracellular stores is a prerequisite for prostaglandin endoperoxide biosynthesis [32,33]. The intracellular location of PES is primarily restricted to the endoplasmic reticulum and nuclear membrane in 3TC fibroblasts [34]. Miyamoto and others have shown that purified PES from ram seminal vesicle has two enzyme activities (Fig. 1) [35-37], a fatty acid cyclooxygenase activity that catalyzes the bis-dioxygenation of arachidonic acid to the hydroperoxy endoperoxide, PGG_2, and a hydroperoxidase that reduces PGG_2 to PGH_2 [38]. During the formation of PGH from arachidonic acid, a number of organic compounds are cooxygenated. Luminol, diphenylisobenzofuran (DPBF) and oxyphenylbutazone are examples of compounds oxygenated by this mechanism [29]. Arachidonic acid dependent cooxidation is inhibited by indomethacin, aspirin, and dimercaptopropanol (potent inhibitors of PES activity). In the absence of arachidonic acid, oxygenation of DPBF and luminol can be triggered by the addition of the hydroperoxy endoperoxide, PGG_2, 15 hydroperoxy-5,8,11,13 eicosatetraenoic acid, cumene hydroperoxide and tert-butyl hydroperoxide, but not by the hydroxyendoperoxide, PGH_2, suggesting that the hydroperoxy group may be essential to the cooxidative process [39]. Furthermore, indomethacin, which inhibits the arachidonic acid dependent cooxygenation by its action on the cyclooxygenase, does not inhibit the reaction when PGG_2 or the other hydroperoxides are used [40]. Zenser et al. have shown cooxidation of FANFT by Tween 20 solubilized kidney inner medullary microsomes [19]. Reconstitution with Mn^{3+}-protoporphyrin IX (which selectively reconstitutes the cyclooxygenase activity and not the hydroperoxidase) did not reactivate the cooxidation of FANFT [19,29]. Thus, it appears that cooxidation of organic compounds by PES are hydroperoxide-dependent oxygenations catalyzed by prostaglandin hydroperoxidase.

The identity of the reactive species in cooxidation is unknown. Oxygen incorporation is apparently not from the hydroperoxide but rather from atmospheric oxygen [39]. Since a variety of antioxidants are potent inhibitors of cooxidation, Marnett has suggested that the oxidation probably occurs by a free radical pathway [29]. Although these oxidations appear to be radical mediated, the exact mechanism will probably vary with each hydrocarbon and differences in cooxidative products are probably due to the different chemistry of each hydrocarbon [29].

NEPHROTOXIC COMPOUNDS

Acetaminophen. Acetaminophen (4-hydroxyacetanilide, paracetamol) is a commonly used analgesic and antipyretic agent. In therapeutic doses it appears to be relatively non-toxic. However, ingestion of large amounts of acetamino-phen, either acutely or chronically, is associated with marked clinical conse-quences. A single large dose may result in acute hepatic necrosis which may be associated with acute tubular necrosis and renal failure. There is also a chronic active hepatitis-like syndrome in the susceptible individual. Finally, chronic consumption may result in papillary necrosis; this usually occurs in patients consuming a combination of analgesics (e.g., acetaminophen and salicylate) [16].

Mitchell et al. and others have shown that acetaminophen-induced tissue damage is apparently not due to the parent compound but occurs subsequent to metabolic activation [41,42]. Acetaminophen may be bioactivated by two systems: Mixed function oxidases are known to metabolize acetaminophen in both the liver and kidney cortex to a metabolite capable of depleting tissue glutathione followed by covalent binding to cellular macromolecules [42,43]. Reactive metabolites produced following low doses of acetaminophen appear to be effectively detoxified by conjugation with glutathione. Only after massive doses is the tissue glutathione critically depleted followed by irreversible binding of the reactive intermediate to cellular macromolecules and possible cellular injury [41-43]. Alternatively, recent evidence by Mohandes et al. have indicated that acetaminophen may be metabolically activated by cooxidation with arachidonic acid by prostaglandin endoperoxide synthetase to a reactive intermediate capable of binding to cellular protein [17].

Metabolism by MFOs. Renal MFOs are located in the renal cortex [10]. In addition, NADPH dependent covalent binding of acetaminophen occurs in the cortex and correlates with the histological lesion observed following an acute dose of acetaminophen indicating that renal metabolic activation of acetamino-phen may proceed by a mechanism similar to that in the liver [44]. Recently Mudge (personal communication) has suggested that the kidney may deacetylate acetaminophen to para-aminophenol, a known nephrotoxicant. McMurtry et al. and Mudge et al. have reported the depletion of renal cortical and papillary glutathione by acetaminophen and subsequent covalent binding to protein [44,45]. Recently, Newton et al. [46] demonstrated dose dependent depletion of cortical glutathione by acetaminophen in the isolated perfused rat kidney. In these studies the renal excretion of some of the major acetaminophen metabo-lites were quantified (Table 4). Excretion of metabolites occurred mainly as the sulfate, glucuronide and the N-acetylcysteine conjugates. Induction of mixed function oxidases by either phenobarbital, 3MC or PBBs have differential effects on acetaminophen induced renal damage. Phenobarbital, as discussed earlier, does not alter rat renal MFOs and accordingly does not alter acetaminophen renal toxicity in rats. Surprisingly, induction of MFOs by 3MC, while increasing the hepatic necrosis, had no effect on renal acetaminophen-induced damage or covalent binding [44]. However, administration of PBBs has been demonstrated to potentiate the renal depletion of glutathione by acetaminophen and increase the excretion of the N-acetylcysteine conjugate of acetaminophen by the isolated perfused kidney (Table 4).

Metabolism by prostaglandin synthetase. In vivo binding studies have shown that the greatest amount of covalent binding of acetaminophen occurs in the renal inner medulla, the location with the least amount of MFO activity [47]. Thus, it was postulated by Duggin that another mechanism might exist for the activation of acetaminophen in the medulla [48]. Zenser et al. demonstrated that acetaminophen could weakly inhibit prostaglandin E_2 and $F_{2\alpha}$ synthesis in rabbit renal inner medulla and later suggested that cooxidation with arachidonic acid by prostaglandin synthetase may be responsible for the covalent medullary protein binding [47,49]. Subsequently, Mohandas et al. have shown arachidonic

TABLE 4.   Effects of polybrominated biphenyls on the excretion of acetamino-phen metabolites in the isolated perfused rat kidney.

Pretreatment	Acetaminophen in Perfusate	Excretion of Acetaminophen Metabolite[a]		
		Sulfate	Glucuronide	N-acetylcysteine
None	3×10^{-5}M	772	272	44
PBB	3×10^{-5}M	571	220	172[b]

[a]ng of conjugate/g kidney/hr. [b]Significantly different from control, $p < .05$. Modified from [46].

acid dependent covalent binding of acetaminophen to renal medullary micro-somes [17].   While compounds like glutathione, ascorbic acid and ethoxyquin inhibited both NADPH and arachidonic dependent covalent binding of acetamino-phen to protein, indomethacin and aspirin inhibited only the arachidonic acid dependent covalent binding.   Organic hydroperoxides such as cumene hydroper-oxide have been shown to initiate cooxidative metabolism of acetaminophen [49].

Thus, the activation of acetaminophen by prostaglandin synthetase appears to be catalyzed by the hydroperoxidase as is the case with luminol and benzo(a)py-rene.   It must be recognized, however, that renal papillary and inner medullary tissue damage is not a common problem following acute acetaminophen admini-stration.   In fact, it usually appears after long-term use and in combination with other analgesics like salicylates which inhibit the prostaglandin synthetase. Thus, the toxicological significance of acetaminophen cooxidation and subse-quent protein binding is not clear.

Chlorinated   hydrocarbons.   Many   of   the   small   aliphatic,   halogenated hydrocarbon solvents require bioactivation prior to producing nephrotoxicity and hepatotoxicity.   It appears that MFOs are necessary for the generation of toxic metabolites   of   solvents   such   as   chloroform   ($CHCl_3$),   carbon   tetrachloride, trichloroethylene and 1,1,2-trichloroethane [7].   The acute nephrotoxicity to $CHCl_3$ is characterized morphologically as necrosis of the proximal tubular cells and functionally as a decrease in organic acid transport and an increase in blood urea   nitrogen   [7,50].   In   addition,   a   chemically   reactive   intermediate   of chloroform metabolism, phosgene, has been identified [51].   Pretreatment of rats and mice with phenobarbital potentiates the hepatotoxicity of $CHCl_3$ but not the renal toxicity.   Alternatively, 3MC has little effect on hepatic CHCl toxicity but markedly reduces renal toxicity.   On the other hand, pretreatment of   mice   with   PBB   potentiates   the   nephrotoxicity   of   chloroform   in   a   dose dependent fashion while pretreatment of mice with polychlorinated biphenyls protects the kidney from $CHCl_3$-induced damage [52].   Environmental contami-nants like PBBs also enhance the nephrotoxicity of other halogenated hydrocar-bons like carbon tetrachloride, trichlorethylene and 1,1,2-trichloroethane [7].

There are no reports to date implicating any role of cooxidation with prostaglandin synthetase of the halogenated hydrocarbons.

RENAL ACTIVATION OF CARCINOGENS

Benzidine, an aromatic amine, causes urinary bladder tumors and nephrotoxi-city in certain species.   It has been suggested that benzidine must be metabolically activated to a reactive intermediate to elicit a toxic response [53]. Recently, Zenser et al. have reported data consistent with the hypothesis that the renal inner medulla is a site for the metabolism of certain chemicals which induce bladder cancer [19]. The hydroperoxidase of prostaglandin synthetase will cooxidize the bladder carcinogens FANFT and benzidine [9,19]. As mentioned earlier, prostaglandin synthetase is in high concentration in the epithelial cells of the collecting duct [18]. Since the urine is greatly concentrated in the presence of antidiuretic hormone and that these cells are in contact with the urine just before entry into the urinary space, the inner medulla is ideally suited for playing a key role in the bioactivation of bladder carcinogens.

ACKNOWLEDGEMENTS

The authors' research is supported by USPHS Grant No. ES00560. We wish to thank D. Hummel for her skillful help in preparing this mansucript.

REFERENCES

1. Ames BN, Durston WE, Yamasaki E and Lee FD, Proc Natl Acad Sci USA 78:2281-2285, 1973.
2. Gillette JR, Mitchell JR and Brodie BB, Ann Rev Pharmacol 14:271-289, 1974.
3. Jones DP, Orrenius S and Jakobson SW, in Extrahepatic Metabolism of Drugs and Other Foreign Compounds. S.P. Medical and Scientific Books, New York, 1980, p. 123-158.
4. Dunkel AE, J Amer Vet Med Assoc 167:838-841, 1975.
5. McCormack KM, Kluwe WM, Rickert DW, Sanger VL and Hook JB, Toxicol Appl Pharmacol 44:539-553, 1978.
6. Dent JG, Environ Health Perspect 23:301-307, 1978.
7. Kluwe WM and Hook JB, Kidney Int 18:648-655, 1980.
8. Marnett LJ, Reed GA and Johnson ST, Biochem Biophys Res Commun 79:569-576, 1977.
9. Zenser TV, Mattammal MB and Davis BB, J. Pharmacol Exptl Ther 211:460-464, 1979.
10. Zenser TV, Mattammal MB and Davis BB, J Pharmacol Exptl Ther 207:719-725, 1978.
11. Fowler BA, Hook GER and Lucier GW, J Pharmacol Exptl Ther 203:712-721, 1977.
12. Dees JH, Coe LD, Yasukochi Y and Masters BSS, Science 208:1473, 1980.
13. Masters BSS, Parkhill LK and Okita RT, Fed. Proc. 40:697, 1981.
14. Zenser TV, Mattammal MB and Davis BB, J Pharmacol Exptl Ther 208:418-421, 1979.
15. Joshi S, Zenser TV, Mattammal MB, Herman CA and Davis BB, J Lab Clin Med 92:924-931, 1978.
16. Duggin GG, Kidney Int 18:553-561, 1980.
17. Mohandas J, Duggin GG, Horvath JS and Tiller DJ, Toxicol Appl Pharmacol (in press).
18. Smith WL and Bell TG, Am J Physiol 235:F451-F457, 1978.
19. Zenser TV, Mattammal MB and Davis BB, Cancer Res 40:114-118, 1980.
20. Liem HH, Muller-Eberhard U and Johnson EK, Mol Pharmacol 18:565-570, 1980.
21. Guengerich FP and Mason PS, Mol Pharmacol 15:154-164, 1979.

22. Orrenius S, Ellin A, Jakobson SW, Thor H, Cinti DL, Schenkman JB and Estabrook RW, Drug Metab Disp 1:350-357, 1973.
23. Okita RT and Masters BSS, Drug Metab Disp 8:147-151, 1980.
24 Ellin A, Jakobson SW, Schenkman JB and Orrenius S, Arch Biochem Biophys 150:64-71, 1972.
25. Sasame HA, Thorgeirsson SS, Mitchell JR and Gillette JR, Life Sci 14:35-45, 1974.
26. Masters BSS, Okita RT, Dees, JH, Yasukochi Y and Parkhill LK, Fifth Intl. Symposium on Microsomes and Drug Oxidations, p. 48, 1981.
27. Uhleke H and Greim H, Naunyn-Schmiedeberg's Arch Pharmak Exp Path 361:152-161, 1968.
28. Rush FG and Hook JB, Fed Proc 40:637, 1981.
29. Marnett LJ, Life Sciences 29:531-546, 1981.
30. Hamberg M and Samuelsson B, Proc Natl Acad Sci USA 70:899-903, 1973.
31. Nugteren DH and Hagelhof E, Biochim Biophys Acta 326:448-461, 1973.
32. Lands WEM and Samuelson B, Biochim Biophys Acta 164:426-429, 1968.
33. Vonkeman H and Van Dorp DA, Biochim Biophys Acta 164:430-432, 1968.
34. Rollins TE and Smith WL, J Biol Chem 255:4872-4875, 1980.
35. Miyamoto T, Ogino N, Yamamoto S and Hayaishi O, J Biol Chem 251:2629-2936, 1976.
36. Vander Oucheraa FJ, Buytenhek M, Nugteren DH and Van Dorp DA, Biochim Biophys Acta 487:315-331, 1977.
37. Ogino N, Ohki S, Yamamoto S and Hayaishi O, J Biol Chem 253:5061-5069, 1978.
38. Ohki S, Ogino M, Yamamoto S and Hayaishi, J Biol Chem 254:836-839, 1979.
39. Marnett LJ and Bienkowski MJ, Biochem Biophys Res Commun 96:639-647, 1980.
40. Marnett LJ, Wlodawer P and Samuelsson B, J Biol Chem 250:8510-8517, 1975.
41. Mitchell JR, Jollow DJ, Potter WZ, Davis DC, Gillette JR and Brodie BB, J Pharmacol Exptl Ther 187:185-194, 1973.
42. Jollow DW, Mitchell JR, Potter WZ, Davis DC, Gillette JR and Brodie BB, J Pharmacol Exptl Ther 187:195-202, 1973.
43. Mitchell JR, Jollow DJ, Potter WZ, Gillette JR and Brodie BB, J Pharmacol Exptl Ther 187:211-217, 1973.
44. McMurtry RJ, Snodgrass WR and Mitchell JR, Toxicol Appl Pharmacol 46:87-100, 1978.
45. Mudge GH, Gemborys MW and Duggin GG, J Pharmacol Exptl Ther 206:218-226, 1978.
46. Newton JF, Kluwe WM and Hook JB, Toxicol Appl Pharmacol 48:A19, 1979.
47. Mattammal MB, Zenser TV, Brown WW, Herman CA and Davis BB, J Pharmacol Exptl Ther 210:405-409, 1979.
48. Duggin GG and Mohandas J, Eighth International Congress of Pharmacology (in press).
49. Zenser TV, Mattammal MB, Herman CA, Joshi S and Davis BB, Biochim Biophys Acta 542:486-495, 1978.
50. Kluwe WM and Hook JB, Toxicol Appl Pharmacol 45:861-869, 1978.
51. Pohl LR, Bhooshan B, Whittaker NF and Kirshna G, Biochem Biophys Res Commun 79:684, 1977.
52. Kluwe WM, McCormack KM and Hook JB, J Pharmacol Exptl Ther 207:566-573, 1978.
53. Miller EC, Cancer Res 38:1479-1496, 1978.

LOCALIZATION OF NADPH-CYTOCHROME P-450 REDUCTASE AND CYTOCHROME P-450 IN ANIMAL KIDNEYS

Jane H. Dees, Linda K. Parkhill, Richard T. Okita, Yukio Yasukochi and Bettie Sue Masters

Biochemistry Department, University of Texas Health Science Center at Dallas, Dallas, Texas 75235, USA

INTRODUCTION

The cytochrome P-450-containing monooxygenase system in kidney cortex microsomes was originally thought to be specialized almost exclusively for the ω and ω-1 hydroxylation of medium chain fatty acids [1]. It is now known that mixed function oxidase enzymes in the kidney are responsible not only for fatty acid hydroxylation, but also for the hydroxylation of steroids, prostaglandins, vitamin D, and a number of exogenous chemical compounds.

It is now accepted that a number of drug- and heavy metal-induced nephropathies may be influenced by cytochrome P-450-mediated metabolic pathways [2,3]. Some of the chemicals thought to cause kidney damage in this manner are: the analgesics, acetaminophen, phenacetin and the salicylates; cephaloridine and the cephalosporin antibiotics; furans and furosamides including 4-ipomeanol; halogenated hydrocarbons including chloroform, carbon tetrachlorides and bromobenzene; and certain carcinogens such as dimethylnitrosamine (DMNA). Many of these compounds cause extensive damage to the proximal tubules, particularly to the pars recta. Other compounds including environmental pollutants such as the polychlorinated biphenyls and polybrominated biphenyls (PCB's and PBB's), tetrachlorodibenzo-p-dioxin (TCDD), and hexachlorobenzene (HCB) are known to induce renal drug metabolism. Alterations in the smooth-surfaced endoplasmic reticulum (SER) can accompany exposure to certain of the nephrotoxins. Therefore, the localization of cytochrome P-450 and NADPH-cytochrome P-450 reductase is of vital importance to the understanding of the mechanisms of nephrotoxicity.

MIXED FUNCTION OXIDASE ENZYMES IN RAT KIDNEY

We have used indirect immunofluorescence to localize NADPH-cytochrome P-450 reductase [4] and cytochrome P-450 in the kidneys of

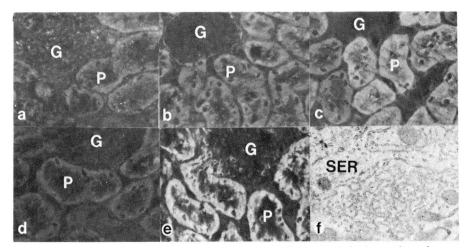

Figure 1. Rat Kidneys. a. non-immune control, normal kidney; b and c.
kidney sections from BNF-pretreated rats stained for NADPH-cytochrome
P-450 reductase and cytochrome P-450$_{kidney}$ respectively; d. normal
kidney stained for cytochrome P-448; e. kidney of BNF-pretreated rat
stained for cytochrome P-448; f. ultrathin section of kidney from a
BNF-pretreated rat showing proliferation of the smooth-surfaced endoplasmic reticulum (SER) in the base of a proximal tubule cell.
Glomerulus, G; proximal tubule, P; smooth-surfaced endoplasmic
reticulum, SER.

control rats, and rats pretreated with either phenobarbital (PB, an
inducer of P-450, 40mg/kg) or beta-naphthoflavone (BNF, an inducer of
P-448, 75mg/kg). We applied rabbit IgG against NADPH-cytochrome P-450
reductase isolated from untreated abattoir pig liver microsomes, or
against cytochrome P-450 isolated from untreated abattoir pig kidney
microsomes (cytochrome P-450$_{kidney}$) as our primary antibodies, and
fluorescein isothiocyanate-conjugated goat anti-rabbit IgG as our
secondary antibody, to frozen sections of rat kidney. In kidneys from
these animals specific fluorescence for NADPH-cytochrome P-450
reductase was present in all segments of the proximal tubules. The
glomerulus and all other segments of the nephron were negative.
Cytochrome P-450$_{kidney}$ stained the P_1 segment of the proximal tubule
weakly, the P_2 segment moderately, and the P_3 segments intensely. No
fluorescence was seen in the inner stripe of the outer medulla or the
inner medulla. We did not detect any appreciable difference in
staining for these two enzymes between control, PB- or BNF-pretreated
rats. However, when we stained for P-448, we saw only weak
fluorescence in the proximal tubules of control kidneys, but intense
fluorescence in the proximal tubules of BNF-pretreated animals.
Electron microscopy shows proliferation of the smooth-surfaced
endoplasmic reticulum (SER) in the proximal tubules of BNF-pretreated
rats. These results are consistent with the fact that phenobarbital
does not induce the mixed function oxidase enzymes in rat kidney, and
that BNF induces P-448, but not the cytochrome P-450$_{kidney}$. Results
in the minipig kidney show similar localization in PB and control
animals but BNF seems to have no effect.

Table 1. Kidney Mixed Function Oxidase Enzymes

	NADPH-cytochrome P-450 reductase (nmol/min/mg)		Cytochrome P-450 (nmol/mg)	
	Control	Test	Control	Test
RAT				
I Control vs PB	61.5	67.8	.34	.37
II Control vs PB	28.2	22.9	.23	.19
III Control vs BNF	44.5	59.2	.40	.95
MINIPIG				
I Control vs PB	28.25	31.8	.53	.53

MIXED FUNCTION OXIDASE ENZYMES IN CONTROL PB OR TCDD-PRETREATED RABBITS

TCDD or 2,3,7,8-tetrachlorodibenzo-p-dioxin, a by-product of the manufacture of a number of commercial chemicals, is an extremely toxic environmental pollutant having an LD_{50} of 3.1×10^{-9} moles/kg in guinea pigs [5]. It is thought to be teratogenic and carcinogenic. It is an inducer of aryl hydrocarbon hydroxylase, being 30,000 times as potent as 3-methylcholanthrene in this respect. In collaboration with Drs. Eric Johnson and Ursula Muller-Eberhard of the Scripps Clinic and Research Foundation, La Jolla, California, we studied the localization of four isozymes of cytochrome P-450 in control rabbits and in rabbits pretreated with PB (0.1% PB w/v in the drinking water) or TCDD (30nmol/kg, i.p.), using indirect immunofluorescence [6]. These isozymes were: Form 2 (LM_2), the major phenobarbital-inducible form in rabbit liver [7]; Form 3 (LM_3), a constitutive form in rabbit liver [8]; Form 4 (LM_4), the major form inducible in adult rabbit liver by beta-naphthoflavone or TCDD [9]; and Form 6 (LM_6), the major form inducible in neonatal rabbit liver by TCDD [10]. We find that Forms 2 and 3 are present in normal rabbit kidney in the proximal tubules of the cortex and outer stripe of the outer medulla, but that immunofluorescence for these two forms is markedly reduced in TCDD-pretreated animals. (Form 2 is induced in phenobarbital-pretreated rabbits.) In contrast, immunofluorescence for Forms 4 and 6 is weak to negative in control rabbit kidneys, but is strong in the kidneys of TCDD-pretreated rabbits where these forms are also induced in the endothelium of the renal vasculature. Thus, we see a shift from Forms 2 and 3 being predominant in normal rabbit kidneys to Forms 4 and 6 becoming predominant in kidneys from TCDD-pretreated rabbits. Johnson, et al. [11] have shown that the different forms of cytochrome P-450 metabolize 2-acetylaminofluorene (AAF) to different extents and by different pathways. Cytochrome P-450 Form 4 catalyzed the N-hydroxylation of AAF (activation), while Forms 3 and 6 catalyzed the ring hydroxylation of AAF (detoxication). Thus, a shift in balance among the multiple forms of cytochrome P-450 present in a tissue may affect the outcome (activation/detoxication) of exposure of that tissue to a given chemical, and has implications in both toxicity and carcinogenesis.

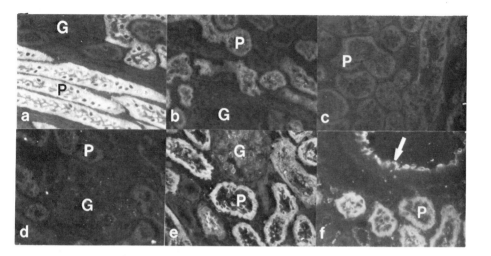

Figure 2. RABBIT KIDNEYS. a. normal kidney stained for cytochrome P-450 Form 2; b. kidney from a TCDD-pretreated rabbit stained for cytochrome P-450 Form 2; c. non-immune control; d. normal kidney stained for cytochrome P-450 Form 4; e and f. kidney sections from TCDD-pretreated rabbits stained for cytochrome P-450 Form 4. Glomerulus G; proximal tubule, P; endothelium, arrow.

CONCLUSIONS

Our immunofluorescence studies have shown that cytochrome P-450 and NADPH-cytochrome P-450 reductase are localized in the proximal tubules of rat, rabbit, and minipig kidneys, particularly the P_3 segment of the proximal tubule, and that no specific fluorescence was seen in the nephron segments in the inner stripe of the outer medulla or the inner medulla under the conditions which we examined. Certain isoenzymes of cytochrome P-450 in the rabbit appear in the endothelium of the renal vasculature following pretreatment of the animal with the Ah inducer, TCDD.

REFERENCES

1. Orrenius S, et al. Drug Metab. Dispo. 1:350-356, 1973.
2. Mitchell JR, et al. Amer. J. Med. 62:518-526, 1977.
3. Hook JR, et al. Revs. Biochem. Toxicol. 53-78, 1979.
4. Dees JH, et al. Science 208:1473-1475, 1980.
5. Poland A and Kende A, Fed. Proc. 35:2404-2411, 1976.
6. Dees JH, Submitted to Cancer Research.
7. Haugen DA, et al. J. Biol. Chem. 250:3567-3570, 1975.
8. Johnson EF, J. Biol. Chem. 255:304-309, 1980.
9. Johnson EF and Muller-Eberhard U, J. Biol. Chem. 252:2839-2845, 1977.
10. Norman RL, et al. J. Biol. Chem. 253:8640-8647, 1978.
11. Johnson EF, et al. Cancer Res. 40:4456-4459, 1980.

RENAL UPTAKE, STORAGE AND EXCRETION OF METALS

Gunnar F. Nordberg

*Department of Environmental Hygiene, School of Medicine, University of Umeå,
S-901 87 Umeå, Sweden*

ABSTRACT

Renal effects may be caused by about 20 metals or their compounds and mechanisms for their uptake in the kidney are thus of
interest. However, only for a limited number of these metals
does the renal effect develop as an early manifestation of poisoning. It is of particular importance to achieve and understanding of renal uptake mechanisms for those metal compounds whose
"critical" effect is excerted on the kidney.

In order to calculate the renal uptake, quantitative data on
distribution, renal uptake and excretion i.e. "the metabolic
model" of the metals in question must be known.

Absorption of metals into the body from exposure media e.g.
industrial air or food must be known. Such absorption factors
vary greatly depending on particle size of airborne metallic
dusts and various nutritional factors for metals that occur in
the diet.

Transport of metals in blood, particularly the proportion of
metal that occurs in the "diffusible" fraction in plasma is of
importance for renal uptake. The renal clearance of several
metals ions, as they occur in blood plasma, is lower than expected from their calculated glomerular filtration rate. A considerable tubular reabsorption thus occurs. Metals bound to
metallothionein(mol. wt. 6500) in plasma are, for example,
efficiently transported to the renal tubules by glomerular filtration and a subsequent almost complete tubular reabsorption.
Excretory mechanisms for metals include also transtubular transport. Excretion rate can in some instances be described as a
biological half-time for the kidney.

To exemplify the use of data on absorption, distribution and
renal uptake for risk estimation, a metabolic model for cadmium
is described. This model involves absorption factors from lung
and gastrointestinal tract, transport to the kidney and biological half-time in this organ. When used in combination with
an estimated "critical" renal cortical level(= 200 ug Cd/g)
exposure levels in industrial air or oral intake levels of
Cd leading to renal dysfunction can be calculated.

INTRODUCTION

A number of metals or their compounds may give rise to renal disease or dysfunction. Ag, Au, Be, Bi, Cd, Cr, Co, Cu, Ge, Hg, In, Mo, Ni, Pb, Pt, Te, Tl, U and V may give rise to such effects in man or experimental animals [1,2]. However, only for a limited number of these metals does the renal effect develop as an early manifestation of poisoning. It is of particular importance to achieve an understanding of renal uptake mechanisms for those metal compounds whose "critical effect" is exerted on the kidneys. An understanding of renal uptake, storage and excretion, i.e. the "metabolic model" allows predictions to be made about exposures that may give rise to undesirable effects if a critical tissue level for development of such an effect is known. Although an understanding of the mechanisms for renal handling of metals and their transport in the body is of great interest, the ultimate aim from the preventive medicine point of view must be to arrive at possibilities to predict the appearance of health effects and in this paper an example of such a metabolic model for cadmium will be given. Before a description and discussion of this example some general remarks will be given on metal uptake from exposure media such as food and inhaled air, and some other factors of general importance for distribution, renal uptake and excretion. Reviews on these aspects have been presented by WHO [3] for substances in general, by the Task Group on Metal Accumulation [4] and by Camner et al. [5] for metals. When specific references are not given in the following text, information is derived from these reviews.

UPTAKE AND ABSORPTION FROM EXPOSURE MEDIA

Metal uptake via the gastrointestinal tract is dependent on a number of factors. It varies greatly among metals and among compounds of the same metal. When metals occur as inorganic salts, their gastrointestinal absorption varies from less than 10% for cadmium, indium, tin and uranium to almost complete absorption (90-100%) for soluble inorganic salts of arsenic, germanium and thallium. The reason for this variation is not easily explained. General theory on the passage of chemical substances across cell-membranes involves the processes of passive diffusion and ultrafiltration. Some molecules which serve an important function in the organism may be carried across cell membranes by means of specialized systems. The diffusion of organic molecules through the cell membranes of the gastrointestinal tract are influenced by the lipid solubility and ionization of the molecule. Inorganic salts of metals are usually not lipid soluble and cannot be absorbed according to the principles mentioned. Metals are dissolved in the fluids of the gastrointestinal tract and subsequently absorbed. There is no generally valid theory concerning the absorption of inorganic metal salts and special systems such as those available for essential metals probably play an important part. For example the absorption mechanism for thallium is supposed to occur by the same system as for calcium and iron[6]. Various inorganic salts of the same metal may differ considerably in absorption. Their varying solubility in the fluids of the gastrointestinal tract may be an important factor as illustrated by various trivalent arsenic compounds.

A number of additional factors have been shown to influence gastrointestinal absorption, for example the magnitude of the dose[7] and the presence of various specific food components in the diet[8].

Inorganic and organometallic compounds of the same metal may differ

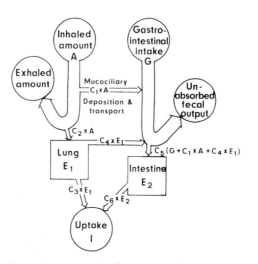

Figure 1 Model for the total (systemic) absorption (= uptake I) resulting from inhalation or gastrointestinal intake of a metal compound. The proportion (C_1) of the inhaled amount(A) that will be deposited on the mucociliary escalator and transferred to the GI tract varies with particle size (see Table 1). This is also the case regarding the proportion (C_2) deposited in the peripheral parts of the lung. The amount retained in these parts (E_1) will be dependent largely on in vivo solubility and the extent of phagocytosis, which processes govern the coefficients C_3 and C_4. The proportion (C_5) of the amount of metal present in the intestinal lumen that will be taken up in the intestinal mucosa (E_2) depends on a number of factors such as solubility and particle size. Retention in the mucosa is dependent on binding characteristics for the metal compound in intestinal cells, and C_6 therefore may vary dependent on, for example, the amount of metallothionein present in the mucosal cell.

From Nordberg and Kjellstrom, Environ Health Perspect 28: 211-217, 1979, Courtesy: National Institute of Environmental Health Sciences, US Dept. of Health, Education and Welfare.

considerably with regard to gastrointestinal absorption. Methyl mercury, for example is almost completely absorbed whereas divalent inorganic(Hg^{2+}) salts of this metal are absorbed only to an extent of about 10%[9].

After gastrointestinal absorption the metal may take various routes. There may be a direct uptake from the gastrointestinal tract into the mucosa and further transfer into the portal blood. A proportion of the metal may then be excreted through biliary excretion and then reabsorbed again from the gastrointestinal tract into the body. Such a recirculation between the gut and the liver i.e. enterohepatic circulation may be of great importance for some metals.

Exposure to metals by inhalation occurs in the form of a metal containing aerosol. The only exception to this is mercury vapour that is possible to inhale in gaseous form. Deposition and absorption of particulates in the respiratory tract has been discussed in relation to metals by the Task Group on Metal Accumulation[4]. Depending on

TABLE 1   Calculation of total absorption into the body as function of two different rates of alveolar absorption and different particle sizes for a specific deposition and clearance model.

Particle size (MMAD) (μm)	Alveolar deposition (%)	Tracheobronchial-nasopharyngeal deposition (%)	Total absorption(%) into body when alveolar absorption is	
			100%	50%
0.1	50	9	50.4	26.7
0.5	30	16	30.8	16.6
2.0	20	43	22.2	12.6
5.0	10	68	13.4	8.6
10.0	5	83	9.2	6.8

Gastrointestinal absorption is assumed to be 5%.
MMAD = mass median aerodynamic diameter.

From Task Group on Metal Accumulation, Environ Physiol Biochem 3:65-107, 1973. Courtesy: Munksgaard International Publishers Ltd.

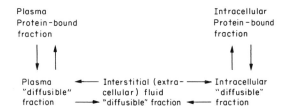

Figure 2.   Model for the exchange of metal between blood and other tissues (from Task Group on Metal Accumulation, Environ Physiol Biochem 3: 65-107, 1973.   Courtesy Munksgaard International Publishers Ltd.

particle size and respiratory rate, particles will be deposited in various parts of the respiratory tract and be absorbed either in the alveoli or depending on their water solubility from the bronchial mucosa.   Tracheobronchial clearance is in this connection of importance, since less water soluble particles that are deposited in the tracheobronchial tract may be transferred to the gastrointestinal tract by this clearance mechanism.

Total absorption.   The systemic uptake of metals includes both the part of metal that is absorbed following gastrointestinal translocation of inhaled particles as well as those amounts of metal that are absorbed from the gastrointestinal tract from food and drink.   Figure 1 demonstrates the pathways by which metals may be absorbed[10].   In table 1 the total absorption (for example cadmium) is shown[4].   Two alternatives for alveolar absorption (50% and 100%) are shown since knowledge about the magnitude of this factor is still uncertain.

TRANSPORT, BIOTRANSFORMATION AND RENAL UPTAKE

The transport of metals from the site of absorption to various organs occurs mainly via the blood. Particularly the binding of metals in blood plasma is of importance for the transport to various organs. The "diffusible fraction" in plasma, interstitial and intracellular fluid, the rate of organ perfusion, the rate of biotransformation and the permeability of cell membranes are important factors that determine the uptake of metals into tissues. Figure 2 demonstrates general pathways of interchange of metals between blood and other tissues. The "diffusible fraction" is of fundamental importance. When metals occur in ionic form in these fluids and do not become bound to any other molecules, an even distribution of the metal in total body water may be expected.

Elements like sodium and potassium which are intimately coupled to water and acid-base balance, are regulated by specialized systems involving active transport. In certain instances such systems may carry non-essential elements. An example is the ionic transport of thallium across cell membranes which occurs through the same mechanism as for potassium[11]. Many metals bind to proteins in plasma and organs and in such cases the distribution will occur in proportion to the availability of binding sites on proteins. Protein binding of metals in plasma is thus of great importance. Such binding varies greatly among metals. Germanium is believed not to be bound to plasma protein[12], beryllium may be transported in the form of a colloidal phosphate absorbed to plasma alpha-globulin[13]. Uranium is partly complexed with bicarbonate in plasma and partly bound to plasma protein[14]. Cadmium and mercury in plasma are protein bound to at least 99%. Since the non-protein bound fraction of metals is usually identical with the "diffusible fraction" which can move freely among various body compartments, protein binding is of great improtance for metal distribution. Whereas protein binding is of importance generally for the distribution of metals, it has special significance for renal uptake of metals. Binding to such proteins and other molecules that are filtrable through the glomerular membrane(mol. wt <30000) may allow excretion and (if combined with tubular reabsorption) renal tubular accumulation of the metal.

Role of metal binding proteins in metal distribution and renal uptake. The low molecular weight protein metallothionein has a specific role when it comes to uptake of metals in renal tissue. This protein has a molecular weight of about 6000 and may bind several metals such as cadmium, mercury, copper, zinc, silver and possibly bismuth and gold[15]. Metallothionein has seven binding sites for metals on its sulfhydryl groups which are abundant as a result of the high cysteine content (more than 30%) of the molecule. Up to 10% w/w of the protein may thus be made up by metal[16]. Metallothionein occurs mainly as an intracellular protein where it binds considerable amounts of metal. For cadmium, the protein is the main pool of intracellular cadmium. If released into blood plasma, metals bound to metallothionein may be very efficiently taken up in the renal tissue as a result of glomerular filtration and subsequent tubular uptake of cadmium[17]. Another example of a transport protein for metals is ceruloplasmin which serves an important transport function for copper. Plasma albumin is a carrier of several metals. For copper, for example, this protein is involved in the initial transfer of copper from the intestine to the liver[18]. Albumin may serve a similar function in relation to cadmium[19]. The iron-binding protein transferrin is another specific metal transporting protein. In addition to iron, indium may be bound to transferrin in plasma.

RENAL EXCRETION OF METALS

Urinary excretion is probably the most important excretory route for metals, although gastrointestinal excretion may in some instances be greater than the urinary one. An understanding of renal excretion mechanisms may make it possible to influence such excretion and thereby speed up the elimination of metals.

Classical renal physiology sometimes does not explain the renal excretion of metals. This is so because of the complex physical chemical state of metals in blood, involving in some instances colloidal solutions, protein binding of various types etc. Classical renal physiology applies only to the "diffusible fraction".

The glomerular ultrafiltrate contains various ions and compounds from plasma ranging in size up to plasma albumin. Only a small proportion of plasma albumin appears in the glomerular filtrate and proteins with larger molecular size are retained in blood. Substances with relatively low molecular weight, such as inulin (Mol. wt. 5000) or metallothionein (Mol wt. 6500) pass the glomerular membrane. Metals bound to such low molecular weight proteins may thus be cleared from plasma into tubular fluid. The filtrable fraction in plasma has been determined for several metals (Table 2)[14,17,20-26]. Measurements of renal clearance have

TABLE 2.   RENAL EXCRETION OF METALS.

Metal	% diffusible in plasma	% tubular reabsorption	Reference
Cu^{2+}	4	99	[20]
Ni^{2+}	41	99	[21]
Zn^{2+}	70	97	[22]
Cd^{2+}	~ 50	95	[17]
Cr^{3+}	5	64	[23]
Tl^{+}	~ 100	~ 50	[24]
U^{6+}	~ 100	~ 0	[14]
Pb^{2+}	~ 3	TT?*	[25]
Hg^{2+}	0,3	TT?*	[26]

* Transtubular transport

found lower values than the calculated glomerular filtration. This may be explained by tubular reabsorption of part of the metal present in tubular fluid. Values for calculated tubular reabsorption is shown in table 2. Cadmium bound to metallothionein, for example, is efficiently reabsorbed from the renal tubular fluid and only a small fraction is excreted in urine. For mercury and lead the role of glomerular filtration is still unclear. It has been suggested that transtubular transport may be involved in the excretory mechanism for these metals[26,25] but no firm evidence for this has as yet been established in mammals. Urinary excretion of beryllium is considered to take place through tubular secretion[13].

Changes in urinary pH may give rise to changes in urinary excretion of lead, indicating that tubular reabsorption is of importance in the renal handling of that metal[4]. With uranium it is known that a low pH in the tubular fluid gives rise to splitting of the uranyl-bicarbonate complex and to an augmented tubular reabsorption of the uranyl ion[14]. The filtrable fraction of metal in plasma may be influenced by some factors i.e. changes in the concentration of some ions and other substances that occur normally in plasma. It was mentioned previously that uranyl ion is transported in plasma complexed with bicarbonate. An increase in plasma bicarbonate will increase the filtrable fraction and also increase the urinary excretion of uranium. The concentration of some amino acids such as cysteine and histidine may increase the filtrable fraction of some metals (mercury, copper or nickel).

Excretion rate - biological half-time. A number of specific processes determine the rate of excretion or clearance of a metal compound from the kidney. When the course of elimination is given only by concentration gradient over a membrane, the process can be represented with reasonable accuracy by a single exponential function[4]. The concentration in the organ under consideration may be expressed as:

$$C_t = C_0 \cdot e^{-b\,t}$$ (Equation 1)

C_t = concentration at time t

C_0 = concentration at time 0.

b = elimination constant

The biological half time, T, may be expressed as:

$$T = \frac{\ln 2}{b}$$ (Equation 2)

T = biological half time

$\ln 2$ = logarithm for 2 = 0.693

The biological half-time varies greatly among metals. When discussing half-time it is customary to talk about the elimination rate from a particular compartment. One may speak for example of the "renal compartment" or some other part of the body. Data on the half-time of a compartment may be obtained by actual measurements of elimination from that compartment. Measurements of metal concentration in renal tissue of living persons may be possible when external scanning methods are used after ingestion of substances labelled with gamma-emitting radioisotopes. In other instances external measurements can be done by prompt gamma-emission techniques. In most instances, however, concentrations have to be inferred from indirect measurements. A description of the variations in excretion rates (i.e. the variation in biological half-time) among various groups in the population is very useful when trying to estimate risk of poisoning. Such information is not yet available for metal compounds with the exception of methylmercury.

METABOLIC MODELS AND THEIR USE IN RISK ESTIMATION

When quantitative data are available to describe the processes of absorption, distribution, excretion and renal uptake, concentrations of the metal in the kidney can be calculated as a function of time and exposure. Together with knowledge about the "critical concentration" for development of renal disease or dysfunction, such calculations may allow estimation of risk for development of adverse effects at specified exposures[27].

One-compartment model. The one-compartment model describes the elimination or accumulation from a single compartment. The mathematical expression for the course of elimination process when there is no further influx is the same as described by equation 1.

When there is a continuous influx the accumulation process may be described by the following equation:

$$A = \frac{a}{b} (1 - e^{-b\,t}) \qquad\qquad \text{(Equation 3)}$$

A = accumulated amount
a = amount of metal entering the compartment
    at each time interval
b = elimination constant
t = time of exposure

One-compartment models have been widely used for calculations involving metals[4]. However, since metals are often bound to proteins and compartmentalized in a number of compartments in the body, the use of one-compartment models often constitutes an oversimplification of the real situation.

Multicompartment models. It has been recognized that an adequate and useful quantitative description of the metabolism of several metals including the nephrotoxic species of cadmium, lead and mercury requires multicompartment models[4]. In order to illustrate the use of a multicompartment model, some data on cadmium metabolism will be discussed including an eight-compartment metabolic model for this metal. As background data for this model, information about urinary excretion

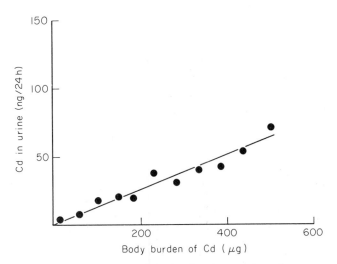

Figure 3.   Relationship between body burden and urinary excretion of cadmium in mice given repeated exposures to radioactive ^{109}CdCl$_2$.

and renal uptake is of importance and some data on these factors will therefore be mentioned.

Relationship between urinary excretion and body burden of cadmium.   In an experiment with mice partly reported previously[19], radioactive cadmium was injected subcutaneously in mice. Body burden was measured by external measurement and urine collected in metabolism cages. Results from these measurements are shown in figure 3.   There is a statistically significant linear relationship between urinary excretion and body burden of cadmium. The urinary excretion (at variance with the fecal excretion) does not seem to be directly related to daily dose. It appears to be directly related to body burden of cadmium. Thus, the urinary excretion of cadmium may be a useful indicator of body burden of cadmium.

Recently, in vivo measurements of cadmium concentrations in liver and kidney of occupationally exposed human beings have been performed[28] and correlated to simultaneously measured cadmium concentrations in urine. These studies in humans have confirmed the conclusions from the animal studies. Concentrations of cadmium in urine are thus used both in environmental and industrial health as an indicator of body accumulation (mainly renal accumulation) of cadmium.

Mathematical model for cadmium metabolism. Based on data on cadmium metabolism obtained in our own studies [16,17,19,29] as well as data available from the literature [30,31], the flow of cadmium among various body compartments can be described. In order to use this information for calculations of cadmium accumulation in the kidney cortex and in other tissues, the flow of cadmium was described by a number of differential equations. Detailed description of the model has been presented by Nordberg and Kjellstrom [10,32]. The first part of this model describes pulmonary and gastrointestinal uptake of cadmium and has

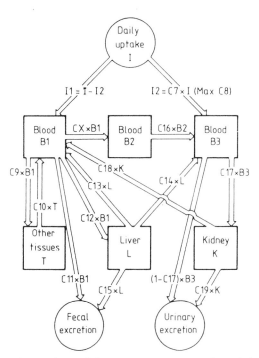

Figure 4.   Flow schema describing the movement of cadmium among various
             compartments (from Nordberg and Kjellstrom, Environ Health
             Perspect 28: 211-217, 1979. Courtesy: National Institute of
             Environmental Health Sciences, US Dept. of Health, Education
             and Welfare.

been presented in Figure 1. Total daily uptake, I, was derived from
this part of the model. The pathways for cadmium after uptake are shown
in Figure 4.   Cadmium is mainly bound to albumin in plasma (blood
compartment B1) immediately after uptake.   Cadmium bound in this way
will be transported mainly to the liver (C12 = 0.25) and other tissues
(C9 = 0.44).   Part (C7 = 0.25) of the daily uptake is bound in plasma
directly to metallothionein. A part (C11 = 0.27) of B1 is excreted in
feces and represents that part of fecal excretion which is dependent on
daily dose. A small part (CX = 0.04) of B1 is transferred to blood
cells (B2). From the blood cells cadmium-metallothionein is released in
relation to blood cell turnover (C16 = 0.012).   B3 is free
metallothionein-bound cadmium in plasma that originates also from the
liver (C14 = 0.00016).   Such cadmium will mainly (C17 = 0.95) be
reabsorbed in the renal tubules and only a small amount will be excreted
in the urine.   Since there is reason to believe that renal tubular
reabsorptive capacity is diminished with age, C17 was made partly
age-dependent on renal accumulation C19xK (C19 = 0.00014).
      Values for cadmium accumulation in the renal cortex by age in persons
with normal cadmium intake in Sweden have been calculated with this
model and compared with empirically found values. As shown in Figure 5
this comparison turns out favourably as does the urinary excretion of
cadmium (Figure 6). As discussed by Nordberg and Kjellstrom [32], other
empirical data, e.g. liver and blood values in persons undergoing

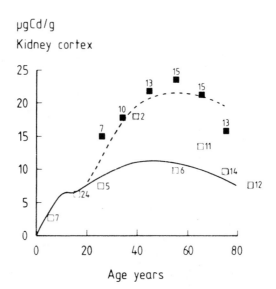

Figure 5.   Calculated and empirical concentrations of cadmium in kidney
cortex by age (Sweden); (———) calculated, nonsmokers; (– – –)
calculated smokers; (□) observed, nonsmokers; (■)
observed, smokers. Figures show number of observations (From
Nordberg and Kjellstrom, Environ Health Perspect 28: 211-217,
1979. Courtesy: National Institute of Environmental Health
Sciences, US Dept. of Health, Education and Welfare.

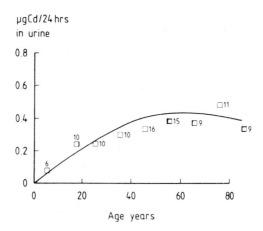

Figure 6.   Calculated and empirical concentrations of cadmium in urine
by age (Sweden):(———) calculated excretion; (□) observed.
(From Nordberg and Kjellstrom, Environ Health Perspect 28:
211-217, 1979. Courtesy: National Institute of Environmental
Health Sciences, US Dept. of Health, Education and Welfare.

surgery for gall bladder operations also fit with the values calculated with this model. Whereas the model seems to give reasonably good results for liver and kidney values under long-term exposure conditions, it is still questionable whether cadmium accumulation in other compartments can be described as well.

Since the critical effect of cadmium is renal tubular dysfunction, calculations of intakes giving rise to certain concentrations in the kidney cortex are of particular interest. The daily intake by the oral route required to reach 200 g/g in the kidney cortex was calculated to be 440 g. For industrial exposure during 25 years, the present model arrives at a concentration in industrial air of approximately 40 g/m^3 to reach 200 g/g in kidney cortex.

Although these estimates are probably quite reasonable because they also fit with epidemiological evidence concerning dose-response relationships, it should be remembered that the present model is based on a number of assumptions concerning pathways for the cadmium flow in the human organism which have only been partly confirmed by experimental data. For example, the model is based on linear kinetics with regard to uptake. Experimental data on cadmium metabolism indicates that the gastrointestinal uptake of cadmium and biological half-time do not display fully linear kinetics [7]. In order to make the mathematical model more generally valid such deviations from linearity should be taken into account in the future.

REFERENCES

1. Friberg L, et al. Handbook on the Toxicology of Metals. Elsevier, Amsterdam, 1979.
2. Daley-Yates PT and McBrien DCH, J Appl Toxicol 1: xi, 1981.
3. WHO, Principles and Methods for Evaluating the Toxicity of Chemicals, Environmental Health Criteria 6, World Health Organization, 1978 Geneva.
4. Task Group on Metal Accumulation, Environ Physiol Biochem 3: 65-107, 1973.
5. Camner P, Clarkson TW and Nordberg GF, In Handbook of the Toxicology of Metals, (L. Friberg et al., eds.). Elsevier, Amsterdam, 1979, pp.65-97.
6. Leopold G, et al, Arch Pharmacol Exp Pathol 263: 275, 1969
7. Engstrom B and Nordberg GF, Toxicology 13: 215-222, 1979.
8. Nordberg GF et al. In Handbook of the Toxicology of Metals, (L. Friberg et al., eds.). Elsevier, Amsterdam, 1979, pp. 143-157.
9. Berlin M, In Handbook of the Toxicology of Metals, (L. Friberg et al., eds.). Elsevier, Amsterdam, 1979, pp. 503-530.
10. Nordberg GF and Kjellstrom T, Environ Health Perspect 28: 211-217, 1979.
11. Gehring PJ and Hammond PB, J Pharmacol Exp Ther 145: 215-221, 1964.
12. Vouk VB, In Handbook of the Toxicology of Metals, (L. Friberg et al., eds.). Elsevier, Amsterdam, 1979, pp.421-428.
13. Reeves AL, In Handbook of the Toxicology of Metals, (L. Friberg et al., eds.). Elsevier, Amsterdam, 1979, pp.329-343.
14. Berlin M and Rudell B, In Handbook of the Toxicology of Metals, (L.Friberg et al., eds.). Elsevier, Amsterdam, 1979, pp.647-658.

15. Nordberg M and Kojima Y, Metallothionein (JHR Kagi and M
    Norberg,eds.). Experientia Suppl 34, Birkhauser Verlag,
    Basel, 1979.
16. Nordberg GF et al. Biochem J 126: 491-498, 1972.
17. Nordberg M and Nordberg GF, Environ Health Perspect 12: 103-108,
    1975.
18. Piscator M, In Handbook of the Toxicology of Metals, (L Friberg et
    al., eds.). Elsevier, Amsterdam, 1979, pp. 411-420.
19. Nordberg GF, Environ Physiol Biochem 2: 7-36, 1972.
20. Walshe JM and Cumings: Wilsons disease. CC Thomas Publ Springfield
    43, 1961.
21. Hendel RC and Sunderman FW, Res Comm Chem Path Pharm 4: 141-146,
    1972.
22. Prasad AS,In Zinc Metabolism (AS Prasad, ed.). CG Thomas
    Springfield: 250-301 1966.
23. Collins RJ et al., Am J Physiol 201: 795-798, 1961.
24. Kazantzis G: In Handbook of the Toxicology of Metals, (L Friberg
    et al.,eds.). Elsevier, Amsterdam, 1979, pp.599-612.
25. Vostal J and Heller J, Environ Res 2: 1, 1968.
26. Berlin M and Gibson S; Arch Env Health 6: 617-625, 1963.
27. Task Group on Metal Toxicity, In Effects and Dose-Response
    Relationships of Toxic Metals, (GF Nordberg, ed.). Elsevier,
    Amsterdam, 1976, pp.10-95.
28. Roels HA et al, Lancet Jan 27: 221, 1979.
29. Nordberg M, Environ Res 15: 381-404, 1978.
30. Friberg L et al, In Cadmium in the Environment, 2nd ed. CRC-press,
    Cleveland, 1974.
31. Friberg L, et al. In Handbook on the Toxicology of Metals,
    (L Friberg et al., eds.). Elsevier, Amsterdam, 1979,
    pp.355-381

32. Kjellstrom T and Nordberg GF, Environ Res 16: 248-269, 1978.

GENERAL PRINCIPLES UNDERLYING THE RENAL TOXICITY OF METALS

Thomas W. Clarkson and Zahir A. Shaikh

Division of Toxicology, University of Rochester School of Medicine, Rochester, New York 14642, USA

ABSTRACT

Heavy metals have special characteristics that play an important role in their renal toxicity. As elements they are indestructible so the kidney cannot detoxify metals like organic chemicals. Renal toxicity of metals may be modified by or expressed through interaction with essential trace elements. Several metal cations may exist in a number of oxidation states; each oxidation state usually differs markedly in renal toxicity. Several metals form organometallic compounds in which the metal is linked covalently to at least one carbon. Such compounds, which may be synthesized or degraded in mammalian tissues, differ from the inorganic form in toxicity to the kidneys.

Perhaps the most important characteristics, common to all metal cations, is their ability to form, reversibly, complexes and chelates with endogenous ligands. Filterable ligands in plasma affect renal uptake, excretion and toxicity of metals such as bicarbonate with uranium and thionein with cadmium. The location of ligands in the cell membrane and cell interior determine the "geographical specificity" of the cellular action of the metal. The synthesis of certain ligands, e.g. thionein, is induced by some metals. Such ligands play a key role in metal toxicity and possibly cellular tolerance to damage.

Keywords: elements, oxidation-state, organometals, ligands, complexes, tolerance.

INTRODUCTION

The clinical history of renal damage due to metal exposure traces back at least into the 19th century. A wide variety of effects have been reported. The first part of this paper will summarize the major types of damage produced by metal action on kidney. The second part of the paper will review the metal action from the perspective of special characteristics of metals. An attempt will be made to explain mechanisms of toxicity wherever possible.

MAJOR TYPES OF RENAL DAMAGE BY METALS

The major effects of metals may be conveniently classified into those occurring after acute and those after chronic exposure to the metal. Acute effects may result from direct action of the metal. Hemolysis caused by arsine is an example of an indirect effect when the products of hemolysis cause kidney damage. Perhaps the most common type of indirect effect occurs with massive acute exposure to toxic metals resulting in cardiovascular shock leading to localized renal ischemia. This results in rupture of the basal membrane preventing orderly regeneration of tubular epithelial cells [1].

The early direct effects of metals on kidney usually manifest themselves as damage to the cells lining the proximal portion of the nephron. In general, the reabsorptive and secretive properties of the proximal convoluted tubule are the first to be affected by short-term metal exposure. Reasons for this selective location of damage will be discussed later. The processes in the proximal convoluted tubule usually affected are the reabsorption of the small molecular weight proteins, amino acids and glucose, and the secretion of uric acid. In the more severe exposures these effects are similar to those seen in the Fanconi syndrome.

The direct effects of metals on the proximal convoluted tubule is often followed by tolerance. The kidney becomes resistant to subsequent doses of the metal. A common mechanism of tolerance to a variety of metals involves the regeneration of new epithelial cells. The destruction of the proximal tubular epithelial cells, followed by exfoliation occurs within a few hours. Subsequently, regeneration of new cells begins on the basement membrane [2]. The regenerated cells differ in shape and structure from the fully developed epithelial cell. They lack microvilli. It is not until several weeks after the initial injury that these cells fully develop to their mature form. During this developmental phase, these cells appear resistant to attack by a number of metals including mercury and uranium.

Chronic effects have been described for a number of metals. Mercury compounds, both organic and inorganic forms, may cause a nephrotic syndrome involving protein excretion and loss of albumin from the plasma compartment resulting in edema. One mechanism of damage involves the formation of auto-immune complexes. Damage to the basement membrane releases tubular epithelial antigen into the circulation resulting in the production of antibodies. The antigen-antibody complex is deposited in the glomerulus, affecting its function [3,4]. Similar effects produced by auto-immune mechanisms have been demonstrated in animals [5].

Chronic exposure to cadmium results in delayed onset of tubular dysfunction. It is similar to that produced by the short-term exposures: the excretion of small molecular weight proteins, amino

acids, glucose, and phosphate is increased [6]. These effects of
cadmium may progress to a chronic interstitial nephropathy as may
have occurred in Itai-Itai disease [7].

In the case of chronic exposure to lead, decreased glomerular
function has been reported in people occupationally exposed for
periods of a year or more [8]. A fascinating aspect of human exposure
to lead is the history of the "Queensland nephropathies". An
unusually high prevalence of chronic nephritis was reported in Queensland, Australia in the late 1920s involving a gradually deteriorating
renal function resulting in death due to uremia at an early age. Most
of these excess deaths were recorded before the age of 40. At the
time, many physicians suspected lead as the cause. Epidemiological
investigation implicated childhood exposure to lead paint used in the
exterior part of the house. The connection with lead has been
documented in some detail since the 1920s [9,10,11]. What has not been
explained is why such nephropathies have not been recorded in other
situations of childhood exposures such as in the inner cities in North
America where exposure has been high enough to cause severe
encephalopathies. No evidence of any kind of renal impairment has been
found in these children despite a careful search [12]. Clearly,
although there is a very strong connection with lead, some other factors must have been involved which, to date, have not been identified.

Chronic occupational exposure to cadmium and lead produces aminoaciduria [13,14,15]. Lead effects probably occur at high exposures
[16].

In general, it would appear that numerous types of damage can be
inflicted by metals on the kidney affecting the vasculature, the
glomerular and basement membranes and the tubular cells both on acute
and chronic exposures. To obtain a deeper understanding of the action
of metals, we should like to view the action of metals from the
properties of the metals themselves. What special characteristics do
the metals possess, from a chemical or biochemical viewpoint, that
might help us understand, at least partially, the action of metals on
the kidneys.

SPECIAL CHARACTERISTICS OF METALS RELATED TO RENAL TOXICITY

Some special characteristics of metals which play a role in renal
toxicity are listed in Table 1.

Table 1. Some Characteristics of Metals

---

1. Elements
2. Oxidation-reduction reactions
3. Organo-metallic compounds
4. Reversible reactions with ligands

Metals as elements. Since metals are elements, they are indestructible and cannot be detoxified like organic chemicals. To protect
itself, renal tissue must eject metals into urine or blood or must
devise means of packaging metals into an inert form. In fact, both
these mechanisms of protection are used by kidney cells. Toxic metals
may interact with other elements, for example, by displacing essential
trace elements such as zinc.

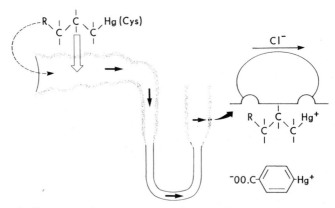

Figure 1. A diagrammatic representation of the transport of an organomercurial diuretic to its site of action in the ascending limb of the loop of Henle. The organomercurial diuretic depicted as $R_C C_C C$ Hg^+ is assumed to bind to a specific receptor site from which it may be displaced by p-mercuribenzoate.

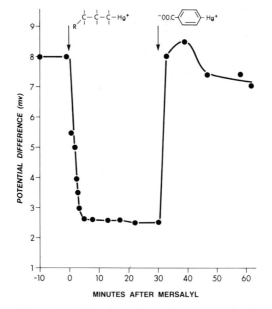

Figure 2. The effect of addition of an organomercurial diuretic (mersaly) on the potential difference across an isolated segment of Henle's loop isolated from a rabbit kidney. The figure also accords the immediate reversal of the potential by addition of p-chlor-mercuribenzoate. Adapted from figure 3 in ref. [20].

Oxidation states of metals. The oxidation state of the metal is an important factor to the kidney. The differences in renal toxicities between elemental mercury vapor, mercurous mercury, and mercuric mercury are dramatic both quantitatively and qualitatively. Similarly, the hexavalent chromium is a great deal more toxic than the trivalent chromium [17].

Organometallic compounds. The ability of metals to form organometallic compounds, that is, to form a covalent bond with a carbon atom is also important in renal toxicity. The organic moiety can play an important role in the renal handling and in the toxicity of the metals.

The most studied example is the work on the organic mercury diuretics [18,19]. The diuretic is illustrated by the structure in the upper left hand corner of Figure 1. The structural requirements for diuretic activity are a mercury atom with one valence attached to a carbon which is a member of a three carbon chain and an organic moiety, usually containing an acidic group, attached at the other extremity of the chain, depicted by R. The organic moiety allows rapid entry of mercury into the renal tubule usually by the acid secretory system. Although the diuretic probably affects cells lining the proximal tubular area, sufficient amounts of the diuretic persist in the tubular fluid to reach the ascending limb of the loop of Henle, depicted in the right hand side of Figure 1. At this point, the diuretic inhibits the active transport of chloride. The organic moiety here is believed to interact with a specific receptor involved in active chloride transport as depicted diagrammatically on the left hand side. Interestingly, other organo materials, not having the required three carbon structure such as parachloromercuric benzoate (PCMB) are able to displace the organomercurial from its receptor and reverse diuresis. The ability of PCMB to inhibit diuresis is dramatically illustrated by data in Figure 2 [20]. The potential difference across the isolated tubule is a measure of active chloride transport across the tubular cells. On addition of the diuretic to the medium, active chloride transport is rapidly inhibited. On addition of PCMB, transport immediately returns to normal rates.

Another important aspect of the organometallic compounds, is the fact that the carbon-metal bond can be cleaved in tissues, resulting in the liberation of the inorganic form of the metal. For example, the rate of breakdown of organo-mercurials differs considerably from one class of mercurials to another. The release of inorganic mercury to the kidney, in turn, may be responsible for renal toxic effects. The build-up of inorganic mercury in the kidney after phenyl mercury compounds is much faster than after methylmercury (Figure 3). An interesting aspect is that inorganic mercury, accumulated either from the phenyl or from the methyl form, reaches levels which are very high compared to toxic levels resulting from a single dose of inorganic mercury. This phenomenon is believed to reflect the tolerance of the kidney to the slow accumulation of inorganic mercury [21].

Metal-ligand complexes. Perhaps the most important property of toxic metals from the viewpoint of understanding their renal toxic action, is the ability of metal cations to form reversible complexes with electron donating groups usually referred to as ligands. The interaction of metals with ligands underlies most of the action of metals on the kidney. In the case of early effects of metals, we are

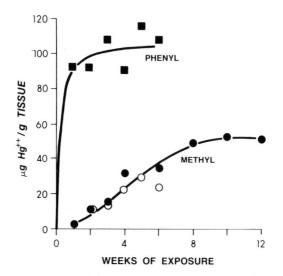

Figure 3. The accumulation of inorganic mercury in rat kidneys
following repeated doses of phenyl or methylmercury compounds.
Adapted from figure 3 of ref. [21].

in a position to understand some examples of selective action along
the renal tubule, sequence of effects on renal cells, and some of
the protective mechanisms developed by kidney tissue. The mechanisms
of the chronic nephropathies is another matter and is still beyond our
understanding in mechanistic details.

The first point to be made is that the degree of association of a
metal with a ligand differs enormously from one ligand to another as
illustrated in the data for methylmercury in Table 2.

Table 2. The association constant (K) for the reversible binding of
electron donating ligand (L) to the methylmercury cation. Adapted
from Clarkson [22].

Ligand (L)	log K approx.	
Cl-	5	$CH_3Hg^+ + L^- \rightleftarrows CH_3HgL$
NH_2 (hist.)	9	
OH-	10	$K = [CH_3HgL] / [CH_3Hg^+] [L^-]$
RS- (CyS-, GS-)	16	

The value of the logarithm of the equilibrium constant K is quoted
for a number of complexes that methylmercury forms. Even the lowest
value of K, in this case five, indicates a substantial interaction
with the chloride anion. The values of K indicate large differences
between chloride, amino groups, hydroxyl and sulfhydryl groups.
Despite high affinity for sulfhydryl groups, interaction of the metal
may occur with other groupings depending upon the relative concentration of the ligands. Thus the possibility exists of formation of

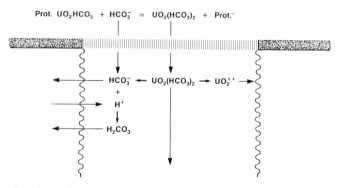

Figure 4. A schematic representation of the role of bicarbonate anions in the renal uptake and excretion of uranium. The uppermost compartment is plasma. The glomerular membrane is depicted as and the membrane of the tubular cells as . Serum albumin is depicted as Prot. Normal chemical symbols apply otherwise.

a variety of complexes in vivo. It should be noted also that other metal cations may have a completely different order of affinities for organic ligands. Uranium, for example, prefers phosphate and carboxylate groups and lead forms stable complexes not only with sulfhydryl but with carboxylate and amino groupings.

We shall discuss the role of metal-ligand interaction in renal toxicity under a variety of sub-headings; first with regard to the importance of ligands in the general circulation and second with regard to ligands associated with the renal tubular cells.

Circulating ligands. The uranyl cation, UO_2^{++}, is present in plasma attached to carboxylate groups of serum albumin and also with bicarbonate groupings (Figure 4). This is subject to equilibria conditions in plasma whereby a small amount of the uranium exists as the diffusible bicarbonate complex itself. This in turn is filtered at the glomerulus. The reabsorption of bicarbonate by the normal acidification mechanisms in the renal tubule, depicted by the reactions on the left hand side of Figure 4, results from the removal of bicarbonate from the tubular fluid and the subsequent dissociation of the uranium bicarbonate complex. This in turn releases the uranyl cation to bind to the surface of the proximal tubular cells resulting in cellular dysfunction such as the inhibition of reabsorption of amino acids, a well-known effect of uranyl cations.

This mechanism explains the dramatic effects of acidosis and alkalosis on the toxicity and urinary excretion of uranium. If sufficient amounts of bicarbonate are given such that the bicarbonate anion persists in the tubular fluid and eventually appears in urine, the uranyl bicarbonate complex will not have the possibility of complete dissociation. One would predict, therefore, that less will be bound to the cells and more excreted in the urine. If, on the other hand, the animal is made acidotic, exactly the opposite is expected: much more release of metal cation, more kidney uptake, and less urinary excretion. This is illustrated by the experimental data given in Figure 5. Cats, treated with bicarbonate, excreted large amounts of UO_2^{++} in urine and only small amounts are bound to kidney. Animals

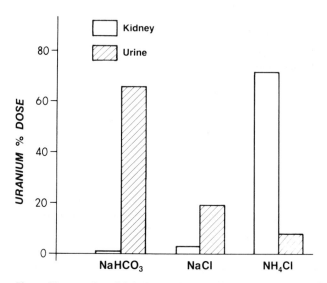

Figure 5.   The effect of acid-base relations on uranium deposition
in cat kidney and urinary excretion.   Animals were injected with 3.37
mg U/kg as uranyl acetate and treated as follows:
  $NaHCO_3$ = infused intravenously with 0.85% $NaHCO_3$ and sacrificed
               at 5 hours.
  NaCl   = infused intravenously with 0.85% NaCl and sacrificed at
               8 hours.
  NH_4Cl = NH_4Cl added to diet to make animals acidotic prior to
               UO_2^{++} dose.   Infused with NaCl and sacrificed at 8 hours.
Data from Neuman [23].

made acidotic with ammonium chloride, bind large amounts to kidney
tissue but excrete small amounts in the urine.   These findings have
led to the use of bicarbonate as an antidote for uranium poisoning.
    Circulating filterable ligands probably play a role in renal
uptake and excretion of other metals.   Clarkson and Vostal [24] have
proposed that mercury enters tubular fluid as a complex with cysteine.
The mercuric ion is liberated when cysteine is reabsorbed in the
proximal tubule.   The highly reactive mercuric ion should immediately
form complexes with chloride ions which are present at high concentrations (0.1M).   The uncharged chloride complex ($HgCl_2$ with Hg^{++}
and R HgCl for organomercurials) should readily pass into the tubular
cells.   It is claimed that this model will explain the increased
renal uptake of mercury when cysteine and other reabsorbed thiols are
given and increased urinary excretion after D-Penicillamine and other
non-resorbable thiols.
    There is indirect evidence that lead enters tubular fluid as a
filterable anionic complex [25].   Ionic lead, once liberated from the
complex is actively reabsorbed [26].   With some metals, the complex
itself may be reabsorbed such as cadmium-thionein [27,28], copper-
histidine [29] and also mercury-thiols [30].

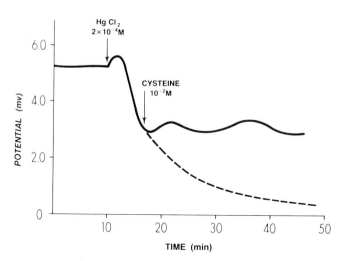

Figure 6. The effect of addition of mercuric chloride to a solution
bathing the mucosal surface of an isolated segment of rat small
intestine. The potential difference is positive with respect to the
serosal side and is due to active transport of sodium ions. A complexing agent (cysteine) was added to the mucosal solution at the time
indicated. Adapted from figure 6-2 in ref. [32].

Interaction of the metals with the cell membrane. Once the metal
cation is released into the tubular fluid, it will react directly with
the epithelial cells. An important concept relating to ligand interaction with the cell has been put forward by Rothstein [31] when he
refers to "geographical specificity" of the metal-ligand interaction.
In other works, the cation approaching the cell will first, in a
geographic sense, react with the outside ligands then with ligands
in the membrane and ultimately with ligands inside the cell. Thus a
sequence of perturbations in cellular function is obtained.
    This sequence of effects is illustrated in the case of an intes-
tinal epithelial cell, when mercury is added to the solution bathing
the mucosal surface (Figure 6). The voltage difference across the
epithelia is taken as a measure of the active transport of sodium
chloride. First, there is an increase in voltage difference due to an
increase in the transport of sodium. This is followed by a decline
in voltage. The initial increase reflects the early interaction of
mercury with the mucosal facing membrane allowing sodium diffusion
from the tubular fluid into the epithelian cell. Experiments reported
elsewhere [32] indicate that mercuric chloride is interacting with
the apical surface of the epithelial cell and once removed by a
complexing agent the normal function is restored.
    The declining phase in the cell function is not reversible. The
addition of a complexing agent stops further deterioration but is
unable to reverse the inhibition (Figure 6). Ionic mercury has
already penetrated the cell and has produced irreversible damage and
probably cell death. Acute mercury effects on renal tubular cells
probably follows a similar course.
    It is possible in isolated cell suspension to illustrate in more

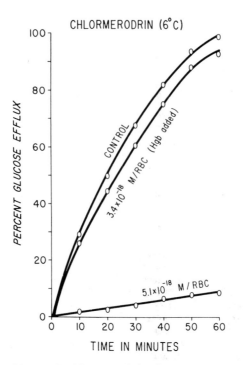

Figure 7. The effect of chlormerodrin (an organomercurial diuretic) binding on glucose efflux from preloaded red blood cells.
The addition of hemoglobin to the saline suspension reduced chlormerodrin binding to 3.4x10⁻¹⁸ moles/cell and almost completely reversed the inhibition of glucose efflux. Adapted from figure 8 in ref. [34].

detail the importance of the geographical location of the ligand and the consequences of metal interaction. Figure 7 is taken from work by Rothstein [31] in which the effect of an organomercurial, chlormerodrin, is studied on glucose transport in a suspension of red blood cells. The control rate of glucose transport is shown by the upper line. On addition of the mercury compound, there is almost complete inhibition. If one adds a non-penetrating complexing agent, in this case, hemoglobin, which can react only with the ligands on the outer surface of the red cell membrane, the glucose transport immediately returns to normal. In other words, in inhibiting glucose transport, mercury reacted only with the external sulfhydryl ligands on the membrane.

The binding characteristics of the mercurial is depicted in the next figure (Figure 8). The binding is plotted according to the Scatchard equation in which the ratio of the bound over the free metal is plotted against the bound. The intercept on the x-axis indicates the number of binding sites in the red blood cell. In this way, it is possible to quantify the number of ligands available on the outer surface of the cell and, indeed, other parts of the membrane depending upon the type of probe that is used to measure the sulfhydryl groupings.

As a result of these types of measurements, it is possible to make a kind of geographical accounting of sulfhydryl groups in the red

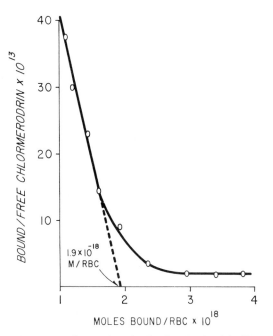

Figure 8. The Mass Law (Scatchard Plot) of the binding of chlormerodrin to human red blood cells. The intercept on the x-axis gives the
number of moles of chlormerodrin bound per cell. Adapted from figure
7 of ref. [34].

blood cell and to associate certain functions with them. This is
summarized in Table 3. It may be seen that a very small fraction of
the total ligands in the cell is associated with the outer part of
the membrane but these ligands are essential to glucose transport.
A slightly higher fraction, but still a very small fraction of the
total sulphur ligands in the cell, is located within the membrane
structure itself and is associated with the permeability to cations.

Table 3. Number, location and function of -SH ligands in red blood
cells[a] .

-SH Ligands (% in cell)	Location	Function
0.06	outer membrane	glucose transport
0.2 to 0.7	membrane matrix	cation transport
5	total membrane	

[a]from Sutherland, Rothstein and Weed [33] and Vansteveninck, Weed
and Rothstein [34].

Although these observations have been made on the red cell, it seems
highly likely that the principle of geographical specificity will apply
to the renal tubular cell: that the metal is interacting at different
stages with ligands located in different regions of the cell and that
the same ligands, sulfhydryl in this case, can be associated with a
number of different functions of the cell.

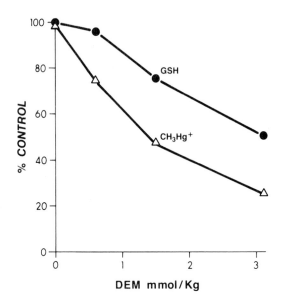

Figure 9. The effect of increasing doses of diethylmaleate (DEM) on kidney glutathione (GSH) and kidney mercury (CH₃Hg⁺) in rats injected (i.p.) with 1.0 mg/kg CH₃HgCl 30 min. after receiving either DEM (i.p.) in propylene glycol or propylene glycol alone and sacrificed 2 hr. later. Adapted from figure 3 in ref. [35].

Intracellular ligands. Interaction of metals with ligands located within the cell is also important to their accumulation within the kidney and their toxic action. To consider first the role of the diffusible ligands inside the cell, the case of mercury interaction with glutathione is a good example. The work of Richardson and Murphy [35] indicates the close parallel between levels of glutathione in kidney cells and the accumulation of methylmercury cations inside the kidney (Figure 9).

The mechanism whereby glutathione is connected with renal accumulation of mercury is not yet understood. It may be concerned with both trans-membrane transport and possibly distribution of mercury to other binding sites within the renal tubular cell.

Intracellular concentrations of reduced glutathione may be important to the earliest toxic effects of inorganic mercury on kidney cells. If animals are pretreated with a reagent that reduces renal-glutathione, $HgCl_2$ is no longer able to inhibit sodium reabsorption [36]. This is probably due to the fact that mercury is not accumulated in tissue with low glutathione.

Present also within the cell are a number of special metal binding proteins which shall be discussed in detail in other papers in this volume. Thionein is known to possess a very high sulfhydryl content and to be involved in the binding of cadmium and mercury. An acidic protein is believed to be involved in the binding of lead. Both these proteins are inducible and a number of different roles for them have been proposed involving both the storage, detoxification, transport, and even some of the toxic effects of the metals. Some recent data

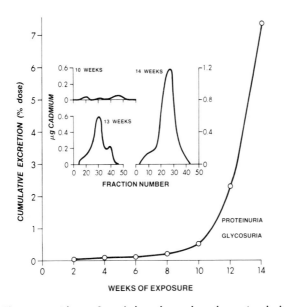

WEEKS OF EXPOSURE

Figure 10. The excretion of cadmium in urine in rats injected
(s.c.) with 5 μmole ^{109}Cd Cl$_2$/kg 5 days per week for up to 14 weeks.
The inserted figures record the results of gel filtration chromatography (0.9x60 cm column packed with Sephadex G-75) on urine
samples collected at 10, 13 and 14 weeks. 1 ml of clear urine was
applied to the column and the Cd content of each fraction collected
from the column is plotted according to fraction number. Cadmium-
metallothioein appears as a peak at about fraction number 30.
Adapted from figures 5 and 6 in ref. [37].

by Shaikh and Hirayama [37] illustrate the importance of special
metal binding proteins (Figure 10). Similar data have been published
earlier by others with regard to effects of cadmium on renal function,
particularly proteinuria and glucosuria. This figure illustrates the
fact that effects of cadmium given in small continuous doses do not
manifest themselves until the completion of a latent period of about
ten weeks, at which point the proteinuria and glucosuria appear. At
this time, cadmium has achieved a critical concentration in kidney
tissue so these effects manifest themselves. On the insert of this
figure is shown the excretion of cadmium in the urine as a function of
its molecular size. After ten weeks exposure, just before the onset
of damage, very little cadmium is seen either as metallothionein or
bound to other ligands. At thirteen weeks and fourteen weeks, when
damage has already occurred, the majority of the cadmium is detected
as metallothionein.
    Amino aciduria, glucosuria, and proteinuria are non-specific
indices of renal tubular damage and could be caused by a variety of
agents. However, the appearance of metallothionein in urine is very
much more specific to the effects of metals, particularly cadmium. A
radioimmunoassay technique has been used to determine metallothionein
in urine of Itai-Itai disease patients [38] as well as those
individuals chronically exposed to cadmium either through the general
or occupational environment [38,39,40].

The mechanism of renal tubular dysfunction in chronic cadmium poisoning is not yet fully understood. It has been shown that cadmium deposited in liver and other tissues is released into the circulation as metallothionein complex [37,41-43]. This complex, due to its low molecular weight, is probably filtered at the glomeruli and reabsorbed subsequently by the renal tubular cells. Such selective accumulation of cadmium in the tubular epithelial cells thus may result in renal tubular dysfunction under chronic exposure conditions [7]. Once this occurs, the urinary excretion of metallothionein is increased along with a number of other filtered nutrients which are otherwise conserved and completely reabsorbed [37,44,45].

Macromolecular ligands inside the cell. Metal cations can react with a wide variety of proteins inside the cell. Unfortunately, the possibilities for such interactions is so great that it has not been possible to follow these in any detail. Clearly, a wide number of enzymes are subject to inhibition by metals inside the cell. Because of the large number of enzymes and the reversible nature of the complexes, very little useful information has as yet been obtained in studies of this kind. Metals may also interact with the nucleic acid macromolecules within the cell. Examples of this are few except in the case of lead [46]. Treatment of animals with a small non-toxic dose of lead produces a dramatic increase in the turnover of DNA in renal tubular cells as indicated by tritiated thymidine labeling (Figure 11). This occurs in a highly uniform fashion and is followed,

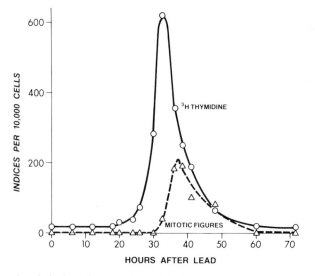

Figure 11. Lead-induced nucleic acid turnover and cell proliferation in the mouse kidney. Mice were given an intra-cardiac injection of lead acetate (5 µg Pb/g. body weight at 0 hr. Each mouse was pulse-labelled with ^{3}H-thymidine for 1 hr. before sacrifice. Mean labelling and mitotic indices per 10,000 cells were determined for proximal tubular epithelian cells from autoradiographs. Each point represents the mean of 5 mice. Mean labelling and mitotic indices for controls were 14 and 3 per 10,000 cells respective. Adapted from figure 4 of ref. [47].

a few hours later, by an increase in the mitotic index of the renal tubular cells, indicating the increase in cellular division. Since these effects are occurring without any visible damage to the cells either under visible or electron microscope, one must assume that this is a specific effect of lead on nucleic acid turnover.

The effects of lead on DNA are intriguing and may be connected with the finding that lead has now been demonstrated to produce renal tumors. [For review, see reference 47]. Recently, methyl-mercury treatment over a period of one year has been shown to produce renal tumors when given in large doses [48].

CONCLUSIONS

Our knowledge of the general principles underlying the renal toxic action of metals is still rather limited. One approach is to examine the role of the properties of the metals themselves with regard to the oxidation states, formation of oranometallic compounds, and the reversible interaction of metals with organic ligands. We have reached the position of being able to explain some of the earliest effects of metals in terms of metal interactions with circulating ligands, changes in the composition of the tubular fluid, the geo-graphical specificity of ligands in the cell membrane and within the cell, and the special metal binding proteins.

At the same time, we must also conclude that an understanding of the long-term nephropathies is still beyond mechanistic explanation. The possibilities that metals can influence turnover of nucleic acids might be related to some of these long-term effects including the production of renal tumors.

ACKNOWLEDGEMENT

The authors appreciate the suggestions and criticisms, during preparation of this manuscript, of Dr. Julius J. Cohen and Dr. Gary L. Diamond.

REFERENCES

1. Oliver J, et al. J Clin Invest 30:1307-1439, 1981.
2. Cuppage FE and Tate A, Am J Pathol 51:405-429, 1967.
3. Kazantzis G, et al. Q J Med N.S. 31:403-418, 1962.
4. Kibukamusoke JW, et al. Br Med J 2:646-647, 1974.
5. Bariety J, et al. Am J Pathol 65:293-302, 1971.
6. Axelsson B and Piscator M, Arch Environ Health 12:360-373, 1966.
7. Friberg L, et al. Cadmium in the Environment, 2nd edit. CRC Press Inc., Cleveland, 1974.
8. Goyer RA, Cur Top Pathol 55:147-176, 1971.
9. Croll DG, Med J Aust 2:144-145, 1929.
10. Nye LJJ, Med J Aust 2:145-159, 1929.
11. Henderson DA, Med J Aust 1:377-386, 1958.
12. Tepper LB, Arch Environ Health 7:76-85, 1963.
13. Clarkson TW and Kench JG, Biochem J 66:361-372, 1956.
14. Cramer K, et al. Br J Ind Med 31:113-127, 1974.

15. Goyer RA, et al. Am J Clin Pathol 57:635-642, 1972.
16. Buchet JP, et al. JOM 22:741-750, 1980.
17. Hunter D, Diseases of Occupations. Little Brown, Boston, 1969.
18. Kessler RH, et al. J Clin Invest 36:656-668, 1957.
19. Weiner IM, et al. J Pharmacol Exp Ther 138:96-112, 1962.
20. Burg M and Green N, Kidney Int 4:245-251, 1973.
21. Clarkson TW, in Handbook on the Toxicology of Metals. (L. Friberg, GF Nordberg and VB Vouk, eds.) Elsevier Press, Amsterdam, 1979, pp.65-97.
22. Clarkson TW, CRC Crit Rev Toxicol 2:203-234, 1972.
23. Neuman WF, in Pharmacology and Toxicology of Uranium Compounds. (C Voegtlin and HC Hodge, eds.) McGraw Hill, New York, 1949, p.701.
24. Clarkson TW and Vostal JJ, in Modern Diuretic Therapy in the Treatment of Cardiovascular and Renal Diseases. (G Wilson and AF Laut, eds.). Excerpta Med Foundation, Amsterdam, 1973, pp.221-232.
25. Vostal J and Heller J, Proc XV Congr Occup Health, Vienna 3: 61-64, 1966.
26. Vander AJ, et al. Am J Physiol 236:373-378, 1979.
27. Nordberg M and Nordberg GF, Environ Health Perspect 12:103-108, 1975.
28. Cherian MG and Shaikh ZA, Biochem Biophys Res Commun 65:863-869, 1975.
29. Neuman PZ and Silverberg M, Nature 210:414-416, 1966.
30. Richardson RJ, et al. Proc Soc Exp Biol Med 150:303-307, 1976.
31. Rothstein A, in Mercury, Mercurials and Mercaptans. (MW Miller and TW Clarkson, eds.). Charles C. Thomas, Springfield, Ill., 1973, pp.68-98.
32. Clarkson TW, in Intestinal Transport of Electrolytes, Sugars and Amino-Acids. (W Armstrong and AD Nunns, eds.). Charles C. Thomas, Springfield, Ill., 1971, pp.110-129.
33. Sutherland RM, et al. J Cell Physiol 68:185-198, 1967.
34. Vansteveninck J, et al. J Gen Physiol 48:617-632, 1965.
35. Richardson RJ and Murphy SD, Toxicol Appl Pharmacol 31:505-519, 1975.
36. Johnson DR, Annual Report, Center for the Study of the Human Environment, Department of Environmental Health, University of Cincinnati, 1979, pp.18-20.
37. Shaikh ZA and Hirayama K, Environ Health Perspect 28:267-271, 1979.
38. Tohyama C, et al. Toxicology 20:289-297, 1981.
39. Tohyama C, et al. Proceedings Third International Cadmium Conference, Metal Bulletin Books, London (In press).
40. Chang CC, et al. Toxicol Appl Pharmacol 55:94-102, 1980.
41. Nordberg GF, et al. Acta Pharmacol Toxicol 30:289-295, 1971.
42. Goyer RA, et al. Proceedings First International Cadmium Conference, Metal Bulletin Books, Ltd., London, 1978, pp. 183-185.
43. Tohyama C and Shaikh ZA, Fundam Appl Toxicol (In press).
44. Norberg GF and Piscator M, Environ Physion Biochem 2, 37-49, 1972.
45. Tohyama C, Shaikh ZA, Nogawa K, Kobayashi E and Honda R, (unpublished results).
46. Choie DD and Richter GW, Lab Invest 30:647-651, 1974.

47. Choie DD and Richter GW, in Lead Toxicity (RL Singhal and JA Thomas, eds.). Urban and Schwarzenberg, Baltimore, MD, 1980, pp.187-212.
48. Mitsumori K, et al. Cancer Let 12:305-310, 1981.

THE EFFECTS OF NUTRITIONAL FACTORS ON THE DEVELOPMENT OF METAL-INDUCED RENAL DAMAGE

I. Bremner

Rowett Research Institute, Bucksburn, Aberdeen AB2 9SB, UK

The development of metal-induced renal damage in man and animals is not determined solely by the degree of exposure to a particular metal but is also influenced by nutritional status and dietary composition. In many cases the absorption or excretion of the toxic metal is affected by these factors, with concomitant changes in the rate at which the metal accumulates and causes functional impairment in the kidneys and other organs. The dietary constituents which can modify the renal accumulation of metals such as cadmium, lead, mercury, zinc and copper include protein, fibre, phytate, vitamins, and a range of major and minor essential elements. The mechanisms whereby these effects occur are not yet completely understood but in some cases the formation of insoluble and non-available metal derivatives in the intestinal tract, the induced synthesis of specific proteins or competition between metals for binding sites on proteins or membranes are involved.

Neonatal and milk-fed animals frequently accumulate a large proportion of their dietary intake of several metals and may develop renal damage at dietary metal concentrations which are relatively innocuous in adult animals.

Keywords: metals; renal damage; nutritional status; diet.

INTRODUCTION

It has become increasingly apparent in the last decade as our knowledge of the toxicity of metals has increased that their effects on man and animals cannot always be described by simple dose-response relationships [1,2]. The amount of a metal that is ingested is obviously a major determinant of whether any toxic reactions will ensue, but other factors such as age, sex, genetic strain and physiological state are equally important. Nutritional status and dietary composition also have a major influence on the development of metal poisoning and in this review, an account will be given of how a variety of nutritional factors can affect the occurrence of metal-induced kidney damage in animals. Knowledge of these effects has already been of considerable value in explaining the occurrence of specific cases of metal toxicosis in man and in domestic animals. Moreover it can aid the identification of population groups which may be at particular risk from metal poisoning and, in addition, it offers both prophylactic and therapeutic means of restricting the toxicity of metals, when exposure to them cannot be avoided.

Impairment of renal function is generally a late manifestation of metal toxicosis and may depend on the prior accumulation of the metal in the kidneys until a certain critical concentration is attained. During this time many other lesions may develop, particularly in experimental animals which frequently receive diets containing relatively large amounts of the toxic metal. It is not uncommon, therefore, for such experiments to be terminated before concentrations of the metal have increased to a level where effects on renal structure and function would be expected. Nevertheless, changes in the concentration of the heavy metal in the kidneys as a consequence of particular dietary treatments may be evident. Since there is often (but not always) a correlation between kidney metal concentration and the onset of kidney damage, it is likely that most nutritional factors which affect renal accumulation of a metal will also affect the development of renal failure. A corollary of this is that any dietary component which affects the absorption of a heavy metal may ultimately also influence its nephrotoxic effects. However this paper will be restricted to cases where a change in dietary composition has affected the reno-toxic effects of a metal or has modified its accumulation or distribution in the kidneys. Where possible, the mechanism whereby these effects occur and their possible relevance to human exposure to metals will also be discussed.

GENERAL EFFECTS

Some indication of the diversity of dietary components which have been shown to modify the effects of metals such as lead, mercury, cadmium, zinc and copper on renal function is given in Table 1. The list is not comprehensive and does not indicate whether the individual dietary components exacerbate or ameliorate the nephrotoxic effect of the metals. Moreover, it gives no quantitative information on the magnitude of the effects which can be obtained. However, it does suggest that the toxicity of individual metals is likely to vary considerably when diets of different type are fed to animals and this has been confirmed in several investigations.

Table 1   Nutritional Factors Affecting the Nephrotoxicity of Metals

Level of Food intake
Protein - concentration and type
Fat, fibre and carbohydrate
Milk or other liquid-based diets
Amino acids and hydroxyacids
Calcium, phosphorus and sulphur
Iron, copper, zinc, selenium and molybdenum
Vitamins
Metal-binding ligands in foodstuffs
Acids and alkalis

For example, differences were found in the toxicity of both cadmium
and lead and in their accumulation in kidneys and other tissues when
rats were given a variety of nutritionally-adequate diets [3,4,5].
Animals receiving balanced semi-purified diets were more affected by
lead than were animals given Purina chow diet and the retention of
both metals was much greater in rats receiving 'human-type' diets
(such as bread, meat and milk) than in animals receiving normal
laboratory diets.   The effects of dietary composition are even more
evident if the diet is deficient in certain nutrients or if the
animals have received such diets prior to the administration of the
toxic metal.   Thus, rats reared on a diet deficient in protein and/or
energy suffered more from the addition of lead to their diet than did
rats reared on the same diet but with added protein and energy [6].
In particular the severity of renal damage was greater in the
malnourished animals, as was indicated by increased urinary excretion
of amino nitrogen and of glucose and by a trend towards increased
activities of fructose-1, 6-phosphatase and of glucose-6-phosphatase
in the kidneys.   These effects were noted in rats which only received
the poor quality diets in the period prior to the supplementation with
lead.   All animals received the same nutritionally-adequate diet
during the period of lead exposure, suggesting that the malnourished
state of the animals rather than the simultaneous consumption of a
poor quality diet was responsible for the increased severity of lead
toxicosis.
     A further example of how consumption of a poor quality diet,
deficient in several nutrients, can exacerbate the toxicity of a metal
is provided by the comparison of the effects of cadmium on rats given
a normal commercial rat diet and those given a fibre-free diet
deficient in protein, calcium and phosphorus [7].   The latter animals
exhibited growth failure and increased urinary excretion of cadmium
and protein, indicating a greater degree of renal damage.   This was
confirmed by histological examination of the kidneys, which revealed
atrophic degeneration and desquamation of epithelial cells in the
proximal tubules.
     These and other related investigations are of some importance since
they confirm the earlier suggestion that the occurrence of Itai-Itai
disease in certain areas of Japan was not caused solely by a high intake
of cadmium [8].   The absence of this disease, which is
characterized by osteomalacia and renal failure, in other areas of
Japan with comparable levels of cadmium contamination of foodstuffs,
strongly suggested that other factors were involved in its aetiology.
One was the physiological state of the affected subjects, who were

mainly multiparous post-menopausal women.   Another was their poor
nutritional status, especially with regard to calcium, protein and
perhaps vitamin D.   As will be discussed later, all those nutrients
can modify the effects of cadmium on the skeleton and the kidneys and
there is little doubt that they were a major contributory cause of
Itai-Itai disease.   The influence of dietary composition on the
toxicity of metals is therefore not merely of academic interest and
demonstrable only under carefully-controlled conditions with laboratory
animals.   It can be of major importance in man and domestic animals
inadvertently exposed to any toxic metal.

EFFECT OF MILK AND OTHER LIQUID-BASED DIETS ON METAL TOXICITIES

The toxicities of several metals can be influenced not only by the
chemical composition of a diet but also by its physical form,
especially if it is given in liquid form to young animals.   For
example, suckling lambs given a milk-substitute diet with yeast as
the sole protein source rapidly developed severe renal lesions because
of excessive accumulation of zinc in their kidneys, with concentrations
in the cortex ranging from 3000-8000 mg zinc/kg dry matter [9].   The
kidneys were pale and enlarged, with dilation of tubules and atrophy
of glomeruli.   Although the diet had a high zinc content (840 mg/kg),
it would not have had any serious effect on weaned animals if given in
solid form, other than to cause a slight reduction in food intake and
growth.   Similar renal lesions occurred in lambs given milk with
comparable amounts of zinc, indicating that the suckling animal is
clearly at increased risk from zinc-induced kidney damage, if the diet
contains excessive amounts of this metal.

This effect is not restricted to zinc or to lambs and it is well-
established that the retention of several metals, including lead,
cadmium, mercury, copper and manganese, is greatly increased in milk-
fed animals of several species [10].   As would be expected, this is
most evident in neonatal animals but increased retention has also been
observed in adult animals given milk, indicating that it is not simply
an age-related phenomenon.   Although a large proportion of the metal
ingested by the neonatal animals is frequently retained by the
intestinal mucosa, uptake by the kidneys and other tissues is also
greatly increased.   The mechanism whereby the absorption of the metals
is stimulated is not completely understood, but there is evidence that
uptake by pinocytosis may be occurring [11,12].   Certainly
administration of cortisone to suckling mice to induce gut closure can
reduce the efficiency of lead absorption and also decrease kidney lead
content to levels found in adult animals [11].

Fortunately the concentrations of heavy metals in milk are generally
quite low and it is unlikely that human infants or neonatal animals
would normally receive sufficient of any metal in their milk to give
rise to metal-induced renal damage.   However, any metal which is
absorbed at this time can still contribute to the body burden in later
life, when signs of metal toxicosis may develop.

EFFECT OF DIETARY PROTEIN ON METAL TOXICITY

Variation in the dietary protein content can have a pronounced
effect on the metabolism of several metals.   For example, the toxicity

of cadmium was exacerbated and kidney cadmium concentrations were
increased in rats given a diet deficient in protein [13,14].   A
similar inverse relationship between protein intake and metal toxicity
was apparent in early studies on lead metabolism, since animals on low-
protein diets frequently had elevated skeletal and tissue lead
concentrations [see 15].   However, Quarterman and his colleagues [15]
have shown that, depending on experimental conditions, feeding low-
protein diets to rats can have variable effects on the carcass retention
of this metal and on its distribution (Table 2).   For example, kidney
lead increased in one experiment when the dietary protein content was
increased from 0 to 40%, which is the opposite of what would have been
expected from earlier studies.   The uptake and distribution of the
metal is apparently affected not only by the protein concentration of
the diet but also by the period for which it is fed, the growth rate
of the animals and by their level of food intake.   Quarterman et al
rationalized their results on the basis that a decrease in dietary
protein content reduces lead retention whereas a reduction in food
intake or growth rate increases it.   Since both food intake and
growth rate are affected by protein deficiency, it is at present
extremely difficult, if not impossible, to predict the specific response
of an animal or of man to variations in dietary protein content.   There
is a need for more controlled research on this topic with care being
taken to ensure that control animals have similar growth rates and
food intakes to the lead-treated animals.

Table 2   Effect of Dietary Protein on the Retention of ^{203}Pb in
the Carcass and Kidneys of Rats

Feeding regime	Protein content of diet (%)	^{203}Pb Activity (% of dose x 10^3)	
		Gut-free Carcass	Kidneys
1. Restricted intake	7.5	17	2.3
	20	22	2.9
2. Restricted intake	0	49	4.4
	5	80	8.0
	20	153	20.5
3. Ad libitum	20	88	10.1
	40	165	19.9

Data taken from Quarterman et al [15].

The nature, as well as the concentration, of dietary protein can
also influence the toxicity of some metals, although comparatively
little attention has so far been paid to this effect.   Marked
differences were noted in the severity of cadmium poisoning induced in
Japanese quail receiving soy-protein isolate, casein-gelatin or egg-
white as protein source [16,17].   Renal structure and function were
not examined but differences in cadmium retention did occur.   Similar
differences in renal cadmium concentrations have occurred in rats given
diets with scallops or casein as protein source [18].

Little information is available on the mechanisms whereby dietary
protein affects the accumulation of heavy metals in the kidneys and
other tissues.   One possibility is that amino acids liberated on
hydrolysis of the protein in the digestive tract could complex with the
metals and so affect their solubility, their availability for absorption

and their subsequent distribution.   Certainly addition of amino acids to the diet of rats was found to have a pronounced effect on the retention and distribution of lead [19].   Some amino acids tended to increase kidney lead uptake whereas others had either little or the opposite effect.   The results were somewhat variable, implying the influence also of other factors such as age, and no definite conclusions could be drawn.   Some of the effects of soy-protein isolate on cadmium toxicity may be attributed to the phytate which is also present in this protein source.   Certain metal phytates are relatively insoluble in the digestive tract and are non-available for absorption.   Little is known of the behaviour of cadmium-phytates but effects of phytate on zinc absorption could also have secondary effects on the toxicity of heavy metals (see below).

EFFECT OF DIETARY SULPHUR ON LEAD AND COPPER TOXICITY

Particular attention was paid at one stage to the effects of sulphur-containing amino acids on the toxicity of some metals, because of their high affinity for thiol groups.   For example, administration of cysteine and other related compounds, greatly increased the nephrotoxicity of a single parenteral dose of cadmium in rats [20]. However the effects of methionine on lead metabolism were not different from those of many other amino acids, suggesting that sulphur-containing compounds have no specific effect on lead toxicity [19].

Nevertheless, inorganic sulphur compounds can greatly modify the toxicity of lead, especially in ruminant animals which convert much of their dietary sulphur into sulphide in the rumen.   Thus, male lambs receiving a low-sulphur diet were more affected by a lead supplement of 200 or 400 mg/kg diet than were animals receiving diets supplemented with inorganic sulphate [21,22].   Growth and food intake were severely reduced and mortality was increased in the low-sulphur animals. Moreover, they showed signs of severe kidney damage, with increased interstitial connective tissue and non-focal lymphocyte infiltration and other changes.   There were also large numbers of nuclear inclusion bodies, consistent with the greatly increased kidney lead concentrations in those animals.   Intact rams were more affected than were male castrates, even though their kidney lead contents were less, which may indicate some additional hormonal effects on lead toxicity.   The reason why dietary sulphate provided considerable protection against lead toxicity was not established but it is possible that combination with sulphide in the rumen to form PbS resulted in a decrease in the availability of lead for absorption.

Increased sulphur intakes can also protect against the renal damage which occurs in the terminal stages of chronic copper poisoning in sheep, although there is an important difference in the pattern of development of copper-induced renal damage compared with that induced by metals such as cadmium and lead.   The uptake of copper by the kidneys occurs very suddenly at the time of the "haemolytic crisis" when much of the stored copper in the liver is liberated into the blood, with resultant haemolysis of erythrocytes [23].   It is only after the haemolytic crisis that blood urea levels increase and that degeneration, necrosis and loss of enzyme activity are evident in the cells from the proximal convoluted tubules, which are loaded with copper, iron and haemoglobin.

The protective effect of sulphur against copper-induced nephrotoxicity is associated with its ability to restrict the accumulation of copper by the liver and so delay the onset of liver damage and the haemolytic crisis.   This effect of sulphur is greatly increased if the dietary molybdenum content is also increased, and combined supplements of molybdenum and sulphur have frequently been used to control copper toxicosis in sheep [24].   If, however, very high levels of molybdenum are used (>25 mg/kg diet) then, somewhat ironically, kidney copper concentrations are increased rather than decreased [25].   Indeed, in extreme cases, concentrations may be as high as those found in sheep with copper-induced renal damage [26], although there is no evidence of renal failure in the molybdenum-treated animals, perhaps because the binding of copper in the kidneys is different from that in copper-poisoned animals.   Much of the renal copper in the latter animals is present as metallothionein [27] whereas in molybdenum-treated sheep the copper is bound with molybdenum to proteins of much higher molecular weight in the cytosol, or in particulate fractions in the kidney [25].   The formation of these copper fractions, which are believed to be relatively non-available, is thought to arise from the formation in the rumen of thiomolybdates, or related compounds, which can affect both the absorption and systemic metabolism of copper [28].

Variations in dietary sulphur intake can also influence the renal accumulation of zinc in sheep.   Thus ewes given a low-sulphur diet (0.4 g/kg) for a period of 6 months had significantly greater kidney zinc concentrations than did animals given the same diet with normal (1.8 g S/kg) or high (3.9 g S/kg) sulphur contents [29].   Zinc concentrations were 258 ± 17, 91 ± 15 and 87 ± 4 $\mu g/g$ dry matter respectively.   Under normal circumstances when renal zinc concentrations are elevated as a result of zinc supplementation, most of the additional zinc is present as the cytosolic sulphur-rich protein, metallothionein [30].   However, this was not the case in the sulphur-deficient sheep, as most of the additional zinc was present in the particulate fractions obtained on subcellular fractionation of the kidneys (I Bremner and B W Young, unpublished observations).   Indeed in one kidney containing about 700 μg zinc/g dry matter, only 0.5% of the total zinc was bound to metallothionein. Since metallothionein is thought to function in the cellular detoxification of several metals [1], it will be of interest to establish whether the renotoxicity of zinc is dependent on its distribution and is therefore affected by dietary sulphur.

EFFECT OF CALCIUM ON THE TOXICITY OF CADMIUM AND LEAD

The renal dysfunction which occurs in cadmium toxicosis in man is frequently accompanied by osteomalacia, with marked decalcification of bones and spontaneous bone fractures [8].   Urinary excretion of calcium is also increased, suggesting that major disturbances in calcium metabolism occur in cadmium poisoning and that individuals of low calcium status might be more susceptible to the effects of cadmium exposure.   As was indicated earlier, this was confirmed by epidemiological studies on Itai-Itai disease, since the women most affected by the disease had a low dietary calcium intake and had severely depleted calcium reserves as a result of repeated pregnancies.

The effects of variation in dietary calcium intake on the development of cadmium toxicity have been confirmed in several studies with laboratory animals.   Rats given diets with only 0.1 to 1 g calcium/kg and water with 25-50 mg cadmium/litre had reduced growth rates, haematocrit and bone mineral content compared with animals receiving the same diet with an adequate calcium content (about 6 g/kg) [31,32]. Concentrations of cadmium were greatly increased in the kidneys and other tissues from the calcium-deficient animals (Table 3) [31-33], which is consistent with the increased severity of renal damage revealed by histological examination of their kidneys [34].   The tubular epithelium was desquamated and vacuolized and many casts were present in the tubules.   In addition, there was necrosis and partial hyalization in the glomerular capillaries.   Adhesions were also present between the Bowman capsule and glomerular capillaries.

Table 3   Effect of Dietary Calcium on Kidney Cadmium Concentrations in Rats

Cadmium Conc. in Water (mg/l)	Duration of Experiment (weeks)	Reference	Kidney Cadmium Content (mg/kg d.m.)	
			Low-Calcium diet	Normal-Calcium diet
25	8	[31]	109	35
25	8	[32]	205	129
50	17	[33]	245	123
50	13	[34]	90	64

Activities of leucine aminopeptidase were significantly decreased in the kidneys of the calcium-deficient rats receiving dietary cadmium and this may have contributed to the proteinuria in these animals [31]. Increased blood urea nitrogen levels in calcium-deficient rats receiving cadmium supplements also indicated greater impairment of renal fraction in these animals [34].   Inulin clearance rates also tended to be lower and could be inversely correlated with kidney cadmium concentrations. Finally, the effects of cadmium on fractional calcium excretion (i.e. urinary calcium excretion/urinary inulin excretion) were more pronounced in the calcium-deficient rats [34].   It is likely therefore that the development of osteomalacia in patients with Itai-Itai disease could indeed result from the combined effects of a low dietary calcium intake and the cadmium-induced disturbances in renal tubular reabsorption of calcium.

Low dietary intakes of calcium also result in a major increase in the toxicity of lead.   This was first demonstrated in rats and since then has been confirmed in several species.   The effects of calcium deficiency on renal accumulation of lead were especially dramatic, concentrations of the metal in the kidneys of calcium-deficient rats receiving 200 mg Pb/l of drinking water being about 20 times greater than those in calcium-adequate animals [35].   Much smaller increases in lead concentration were found in the femur and blood of the calcium-deficient animals.   The pathological effects of lead were also greatly enhanced in the calcium-deficient rats.   Urinary excretion of δ-ALA and of amino acids was increased, indicating effects on haematopoiesis

and on renal function respectively.   The latter was confirmed by the
increased incidence of intranuclear inclusion bodies in the kidneys of
the calcium-deficient rats.

The importance of dietary calcium in modulating the effects of lead
on renal function has also been demonstrated in lambs [21].   When
castrated male lambs were given diets with 2.8 or 8.3 g calcium/kg and
400 mg lead/kg the mortality rate was much greater in the low-calcium
animals.   Food intakes and growth rates were reduced to a greater
extent and the severity of the lead-induced renal lesions was also
greatly enhanced in these lambs.   Although kidney cortical tissue
appeared normal in the calcium-adequate animals, the renal tubular
epithelial cells in the calcium-deficient lambs were necrotic and
contained nuclear inclusion bodies.   Kidney lead concentrations were
also greatly increased in the calcium-deficient lambs.

If similar results are obtained in man, then these effects of calcium
status on the toxicity of lead and cadmium could clearly be of
considerable importance in determining the hazard associated with a
certain level of exposure to those toxic metals.   It is noteworthy
that similar increases in renal lead accumulation were obtained in the
rat by decreasing the calcium content of the diet from 7 to 1 g/kg
as by increasing its lead content 16-fold to 200 mg/kg [36].   Increased
renal uptake of lead has even been observed in rats whose dietary
calcium intake is reduced to only half of the recommended dietary
allowance [36].   Such a reduction in calcium supply is not uncommon
in malnourished humans.   Increasing the calcium intake of these
subjects might therefore have a beneficial effect in restricting the
accumulation of toxic metals in the kidneys and other tissues.
However, any further increase in dietary calcium intake to levels in
excess of the normal recommended allowance will not necessarily have
any additional effect on cadmium accumulation and it may in fact
reduce the rate of loss of lead from the body [37].

The mechanisms whereby calcium deficiency increases the concentrations
of certain metals in the kidneys have not been firmly established.
However, there is evidence that the intestinal absorption of cadmium
is increased in these circumstances, since variation in dietary calcium
content only influenced the tissue retention of orally administered
^{109}Cd [38].   The retention of parenterally-administered ^{109}Cd was
unaffected.   This increase in cadmium absorption may be mediated by
intestinal calcium-binding protein, which binds cadmium almost as
effectively as it does calcium and whose synthesis is inversely related
to calcium supply.   Washko & Cousins [31] reported increased binding
of ^{45}Ca and ^{115m}Cd to intestinal calcium-binding protein in rats
receiving low-calcium diets and suggested that this protein might aid
the uptake of cadmium as well as of calcium.

Although it has been suggested that the absorption of lead is also
influenced by calcium deficiency, most studies have in fact only
demonstrated that the retention of the metal is affected, without
distinguishing between changes in its absorption and excretion.   Recent
studies indicated, however, that the principal effect of calcium was
indeed on lead excretion [39].   Calcium-deprived animals did not
absorb more lead although increased intraluminal calcium concentrations
did reduce lead absorption in a dose-related manner.

EFFECT OF VITAMINS ON METAL TOXICITIES

There have been several reports that the toxicity of metals in man and animals is also influenced by their vitamin status. For example, summer outbreaks of paediatric lead poisoning have been attributed to changes in vitamin D metabolism. The effects of this vitamin on lead and cadmium poisoning have attracted particular attention because of its important role in the regulation of calcium metabolism and the effects described above of calcium on metal toxicities. Recent studies by Barton et al [40] show that both vitamin D deficiency and excess stimulate the intestinal absorption of lead in the rat, these effects arising primarily from a decrease in gastrointestinal motility. The whole-body retention of parenterally-administered ^{203}Pb was also decreased by both these treatments, although accumulation of the metal in the kidneys was increased by about 25%.

Early work with rachitic chicks indicated that vitamin D administration also increased cadmium uptake and this was confirmed by direct measurement of intestinal ^{109}Cd absorption [41]. However, no changes in kidney cadmium levels were observed in other experiments when vitamin D was given to calcium-replete rachitic chicks [42].

Dietary supplementation with large amounts of vitamin C can ameliorate the effects of metals such as cobalt, selenium, vanadium, cadmium and copper on the growth of chicks. Ascorbic acid has also prevented the anaemia and the disturbances in trace element metabolism which occur in rats and Japanese quail receiving cadmium-supplemented diets [43]. Although there are no reports of this vitamin being used to prevent cadmium-induced renal damage, renal accumulation of oral ^{109}Cd was reduced in Japanese quail given a diet supplemented with 0.5% ascorbic acid [43]. This protective effect of ascorbic acid against cadmium toxicity is achieved not by direct inhibition by the vitamin of cadmium absorption but as a consequence of an increase in the absorption of dietary iron, perhaps through reduction of iron in the g.i. tract to the more available ferrous form [43]. As will be described below, changes in the iron status of animals can have a pronounced effect on the accumulation of cadmium and other metals.

Ascorbic acid may also influence the metabolism of lead, as was shown by the two-fold increase in the absorption of the metal from duodenal loops of rat intestine when ascorbic acid was added to the incubation medium [44]. Addition of large amounts of ascorbic acid to rat diets (1%) did not affect however the development of lead toxicity or affect kidney lead concentrations, although administration of both iron (400 mg/kg diet) and ascorbic acid had a protective effect [45].

EFFECT OF IRON ON CADMIUM AND LEAD TOXICITY

A common symptom of chronic cadmium toxicosis in industrial workers and experimental animals is the occurrence of a hypochromic, microcytic anaemia, with depletion of iron stores. Dietary supplementation with iron prevents the development of this iron deficiency state and, in addition, eliminates other symptoms of cadmium poisoning, such as growth failure and disturbances in the metabolism of essential elements like copper and zinc [43]. Kidney cadmium concentrations are also reduced in cadmium-treated rats given dietary supplements of iron and ascorbic acid (Table 4).[46]. Although there are no reports of iron preventing

cadmium-induced renal dysfunction, this is merely a reflection of the
short duration of most experiments on the cadmium-iron interaction.

Table 4   Effect of Dietary Iron Intake on Accumulation of
          Cadmium and Lead in Kidneys

Species	Reference	Dietary Fe Content (mg/kg)	Kidney Cd (% of control value)	Kidney Pb (% of control value)
Mouse	[48]	4	427	
		120	100	
Japanese quail	[43]	25	100	
		100	54	
Rat	[36]	10		706
		40		100
		100		59
Rat	[45]	not given		100
		400		49

This effect of iron on cadmium accumulation results primarily from
reduced intestinal absorption of the metal, probably because the two
metals share common pathways for their mucosal uptake and transfer to
the plasma [47].   Any physiological state which induces increased iron
absorption may therefore also increase the absorption of cadmium.   Thus,
absorption of oral ^{115m}Cd by iron-deficient was greater by 40% than that
by iron-adequate animals [48].   The accumulation of cadmium by the
kidneys was particularly enhanced, concentrations in the kidneys of the
iron-deficient animals being 4 times greater than that in control
kidneys (Table 4).

Similar effects of iron deficiency have been noted in studies on
cadmium absorption by humans [48].   Subjects with reduced iron stores,
as indicated by low serum ferritin levels, absorbed 8.9% of a test dose
of 25 μg of ^{115m}Cd, whereas patients with normal serum ferritin levels
only absorbed 2.3% of the dose.   Significantly, none of the human
subjects showed any clinical signs of anaemia and blood haemoglobin
concentrations were normal.   Since mild iron deficiency is not uncommon
in human populations, especially in women, this could have an important
influence on the extent to which cadmium is absorbed and accumulated in
the kidneys of individuals exposed to cadmium, with eventual onset of
renal dysfunction.

Iron-deficient humans may also be at greater risk of lead poisoning,
since it has been shown that iron-deficient rats are more severely
affected by lead than are animals with an adequate iron intake [36].
In particular, renal and femur lead concentrations may be increased up
to 7-fold in animals receiving iron-deficient diets (Table 4).
Conversely, increasing dietary iron concentrations to levels beyond
those regarded as nutritionally-adequate can also provide protection
against lead toxicity.   Thus, a dietary supplement of 400 mg iron/kg
eliminated lead-induced kidney hypertrophy, decreased kidney lead
content and prevented the growth failure and anaemia which occurred in
rats given a diet containing 500 mg lead/kg [45].   However, dietary
iron did not affect the excretion of lead already accumulated in the

body or given parenterally, indicating that the interaction between the metals occurs principally in the intestine. This has been confirmed by the finding that lead and iron, like cadmium and iron, share common absorptive pathways in the intestinal mucosa [49].

EFFECT OF DIETARY ZINC AND COPPER ON METAL TOXICITY

Zinc is another metal which shares the same absorptive pathway as iron and, in addition, interacts with a range of essential and non-essential elements. For example, excessive zinc intakes can seriously disturb copper metabolism and induce copper deficiency in animals. However, dietary supplementation with zinc can also be used to provide protection against copper toxicosis in sheep [50]. Thus increasing the dietary zinc content of lambs to 420 mg/kg diet prevented or delayed the onset of liver damage, the haemolysis of red cells and the renal failure which is thought to be the cause of death in copper poisoned animals. Although it is possible that the inhibitory effect of zinc against lipid peroxidation helped to stabilize lysosomal and erythrocyte membranes and so prevent haemolysis, the main effect of zinc was probably to restrict the hepatic accumulation of copper which is the first step in the development of this disease. This was probably achieved by reduction in the efficiency of copper absorption, possibly through zinc-induced synthesis of intestinal metallothionein, as has been demonstrated in rats [51].

Effects of zinc on metallothionein synthesis are also thought to be responsible for the protection which parenterally-administered zinc affords against acute cadmium toxicity [see 52]. Thus prior injection of zinc has prevented the occurrence of testicular necrosis, placental haemorrhage and impaired hepatic function in cadmium-injected rats. The incidence of chronic cadmium toxicity is also affected by the zinc status of animals. Zinc deficiency exacerbates susceptibility to this disease and zinc supplementation prevents the development of certain lesions, such as growth failure and impaired glucose tolerance, in cadmium-treated rats [53]. However, no investigations appear to have demonstrated that zinc can provide protection against cadmium-induced renal damage in animals. This is probably again a reflection of the relatively short duration of most experiments and the resultant failure to increase renal cadmium concentrations to critical levels. Nevertheless, zinc supplementation can decrease renal cadmium accumulation in rats receiving cadmium-containing diets, as was shown by the decrease by 50% in kidney cadmium when the zinc intake was increased from 30 to 300 mg/kg diet [54].

A similar reduction in renal cadmium content was obtained in rats by increasing the dietary copper content from 2.6 to 7.8 mg/kg, suggesting that slight variations in copper intake could also influence the eventual development of renal damage [54]. Jacobs et al [55] also reported that the renal accumulation of cadmium by Japanese quail could be reduced by a third simply by increasing copper, zinc and manganese intakes from near the estimated requirement level to only double these amounts. Significantly, this effect was obtained at very low dietary cadmium intakes (20-1000 µg/kg), similar to those found in human diets.

Zinc and copper can also modify the toxicity of lead in animals. Thus, increasing the zinc content of a lead-containing diet from 8 to 200 mg/kg decreased lead concentrations in the kidneys and other tissues of rats, and also decreased the inhibition of kidney -aminolevulinic dehydratase activity [56].   Excretion of urinary δ-aminolevulinic acid (ALA) and accumulation of free erythrocyte porphyrins were also decreased by this treatment, indicating a protective effect of zinc against lead toxicity.

In contrast, dietary supplementation with copper (20 mg/kg diet) tended to exacerbate the toxicity of lead, since urinary ALA excretion was increased and kidney lead concentrations were 50% greater than those in rats given a diet with only 1 mg copper/kg [57].

EFFECT OF SELENIUM ON CADMIUM AND MERCURY TOXICITY

The toxicity of some metals is also influenced by variations in selenium intake, as is illustrated by the prevention of acute mercury-induced kidney damage in rats by administration of selenite [58]. Injection of selenite also prevents many manifestations of acute cadmium toxicity, such as testicular and placental necrosis [58]. However the effects of variation in dietary selenium supply on the renal failure which develops on chronic exposure to these metals are not so well established.

Supplementation of rat diets with selenite (5 mg Se/kg diet) prevented the growth failure and kidney hypertrophy in rats given a diet with 40 mg inorganic mercury/kg [59].   Kidney mercury concentrations were decreased by over 60% by this selenium treatment although at higher mercury intakes (400 mg/kg diet), selenite increased kidney mercury levels by this same amount.   Inclusion of selenate in the drinking water of rats (5-15 mg Se/litre) also had a marked protective effect against the renal damage induced by inorganic mercury (50 mg/litre water) [60].   It eliminated the proteinuria and reduced the incidence of swollen tubular cells and epithelial proliferation of Bowman's space in the kidneys.   However, there was a large increase in the numbers of inclusion bodies containing selenium in the proximal convoluted tubules.   Kidney mercury concentrations were also increased in the selenium-treated rats, despite the reduction in the degree of renal damage, suggesting an abnormal distribution of the metal.   An inverse relationship between selenium intake and kidney mercury concentrations was also evident when selenium-deficient rats were given mercury in their drinking water, since kidney mercury was increased 4-fold compared with that in rats given adequate dietary selenium [61].

Increasing dietary selenium concentrations to 1.0 mg/kg diet increased kidney lead concentrations in rats.   Since this was associated with increased urinary excretion of δ-ALA, it appears that the toxicity of lead may have been exacerbated by these high selenium intakes [62].   In contrast, lower selenium intakes (up to 0.5 mg/kg) had a mildly protective effect.

The mechanisms whereby selenium modifies the reno-toxicity and renal accumulation of these metals has not been established but studies involving the parenteral administration of selenium and mercury or cadmium have shown that the distribution of the metals between and within tissues is affected by selenium.   Of particular interest are the findings that selenium often increases the concentration of the metals in critical organs, even though it is preventing tissue damage [58], and that selenium and the metals are frequently associated with the same protein fractions [63,64].

CONCLUSIONS

This review has highlighted how the nephrotoxicity of metals in domestic and laboratory animals can be influenced by a wide range of nutritional factors. It has also drawn attention to factors which can influence the renal accumulation of these metals and may therefore, under more appropriate experimental conditions, also affect the incidence of metal-induced renal damage.

Although relatively little data are available from human studies, it seems likely that the toxicity of these metals to man would be subject to the same controlling influences. Even though humans enjoy more varied diets than do most experimental animals, nevertheless, there is ample evidence that nutritional deficiencies are prevalent in both developed and underdeveloped countries. Considering only essential elements it has been estimated that dietary intakes of zinc and copper in the United States are frequently close to the recommended daily allowances for these elements, iron deficiency occurs frequently in pregnant and menstruating women throughout the world, calcium intakes in Asian children are often sub-optimal, and the selenium status of the inhabitants of New Zealand and other countries is remarkably low. It should be recognized also that the poorer communities which are perhaps most likely to be exposed to excessive amounts of heavy metals, because of lack of environmental protection measures or because of socio-economic conditions, may also be those most likely to be consuming poor quality diets. There is an urgent need therefore for more investigations into the importance of nutritional status in influencing the nephrotoxicity of heavy metals to man.

It is important also that experiments with laboratory animals should look more closely at the effects of marginal deficiencies of nutrients on the toxicity of metals, since severe deficiencies of the type used in many experimental studies carried out to date are relatively rare.

In addition, the dietary concentrations of the toxic metals should relate more closely to those encountered in human diets. However, this will necessitate the development of better techniques for the detection of sub-clinical effects on renal structure and function. In many of the reports cited in this review, only cursory attempts have been made to determine whether the dietary treatments have affected the reno-toxic effects of the metal under examination. Consequently, it has been necessary to attach a great deal of reliance to changes in the renal accumulation of the metals, although this does not necessarily give a valid indication of susceptibility to kidney damage. This is particularly so when dietary treatments modify the distribution of the metal in tissues, as was described for molybdenum-copper and mercury-selenium interactions.

This highlights another area worthy of further examination, since the mechanisms whereby the nephrotoxicity of metals is affected by various dietary components is still largely unknown. On occasion, the primary effect is on the intestinal absorption of the metal. In other cases, the toxic metal appears to share a particular pathway with an essential element, with the result that homeostatic regulation of the metabolism of the latter also affects the uptake, distribution or excretion of the former. Another possibility is that particular dietary treatments favour the introduction of novel metal-binding sites into proteins, with resultant effects on the distribution and toxicity of the heavy metal.

Considerable benefits may accrue from the extension of our knowledge
of these biological processes, since the information gained should
facilitate the development of suitable methods for the control of
metal-induced nephrotoxicity, if or when environmental control measures
should fail.

REFERENCES

1. Bremner I, Q Rev Biophys 7:75-124, 1974.
2. Nordberg GF, et al. Environ Health Perspect 25:3-41, 1978.
3. Mylroie AA, et al. Environ Res 15:57-64, 1978.
4. Kostial K and Kello D, Bull Environ Contam Toxicol 21:312-314, 1979.
5. Rabar I and Kostial K, Arch Toxicol 47:63-66, 1981.
6. Wapnir RA, et al. Am J Clin Nutr 33:1071-1076, 1980.
7. Muto Y and Omori M, J Nutr Sci Vitaminol (Tokyo) 23:349-360, 1977.
8. Friberg L, et al. Cadmium in the Environment, 2nd ed. CRC Press,
     Cleveland, Ohio, 1974. ISBN 0-87819 018X.
9. Davies NT, et al. Br J Nutr 38:153-156, 1977.
10. Kostial K, Environ Health Perspect 25:81-86, 1978.
11. Keller CA and Doherty RA, Am J Physiol 239:G114-G122, 1980.
12. Sasser LB and Jarboe GE, J Nutr 110:1641-1647, 1980.
13. Suzuki S, et al. Ind Health 7:155-159, 1969.
14. Omori M and Muto Y, J Nutr Sci Vitaminol 23:361-373, 1977.
15. Quarterman J, et al. Environ Res 17:68-77, 1978.
16. Fox MRS, et al. Environ Health Perspect 28:107-114, 1979.
17. Fox MRS, et al. Fed Proc 32:924, 1973.
18. Lagally HR, et al. Nutr Rep Int 21:351-364, 1980.
19. Quarterman J, et al. Environ Res 23:54-67, 1980.
20. Gunn SA, et al. J Pathol Bacteriol 96:80-96, 1968.
21. Quarterman J, et al. J Comp Pathol 87:405-416, 1977.
22. Morrison J, et al. J Comp Pathol 87:417-429, 1977.
23. Gopinath C, et al. Res Vet Sci 16:57-69, 1974.
24. Suttle NF, Anim Feed Sci Technol 2:235-246, 1977.
25. Bremner I and Young BW, Br J Nutr 39:325-336, 1978.
26. Van Ryssen JBJ and Stielau WJ, Br J Nutr 45:203-210, 1981.
27. Bremner I and Young BW, Chem Biol Interact 19:13-23, 1977.
28. Mills CF and Bremner I, in Molybdenum and Molybdenum-Containing
     Enzymes (M Coughlan, ed) Pergamon Press, Oxford, 1980,
     pp 517-542. ISBN 0-08-024398-3.
29. Abdel-Rahim AG, Dietary factors affecting selenium utilization by
     animals, PhD Thesis, University of Aberdeen, 1980.
30. Whanger PD, et al. J Nutr 111:1196-1215, 1981.
31. Washko PW and Cousins RJ, J Nutr 107:920-928, 1977.
32. Larsson S-E and Piscator M, Israel J Med Sci 7:495-498, 1971.
33. Itokawa J, et al. Arch Environ Health 28:149-154, 1974.
34. Kawamura J, et al. Nephron 20:101-110, 1978.
35. Six KM and Goyer RA, J Lab Clin Med 76:933-940, 1970.
36. Mahaffey KM, et al. Ann New York Acad Sci 355:285-297, 1980.
37. Quarterman J, et al. Environ Res 17:60-67, 1978.
38. Washko PW and Cousins RJ, J Toxicol Environ Health 1:1055-1066, 1976.
39. Barton JC, et al. J Lab Clin Med 91:366-376, 1978.
40. Barton JC, et al. Am J Physiol 238:G124-G130, 1980.
41. Koo SI, et al. J Nutr 108:1812-1822, 1978.
42. Cousins RJ and Feldman, SL, Nutr Rep Int 8:363-369, 1973.

43. Fox MRS, et al. Ann New York Acad Sci 355:249–261, 1980.
44. Conrad ME and Barton JC, Gastroenterology 74:731–740, 1978.
45. Suzuki T and Yoshida A, J Nutr 109:1974–1978, 1979.
46. Maji T and Yoshida A, Nutr Rep Int 10:139–149, 1974.
47. Hamilton DL and Valberg LS, Am J Physiol 227:1033–1037, 1974.
48. Flanagan PR, et al. Gastroenterology 74:841–846, 1978.
49. Flanagan PR, et al. Gastroenterology 77:1074–1081, 1979.
50. Bremner I, et al. Br J Nutr 36:551–561, 1976.
51. Hall AC, et al. J Inorg Biochem 11:57–66, 1979.
52. Bremner I, World Rev Nutr Diet 32:165–197, 1978.
53. Petering HG, et al. Arch Environ Health 23:93–101, 1971.
54. Bremner I and Campbell JK, Ann New York Acad Sci 355:319–332, 1980
55. Jacobs RM, et al. J Nutr 108:22–32, 1978.
56. Cerklewski FL and Forbes RM, J Nutr 106:689–696, 1976.
57. Cerklewski FL and Forbes RM, J Nutr 107:143–146, 1977.
58. Parizek J, et al. in Newer Trace Elements in Nutrition (W Mertz and
    WE Cornatzer, eds). Marcel Dekker Inc, New York, 1971, pp 85–120.
    ISBN 0-8247-1110-6.
59. Potter S and Matrone G, J Nutr 104:638–647, 1974.
60. Groth DH, et al. in Trace Substances in Environmental Health
    Vol VI (DD Hemphill, ed) University of Missouri, Columbia, 1973,
    pp 187–189.
61. Burk RF, et al. Toxicol Appl Pharmac 40:71–82, 1977.
62. Cerklewski FL and Forbes RM, J Nutr 106:778–783, 1976.
63. Burk RF, et al. Proc Soc Exp Biol Med 145:782–785, 1974.
64. Gasiewicz TA and Smith JC, Biochim Biophys Acta 428:113–122, 1976.

ROLE OF METALLOTHIONEINS AND OTHER BINDING PROTEINS IN THE RENAL HANDLING AND TOXICITY OF METALS

M. Webb

Toxicology Unit, MRC Laboratories, Woodmansterne Road, Carshalton, Surrey SM5 4EF, UK

ABSTRACT

Metallothioneins, in which zinc and/or copper cations are the principal bound metallic ions, are normal foetal-neonatal proteins and also are synthesized under normal physiological conditions in the adult to regulate the metabolism of these ions in response to variations in nutritional status. Certain non-essential, toxic metallic ions also cause the induction of metallothionein synthesis either directly, or indirectly through their interactions with either the essential zinc, or copper cation.

Aspects of the chemistry and biochemistry of these metalloproteins, that are relevant to their functions in metal homoeostasis and detoxification in the kidney, are reviewed. Evidence is given to show that other low molecular weight binding proteins, which function in the renal handling of certain metallic ions, also are metallothioneins. An alternative mechanism of detoxification, particularly for lead and bismuth, which is provided by the formation of intra-nuclear inclusion bodies, is discussed.

The functions and limitations of the soluble metallothioneins and insoluble inclusion bodies in detoxification are considered in relation to human exposure to industrial and environmental metal pollutants, the use of various metallic salts and complexes as therapeutic agents and in disorders of essential metal metabolism.

Key words: Metal-binding-proteins; Metallothioneins; Metal homoeostasis; Detoxification.

METALLOTHIONEINS AND OTHER METAL-BINDING PROTEINS

History and properties. Since the cadmium ion is cumulative and its transfer through the food chains cannot be avoided, long lived animal species, even in uncontaminated environments, can accumulate appreciable body-burdens of the metal during their life-times. Most of this cadmium is stored in the liver and kidneys as a soluble, low molecular weight metalloprotein. The first preparation of this metalloprotein was isolated from horse kidneys by Margoshes & Vallee [1] in 1957 and characterized by Kagi & Vallee [2,3]. It contained zinc and some copper, in addition to cadmium and had an exceptionally high content of cysteinyl sulphur. Because of these characteristics, Kagi & Vallee [2] named the metalloprotein "metallothionein", i.e. the metallo derivative of the sulphur-rich protein, thionein. Later it was found that thionein was inducible and its synthesis in the liver and/or kidney followed the administration to the experimental animal of various other cations, in addition to cadmium. The discovery that synthesis of usually short-lived metallothioneins, in which zinc and copper were the major bound metals, also occurred when the intakes or body burdens of these essential elements were excessive, established that the function of thionein was not confined to the metabolic control of toxic metals such as mercury and cadmium (see ref. 4). Indeed there is now good evidence that thionein is a normal foetal protein, which functions in copper and zinc homoeostasis during gestation and early neonatal life. The capacity for this synthesis is retained in the adult and can provide a control mechanism when serious disturbances occur in zinc or copper metabolism [5]. Synthesis of metallothionein in response to a toxic and unessential metal, therefore, probably reflects nothing more than the ability of this metal to interact, either directly or indirectly, with the normal homoeostatic processes. Nevertheless, much of the early work on metallothioneins was concerned with their toxicological significance and developed from Piscator's [6] observation of the progressive accumulation of the cadmium ion in such protein-bound form in the livers and kidneys of rabbits in response to repeated doses of cadmium chloride. At this time there was much evidence that environmental cadmium pollution was the cause of the Japanese itai-itai disease (see ref. 7) and was a probable hazard to human health in other industrialised countries (see ref 8). Understandably, therefore, Piscator's [6] hypothesis that the inducible synthesis of metallothionein formed a defence mechanism against this toxic cation, led to much effort to validate it (see ref. 4).

Fortunately, this interest in one potential biological function also stimulated developments in the chemistry and biochemistry of the metallothioneins. In these fields evidence accumulated on the existence of multiple forms (isometallothioneins) of the metalloprotein in different species, the amino acid compositions of many, as well as the sequences of certain of them, their physico-chemical properties, the participation of all of their sulphydryl groups in metal coordination and the conservation of the positions of the cysteinyl residues in their polypeptide chains (see refs 4 and 9). Some of these findings that are relevant to the present discussion are illustrated in the following figures. The first (Fig. 1) shows the isolation of metallothionein by gel-filtration of the soluble fraction from the livers of cadmium exposed rats and the second (Fig. 2), the separation of the initial crude preparation into the isometallothioneins by ion-exchange chromatography. Similar separations, which exploit the

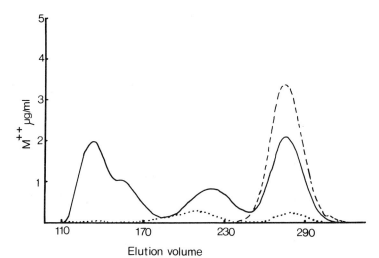

Elution volume

Fig.1.   Isolation of cadmium-induced metallothionein from the soluble
         fraction of rat liver (7g wet weight tissue; 24 μg Cd/g) by gel
         filtration on a column (90 x 2.5 cm) of Sephadex G75 with 10mM
         Tris-HCl buffer, pH 8.0 at a flow-rate of 20 ml/h. as eluant.
         Elution profiles of Cd^{2+} (---), Zn^{2+} (——) and Cu^{2+} (....) are
         shown.   The fraction volume was 3.0 ml. (unpublished results
         of K. Cain and BL Griffiths).

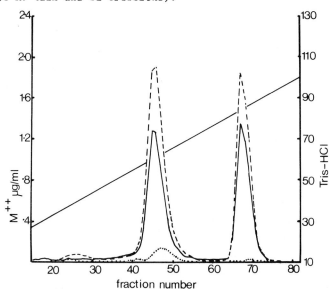

fraction number

Fig.2.   Separation of the isometallothioneins of rat liver by ion
         exchange chromatography.   The crude metallothionein was
         isolated by gel filtration as in Fig. 1 and was chromatographed
         on a column (40 x 1.5 cm) of DE-52 cellulose with a linear
         gradient of 10-200 mM Tris-HCl buffer, pH 8.0 (400 ml), as
         eluant.   Elution of profiles of Cd^{2+} (----), Zn^{2+} (——) and
         Cu^{2+} (....) are shown.   (Unpublished results of K Cain and BL
         Griffiths).

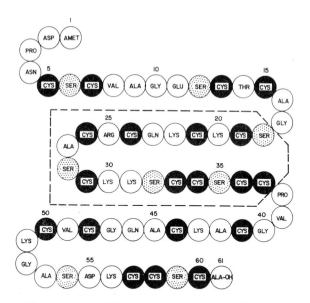

Fig.3. Amino acid sequence of horse kidney isometallothionein 1B.
Reproduced from 'The Chemistry, Biochemistry and Biology of
Cadmium', (M. Webb, Ed), by permission of the publishers.

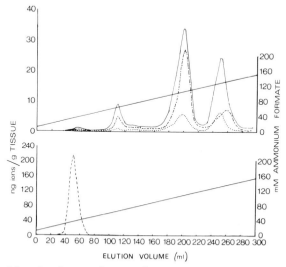

Fig.4. Resolution by ion exchange chromatography of cadmium-induced
rat kidney metallothionein (a) before and (b) after treatment
with mercuric mercury. Elution profiles of Cd^{2+} (——), Zn^{2+}
(......), Cu^{2+} (—·—·—) and Hg^{2+} (----) are shown. The
experimental procedure was as described in the legend to Fig.2
and the fraction volume was 3 ml. (Reproduced from Holt et al;
Chem-Biol Interactions 32:125-135, 1980, by permission of the
publishers).

charge differences of the multiple forms, can be achieved by
electrophoresis and isoelectric focussing (see ref. 4). Fig. 3
illustrates the amino acid sequence of one of the isometallothioneins
of horse kidney and, in particular, the positions of the cysteine
residues in the polypeptide chain.

All of the cysteine residues are involved in cation binding.
Although the structural arrangements at the metal-binding sites
are not fully understood, there is appreciable evidence that zinc
and cadmium cations are bound to thiolate groups in tetrahedral
configuration. Some of the sulphur atoms, therefore, must act as
bridging ligands, since there are seven metal atoms in a (cadmium
zinc)-metallothionein molecule, but only 20 cysteine residues.
Thus each metal cluster in such a metallothionein has a net negative
charge. The total charge on the molecule, however, will be influenced
by the presence of other charged groups in the protein and thus may
vary between isometallothioneins of different amino acid compositions.
The total charge also will alter when cations of different complex
geometry occupy the cation binding sites. After complete substitution
of mercuric mercury for the native cations in a preparation of cadmium
induced rat renal metallothionein in vitro, for example, the isoforms
cannot be separated by ion-exchange chromatography [10]. The major
forms behave as essentially uncharged molecular species and elute from
the column as a single peak with the initial buffer (Fig. 4).

Further problems occur when the metallothionein molecule contains
appreciable amounts of copper. The chemistry of the interaction of the
cupric ion with simple monothiol compounds is complicated not only by
the change in the valency state of the cation, but also by the
susceptibility of the cuprous chelate to oxidation (see e.g. ref. 11).
Metallothionein-bound copper also is in the cuprous form [12]. Whilst
it has yet to be established whether reduction of the cupric ion occurs
before, or is due to, its interaction with the thionein molecule, it is
known that copper-rich metallothioneins are very sensitive to oxidation
and, in air, yield both intra- and inter-molecular disulphides and, in
the presence of peroxides, also sulphinic and sulphonic acids [13].
Such metallothionein molecules, unless isolated and kept under
anaerobic conditions, therefore, not only aggregate readily to
insoluble polymers, but also may have increased negative charge. The
insoluble mitochondrocuprein of neonatal liver [14], for example,
appears to be a polymeric form of copper-thionein, possibly derived
from a (copper,zinc)-thionein by loss of zinc and oxidation of free
thiol groups [15,16]. In 1975, however, it was reported that the low
molecular weight metalloprotein, isolated from the livers and kidneys
of copper-loaded rats, rabbits and chickens contained aromatic amino
acids and had a cysteine content much lower than that of metallothionein [17.18]. This metalloprotein, termed copper-chelatin, bound
irreversibly to DE-cellulose; a property also consistent with the
formation of highly negatively charged species by oxidation of
copper-thionein. Indeed, according to Bremner [19] chelatin is an
artefact of the isolation procedure and, when this is controlled to
prevent oxidation, metallothionein is the only demonstrable
copper-binding protein.

Unfortunately the advent of chelatin cast doubts on the identities
of the metal binding proteins, induced in the kidneys of rats by
exposure to mercury, gold and bismuth and led to the proposal [20] that
these metalloproteins, previously designated "metallothionein-like-
proteins" should be termed "renal metal-binding-proteins". Neither the

alteration in terminology, nor the separation of these metalloproteins into a different family, however, seems justified. The amino acid compositions of the three renal metal binding proteins that are induced in the rat by mercury, for example, characterize them as isometallothioneins [21]. These mercury-induced isometallothioneins, as well as the renal metal-binding proteins induced by gold and bismuth in the rat invariably contain a lot of copper; a probable cause of difficulties in their isolation and purification. Also, copper could be an important factor in their induction and, in this connection, it is unfortunate that most of the work on these metalloproteins has been done with the rat as the experimental animal. In this species, as in the guinea-pig, the hepatic metallothionein that is induced by cadmium is essentially a (Cd,Zn)-metalloprotein, whereas that induced in the kidney contains mainly cadmium and copper. In the mouse, hamster and rabbit, however, chronic cadmium-exposure does not affect the renal concentration of copper, but leads to the accumulation of a (Cd,Zn)-metallothionein [22].

Similar species differences in the redistribution of copper and in renal metalloprotein synthesis are observed after administration of gold [23]. For the rat, at least, there is good evidence that this metalloprotein is a metallothionein. In kidneys of this species, as in the guinea pig, however, the metallothionein induced by gold contains much more copper than the inducing metal; 7 times as much after one dose of 1.0 mg gold/kg body weight. Furthermore the binding of gold in this form is highly correlated with the binding of copper [24]. In the mouse, hamster and rabbit, however, injections of gold neither increase the concentrations of copper or zinc in the kidneys, nor cause the synthesis of a renal metallothionein [23]. Thus the species dependent renal synthesis of metallothionein in response to gold seems to be linked to changes in the kidney concentration of copper.

Renal low molecular weight binding proteins, termed chromochelatins because of their colour and apparent differences from metallothionein in cysteine content and immunological properties, are considered by Piotrowski's group [25-28] to play a key role in the binding of bismuth. The evidence that these proteins are not metallothioneins, however, is equivocal. Bismuth, when given as multiple doses to the rat accumulates, albeit in low concentration, in the liver as a (Zn,Bi)-metallothionein. This metalloprotein has been isolated and characterized; there is no doubt about its identity [27]. As might be expected, the analogous metalloproteins from the kidney are copper, bismuth complexes. The finding that the cysteine contents of the protein moieties of these complexes are about half that of the hepatic metallothionein [27], therefore, could be an artefact; extremely low recovery of cysteine has been a feature of many analyses of authentic copper-metallothioneins (see ref. 4). Also, according to the recent results of Bremner, et al [29], the cysteine contents of the endogenous metallothioneins of rat kidney are about 33% less than those of the liver proteins.

Since the synthesis of metallothioneins, which lack aromatic amino acids and show only minor differences in amino acid sequence, seems to be common to all mammalian species, these metalloproteins are not good antigens. Also it is relevant that, in metal allergy, the immune response appears to be directed more towards the alteration in conformation of autologous proteins caused by metal binding, than towards the substituent metallic ion [30]. It seems significant, therefore, that antisera from rabbits, injected with rat kidney

chromochelatins, cross react with the isoforms of rat renal (Cd,Cu)-,
(Hg,Cu)- and (Bi,Cu)-metal binding proteins, but not with the hepatic
(Cd,Zn)-isometallothioneins [28]. Thus all of the immunoreactive
metalloproteins contain copper and two of them, i.e. those induced by
cadmium and mercury, are known to be metallothioneins. It is likely,
therefore, that chromochelatins, as well as chelatins, are metallothioneins. Thus metallothioneins probably are the only soluble binding
proteins that, through their inducible synthesis, function in the renal
handling and detoxification of certain metals. The significant word
here is "soluble". Insoluble metal-protein complexes, the intranuclear
inclusion bodies, which are discussed later, may be important in the
intracellular metabolism of lead and bismuth.

Functions in metal detoxification. It is assumed that toxic metals,
when bound firmly by the multiple thiol groups of thionein, are
unavailable for interaction at other functional metal-sensitive sites.
Metals that have to be considered in relation to this detoxification
function are not only limited in number, but can be divided into three
groups according to their "hazard-potential" to human health. The
first group includes those metals that, as a result of man's activities
are potentially dangerous to large numbers of people, either through
industrial or environmental exposure. The second contains those that,
through their use as therapeutic agents, may affect smaller numbers,
whilst the third is restricted to essential metals which, through
defects in their metabolism, are associated with specific diseases in
some individuals. In the following discussion it seems appropriate to
consider these groups in reverse order.

The normal function of metallothionein in the regulation of zinc and
copper metabolism, like other biological functions, might be expected
to "go wrong" occasionally. Disorders of zinc metabolism, as in
Acrodermatitis enteropathica and coeliac and Crohn's diseases are due
to congenital or acquired abnormalities in the absorption of this
cation and, although they probably involve metallothionein, are outside
the scope of this meeting. Disorders of copper metabolism are common
to Wilson's disease, Indian childhood cirrhosis and Menkes' disease.
In the last of these, for which a brindled mouse mutant provides an
ideal animal model (see refs 31, 32) the metabolic defect is manifest
by the accumulation of copper, particularly in the kidneys and
intestinal mucosa and a fatal copper-deficiency in the liver. In the
mutant mice, copper trapped in the kidney seems to be stored
irreversibly [32] as the cytoplasmic metallothionein [33]. Prins & Van
den Hamer [33] consider that, as discussed earlier by Danks [31], the
synthesis of this metallothionein is abnormal, and suggest that either
the translation of thionein m-RNA is unrestrained or, as a result of a
defect in renal copper reabsorption, thionein is induced to sequester
the accumulated cation. Mann et al. [34] regard the first of these
alternatives as "probably too simple" and favour the superinduction of
metallothionein, secondary to some other disturbance in the normal
process of intracellular copper transport. This suggestion, which
neglects the cause of the disturbance in the normal transport process,
seems in accord with evidence from other systems that metallothionein
synthesis is determined by an increase in the intracellular
concentration of the inducing metallic ion above a certain critical
threshold (see ref 4). It is known, however, that dexamethasone, in
common with certain other glucocorticoids, can act as a primary inducer
of thionein synthesis in the absence of increased metal uptake [35,36].

Under certain conditions, therefore, metal accumulation may be a consequence of thionein synthesis, not its cause. Any postulate of the hormonal control of thionein synthesis in Menkes' disease, however, would leave unexplained the organ specificity of copper accumulation.

Metallic ions that are used therapeutically, accumulate as metallothioneins in the kidneys and can be nephrotoxic, seem to be limited to gold and bismuth. Platinum binds only to particulate components of the renal tissue; none is found in the soluble fraction, even after treatment of homogenates with reducing agents that are known to liberate particulate-bound metallothioneins (M. Webb, unpublished observations). Gold, at least when administered to experimental animals, either as sodium chloroaurate, which yields monovalent gold by reduction [37], or as aurothiomalate, which liberates the same ion by cleavage and metabolism of the organic part of the molecule [38], causes the synthesis of metallothionein in the kidneys of some species, but not of others [23,24]. Obviously, therefore, this synthesis is not a general mechanism for the renal handling of gold. Furthermore, metallothionein synthesis, in those species in which it occurs, seldom accounts for more than 10% of the total gold in the kidneys and does not seem to have any protective effect. After one dose of 1.0 mg gold/kg body weight the histological changes in the kidneys are the same in the rat and guinea pig, species that synthesize the renal (Cu,Au)-metallothionein, as in those, the hamster and rabbit, that do not [23].

The therapeutic use of organic and inorganic salts of bismuth (e.g. the subgallate, subnitrate and dicitrato-bismuthate) in the treatment of peptic ulcer and colostomy and ileostomy patients can lead to kidney damage [39] in addition to encephalopathy [40]. No attempts seem to have been made, however, to investigate nephrotoxicity in relation to metallothionein synthesis in the bismuth-exposed animals. At present evidence for the synthesis of a renal (Cu,Bi)-metallothionein, on repeated administration of high doses of bismuth, is restricted to the rat. If, as seems probable, species differences in response, similar to those with gold, also occur with bismuth, the induction of thionein synthesis by this metal in the rat may be of academic interest, but is not of general significance.

Ions of a number of metals, for example, nickel, silver, lead, beryllium, tin and chromium, industrial exposure to which may be accompanied by renal problems [41-43], do not, themselves, induce metallothionein synthesis in either the liver or kidney (see ref. 4). Certain of them, however, when administered in high doses to experimental animals may increase the hepatic content of zinc and, perhaps, the renal concentration of copper and thus cause the formation of zinc- or copper-thioneins (see e.g. ref. 44). Thereafter, the administered cation may bind to these metalloproteins. Such interactions, therefore, could be dependent on the essential metal status; variations in zinc status, for example, may explain why Winge et al. [45], in contrast with Chen et al. [46], observed synthesis of a (Zn,Ag)metallothionein in response to a high dose of silver in the rat. There are no reports, however, that chronic exposure to silver leads to the binding of this metal to metallothionein in either the liver or kidney. If a metallothionein (e.g. zinc-thionein) pre-exists in either of these organs, it does not follow that a foreign cation will bind to it, even if such binding occurs with the isolated metalloprotein in vitro. Thus although lead will bind to presynthesized metallothionein [47, 48], about 90% of the lead in the

kidney of the living animal is likely to be associated with
intranuclear-inclusion bodies [49, 50], not with metallothionein.
These bodies may contain up to 5% lead, bound to an acidic protein
component of the nucleus and, even when the renal lead content is
insufficient to cause the formation of discernible structures, most of
the metal can be found to be complexed to the nuclear protein [42].
Whilst little is known about either "the cost in terms of cellular
function ..., or the source and specificity of these acidic proteins",
it seems that the formation of these bodies "enhances tolerance to a
number of environmentally ubiquitous metals" [42]. Of these metals
lead probably is the most important, although formation of inclusion
bodies, which may persist in man for up to 30 years after cessation of
therapy [51] also is a significant response to bismuth.

    Bremner et al. [29] have shown that the renal metabolism of copper
is subject to hormonal influence and the age-related increases in total
and thionein bound copper are greater in the kidneys of female than of
male rats. A similar sex-difference is apparent in mercury-binding to
renal metallothionein in normal and cadmium-pretreated rats [52]. Also
the increases in the kidney concentrations of cadmium and copper, that
result from the oral administration of cadmium, are greater in females
than in males [53]. These differences provide additional evidence,
therefore, that the renal accumulation of thionein-bound cadmium or
mercury occurs not as a result of specific detoxification mechanisms,
but because these metals interact with normal homoeostatic processes.
Furthermore, too much significance should not be attached to the
thionein-binding of mercury; the absolute amount of mercury in this
form is small. Thus in the male rat less than 2% of the total renal
content is thionein-bound at 24 h after a dose of 0.5 mg Hg^{2+}/kg,
(Table 1). This dose is sufficient to cause extensive necrosis in

Table 1. Kidney concentrations of total and thionein-bound mercury in
          normal and cadmium-pretreated male and female rats at 24 h
          after the intraperitoneal administration of $HgCl_2$.

Sex	Pretreatment	Hg dose (mg/kg body wt)	Total Hg	Thionein-bound Hg	Non-thionein bound Hg
				μg/g wet wt tissue	
Male	None	0.5	17.6	0.3	17.3
		1.0	23.9	0.7	23.2
		1.5	30.9	3.7	27.2
Male	Cd	0.5	34.7	3.8	30.9
		1.0	27.7	5.6	22.1
		1.5	31.4	5.2	26.2
Female	None	0.5	26.7	1.1	25.6
		1.0	27.2	2.2	25.0
		1.5	26.7	3.7	23.0
Female	Cd	0.5	37.1	4.1	33.0
		1.0	44.8	12.6	32.2
		1.5	48.4	16.9	31.5

The results shown are mean values, calculated from the data of Webb
and Magos [52].

the proximal tubules of the male, but is not nephrotoxic in the female rat, although it results in higher concentrations of total, thionein-bound and non-thionein-bound mercury (Table 1). At a dose level of 1 mg Hg^{2+}/kg, the concentration of non-thionein bound mercury in the female remains essentially the same as that after the lower dose, since thionein-binding is increased. This increased binding, however, is not protective; tubular damage being extensive at this dose level [54].

Cadmium pretreatment protects against the nephrotoxicity of all of these mercury doses in the female rat, but only against the lowest dose in the male [54]. Although this difference seems to parallel the sex differences in thionein-binding of mercury in the pretreated rats, incorporation of mercury into all other components of the kidney also is increased, relative to the control, by the pretreatment. It appears, therefore, that neither endogenous, nor cadmium-induced metallothionein confers protection against mercury-nephrotoxicity; a conclusion which, of course, is understandable if the renal damage results from extra-tubular or membrane interactions. Alterations in membrane structure similar to those that occur after a low dose of mercury [55], for example, may underlie the protective effect of cadmium-pretreatment. Nevertheless, thionein binding of mercury could be relevant to the increased tolerance of newborn animals to this metal. Both the intestinal copper-complex and hepatic zinc-thionein of the neonate provide additional high-affinity binding sites for mercury and can influence the absorption and distribution of the latter. Thus, although the liver and gastrointestinal tract are not subjects of this symposium, they may be important factors, in addition to the functional and biochemical immaturity of the kidneys, in the resistance of the newborn animal to mercury nephrotoxicity [56].

As there seems to be no information about the thionein-binding of mercuric mercury in the kidneys of animals after prolonged low level ingestion of the cation from food or water, it can only be inferred that such exposure would not lead to appreciable accumulation of the metallothionein. Although mercury binds much more strongly than cadmium to thionein [2], in vivo thionein-bound mercury is cleared from the kidney much more rapidly than thionein-bound cadmium. This is apparent in normal rats and in cadmium-pretreated animals, in which the retention-time of mercury appears to be increased [57]. In both groups, however, the clearance curves for total mercury and thionein-bound mercury parallel one another. Thus all forms of intracellular mercury are in equilibrium. Metallothionein, therefore, acts as a metal ion buffer and the intracellular distribution of a particular cation between this and other proteins at a given time, will depend upon its relative affinities for all binding sites, not on its absolute affinity for thionein. If, for example, mercury is added in an amount equivalent to the total content of thionein-bound metallic ions in a preparation of the soluble fraction from the kidneys of cadmium-exposed rats, most (70%) of the mercury binds to the high molecular weight proteins, not to the metallothionein (Fig. 5). Furthermore, if a preparation of renal (Cd,Hg)-metallothionein is mixed with the high molecular weight protein fraction from the cytosol of the normal rat kidney, an appreciable amount of mercury is transferred from the former to the latter. Intermolecular hybridization between the large proteins and the incompletely metal-saturated metallothionein, which is shown by the apparent transfer of a small amount of cadmium under these conditions, is insufficient to explain the redistribution of mercury.

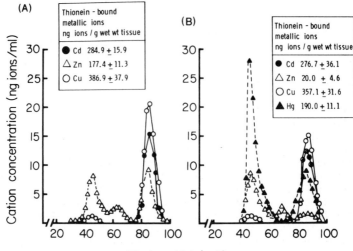

Fig.5.   Gel filtration of the soluble fraction from the kidneys of
         cadmium-treated rats (a) before and (b) after the addition of
         mercury equivalent to the sum of the initial contents of
         thionein-bound cations. The experimental procedure was as
         described in the legend to Fig.1 except that an 80 x 2.5 cm
         Sephadex column was used and 5 ml fractions were collected.
         (Reproduced from Webb et al; Chem-Biol Interactions 32:137-149,
         1980, by permission of the publishers).

If, therefore, elimination of these metallic ions from the kidney is a
function of their concentrations in the non-thionein pool, the rate of
loss of cadmium would be expected to be considerably less than that of
mercury, since its relative affinity for thionein is much greater.

Kidney damage is not a normal response to a single acute dose of
cadmium alone since, under these conditions, accumulation occurs mainly
in the liver and renal uptake is small [58]. The distribution of
cadmium between the liver and kidney, however, can be altered by the
administration of an excess of a suitable chelating agent
simultaneously with the cation. At 1 h after the injection of 10 μmol
cadmium chloride (1.12 mg Cd^{2+}) and 5 m mol cysteine/kg body weight
into the JCL-rat, for example, the hepatic concentration of cadmium is
less, but the renal concentration is 30 times greater than that after
the injection of cadmium chloride alone. In the Wistar rat under the
same conditions the maximal renal concentration is similar to that in
the JCL-rat, but is not attained until 2-4 h after dosing. In these
rats, treatment with 1 μmol cadmium chloride in combination with the
same dose of cysteine leads to a kidney concentration of 5-6 μg
cadmium/g. wet weight without tubular damage. In contrast, rats of
both strains, treated with 10 μmol cadmium chloride and cysteine
develop severe renal damage. Even by light microscopy, the onset of
this is clearly apparent by 4 h and, by 7 h, is extensive. Thus
nephrotoxicity can result from a small renal burden of cadmium,
certainly less than 20, but more than 6 μg/g wet weight, provided this
is accumulated rapidly. The appreciable synthesis of metallothionein,
which occurs in the kidneys of these animals between 2 and 7 h after

the administration of the high dose, occurs after the damage has been done and clearly has no protective effect.

In contrast, prolonged low level dietary administration of cadmium, for which the cadmium-cysteine combination does not provide an ideal short-term experimental model [58], is accompanied by the synthesis of metallothionein in parallel with the renal uptake of the cation. If it is accepted that at any time, at least before the onset of spontaneous nephropathy associated with aging, about 80% of the cadmium in the kidney will be bound as the metallothionein, at the critical concentration, usually regarded as 200 μg/g wet weight [8], the concentration of non-thionein bound cadmium would be approximately 40 μg/g wet weight. This is similar to, but still about twice that observed in the damaged kidneys after administration of the cadmium-cysteine combination. These figures for the concentrations of total and thionein-bound cadmium, of course, are unlikely to reflect accurately those in the tubules or, more specifically, in those tubular cells that suffer damage and thus no great significance should be attached to them. It is possible, however, that metallothionein concentrations, as determined by the analysis of renal soluble fractions only, are too low. Sato [59], for example, has shown that renal mitochondria from cadmium-exposed rats contain a (Cd,Zn)-metallothionein. This could explain why such mitochondria, which may contain what should be an inhibitory concentration of cadmium, not only metabolize pyruvate and succinate at the same rates as control preparations, but also are more resistant than the latter to inhibition by the free cation in vitro (K. Cain & M. Webb unpublished observations).

In the normal animal it is clear that the kidney can tolerate a large amount of this cation because much of it is bound as the metallothionein. As mentioned earlier, however, this binding, is not a specific detoxification mechanism. Indeed, evolution surely would have favoured the development of a defence mechanism that either limited the uptake, or enhanced the elimination of a toxic metal, rather than one that led to its retention. Furthermore, retention of cadmium as the metallothionein is not confined to the kidney, but occurs also in the liver. As the biological half-time of cadmium in the liver is less than that in the kidney, there is a slow transfer of the cation from the former to the latter organ (see e.g. ref 60). The controversy whether this transfer occurs through the liberation of hepatic cadmium either as the "free" cation or as the metallothionein is immaterial, since the rate of transfer is extremely slow. The important fact is that transfer does occur and, at least in the experimental animal that already contains an appreciable renal burden of cadmium, may increase the kidney concentration to above the critical level at some considerable time after the termination of exposure [61]. Since no-one has found a mammalian species that is unable to synthesize metallothionein, it is not possible to answer the question "would cadmium accumulate and be retained in the livers and kidneys if this synthesis did not occur?"

REFERENCES

1. Margoshes M and Vallee BL. J Am Chem Soc 79:4813-4814, 1957.
2. Kagi JHR and Vallee BL. J Biol Chem 235:3460-3465, 1960.
3. Kagi JHR and Vallee BL. J Biol Chem 236:2435-2442, 1961.

4. Webb M. in The Chemistry, Biochemistry and Biology of Cadmium. (M Webb, Ed). Elsevier/North Holland, Amsterdam, 1979, pp.195-266. ISBN 0-444-80109-X.
5. Webb M and Cain K. Biochem Pharmacol. In press.
6. Piscator M. Nord Hyg Tidskr 45:76-82, 1964.
7. Tsuchiya K (Ed). Cadmium Studies in Japan - A Review. Elsevier/North Holland, Amsterdam, 1978 pp. 1-376. ISBN 0-444-80049-2.
8. Friberg L, et al. Cadmium in the Environment. CRC Press, Cleveland, Ohio 1974, pp.1-248. ISBN 0-87819-018-X.
9. Kagi JHR and Nordberg M (Eds). Metallothionein. Experientia Suppl 34, 1979, pp.1-378. ISBN 3-7643-1036-7.
10. Holt D, Magos L and Webb M. Chem-Biol Interactions 32:125-135, 1980.
11. McCall JT, et al. In Trace Substances in Environmental Health - II. Univ Missouri, Columbia, 1968, pp.127-139.
12. Weser U and Rupp H. In The Chemistry, Biochemistry and Biology of Cadmium. (M Webb, Ed). Elsevier/North Holland, Amsterdam, 1979, pp. 267-283. ISBN 0-444-80109-X.
13. Weser U and Rupp H. In Metallothionein. (JHR Kagi and M Nordberg, Eds). Experientia Suppl. 34, 1979, pp.221-230. ISBN 3-7643-1036-7.
14. Porter H and Folch J. J Neurochem 1:260-271, 1957.
15. Porter H. Biochem Biophys Res Commun 56:661-668, 1974.
16. Rupp H and Weser U. FEBS Lett 44:293-297, 1974.
17. Winge DR, et al. Arch Biochem Biophys 170:253-266, 1975.
18. Premakumar R, et al. Arch Biochem Biophys 170:278-288, 1975.
19. Bremner I. In Biological Roles of Copper. Ciba Foundation Symp 79. Excerpta Med 1980, pp.23-38. ISBN 90-219-4085-X.
20. Piotrowski JK, et al. In Metallothionein. (JHR Kagi and M Nordberg, Eds). Experientia Suppl 34, 1979, pp.363-371. ISBN 3-7643-1036-7.
21. Zelazowski AJ and Piotrowski JK. Abst. 2nd Internat. Metallothionein Meeting, Univ. Aberdeen, 4-5 April 1981.
22. Suzuki KT. Arch Environ Contam Toxicol 8:255-268, 1979.
23. Mogilnicka EM and Webb M. J Appl Toxicol 1:42-49, 1981.
24. Mogilnicka Em and Webb M. J Appl Toxicol. In press.
25. Szymanska JA, Mogilnicka M and Kaszper BW. Biochem Pharmacol 26:257-258, 1977.
26. Szymanska JA, et al. Arch Toxicol 40:131-141, 1978.
27. Szymanska JA and Piotrowski JK. Abst. 2nd Internat. Metallothionein Meeting, Univ. Aberdeen, 4-5 April 1981.
28. Zelazowski AJ, Szymanska JA and Cierniewska CS. Chem-Biol Interactions 33:115-125, 1980.
29. Bremner I, Williams RB and Young BW. J Inorg Biochem 14:135-146, 1981.
30. Dewdney JM and Edwards RG. Chem Br 16:600-615, 1980.
31. Danks DM. Inorg Perspect Biol Med 1:77-100, 1977.
32. Prins HW and Van den Hamer CJA. J Inorg Biochem 10:19-27, 1979.
33. Prins HW and Van den Hamer CJA. J Nutr 110:151-157, 1980.
34. Mann JR, et al. Biochem J 196:81-88, 1981.
35. Karin M, Herschman HR and Weinstein D. Biochem Biophys Res Commun 92:1052-1059, 1980.
36. Karin M and Herschman HR. Eur J Biochem 113:267-272, 1981.
37. Sadler PJ. Struct Bonding 29:171-214, 1976.
38. Jellum E and Munthe E. Ann Rheum Dis 39:155-158, 1980.
39. Randall RW, et al. Ann Intern Med 77:481-490, 1972.

40. Thomas DW, et al. In Clinical Chemistry and Chemical Toxicology of
    Metals. (SS Brown, Ed). Elsevier/North Holland, Amsterdam, 1977,
    pp.293-296. ISBN 0-444-41601-3.
41. Just J and Szniolois A. J Am Water Works Assoc 28:492-495, 1936.
42. Goyer RA and Cherian MG. In Clinical Chemistry and Chemical
    Toxicology of Metals. (SS Brown, Ed). Elsevier/North Holland,
    Amsterdam, 1977, pp.89-103. ISBN 0-444-41601-3.
43. Norseth T. In Trace Metals: Exposure and Health Effects. (E Di
    Ferranti, Ed). Pub for CEC by Pergamon Press, Oxford, 1979,
    pp.135-146. ISBN 0-08-0224466.
44. Suzuki Y and Yoshikawa H. Ind Health 14:25-31, 1976.
45. Winge DR, Premakumar R and Rajagopalan KV. Arch Biochem Biophhys
    170:242-252, 1975.
46. Chen RW, Whanger PD and Weswig PH. Biochem Med 12:95-105, 1975.
47. Ulmer DD and Vallee BL. In Trace Substances in Environmental
    Health. (DD Hemphill, Ed). Univ Missouri Press, Columbia, Miss.
    1968, pp.7-27.
48. Mogilnicka EM, Piotrowski JK and Trojanowska B. Med Pracy
    26:147-155, 1975.
49. Goyer RA, et al. Arch Environ Health 20:705-711, 1970.
50. Goyer RA, et al. Lab Invest 22:245-251, 1970.
51. Beaver DL and Burr RE. Am J Pathol 42:609-617, 1963.
52. Webb M and Magos L. Chem-Biol Interactions 14:357-369, 1976.
53. Murthy L, Rice DP and Petering HG. In Trace Element Metabolism in
    Man and Animals - 3. (M Kirchgessner, Ed). Arbeitsgemeinschaft fur
    Tierernahrungsforschung, Freising-Weihenstephan, 1978, pp.557-560.
54. Magos L, Webb M and Butler WH. Br J Exp Path 55:589-594, 1974.
55. Zalme RC, et al. Virchows Arch B 22:197-216, 1976.
56. Webb M and Holt D. Arch Toxicol. In press.
57. Webb M, Magos, L and Holt D. Chem-Biol Interactions 32:137-149,
    1980.
58. Murakami M and Webb M. Br J Exp Path 62:115-130, 1981.
59. Sato M. Abst US-Japan Workshop on Metallothionein. Cincinnati,
    Ohio, 23-26 March, 1981.
60. Webb M. In Kadmium Symposium Jena 1977. Friedrich-Schiller
    Universitat Jena, 1979, pp.101-107.
61. Kawai K and Kimura M. Ind Health 13:261-265, 1975.

CADMIUM-ASSOCIATED RENAL DAMAGE

F. W. Bonner and B. A. Carter

Robens Institute of Industrial and Environmental Health and Safety, and Department of Biochemistry, University of Surrey, Guildford, Surrey GU2 5XH, UK

ABSTRACT.   The kidney is regarded as a target organ for cadmium toxicity after long term exposure and the metal, mainly bound to metallothionein, accumulates to its highest concentration in this tissue.   In order for the metal to produce nephropathy, an interaction with some functional or structural component of the cell is necessary.

Experimentally, the cadmium-induced lesion is characterised by proteinuria (high and low molecular weight proteins) and an excessive loss of other substances into the urine including enzymes, amino acids, glucose and trace metals.   Morphological effects such as degeneration of the proximal tubule and thickening of the glomerular capsule have been reported. Biochemical changes in the kidney are ill-defined but may include disturbances in enzyme activities, essential metal homeostasis and membrane transport processes.   In humans exposed to high concentrations of cadmium in the environment (Itai-Itai disease), renal damage was manifested as a classical tubular type of proteinuria, but a mixed type of proteinuria has been observed in workers exposed to the metal.   Despite the recognition of the cadmium-induced nephrotoxicity for some considerable time, the molecular events underlying the effect are not well understood.

KEYWORDS.   Cadmium, kidney, metallothionein, proteinuria, critical concentration.

INTRODUCTION

Our awareness of the potential toxicity of cadmium can be traced to the 19th century. The first known case of acute poisoning in humans was reported in Belgium in 1858 and resulted from the inhalation of cadmium dust [1], while in 1867 and 1896 are published some of the earliest descriptions of a cadmium-induced renal lesion in experimental animals [2]. The problem did not receive significant attention however until around 1948 when two separate events prompted further investigations. Firstly, a type of osteomalacia which was associated with renal damage, was diagnosed in certain regions of Japan which were heavily contaminated with cadmium. This syndrome which became known as Itai-Itai disease, occurred predominantly in post-menopausal, multiparous women and was characterised by proteinuria and severe pain in the bones and joints. It is now apparent that nutritional deficiencies of calcium, protein and vitamin D were important in the aetiology of the disease [3]. Also in 1948, Friberg [4] found proteinuria to be a common symptom of workers exposed to cadmium during the manufacture of alkaline batteries. Since then a vast literature describing the uptake of the metal into the kidney and the resultant toxic effects has been published, and this is briefly reviewed.

CADMIUM EXPOSURE AND RENAL UPTAKE

Cadmium is a natural component of the lithosphere and therefore once mobilised, exposure is unavoidable. Mobilisation may occur via both natural (eg. volcanic action) and artifical (eg. mining) processes, though the latter is now of much greater significance. Human exposure to cadmium may occur during production of the metal (occupational exposure), during the utilisation of cadmium-containing products (consumer exposure), and through contaminated foodstuffs as a consequence of the concentration and accumulation of the metal along food chains (environmental exposure). Uptake by inhalation may be significant for persons living close to cadmium-emitting industries. Once exposure has occurred, cadmium is rapidly removed from the blood and deposited in various organs. In this respect, cadmium, like many metals, shows distinct organ specificity, since although most tissues take up cadmium, about 50-75% of the administered metal concentrates in the liver and kidneys [5]. With time however the ratio of metal in the liver compared to kidney decreases which is consistent with the view that transfer from hepatic to renal tissue can occur. After long term exposure however, the highest concentration of cadmium in any tissue occurs in the renal cortex. The kidney is thus regarded as a major target organ.

RENAL EFFECTS OF CADMIUM AFTER CHRONIC EXPOSURE

In experimental animals, the rate of absorption of cadmium is greater via the lung than the gut [6], but regardless of route of exposure, the metal eventually accumulates in the kidney, in association with metallothionein until such time as the concentration becomes critical. Thereafter a wide range of morphological and functional changes may be produced, and these are summarised in Table 1. Many of the effects such as proteinuria and amino aciduria have been shown to occur in humans.
One of the earliest and perhaps most prominent manifestations of

Table 1: Chronic renal effects of cadmium in experimental animals.

Biochemical and Functional Changes

i) Kidney
- decreased activity of leucine
  aminopeptidase
- increased activity of
  gluconeogenic enzymes
- changes in essential metal
  concentrations (Zn, Cu, Fe)

ii) Urine
- increased excretion of
  proteins, amino acids, glucose,
  enzymes, trace metals, calcium,
  phosphate, sodium, potassium,
  cadmium.
- decreased concentrating
  capacity

Morphological Changes

- degeneration of proximal tubules
- thickening of glomerular capsule
- fibrosis of basement membrane
- constriction of renal arteries
- diffuse fibrosis of capillaries

- dilation/proliferation of
  endoplasmic reticulum
- nuclear enlargement
- mitochondrial swelling
- increased numbers of lysosomes
- cytoplasmic oedema

cadmium nephropathy is proteinuria. Traditionally, the proteinuria has been regarded as of tubular origin, ie. a preponderance of low molecular weight proteins derived from the serum such as β_2-microglobulin, retinol-binding protein, lysozyme, ribonuclease etc., and has been observed in both cadmium-exposed workers [7] and experimental animals [8]. An excessive excretion of β_2-microglobulin into the urine was a common finding in Itai-Itai patients [9] and it has been suggested that the determination of this protein may serve as a useful monitor of cadmium-induced renal damage [10]. Such findings support the idea that cadmium exerts its effect upon the kidney by disturbing reabsorption of these low molecular weight compounds by the proximal tubules.

The components of cadmium-proteinuria have been studied by a variety of techniques but more recently, using electrophoresis and quantitation of the proteins, Bernard and co-workers have also demonstrated the excretion of larger amounts of high molecular weight proteins such as albumin and transferrin, in cadmium-exposed workers [11,12]. This infers that cadmium may also disturb the mechanisms regulating the excretion of high molecular proteins in the glomerulus and/or the tubule. A mixed type of proteinuria (ie. both low and high molecular weight components) has also been demonstrated to occur in female rats after repeated parenteral administration of cadmium [13]. Further investigation showed that dietary administration of cadmium produced a proteinuria characterised only by high molecular proteins, especially γ-globulins [14]. Thus, the mode of administration of the cation appears to be an important factor in determining the nature of the proteinuria.

The development of proteinuria is also accompanied by a leakage of other components from the kidney into the urine, including enzymes and trace metals. Figure 1 shows the urinary excretion of cadmium, zinc, copper, iron and alkaline phosphatase after the repeated parenteral administration of cadmium to rats (1.5mgCd/kg/day) [15,16]. Initially

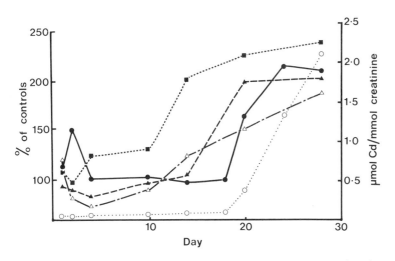

Figure 1. The urinary excretion of alkaline phosphatase (●), cadmium
(○), zinc (▲), copper (■) and iron (△) after the repeated
parenteral administration of cadmium to rats (1.5mgCd/kg/day).
All results are expressed as % of controls except for cadmium excretion
which is expressed as μmol/mmol creatinine.

cadmium excretion is low due to efficient reabsorption through the
proximal tubule but with continued exposure to the metal, a sudden and
dramatic increase in the urinary cadmium occurs.   This is thought to
reflect the onset of renal damage [17].   There is a similar loss of
other metals such as zinc, copper and iron, and also enzymes such as
alkaline phosphatase, probably representing spillage of the
intracellular content of these substances from damaged kidney cells.
    The release of kidney enzymes into the urine may reflect the
development of nephropathy and this has been studied experimentally.
Experiments have shown that in rats given repeated injections of cadmium
(1.5mgCd/kg/day), the appearance of enzymuria was biphasic. An initial
transitory peak of enzymes (eg. alkaline phosphatase, leucine
aminopeptidase, γ-glutamyl transpeptidase) occurred around 24-48 hours
after dosing commenced, the extent of which was dose-related.   As
cadmium treatment continued, this was followed by a second, persistent
phase of enzyme loss, the onset of which was dose-related [18].
Pretreatment with zinc at doses known to induce the synthesis of
zinc-thionein abolished the initial phase but had no effect upon the
second phase of enzymuria [19] (Table 2).   This would suggest that in
the absence of adequate amounts of thionein, eg. before synthesis of the
protein is maximally induced, or after the critical concentration is
reached, cadmium has the potential to produce cell damage.

THE CRITICAL CONCENTRATION AND CADMIUM NEPHROPATHY

    The critical concentration has come to be a useful concept in
explaining the toxic effects of cadmium. By definition, the critical
concentration for a cell is the concentration at which undesirable (or
adverse) functional changes, reversible or irreversible, occur in the
cell [20].   Such a concept obviously has important implications when

Table 2. Urinary excretion of alkaline phosphatase after repeated parenteral administration of cadmium (1.5mgCd/kg,daily) in rats.

	Day			
	2	10	20	28
controls	9.7 ± 0.3	9.4 ± 0.3	7.8 ± 0.2	9.2 ± 0.2
Cd-treated	14.2 ± 0.4[a]	11.9 ± 1.1	14.0 ± 0.5[a]	18.5 ± 0.7[a]
Cd-treated (Zn supplement*)	9.3 ± 0.2	11.2 ± 0.5	14.4 ± 0.6[a]	17.9 ± 0.7[a]

*Zinc supplement (2,000 ppm Zn in diet) for 7 days prior to commencement of cadmium injections.

Enzyme excretion expressed as U/mmol creatinine, mean ± SEM of 5 animals. Statistically significant differences ($p < 0.01$) between groups and controls are denoted by a.

discussing the development of renal damage. Before the critical concentration is reached, metallothionein appears to be synthesised at such a rate as to have sufficient capacity to bind all available cadmium. The protein is thus acting in a detoxifying role. With continued exposure to cadmium, the rate of synthesis of thionein becomes inadequate and the critical concentration is reached. At this stage, it can be envisaged that either the ratio of unbound: thionein bound metal increases, or the ratio of cadmium bound to other protein components: thionein bound metal increases. Alternatively, the concentration of cadmium-thionein in the kidney reaches a level where the metal-protein complex becomes toxic. In either case, cellular damage is the result.

However, this raises the question: what is the toxic agent in cadmium induced nephropathy? It has been shown that cadmium, when bound to thionein is 7 to 8 times more toxic in the rat compared to ionic cadmium [21], and it is postulated that the cadmium-thionein complex produces the damage during the process of entering the cell [22]. Conversely, zinc-thionein is relatively non-toxic [21], and the pre-induction of cadmium-thionein prevents the toxicity due to a subsequent acute dose of the cation [23]. The demonstration that the degree of renal tubular necrosis correlated with the cadmium content in the thionein, but not with the amount of thionein is perhaps the most significant evidence supporting the idea that the cation is the toxic agent [24].

POSSIBLE ROLE OF THE LYSOSOME IN THE RENAL EFFECTS OF CADMIUM

The protein moiety of cadmium-thionein may be broken down to acid-soluble products, in vitro, by kidney cortex homogenate containing enzymes which are probably of lysosomal origin [21], and differential centrifugation techniques have demonstrated a significant uptake of cadmium by lysosomes following intravenous administration of cadmium-thionein to rats [25]. The number of lysosomes in rat kidney proximal tubules has also been shown to increase in relation to the amount of cadmium ingested [26]. Thus, it is reasonable to assume that metallothionein is catabolised within lysosomes in the same way that other low molecular weight proteins are taken up by tubular cells and catabolised within these structures [27].

A cycle of catabolism and re-synthesis of thionein may be envisaged as follows:-

i)   Cadmium is taken up by proximal tubule cells, either as the free ion (by processes not clearly defined), or as thionein-bound (by endocytotic processes).

ii) In the cytosol, free cadmium ion stimulates the synthesis of thionein and is subsequently bound by the protein.

iii) Cadmium-thionein is taken up by the lysosome and undergoes digestion, releasing the free metallic ion.

iv) The liberated cation stimulates further thionein systhesis in the cytosol, and the process of uptake and degredation re-commences.

Thus, the protein exhibits a continual turnover with a half-life of about 3.6 days [28], though it has been suggested that the ratio of cadmium to other bound cations may be a controlling factor in the rate of degradation of the protein [29]. Overall, therefore, cadmium remains protein bound, until such time as the critical concentration is reached, at which time the cation, in excess, becomes available to interact with sensitive cellular targets. Such a view is consistent with the increased toxicity of parenterally administered cadmium-thionein compared to cadmium chloride, since it is known that renal uptake of the former is much more efficient than the latter [30], and hence more cation is liberated following lysosomal degradation.

TARGETS OF CADMIUM TOXICITY

The cell contains abundant electron donor atoms in the form of sulphydryl, hydroxyl, carboxyl, amino groups etc. with which the cadmium ion may react to form ionic or covalent complexes. Any effect of cadmium may be either direct or indirect. Direct effects imply an interaction with some functional or structural component of the cell. Indirect effects may occur for instance as a result of a disturbance in essential metal homeostasis. Some of the potential targets of cadmium toxicity are summarised.

Essential metal homeostasis. By virtue of the similarity in the valency shell electronic structures, interactions between Cd^{2+}, Zn^{2+} and Cu^{2+} may be expected. As a consequence of their isomorphous replacement, cadmium may interfere with the normal biological functions of these essential metals. Cadmium may also alter zinc and copper homeostasis due to the binding of these ions by metallothionein [31]. The effects of cadmium upon zinc, copper and also iron which is depleted in the kidney after chronic cadmium exposure, has been reviewed in relation to the development of cadmium toxicity, experimentally [32]. Cadmium and calcium also have very similar ionic radii which may portend some disturbance in the normal function of the latter ion, and in addition, it has been suggested that cadmium may inhibit the renal hydroxylation of 25-hydroxycholecalciferol which is required to stimulate the synthesis of the calcium-binding protein in the gut [33].

Cell membrane. Cadmium may affect both structural integrity and transport processes of the cell membrane. Cd^{2+} is known to interact directly with phospholipids such as phosphatidylcholine [34], and since both zinc and calcium have vital functions, eg. prevention of membrane lipid peroxidation, the inter-relationship of cadmium with such metals may be important. Cellular transport of both organic and inorganic substances may be affected [35].

Enzyme function. Cadmium is known to inhibit or stimulate a large variety of enzymes [36], and this may be partly explained by displacement of functional cations from enzymic active sites. Enhanced activities of renal gluconeogenic enzymes have been reported in rats after cadmium treatment, and it is suggested that such an effect upon carbohydrate metabolism may be mediated via increased levels of cyclic AMP [37].

Nucleic acids. From physico-chemical considerations, cadmium reacts with purine and pyrimidine bases of nucleic acids, as would be expected of a soft ion [38], though in vivo it has been shown that soon after parenteral administration, cadmium may penetrate the cell nucleus and small amounts associate with DNA [39]. Several metalloenzymes are essential for the synthesis and function of nucleic acids, of which thymidine kinase which is zinc-containing may be a potential target, but those enzymes containing functional sulphydryl groups may be more important. Evidence supporting an effect of cadmium upon such processes is derived from the liver and further investigations with the kidney are needed.

Ribosomes. It has been demonstrated that after the acute parenteral administration of $CdCl_2$ to rats, the ribosomal RNA content of purified kidney ribosomes was decreased and there was a significant increase in bound ribosomes relative to free. The activity of the ribosomes was significantly increased. Chronic cadmium treatment produced similar, though less significant results [40]. These authors suggest that such effects may be due to either an increased translational activity in response to thionein synthesis, or a generalised response resulting from repair of damaged cells. These results contrast to those observed in the kidney after mercury administration and in the liver after cadmium treatments, where dilation and fragmentation of the rough endoplasmic reticulum has been shown [41]. Again further investigation is required to elucidate the potential of cadmium to affect ribosomal activity and protein systhesis.

Mitochondria. In vitro, cadmium may uncouple oxidative phosphorylation in isolated renal mitochondria at relatively low concentrations [42], though much higher concentrations of the metal in the kidney have not been observed to produce a similar effect in vivo [41]. Ultrastructural changes have however been demonstrated in cadmium-treated animals [43]. In addition, energy production may be distrubed via an effect of cadmium upon the organelle membrane. Evidence from the liver suggests that the mitochondrion may be another sensitive target but evidence regarding the kidney is once again scarce.

MOLECULAR BASIS FOR CADMIUM-INDUCED NEPHROTOXITY

The development of renal injury as a result of cadmium accumulation can be envisaged as a two-stage process. During the first stage, exposure to the metal stimulates thionein synthesis which sequesters the cation.   Metallothionein may be regarded as fulfilling a protective function. Thionein synthesis however will also increase the biological demand for zinc and copper, and the cadmium-exposed organism will attempt to maintain intracellular concentrations of these two ions which are required for essential processes by normal homeostatic controls such as increased uptake from the gut, decreased excretion and mobilisation from other tissues.   In the second stage, as exposure to cadmium continues, the concentration of metal in the kidney becomes critical and cellular damage occurs as a result of some interaction with a sensitive target.

At the present time an explanation for this interaction at the molecular level remains obscure.   One mechanism has been proposed involving an exchange between cadmium and zinc in renal leucine aminopeptidase which functions in the renal handling of proteins.   Such an interaction would result in an altered catalytic activity and disturb the reabsorption and catabolism of proteins, thereby leading to proteinuria [44].

A decreased activity of renal leucine aminopeptidase has been demonstrated experimentally after cadmium-treatment [45], however this effect is not specific.   Other enzymes such as alkaline phosphatase and γ-glutamyl transpeptidase also show a similar response but this is probably associated with excessive loss of the enzymes into urine due to renal cell damage rather than to a direct inhibitory action of cadmium upon the enzyme.   The ultimate cause of the tissue injury produced by cadmium therefore remains unknown.

It is clear though that a multiplicity of metabolic targets is readily identifiable, and it is also evident that the potential toxicity of any metal is influenced by factors such as uptake and distribution among organs and availibility of the toxic agent to interact with a cellular ligand.   Availability in turn is mainly dictated by protein binding of the cation, especially by metallothionein.   Since much of the available data are derived from in vitro experiments, it is difficult to assess the toxicological significance of many of the possible interactions of cadmium with metabolic processes and therefore some suggestions remain speculative at present.

CONCLUSIONS

The kidney is undoubtedly an important target of cadmium toxicity. However, in order to evaluate the possible implications for human health due to an increasingly contaminated environment or after occupational exposure, several important areas need to be investigated.

Firstly, the validity of the critical concentration of cadmium in renal cortex for humans has been questioned [46], and our knowledge of the kinetics of thionein synthesis and the properties of the protein in humans is very limited.   It should also be considered that there are tremendous differences in the functional capacity of the kidney between species, especially rat and man, yet much of our data on which concepts are based have been established using animal models.   Such experimental systems do provide useful information but from a relatively homogeneous population under restricted and well defined conditions.   This is obviously dissimilar to the human situation where persons exposed to cadmium may incur simultaneous exposure to other metals, industrial and environmental chemicals, drugs etc., or be suffering from a nutritional deficiency, disease state, genetic abnormality etc. Thus an adequate assessment of risk requires a full consideration of the many interacting factors that may influence cadmium deposition and toxicity. Finally, it is vital to understand the molecular mechanisms of cadmium-toxicity. Together, such information may be useful in the prediction of human health effects and identification of high risk groups in the population.

REFERENCES

1. Lauwerys RR, In The Chemistry, Biochemistry and Biology of Cadmium, (M Webb, ed.). Elsevier/North Holland Biomedical Press, Amsterdam, 1979, pp. 433-455. ISBN 0-444-80109-X.
2. Samarawickrama GP, In The Chemistry, Biochemistry and Biology of Cadmium, (M Webb, ed.). Elsevier/North Holland Biomedical Press, Amsterdam, 1979, pp.341-421. ISBN 0-444-80109-X.
3. Friberg L, et al. In Cadmium in the Environment. CRC Press, Cleveland, Ohio, 1974, pp. 137-195. ISBN 0-8493-5020-4.
4. Friberg L, J Ind Hyg Toxicol 30: 32-36, 1948.
5. Webb M, Br Med Bull 3: 246 -250, 1975.
6. Friberg L, et al. In Handbook on The Toxicology of Metals, (L Friberg et al. eds.). Elsevier/North Holland Biomedical Press, Amsterdam, 1979, pp. 355-381. ISBN 0-444-80075-1.
7. Piscator M, Arch Environ Hlth 12: 335-344, 1966.
8. Nordberg GF and Piscator M, Environ Physiol Biochem 2: 37-49, 1972.
9. Kjellstrom T et al. Environ Res 13: 318-344, 1977.
10. Piscator M, In Clinical Chemistry and Chemical Toxicology of Metals, (SS Brown, ed.). Elsevier/North Holland Biomedical Press, Amsterdam, 1977, pp. 143-155. ISBN 0-444-41601-3.
11. Bernard A et al. Int Arch Occup Environ Hlth 38: 19-30, 1976.
12. Bernard A et al. Eur J Clin Invest 9: 11-22, 1979.
13. Bernard A et al. Toxicology 10: 369-375, 1978.
14. Bernard A et al. Toxicology 20: 345-357, 1981.
15. Bonner FW et al. Chem-Biol Interact 27: 343-351, 1979.
16. Bonner FW et al. Toxicology 19: 247-254, 1981.
17. Nordberg GF, Environ Physiol Biochem 2: 7-36, 1972.
18. Bonner FW et al. Environ Res 22: 237-244, 1980.
19. Bonner FW et al. Toxicology Lett 6: 369-372, 1980.
20 Task Group on Metal Toxicity. In Effects and Dose-Response Relationships of Toxic Metals, (GF Nordberg, ed.). Elsevier, Amsterdam, 1976, pp. 10-13. ISBN 0-444-41370-7.
21. Webb M and Etienne AT, Biochem Pharmacol 26: 25-30, 1977.
22. Cherian MG, Biochem Pharmacol 27: 1163-1166, 1978.
23. Terhaar CJ et al. Toxicol Appl Pharmacol 7: 500, 1965.
24. Suzuki KT et al. Arch Environ Contam Toxicol 8: 85-95, 1979.
25. Squibb KS et al. Environ Hlth Perspect 28: 287-296, 1979.
26. Nishizumi M, Arch Environ Hlth 24: 215-225, 1972.
27. Strober W and Waldmann TA, Nephron 13: 35-66, 1974.
28. Feldman SL et al. J Toxicol Environ Helth 4: 805-813, 1978.
29. Cain KC and Holt DE, Chem-Biol Interact 28: 91-106, 1979.
30. Tanaka K et al. Toxicol Appl Pharmacol 33:258-266, 1975.
31. Webb M, In the Chemistry, Biochemistry and Biology of Cadmium, (M Webb, ed.). Elsevier/North Holland Biomedical Press, Amsterdam, 1979, pp. 195-266. ISBN 0-44-80109-X.

32. Bonner FW, In Studies on the Toxicity of Cadmium. PhD Thesis, University of Surrey, Guildford, 1980.
33. Feldman SL and Cousins RJ, Nutr Rep Int 8: 251-260, 1973.
34. Belmonte AA et al. Lipids 7:490-491, 1972.
35. Webb M, In the Chemistry, Biochemistry and Biology of Cadmium, (M Webb, ed.). Elsevier/North Holland Biomedical Press, Amsterdam, 1979, pp. 267-340. ISBN 0-444-80109-X.
36. Vallee BL and Ulmer DD, Ann Rev Biochem 41: 103-109, 1972.
37. Singhal RL et al. Science 183: 1094-1096, 1974.
38. Jacobson KB and Turner JE, Toxicology 16: 1-37, 1980.
39. Hidalgo H and Bryan SE, Toxicol Appl Pharmacol 42: 319-327, 1977.
40. Kuliszewski MJ and Nicholls DM, Chem-Biol Interact 33: 307-318, 1981.
41. Hoffmann EO et al. Lab Invest 32: 655-670, 1975.
42. Southard JP et al. Fed Proc 33: 2147-2153, 1974.
43. Gonick HS et al. Current Probl Clin Biochem 4: 111-118, 1975.
44. Friberg L et al. In Cadmium in the Environment. CRC press, Cleveland, Ohio, 1974, pp. 93-130. ISBN 0-8493-5020-4.
45. Cousins RJ et al. J Nutr 103: 964-972, 1973.
46. Nomiyama K, J Toxicol Environ Hlth 3: 607-609, 1977.

INTRACELLULAR REDISTRIBUTION OF CADMIUM-THIONEIN FOLLOWING ITS UPTAKE INTO THE RENAL CORTEX

M. Dobrota, F. W. Bonner and B. A. Carter

Robens Institute of Industrial and Environmental Health and Safety, and Department of Biochemistry, University of Surrey, Guildford, Surrey GU2 5XH, UK

INTRODUCTION

Following injection or oral administration of Cd^{2+}, the metal, bound to serum proteins [1] is taken up primarily into the liver. The uptake results in the induction of a specific Cd-binding protein, metallo-thionein. The subsequent slow shift of Cd-thionein from the liver to the kidney is thought to occur because hepatic Cd-thionein is released into the circulation [2, 3] and following filtration in the glomerulus is taken up into the cells of the proximal tubule [4]. Parenterally administered Cd-thionein is rapidly cleared from the blood by filtration and reabsorption in the proximal tubule. The uptake of Cd-thionein appears to be analogous with the well-established fate of circulating low molecular weight proteins and their catabolism [5]. The subcellular Cd-thionein distribution, after IV injection, indicates a significant association with lysosomes and other membranous organelles [4] of the proximal tubule cells.

In this work we have examined the subcellular distribution of Cadmium at various time intervals after IV injection of ^{109}Cd-thionein with the aid of subfractionation techniques developed specifically for studying the heterogeneity of kidney cortical lysosomes [6]. In order to investigate the uptake and intracellular transport of Cd-thionein the dose of thionein was carefully chosen not to cause significant cellular changes.

MATERIALS AND METHODS

Hepatic (Cd, Zn)-thionein was isolated from male Wistar Albino rats injected subcutaneously with 1.5 mg Cd^{2+}/kg/day (5 x per week for 4 weeks). This thionein was incubated with carrier-free $^{109}CdCl_2$ (1.5 mg thionein, 50 µCi $^{109}CdCl_2$ at 4^0 for 16 h) and purified by chromatography on Sephadex G-25. Male rats were injected intravenously (via Jugular vein) with ^{109}Cd thionein (5 µCi, 0.3 mg thionein per rat, equivalent to a dose of 0.1 mg Cd^{2+}/kg). After 0.5, 1.5 and 24 h the kidney cortices of 5 rats were excised and homogenised in 0.25 M sucrose containing 5 mM, pH 7.4 tris-HCl. The homogenate was filtered through a coarse sieve (tea strainer) and subfractionated by classical differential pelleting. The 'ML' fraction was further subfractionated by rate sedimentation in a zonal HS rotor (MSE Scientific Instruments Ltd.) exactly as previously described [6]. The classical subfractions and the zonal fractions were analysed for protein [7], various marker enzymes [8, 9] and [109]Cd counts.

RESULTS

The % recoveries of [109]Cd, protein and the marker enzymes, presented in Table 1, give a clear indication of the distribution of Cd-thionein amongst the classical subfractions. 30 min after injection of [109]Cd thionein there is a considerable proportion of the label in the particulate fractions (N, Ml, Mic = 51%). However, with increasing time there is a redistribution of the label from the membranous organelles into the cytosol. This increase in cytosolic [109]Cd is very similar to that reported by Squibb *et al.* [4]. The distribution of marker enzymes, especially acid hydrolases, does exhibit some differential changes with increasing time after Cd-thionein injection and when compared with the control values. In comparison with control animals the acid β-glycerophosphatase distribution in the Cd-thionein treated animals is virtually unchanged whilst acid β-galactosidase shows significant redistribution from the particulate fractions into the cytosol.

The subfractionation of the cortical 'ML' fraction by rate-zonal sedimentation, as well as separating different populations of lysosomes also achieves the separation of 'microsomes', mitochondria and brush-border membranes. The distribution patterns of various marker enzymes (Fig. 1) show no significant changes between the different time intervals of Cd-thionein treatment. However, the peak of protein droplets (lysosomes involved in the catabolism of reabsorbed protein) shows considerable [109]Cd activity at 0.5 and 1.5 h whilst at 24 h almost all the activity is lost.

Kidney cortex from animals treated with Cd-thionein for 24 h examined by electron microscopy showed some proximal tubule cells with degeneration of the endoplasmic reticulum, particularly near to the brush border. However, the majority of tubular cells appeared normal.

DISCUSSION

The % recovery of [109]Cd in the classical fractions indicates that 30 min after injection of [109]Cd-thionein 51.0% of the label is organelle associated whilst only 37.6% is cytosolic. This suggests that an active receptor for thionein is located in the membranous fraction. Two distinct binding sites for Cd-thionein have been found in the renal brush border membranes [10]. With time considerable amounts of the organelle associated [109]Cd are released and transferred to the cytosol (65.7% at 24 h) by an unknown and possibly unique mechanism.

From the distribution patterns of [109]Cd after further subfractionation of the 'ML' fraction it is quite clear that [109]Cd is present in protein droplets (large lysosomes of the proximal tubule cells) 30 min after Cd-thionein injection but is lost 24 h after injection. Since during this loss of lysosomal [109]Cd other organelles do not gain [109]Cd it appears that the cadmium is released from lysosomes into the cytosol. Thus it seems likely that the route of Cd-thionein transport from the glomerular filtrate to the intracellular cytosol follows the path: brush

Table 1. % Recoveries of [109]Cd, protein and marker enzymes in the
classical subfractions of the rat kidney cortex after IV injection of
[109]Cd-thionein. The control values are averages of 12 observation
whilst the three time point values are from single experiments. The
% recoveries are the original observations and are not corrected for
100% in each column.

CONTROL

	[109]Cd	PROTEIN	ACID P'	β-GALACT.	NAG	AMP'	G-6-P'	SDH
N	-	17.0	12.9	13.7	20.8	18.1	19.0	12.9
ML	-	27.2	36.9	41.0	41.9	26.3	20.0	66.4
MIC	-	18.8	22.8	11.5	24.9	39.5	53.6	18.7
SUP	-	36.8	27.3	36.9	12.3	16.0	7.5	6.3

0.5h

N	16.4	17.1	13.6	11.9	18.6	13.2	36.1	18.1
ML	21.5	19.9	24.0	19.6	28.5	11.7	13.8	58.4
MIC	13.1	18.0	15.8	9.5	26.4	37.4	44.7	17.3
SUP	37.6	30.8	22.3	42.9	5.1	2.2	4.0	<1

1.5h

N	8.8	13.0	9.6	10.2	18.3	11.9	18.9	15.4
ML	18.5	22.7	31.2	25.5	36.2	12.8	11.6	56.2
MIC	13.7	21.0	20.9	10.6	29.6	52.1	50.2	20.3
SUP	51.9	33.7	22.2	40.9	10.0	8.5	5.1	<1

24h

N	5.5	9.9	9.5	6.6	10.1	7.9	16.5	9.2
ML	10.3	28.0	36.1	23.9	37.2	14.9	27.0	69.7
MIC	8.5	18.0	17.0	9.7	25.6	42.1	35.8	12.2
SUP	65.7	39.7	22.2	47.0	10.1	6.7	1.7	3.4

(Acid P : Acid β-glycerophosphatase, β-galact : Acid β-galactosidase,
 NAG : Acid N-acetyl β-D glucosaminidase, AMP : 5'-nucleotidase,
 G-6-P : Glucose-6-phosphatase, SDH : Succinic dehydrogenase).

Subcellular Fractions are denoted; N:nuclear, ML:mitochondrial,
MIC:microsomal, SUP:supernatant.

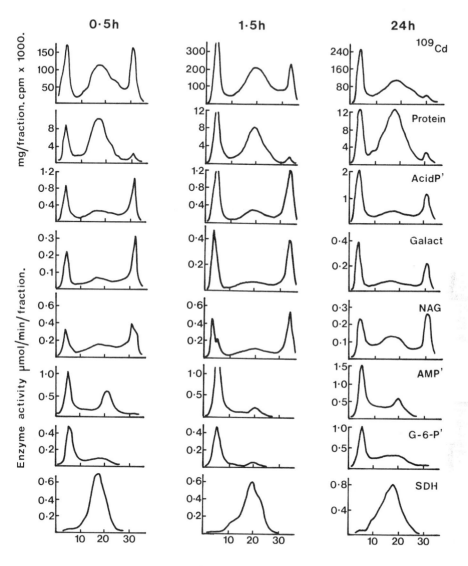

Fraction number

Fig 1. Distribution patterns of [109]Cd, protein and marker enzymes after subfractionation of the rat kidney cortex 'ML' fraction by rate zonal sedimentation. The [109]Cd counts, mg protein and enzyme activities are presented as total/fraction. The protein and enzyme values have not been corrected for the inhibitory effect of sucrose.

border → endocytic vesicles → secondary lysosomes → cytosol. The first steps of such a pathway are well established as the catobolic route of reabsorbed low mol. wt. proteins. However, the appearance of ^{109}Cd in the cytosol may be explained by the rapid intralysosomal breakdown of thionein [11] and the sequestration of released Cd^{2+} by cytosolic Zn-thionein. It is also possible that Cd^{2+} release may be due to the intra-lysosomal acid pH. Although there is no reliable data on the levels of endogenous cytosolic Zn-thionein in the kidney, our results would suggest that the level is quite sufficient to sequester the amount of Cd^{2+} released during the early time points and under our experimental conditions. Preliminary examination of the 30 min cytosol indicates that all ^{109}Cd is thionein associated.

Whilst with time ^{109}Cd label is lost from the protein droplets it is not clear why during the same time the distribution of ^{109}Cd in the slower sedimentation regions of the subfractionated 'ML' (Mitochondria - SDH peak, Brush border — AMP'ase region, Small lysosomes — early acid hydrolase peak) remains virtually unaltered. This is most likely due to non-specific binding of Cd-thionein to membranous organelles. However, the non-specific binding cannot explain the net loss of ^{109}Cd from all membranous particulates. The redistribution of particulate ^{109}Cd to cytosolic does therefore support the idea of active transport.

Data from the Table of Recoveries of marker enzymes indicate that some subtle subcellular changes have occurred as a result of the Cd-thionein administration. The differential changes with time of the three acid hydrolases suggest that only specific lysosomal populations may be affected. However, there is very little increase in cytosolic acid hydrolases in comparison with control animal suggesting virtually no increase in lysosomal fragility. This is supported by the morpholo-gical examination with normal appearance of small and large lysosomes in the proximal tubule cells. The slight redistribution of AMP'ase from the control 'ML' to the Cd-thionein treated 'microsomes' indicates some alterations in the brush border membranes which are possibly associated with the membrane located binding sites for Cd-thionein.

REFERENCES

1. Watkins SR, et al. Biochem Biophys Res Comm 74:1403-1410, 1977.
2. Nordberg GF, Environ Physiol Biochem 2:7-36, 1972.
3. Tanaka K, et al. Toxicol Appl Pharmacol 33: 258-266, 1975.
4. Squibb KS, et al. Environ Health Pespect 28: 287-296, 1979.
5. Strober W and Waldman TA Nephron 13: 35-66, 1974.
6. Andersen KJ, et al. Biochem Soc Trans 8:597-598, 1980.
7. Hinton RH and Norris KA Anal Biochem 48: 247-258, 1972.
8. Dobrota M and Hinton RH Anal Biochem 102, 97-102, 1980.
9. Hultberg B and Öckerman PA Clin Chim Acta 39: 49-58, 1972.
10. Selenke W and Foulkes EC Proc Soc Exp Biol Med 167: 40-44, 1981.
11. Cherian MG and Shaikh ZA Biochem Biophys Res Comm 65: 863-869, 1975.

MERCURY INDUCED NEPHROTOXICITY

L. Magos

Toxicology Unit, MRC Laboratories, Woodmansterne Road, Carshalton, Surrey SM5 4EF, UK

ABSTRACT

Diffuse proximal tubular damage, mainly in the middle and the end part of the proximal tubular cells is the characteristic renal response to a single dose of $HgCl_2$. Conditions which alter the sensitivity of the proximal tubular cells to the toxic effect of mercurials or differences in the ability of various mercurials to damage the proximal tubules are best compared after the administration of a single dose, because – at least until the completion of regeneration – the damaged tubular cells are tolerant to subsequent doses.

Tolerance can be induced by nephrotoxic agents which do not induce thionein and it is not conditional on a decrease in the kidney content of mercury, but it may be linked to a reduction in the rate of initial renal mercury uptake. The order of initial mercury uptake for different mercurials is the same as the order of renotoxicity, that is:

$$MeHg^+ < EtHg^+ < PhHg^+ < MeOEtHg^+ < Hg^{2+}$$

The order of initial mercury uptake for organomercurials may only reflect their decomposition rates because any increase in the inorganic proportion of blood mercury must accelerate renal uptake. Though the conversion of mercury vapour to Hg^{2+} is faster than the decomposition of any organomercurial, the diffusion of elemental mercury into extrarenal tissues limits the initial renal mercury accumulation and consequently renal toxicity.

Key words: mercurials, renal uptake, renotoxicity,
            proximal tubular cells, regeneration, tolerance.

In acute renal failure some important clinical and pathological features are independent of the aetiology. Oliver, McDowall and Tracy [1] emphasized that both in traumatic injury and severe sublimate intoxication an episodic collapse in general circulation precipitates a common chain of events: renal ischemia, anuria, uremia and death. Renal ischemia is responsible for the focal disruptive tubular lesions, which are mainly localized in the cortico-medullary junction. The key role of renin release and the activation of preglomerular angiotensin in renal ischemia and in the development of acute renal failure can be reasoned on the following grounds. Firstly, in many cases of acute renal failure the concentration of plasma renin is increased [2] and secondly, the suppression of renal renin by salt loading protects against renal failure [3,4]. However, while in traumatic shock the release of renin is most likely precipitated - at least in the early phase - through the renal baroreceptors [5] (and also see review on renin by Keeton and Campbell) [6], some other mechanisms must be responsible for the release of renin when the dose of $HgCl_2$ is not high enough to precipitate a fall in blood pressure. Thiel et al. [7] proposed that in this case renin is discharged by the diuretic-like inhibitory effect of $HgCl_2$ on the reabsorption of NaCl. The resulting preglomerular ischemia is supposed to be responsible for the characteristic nephrotoxic lesion: diffuse proximal tubular damage. However, there are observations which point to the role of factors other than renal ischemia in the development of proximal tubular damage. Firstly there is a correlation between the site of morphological damage and the renal localization of mercury: both are found mainly in the middle to end portions of the proximal tubules [8]. Secondly, there is a $HgCl_2$ dose range which does not decrease but increases urine flow and in spite of this the proximal tubules are damaged [9]. Thirdly, in salt loaded rats $HgCl_2$ can cause severe tubular necrosis while renal function is maintained [3] and the cortical blood flow decreases only temporarily [10].

Based on these arguments it would be plausible to conclude that acute renal failure and proximal tubular damage are precipitated by $HgCl_2$ through two distinctly different mechanisms. Acute renal failure is mediated through the release of renin and consequently can be prevented by renin depletion, while proximal tubular necrosis seems to be the consequence of the localised effect of $HgCl_2$ on those parts of the nephron where this corrosive compound accumulates. Therefore the relationship between proximal tubular damage and renal mercury accumulation can be the subject of discussion without extending it to acute renal failure. This approach is justified even when one considers that proximal tubular damage, like renal failure, is an acute effect. The acuteness of diffuse proximal tubular damage explains why differences in renal morphology cannot be used to grade the renotoxic potential of mercurials, when - like in the widely quoted comparative study of Fitzhugh et al. [11] - the mercurials (inorganic and phenyl mercury) were given for a long time: damage caused by individual doses induced tolerance and tolerance mitigated the effects of subsequent doses. Thus the measure of renotoxic potential, when different mercurials are compared, is the renal reaction after a single dose.

The following discussion will focus on the two problems just mentioned: tolerance and differences in the toxicity of inorganic and organic mercurials, both in conjunction with the renal accumulation of mercury. However, firstly, it must be pointed out that in the toxic

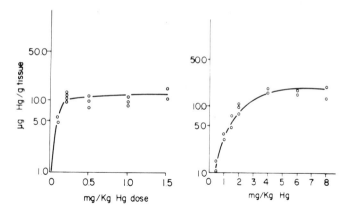

Fig. 1. The effect of a single i.v. (left hand graph) or oral
(right hand graph) dose of HgCl$_2$ on the kidney concentration
of mercury 48 hr after injection.

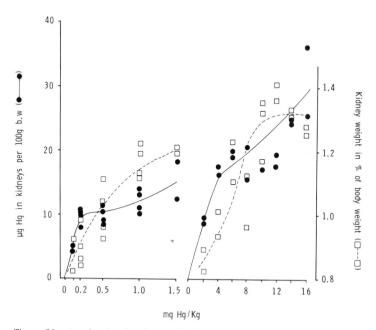

Fig. 2. The effect of single i.v. (left hand graph) or oral (right hand
graph) dose of HgCl$_2$ on the kidney content of mercury (solid
circles) and on the kidney weight (open squares) 48 hr after
injection.

dose range the renal concentration of mercury is not an indicator of renal mercury uptake. Thus 48 hr after i.v. or oral administration of increasing doses of sublimate the kidney concentration of mercury levels off at 0.5 mg Hg/kg and 4.0 mg/kg doses respectively (see Fig. 1). This levelling off does not indicate a saturation point, but it indicates two important toxic effects: increase in kidney weight and the release of mercury with or without cell debris. The effect of kidney weight is eliminated when the kidney content of mercury is expressed per 100g body weight or in % of the dose. When the experimental points are plotted this way, the plateau is converted to a slope which is gentler than the slope of the first part of the curve (see Fig.2). The difference in the steepness of the first and the second part of the curve probably depends on the extent of mercury loss with cell constituents from the damaged proximal tubular cells.

TOLERANCE

Pretreatment of mice with a non-lethal dose of $HgCl_2$ gives protection against an otherwise lethal dose given 24-48 hr later [12] by increasing the LD_{50} [13]. Prolonged treatment could also produce tolerance to $HgCl_2$. In spite of the continuance of treatment the entire tubular epithelium of rats which survives the first few days of daily treatment with $1.8 - 2.0$ mg/kg $HgCl_2$ regenerates with little signs of necrosis [14,15].

The most logical explanation for the mechanism of tolerance is an increase in the neutralization of renal mercury deposits by metallothionein synthetized in response to the previous treatment. In agreement with this assumption, pretreatment with a good thionein inducer, like cadmium, decreased the sensitivity of kidneys against a subsequent dose of mercury [16] . However, at doses where the protection was the most prominent, the non-thionein mercury content of kidneys increased more than the thionein bound (see Table 1) [17].

Table 1. The effects of cadmium pretreatment in rats on the total and thionein bound mercury contents of kidneys 24 hr after the i.p. injection of $HgCl_2$.

dose[a] in mg Hg/kg	sex	pretreatment	renal Hg^{2+} in µg/100g b.w.		A-B
			total (A)	thionein bound (B)	
0.5	m	−	15.2	0.3	14.9
0.5	m	+	28.1	1.7	26.4
1.0	f	−	26.0	1.5	24.5
1.0	f	+	34.6	4.3	30.3

[a] The most prominent protection [16,17] was observed at doses shown in Table.

Protection in spite of increased mercury uptake is not restricted to cadmium pretreatment but was observed by Surtshin and Parelman [18] after 3 intraperitoneal injections of 16 ml 6% albumin. In albumin pretreated rats the sum of renal mercury content and 24 hr urinary mercury excretion was less than in controls, but the kidneys of albumin treated rats contained more mercury because they lost significantly less into urine as Table 2 shows. If the same rule applies to cadmium pretreated rats, it is possible that the rate of initial mercury

Table 2. The effect of albumin pretreatment on the urinary excretion and renal contents of mercury 24 hr after the i.v. injection of 2.2 mg/kg mercury as $HgCl_2$ [18].

Pretreatment	Hg^{2+} in $\mu g/100g$ b.w.		A + B
	in kidney (A)	in urine (B)	
—	35.6	29.1	64.7
+	46.0	12.6	58.6

accumulation was slower in tolerant than in normal kidneys. Higher challenging dose or longer time interval between the administration of $HgCl_2$ and sacrifice may disguise this effect. Thus 48 hr after the administration of 1.1 mg Hg^{2+}/kg the kidneys and urine of rats pretreated with sodium chromate 3 days earlier contained slightly more mercury than the kidneys and urine of controls (see Table 3).

Table 3. The effects of sodium chromate given 3 days before the i.p. injection of $HgCl_2$ or mercury penicillaminate [19,20] on the 48 hr urinary excretion and renal contents of mercury.

Hg^{2+} dose in mg/kg	Form of Hg	Pretreatment	Hg in $\mu g/100g$ b.w.		A+B
			in kidneys (A)	in urine (B)	
1.1	$HgCl_2$	—	15.6	16.5	32.2
1.1	"	+	17.4	22.1	39.5
0.5	"	—	9.0	9.7	18.7
0.5	"	+	3.8[a]	4.4[a]	8.2[a]
0.5	$Hg(Pen)_2$	—	8.8	10.2	19.0
0.5	"	+	6.0[a]	4.6[a]	10.6[a]

[a] Significantly different from controls, $P < 0.05$; N=4.

Table 4. The effects of pretreatment with nephrotoxic agents on the urinary excretion of mercury in male rats given 1.1 mg Hg/kg as $HgCl_2$ 7 days after pretreatment [14].

Pretreatment	N	Daily urinary Hg excretion in $\mu g/100$ g b.w.		
		1st day	2nd day	3rd day
—	19	13.6	1.4	0.9
chromate	5	12.8	7.3[a]	3.6[a]
p-aminophenol	5	20.6[a]	7.7[a]	3.5[a]
maleate	5	14.5	8.2[a]	4.8[a]

[a] significantly different from the control, $P < 0.05$

Pretreatment with p-aminophenol or sodium maleate caused even larger
increases, though as Table 4 shows the increase in the urinary excretion
of mercury, like in the case of chromate pretreatment, was more
pronounced after the first 24 hr [19]. However, pretreatment with
chromate decreased both the kidney content and urinary excretion of
mercury (see Table 3) when the dose of mercury was reduced to 0.5
mg/kg. Whether mercury was injected as chloride or complexed with
penicillamine it made no difference. When mercury is administered with
a thiol compound the renal uptake of mercury peaks within 3 hours and
therefore offers a sensitive and rapid way to estimate the rate of
uptake. Table 5 shows that while the liver contents of mercury were
lower in control rats, the kidney uptake of mercury proceeded at a
slower rate in chromate pretreated rats. Even when mercury was given 7
days after chromate, the rate of initial renal mercury uptake did not
reach the control level [20].

Table 5.   Effect of chromate pretreatment on the kidney contents of
           mercury 150 min. after the i.p. administration of 0.5 mg/kg Hg
           as Hg-penicillaminate[20].

Pretreatment	Hg in µg/100 g b.w.		
	kidneys (A)	liver (B)	$\frac{A}{B}$
none	30.0 (60%)	3.0	10.0
7 days earlier	22.5 (45%)	4.5	5.0
3 days earlier	16.0 (32%)	6.0	2.6

Histological examination of the kidneys of rats made tolerant to
$HgCl_2$ by pretreatment with a nephrotoxic agent revealed that the
population of those tubular cells which survived the pretreatment with
intact brush border were the target of $HgCl_2$, while regenerating cells
were the resistant ones [19]. Whether this selective protection is the
result of unequal mercury distribution between intact and regenerating
cells or differences in the sensitivity of these cells to $HgCl_2$ is not
known, but it has been reported that the sensitivity of young rats to
the renotoxicity of mercury reaches the adult level when they are 3
weeks old, that is with the acquisition of differentiated brush border
and the ability to store vital dyes [21,22,23]. Thus it might be a link
between the ability of a compound to cause damage and therefore less
differentiated proximal tubules and its ability to induce tolerance to a
nephrotoxic agent which acts on the same part of the nephron.
     Proteins might be no exception to this rule. Proteins are taken up
by the proximal tubules by endocytosis where, depending on the load, the
protein is either found in vacuoles and lysosomes [24] or as droplets of
high thiol content attached to mitochondria [25]. As reabsorption of
homologous serum proteins is a continuous process, it seems likely that
the conditions of protection is a protein load which, like in the
experiments of Reber [26], results in mitochondrial swelling,
aggregation and depletion. The role of storage induced proximal tubular
changes in the development of tolerance is supported by the following
observations. Firstly, albumin given concomittantly with $HgCl_2$ does not

decrease but increases the toxicity of HgCl$_2$ [27]. Secondly, sucrose, which is taken up and stored by the proximal tubules has similar effects on mitochondria [28] and on HgCl$_2$ toxicity as albumin [26].

THE COMPARATIVE RENOTOXICOLOGY OF MERCURIALS

The observation that damaged or regenerating cells are tolerant to the renotoxic insult means that after repeated daily doses one cannot expect correlation between the number of necrotic proximal tubular cells and the renotoxic potential of a chemical. Thus in the long term experiment of Fitzhugh et al. [11], who fed phenylmercury or inorganic mercury to rats, necrosis or sloughing of the proximal tubular cells was only occasionally seen. Consequently the grading of renotoxicity was based on non-specific kidney lesions, seen also in control rats. Treatment with the two mercurials only intensified these lesions in time and degree. Based on this criterion dietary phenylmercury which resulted in 10 to 20 times higher organ concentrations than the same exposure to Hg^{2+}, was 10 to 20 times more renotoxic than inorganic mercury. However the same criterion also indicated that male rats were less sensitive to inorganic mercury than females, though the opposite is true after a single parenteral dose [29]. To avoid differences in gastrointestinal absorption and the interfering effect of tolerance, the renotoxicity of mercurials is best compared after a single parenteral injection. When the mercurial is administered orally and/or repeatedly, the interpretation of the results is hardly possible without knowing the renal effect of a single parenteral dose. Moreover it is an advantage to use a dose below the threshold for acute renal failure, because the acute lethality of mercurials may not solely depend on their direct effect on the kidneys and within the kidneys on the proximal tubular cells. However it must be pointed out that in mice the LD$_{50}$ values for a single oral dose, as tabulated by Swensson and Ulfvarson [30] seems to follow the order of renotoxic potential.

(a) Phenylmercury. Mercury given i.p. in a single dose of 0.5 mg Hg/kg or 1.0 mg Hg/kg as HgCl$_2$ to male rats increased the urinary excretion of alkaline phosphatase from the control base line level (33 mU/100 g body weight) by six-fold and sixty-fold respectively. Identical doses of phenylmercury did not increase the excretion of alkaline phosphatase at all, at least up to 48 hours. There was a lack of correlation between the urinary excretion of alkaline phosphatase and morphological proximal tubular damage. In phenylmercury treated rats there was no increase in the excretion of this enzyme, nevertheless they developed proximal tubular damage though the extent of damage was less than in HgCl$_2$ treated rats. At 24 hr there were cytoplasmic metachromasia, vacuolation and a slight sloughing of the tubular epithelium, mainly in the pars recta, of rats treated with 1.0 mg Hg/kg as phenylmercury, while in HgCl$_2$ treated rats approximately the same degree of damage developed by the administration of 0.5 mg Hg/kg [31].

The more pronounced damage in HgCl$_2$ treated rats resulted in higher urinary mercury contents in the first 24 hr period and, in spite of the increased urinary mercury excretion, higher renal mercury contents. Thus in this period identical inorganic and phenylmercury doses presented the kidneys with different levels of mercury exposure (see Table 6). The differences in renal mercury contents were even higher at 12 hr, when at the two dose levels inorganic mercury treated rats had in

Table 6.   The renal and urinary contents of mercury 24 hr after i.p.
treatment with $HgCl_2$ or phenyl mercuric chloride [31].

form of Hg	dose in mg Hg/kg	μg Hg/100 g b.w. kidneys (A)	urine (B)	A+B
Hg^{2+}	0.5	13.1	4.1	17.2
$PhHg^+$	0.5	11.9	1.3	13.2
Hg^{2+}	1.0	19.0	11.8	30.8
$PhHg^+$	1.0	15.3	4.9[a]	20.2[a]

[a] $p < 0.05$ with two tailed Mann Whitney U-test, N=4.

their kidneys 15.1 and 25.5 μg Hg/100 g body weight and phenylmercury
treated rats 10.0 and 18.1 μg Hg/100 g body weight respectively. From
12 hr onward the difference between inorganic and phenylmercury treated
rats progressively declined [31] but, as it seems, the extent of
proximal tubular damage was already determined by the initial rate of
slower renal mercury uptake.

(b) Methoxyethylmercury.   Compared with phenylmercury [32], the
decomposition of methoxyethylmercury [33] is faster and therefore one
expects that the renotoxicity of methoxyethylmercury will be between the
renotoxicities of mercuric chloride and phenylmercury.   This assumption
seems to be correct, if one considers that 1.0 mg Hg/kg given as
methoxyethylmercury increased the urinary excretion of gamma glutamyl
transferase in the second, but not in the first 24 hr period after
treatment [34].   Though the relationship between dose and toxic effects
is unknown for most of the reported occupational cases of intoxication,
it might be of some significance that while reviewers of phenylmercury
were unable to find definite cases of renal injury [35,36,37], in severe
cases of intoxication caused by exposure to methoxyethylmercury the
signs of renal injury are part of the clinical entity [38,39].

The uptake of mercury by kidneys in the first 6 hours is only
slightly more in methoxyethylmercury than in phenylmercury treated rats,
though a higher proportion of the mercury is in the inorganic form.   The
difference in the i.v. distribution is enlarged when the kidney Hg to
liver Hg ratios are compared (see Table 7) which twenty-four hours after
administration significantly differed for the two organomercurials.

Table 7.   The kidney and liver contents of mercury 24 hr after the s.c.
administration of inorganic, phenyl- and methoxyethylmercury.

form of Hg	dose in mg Hg/kg	Hg in % of dose kidneys (A)	liver (B)	$\frac{A}{B}$
Hg^{2+}	1.0	19.0	4.1	4.6[a]
$PhHg^+$	1.5	15.2	22.2	0.7 [32]
$MeOEtHg^+$	0.95	15.0	4.8	3.1 [33]

[a] own laboratory (unpublished)

(c) Alkylmercurials. Even alkylmercurials which decompose slower than phenylmercury can produce kidney injury depending on the level of exposure and the type of alkyl radical. Thus in the victims of the ethylmercury epidemics in Iraq polyuria or oliguria with urinary casts and albumin were not infrequent [40,41]. In the largest methylmercury epidemics the kidneys of even the most severely affected persons were spared [42], probably because methylmercury is more stable than ethylmercury [43,44]. Nevertheless in rats methylmercury can be renotoxic, though to a lesser extent than either phenyl- or methyoxyethylmercury. The renal damage in male rats treated daily for five days with 2.0 mg Hg/kg or 10.0 mg Hg/kg methylmercury was restricted to mild proteinuria of plasma origin and foci of swollen vacuolated tubular epithelial cells with signs of regenerations as early as 6 days after the last treatment day [45]. The moderate renal injury can be contrasted with the relatively high renal mercury concentrations: even the lower dose increased not only the total mercury but also the inorganic mercury concentration above levels found after a single moderately renotoxic dose of $HgCl_2$.

After longer treatment with smaller daily doses the characteristic renal histological features are flattened basophilic proximal tubules with occasional mitotic figures surrounded by inflammatory reaction [46,47]. While male rats are more sensitive to the renotoxic effect of mercuric chloride than female rats [27] the opposite is true for the renotoxicity of methylmercury [48]. While it is possible that the lower sensitivity of females to the first few treatments is responsible for the inferior tolerance later, it must be emphasised that female rats are also more sensitive to the neurotoxic effects of methylmercury than males [49].

In agreement with their inferior renal toxicity, alkylmercurials are taken up rather slowly by the kidneys. Within a wide dose range and 2 hr after i.v. administration the mercury concentrations in the kidneys of mercuric chloride treated rats were approximately 7.5 times higher than in methylmercury treated rats [50]. As Table 8 shows at 24 hr the difference between alkylmercury and inorganic mercury treated rats decreased only slightly and the kidney Hg to liver Hg ratios remained

Table 8. The kidney and liver constants of mercury 24 hr after the administration of alkylmercurials or inorganic mercury.

form of Hg	dose in mg Hg/kg		Hg in % of dose kidneys (A)	liver (B)	$\frac{A}{B}$	
Hg^{2+}	1.0	(s.c.)	19.0	4.1	4.6[a]	
Hg^{2+}	1.0	(i.p.)	23.6	9.4	2.3	[16]
$EtHg^+$	0.95	(i.p.)	7.2	22.3	0.32	[51]
$EtHg^+$	10.0	(s.c.)	3.9	6.7	0.58	[52]
$MeHg^+$	0.2	(s.c.)	4.6	5.9	0.78	[53]
$MeHg^+$	0.8	(s.c.)	4.5	8.8	0.51	[54]
$MeHg^+$	1.0	(i.v.)	6.0	7.5	0.80	[55]

[a]own laboratory (unpublished)

below one. The table also shows that methylmercury and ethylmercury behaved similarly. In piglets — at least up to 14 days — the renal mercury concentrations were always less in methyl- or ethylmercury treated animals, than in inorganic mercury treated ones [56,57]. The kidney Hg to liver Hg ratios are smaller in ethylmercury than in methylmercury treated mice, but this difference is caused mainly by the significantly higher mercury contents in the liver of ethylmercury treated mice [58].

(d) The decomposition of organomercurials and renotoxicity. The order of Hg^{2+} formation from organomercurials, that is the order of decomposition is:

$$MeHg^+ < EtHg^+ < PhHg^+ < MeOEtHg^+$$

As renotoxicity depends on the rate of mercury uptake and both renotoxicity and the initial rate of mercury uptake is influenced by the proportion of inorganic mercury to total mercury, the following order for renal toxicity and the rate of initial uptake is a logical conclusion confirmed by experience:

$$MeHg^+ < EtHg^+ < PhHg^+ < MeOEtHg^+ < Hg^{2+}$$

Decomposition may influence renotoxicity not only through its effect on the renal uptake of mercury, but in equivalent renal concentration an organomercurial is probably less toxic than inorganic mercury. That, in the case of organomercurial diuretics, diuresis depends on the inorganic mercury and not on the total mercury concentration in the kidneys has been shown by Clarkson and Greenwood [59]. They found that even the non-diuretic p-chloromercurybenzoate can produce diuresis when the dose is adjusted to give 35 µg of mercuric ion per g wet weight renal tissue. The comparison of Table 7 and 8 clearly indicates that at 24 hr after administration the largest difference in the kidney contents of mercury is between inorganic mercury and alkylmercurials. Phenyl- and methoxyethylmercury occupy an intermediate position. However when the kidney Hg to liver Hg ratios are compared, methoxyethylmercury seems to behave like inorganic mercury, and phenylmercury like alkylmercurials because only the decomposition of phenylmercury but not the decomposition of methoxyethylmercury is slow enough to influence significantly the relative organ distribution of mercury at that time. However, when distribution is measured 2 hr after the injection of methyoxyethylmercury, when less than 50% of the kidney mercury is in the inorganic form [33], the kidney content of mercury or the kidney Hg to liver Hg ratio is very much less than in inorganic mercury treated rats. Table 9 shows that 1 to 2 hr after their injection all the organomercurials form a group distinctly different from inorganic mercury indicating that in the previous period renal mercury uptake was mainly influenced by the original mercury molecule. Thus the lower renotoxicity of organomercurial may depend not only on the renal accumulation rate, but in the form in which mercury accumulates.

(e) Mercury vapour. In acute inhalation experiments mercury vapour exposure which produced kidney damage in rabbits, also produced damage in the heart, brain and lung [61]. Rabbits exposed 7 hr per day to 0.86 mg Hg/m^3 showed signs of kidney damage as early as the third week, but in some of the experimental animals liver, brain and heart were also damaged. The renal damage was mild and reversible. Although Ashe et al [61] did not give the localization and nature of damage, it is clear

Table 9.   The kidney and liver contents of mercury 1 or 2 hr after the
            administration of different mercurials.

form of Hg	dose in mg Hg/kg		time in hr	Hg in % of dose kidneys (A)	liver (B)	$\frac{A}{B}$	
Hg^{2+}	1.5	(i.p)	1	18.0	12.5	1.4	[60]
$PhHg^+$	1.5	(i.p)	1	4.5	15.1	0.3	[60]
$EtHg^+$	0.95	(i.p)	1	5.2	14.3	0.36	[51]
Hg^{2+}	1.0	(i.v)	2	45.0	13.5	3.3	[50]
$MeHg^+$	1.0	(i.v)	2	6.0	13.5	0.45	[50]
$PhHg^+$	1.48	(s.c)	2	4.8	5.8	0.83	[32]
$MeOEtHg_2^+$	0.95	(s.c)	2	7.4	9.5	0.78	[33]

that experimentally some type of kidney damage can be produced by
mercury vapour, when the exposure is high enough to affect not only the
nervous system, but also other organs. The renal damage might not be
the same as after a single dose of $HgCl_2$.

Certainly in human cases of mercury vapour intoxication, the
importance of renal damage is small compared with the disorders of the
nervous sytem. Proteinuria is mild and transient and does not show any
relationship with tremor [62] or the severity of exposure [63]. The
urinary protein is not tubular but glomerular and indicate membranous
glomerulopathy which is usually responsible for the nephrotic
syndrome: albuminuria with or without hypoproteinaemia and oedema which
clears fast after the cessation of exposure [63–66].

Compared with the decomposition of organomercurials to Hg^{2+} and to
the organic radical, the oxidation of elemental mercury (Hg^0) to Hg^{2+} is
extremely fast and it is nearly complete within 1 min [67]. However
compared with Hg^{2+}, the blood clearance of elemental mercury, unlike the
clearance of organomercurials, is also fast. This fast clearance
permits the distribution of blood mercury in the elemental form [67]
without interference from the preferential renal uptake mechanism for
Hg^{2+} (see Table 10). As oxidation of Hg^0 takes place not only in blood
but in other tissues [68] and the re-entry of extravascularly oxidized
Hg^{2+} into plasma is slowed down by its diminished diffusibility, the

Table 10.   Differences in the blood and kidney contents of mercury in
             rats after the i.v. injection of elemental mercury or $HgCl_2$
             [67].

Form of Hg	time in min	Hg in % of dose/g tissue blood	kidneys
Hg^0	0.5	0.33	1.10
Hg^0	2.0	0.29	1.26
Hg^0	5.0	0.30	1.33
Hg^{2+}	0.5	3.68	1.77
Hg^{2+}	2.0	2.52	2.99
Hg^{2+}	5.0	2.33	4.25

renal accumulation is further delayed. One day after a single 4 to 5 hr vapour exposure the kidneys of mice contained 34% [69] and the kidneys of rats 24% less mercury [70,71] than the kidneys of animals which had the same initial body burden by the i.v. injection of a single dose of $HgCl_2$.

REFERENCES

1. Oliver J, MacDowell M and Tracy A. J Clin Invest 30:1307-1440, 1951.
2. Brown JJ, et al. Brit Med J 1:253-258, 1970.
3. DiBona GF, et al. Nephron 8:205-220, 1971.
4. Flamenbaum W, et al. Am J Physiol 224:305-311, 1973.
5. Dunnil MS. J Clin Pathol 27:2-13, 1974.
6. Keeton TK and Campbell WB. Pharmacol Rev 31:81-227, 1981.
7. Thiel G, et al. J Urol Nephrol, (Paris) 79:976-977, 1973.
8. Taugner R, Winkel K and Iravani J. Virchows Arch (Pathol Anat) 340:369-383, 1966.
9. Kempson SA, Ellis BG and Price RG. Chem Biol Interact 18:217-234, 1977.
10. Hsu CH, et al. Nephron 18:326-332, 1977.
11. Fitzhugh OG. Arch Ind Hyg Occup Med 2:433-442, 1950.
12. Yoshikawa H. Ind Health (Japan) 8:184-191, 1970.
13. Jones MM, Schoenheit JE and Weaver D. Toxicol Appl Pharmacol 49:41-44, 1979.
14. Dieckmann W and Butler WH, in The Correlation of Adverse Effects in Man with Observations in Animals. Excerpta Medica, Amsterdam, 1971, pp.247-252. ISBN 90-219-0295-5.
15. Prescott LF and Ansari S. Toxicol Appl Pharmacol 14:97-107, 1969.
16. Magos L, Webb M and Butler WH. Br J Exp Pathol 55:589-594, 1974.
17. Webb M and Magos L. Chem Biol Interact 14:357-369, 1976.
18. Surtshin A and Parelman AG. Am J Physiol 190:278-280, 1957.
19. Tandon SK, Magos L and Cabral JRP. Toxicol Appl Pharmacol 52:227-236, 1980.
20. Tandon SK and Magos L. Br J Ind Med 37:128-132, 1980.
21. Wachstein M and Robinson M. Fed Proc 24:619, 1965.
22. Wachstein M and Bradshaw M. J Histochem Cytochem 13:44-56, 1965.
23. Baxter JJ and Yoffey JM. J Anat 82:189-197, 1948.
24. Maunschbach AB. J Ultrastruct Res 15:197-241, 1966.
25. Oliver J, et al. J Exp Med 99: 605-620.
26. Reber K. Schweiz Z Allg Pathol 16:755-771, 1953.
27. Lippman RW. Proc Soc Exp Biol Med 72:682-687, 1949.
28. Zingg W. Schweiz Z Pathol Bakt 14:1-16, 1951.
29. Harber MH and Jennings RB. Arch Pathol 79:218-222, 1965.
30. Swensson A and Ulfvarson E. Occup Health Rev 15:5-11, 1963.
31. Magos L, Sparrow S and Snowden RT. Publication in preparation.
32. Daniel JW, Gage JC and Lefevre PA. Biochem J 129:961-967, 1972.
33. Daniel JW, Gage JC and Lefevre PA. Biochem J 121:411-415, 1971.
34. Burgat V, et al. Bull Schweiz Ges Klin Chem 21:114-117, 1980.
35. Ladd AC, Goldwater LJ and Jacobs MB. Arch Environ Health 9:43-52, 1964.
36. Goldwater LJ. Occup Med 6:227-228, 1964.
37. Massman W. Zentralbl Arbeitsmed Arbeitsschutz 7:9-13, 1957.

38. Wilkening H and Lutzner S. Dtsch Wochenschr 77:432-434.
39. Derebert L and Marcus O. Ann Med Leg 36:294-296, 1956.
40. Jalili MA and Abbasi AH. Brit J Ind Med 18:303-308, 1961.
41. Damluji S. J Fac Med Baghdad 4: No.3 83-103, 1962.
42. Bakir F, et al. Science 181:230-241, 1973.
43. Suzuki T, et al., in Mercury, Mercurials and Mercaptans. (MW Miller and TW Clarkson, eds.). Charles C Thomas Publ. Springfield, 1973, pp.209-231, ISBN 0-398-02600-9.
44. Fang SC and Fallin E. Chem Biol Interact 9:57- , 1974.
45. Klein R, et al. Arch Pathol 96:83-90, 1973.
46. Magos L and Butler WH. Food Cosmet Toxicol 10:513-517, 1972.
47. Magos L and Butler WH. Arch Toxicol 35: 25-39, 1976.
48. Fowler BA. Amer J Pathol 69:163-174, 1972.
49. Magos L, et al. Arch Toxicol, 1981. In press.
50. Klaassen CD. Toxicol Appl Pharmacol 33:356-365, 1975.
51. Takahashi T, et al. Eisekagaku (Japan) 17:93-107, 1971.
52. Takeda Y, et al. Toxicol Appl Pharmacol 13:156-164, 1968.
53. Magos L and Webb M. Arch Toxicol 38:201-207, 1977.
54. Farris FF, Poklis A and Griesmann GE, in Biological Implications of Metals in the Environment. ERDA Symposium Series No.42, 1977, pp.465-477.
55. Norseth T and Clarkson TW. Arch Environ Health 21:717-727, 1970.
56. Platonow N. Occup Health Rev 20:108, 1968.
57. Platonow NA. Occup Health Rev 20:9-19. 1968.
58. Suzuki T, Miyama T and Katsunuma H. Jap J Exp Med 33:277-282, 1963.
59. Clarkson TW and Greenwood M. Brit J Pharmacol Chemother 26:50-55, 1966.
60. Canty AJ and Parsons RS. Toxicol Appl Pharmacol 41:441-444, 1977.
61. Ashe WF et al. Arch Ind Hyg Occup Med 7:19-43, 1953.
62. Suzuki T. Ind Health (Japan) 15:77-85, 1977.
63. Friberg L, Hammerstrom S and Nystrom A. Arch Ind Hyg Occup Med 8: 149-153, 1953.
64. Goldwater LJ. Arch Indust Hyg 8:588, 1953.
65. Kazantzis G. Q J Med 31:303-418, 1962.
66. Kazantzis G. Ann Occup Hyg 8:65-71, 1965.
67. Magos L. Brit J Ind Med 25:315-318, 1968.
68. Magos L, Clarkson TW and Greenwood MR. Toxicol Appl Pharmacol 26: 180-183, 1973.
69. Berlin M, Jerksell LG and Ubisch H. Arch Environ Health 12:33-44, 1966.
70. Rothstein A and Hayes AD. J Pharmacol Exp Ther 130:166-176, 1960.
71. Hayes AD and Rothstein A. J Pharmacol Exp Ther 138:1-10, 1962.

THE NEPHROTOXIC EFFECTS OF LEAD

Robert A. Goyer

National Institute of Environmental Health Sciences, Research Triangle Park, North Carolina, USA

Nephrotoxicity has long been recognized as a possible effect of chronic exposure to lead. Experimental studies have demonstrated pathologic changes extending from initial functional and morphologic abnormalities in proximal tubular lining cells to a progressive fibrosing interstitial nephropathy. The early changes are seen in children with acute lead toxicity and in recently employed adults with heavy occupational exposure. The proximal tubular dysfunction, characterized by glycosuria, aminoaciduria and hyperphosphaturia, is thought to be related to impaired transport due to lead effects on cellular respiration. Also present are well-defined nuclear inclusion bodies composed of lead-protein complexes. Chronic nephropathy has been seen in workmen with prolonged and excessive exposure and consists of both tubular atrophy and tubular cell hyperplasia. Renal adenoma and adenocarcinoma occur in rats in the later stages of lifetime (two years) exposures in rats but the carcinogenicity of lead in man is unclear. Reduction in glomerular filtration rate occurs in chronic nephropathy which has progressed to interstitial fibrosis. There is need to determine the level of lead exposure that will result in significant reduction in glomerular filtration rate (GFR) but study is complicated by changes in GFR with aging and intercurrent renal diseases. Other metabolic effects of lead related to nephrotoxicity include a possible decreasing ability to excrete sodium and increase in plasma renin activity. Persons with lead nephropathy often have increased blood uric acid levels perhaps related to reduced renal excretion of urate.

Key words: Lead, kidney, inclusions, glomerular tubular function.

INTRODUCTION

Of the major clinical effects of lead--neural, hematologic, and renal--it is the effects on the kidney that have received the least attention. A major reason for this is that neural effects of lead are much more overt clinically and hematologic effects of lead are easily measured in the laboratory and serve as effective indicators of severity of lead exposure. Renal effects of lead, on the other hand, are not easily recognized and may only occur after many years of exposure to excessive lead. If one goes back to some of the observations about lead toxicity that were made a century or more ago, renal effects seem to have been first recognized by pathologists but the clinical relevance of lead nephropathy was not appreciated until some years later. The Treatise on Lead Diseases by Tanqueral des Planches [1], a clinician, cites in 1848 that colic arthralgy, paralysis and encephalopathy are "primary effects" and are "precursors of all forms of lead disorder." Although problems in micturation and peculiarities of urine colic referred to as "neuralgia of the digestive and urinary organs" are described, there is no direct reference to chronic lead nephropathy.

Only a few years later in 1881, Charcot and Gombault (cited in Aub [2]) described the diffuse interstitial fibrosis in the kidney that follows prolonged excessive exposure to lead as "epithelial cirrhosis of the kidney." The term implies primary involvement of the tubular epithelial cell, the major feature of acute renal effect of lead, and the shrunken hardness of the contracted fibrotic kidney characteristic of end-stage renal disease. Sir Thomas Oliver in his book on lead poisoning [3] published in 1914 recognized that "lead absorbed into the system cannot circulate in the blood without inflicting injury upon such eliminating organs as the kidneys and liver." He also comments that "interstitial nephritis or contracted kidney is the most common pathological event in chronic plumbism" and "it is undoubtedly the lesion of chronic lead poisoning; it is found in persons who have worked in lead for years."

Of major concern for the industrial physician today is that late effects of lead on the kidney are irreversible. Although much is known about the early or reversible renal effects, there is no obvious measure of renal function or measurable biochemical parameter of lead toxicity or measure of renal function that will serve to indicate when lead exposure is likely to be associated with irreversible effects. The comments in this short presentation will identify what is known about lead on the kidney at the cellular level and review recent clinical studies on chronic lead nephropathy.

RENAL EXCRETION OF LEAD

Renal excretion of lead may occur by two routes, glomerular filtration and renal tubular secretion. Since more than 90 percent of blood lead is bound to red blood cells, only lead in plasma bound to filtrable ligands is filtered by the glomerulus. A portion of filtered lead may be absorbed by the renal tubule. Also, renal secretion of lead may occur by transtubular transport from peritubular capillaries and secretion into tubular lumen [4]. However, transtubular transport and excretion of lead probably only occurs with excessive lead exposure.

With increased exposure to lead, one of the earliest identifiable effects is formation of lead-protein complexes or inclusion bodies

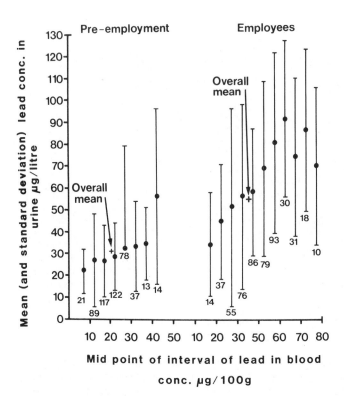

Figure 1. Comparisons of lead in blood and lead in urine
in persons prior to and after occupational exposure to lead
(from Barry, 1972 [7]).

within renal tubular cells [5]. These bodies are probably formed in the
course of transtubular flow of lead (see Acute Renal Effects). The
bodies account for the major fraction of intracellular lead and are
excreted in urine during occupational exposure [6] and may, in fact,
account for the higher urine lead content that has been observed in
occupational exposure as compared to non-occupationally exposed persons
with similar blood lead levels (Figure 1) [7].

Recent studies have shown in the dog, using stop flow analysis, that
either net reabsorption or secretion could occur and that fractional
(excreted/filtered) excretion of lead was lowest in dogs undergoing
metabolic acidosis, highest during metabolic alkalosis, and intermediate
in dogs with normal acid-base status. Also, the site for maximal reabsorption of lead in the distal nephron was almost identical to that for
sodium, chloride and calcium reabsorption but is at least partly independent [8].

ACUTE RENAL EFFECTS OF LEAD

The focus of acute renal effects of lead is the proximal portion of
the renal tubule and is characterized by at least three pathological and

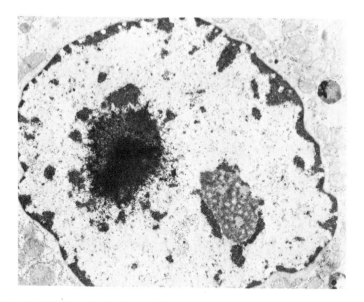

Figure 2. Inclusion body in nucleus of renal tubular
lining cell of rat with lead toxicity.

functional alterations. These are the formation of nuclear inclusion
bodies, the development of functional and ultrastructural changes in
mitochondria and impairment of absorption of amino acids, glucose and
phosphate [9].
     The formation of nuclear inclusion bodies in renal tubular lining
cells is a distinguishing histologic feature of lead toxicity. They
occur most frequently in the proximal portion of the tubule (pars recta)
and by light microscopy appear as dense spherical eosinophilic bodies.
They can be differed from viral inclusion by being acid-fast when
stained with the Ziehl-Neelsen's technique. By electron microscopy,
the inclusions consist of a dense central core and outer fibrillary
zone. They vary considerably in size and the fibrils do not have
periodicity (Figure 2).
     Study of the lead-induced inclusion bodies in experimental animals
has provided some insight into their composition and role in lead
poisoning. The formation of these bodies appears to be a universal
response to excessive body burden of lead and they are particularly
common in kidney and liver, but have also been found in osteoclasts
and astrocytes of animals given large doses of lead. They have been
found to be composed of a lead-protein complex and most of the lead
in the kidney is sequestered in the inclusion bodies [10]. In fact, it
has been found that lead is complexed to proteins in nuclei of control
rats and presumably in nuclei of other species even when tissue lead
is not sufficient to form discernible inclusion bodies. The bodies
may be isolated by differential centrifugation and the protein has
been found to be a non-histone acidic protein, rich in glutamic and
aspartic acids and glycine and may actually be a mixture of acidic
proteins with similar physiochemical properties. The proteins are

probably denatured and insoluble aggregates are built up until bodies are formed [11].

It has also been observed that mitochondria in proximal tubular lining cells of kidneys in persons with excessive exposure to lead are morphologically and functionally abnormal [12]. The mitochondria var: in shape, have a bizarre arrangement of cristae and even show a tendency for budding. When mitochondria are isolated from kidneys of lead toxic rats they show some impairment in oxidative and phosphorylative abilities when compared to mitochondria from control rats [13]. The relationship o: the mitochondrial effect of lead to the clinical symptomatology of lead toxicity is only speculative at the present time but there is reason to believe that the mitochondrial effect of lead is related to both the hematopoietic and renal effects of lead [14]. The lead affects heme bio-synthesis at more than one site. This effect may be a reflection of the action of lead on the mitochondria in hematopoietic cells. Lead impairs aminolevulinic acid dehydratase activity resulting in increased excre-tion of the heme precursor ALA in the urine. It inhibits ferrochelatase, the enzyme responsible for incorporation of iron in the porphyrin ring. The other possible effects of lead on heme biosynthesis are less well known but many of the enzymes involved in heme synthesis are located within mitochondria or are dependent on normal mitochondrial function.

In the kidney, transport functions, particularly in the proximal tubular lining cells, depend on energy derived from oxidative processes in the mitochondria. The decrease in reabsorption of amino acids by the renal tubule that occurs in lead poisoning may be related to the effect of lead on mitochondria in these cells. A difficulty with this inter-pretation is that most of the energy in the proximal tubular lining cells is believed to be used for sodium transport and there is no direct evidence that lead produces any imbalance in the transport of this ion. However, a mild impairment may be compensated for by activity in another portion of the tubule. Some indirect evidence for an effect of lead on sodium transport is found in the clinical observation that lead intoxi-cation has an effect on the renin-aldosterone response to sodium deprivation [15].

With further regard to the role of the inclusion body in the metabo-lism and cellular toxicity of lead, it has been shown that the largest increase in lead within cells in lead poisoning is in nuclei where most of it is concentrated in the inclusion bodies. The increase in lead content of mitochondria in lead poisoned rats as compared to control rats is small. It has been shown that lead intoxication results in a partial impairment of the respiratory and oxidative abilities of kidney mitochondria in lead-poisoned rats. In fact, lead is very toxic to mitochondria and the ADP-stimulated respiration of mitochondria isolated from kidneys of normal rats is completely inhibited when incubated *in vitro* for ten minutes with 0.15-0.20 µg Pb/mg of mitochondrial protein. This is approximately the amount of lead found in the mitochondria of the lead-poisoned rats. It appears, therefore, that no matter how much lead is present in the rat kidney, the mitochondrial content of lead must be restricted to these levels or lower if the cells are to stay viable. This relatively low concentration of mitochondrial lead can be accom-plished by binding lead in a non-diffusible or nontoxic form within the intranuclear inclusion body in the excretion and pathobiology of lead toxicity [15].

As mentioned earlier, excretion of lead, particularly in the presence of elevated blood levels, may be transtubular from peritubular capil-laries to tubular lumen. In the course of the transtubular flow of lead, a portion of the lead enters the cell where it forms a lead-protein complex and is no longer diffusible. The inclusion bodies may actually be formed within the cytoplasm initially and then transported into the nucleus by invagination of nuclear membranes (Figure 3).

Reversal of this process, that is, extrusion of inclusion bodies by evagination of nuclear membranes occurs following chelation therapy (Figure 4) [17]. Support for the cytoplasmic formation of inclusion bodies is found in studies showing that the administration of lead to primary cultures of rat kidney epithelial cells results in formation of typical inclusion bodies in the cytoplasm within four hours, and that the inclusion bodies become relocalized in the nucleus by twenty-four hours [18]. This mechanism, therefore, has the effect of maintaining a relatively low cytoplasmic concentration. Hence, the cytoplasmic contents of the cell, particularly the mitochondria, are spared from exposure to large concentrations of lead. This proposed role for the nuclear complexing of lead is only an hypothesis but it does provide a functional explanation of a morphological phenomenon.

CHRONIC RENAL EFFECTS OF LEAD

A difference between early or acute renal effects of lead and chronic lead nephropathy is that the early changes, confined to renal tubular epithelial cells, are reversible. Progression from the acute tubular cell effects to interstitial fibrosis can be demonstrated in experimental models and the histologic appearances of acute and chronic renal effects of lead have been described in lead workers with brief (weeks) versus prolonged (months/years) of excessive lead exposure. Chelation therapy removes the inclusion bodies and the altered mitochondrial morphology and function is reversed; also, renal tubular function returns to normal [17]. However, it is not possible to reverse the interstitial fibrosis that is present in chronic lead nephropathy. Progression may perhaps be arrested or delayed but the fibrosis cannot be removed. This raises the most important question regarding the renal effects of lead that is yet to be answered, that is, how can the transition from acute to chronic renal effects of lead be recognized clinically without a biopsy. There is great need for a clinically applicable test that is non-invasive that will identify the onset of interstitial fibrosis.

There have been a number of clinical studies of renal function in persons with excessive occupational exposure to lead in recent years and much has been learned. However, it is still not certain how to determine what, if any, renal lead effect is present in any particular person prior to the onset of advanced irreversible kidney disease. Of course, a renal biopsy will go a long way in providing this information but this is not a practical method for surveillance of the person with possible excess lead exposure.

Five of the most recent studies of renal function in persons with occupational exposure to lead have been selected for comment. Although no two of these studies employed the same battery of tests, there is some overlap and each study does provide some information relevant to lead effects on the kidney.

The study by Cramer, et al. [12], of seven heavily exposed shipwreckers in Sweden correlated renal biopsy findings with parameters of lead exposure and renal function. This study confirmed in human subjects that the histologic features of early and chronic exposure to lead

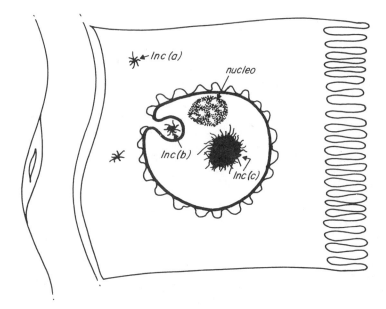

Figure 3. Scheme for cytoplasmic nuclear migration of inclusion bodies.

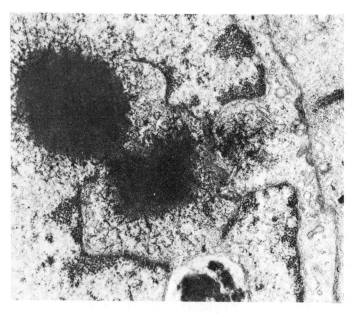

Figure 4. Extrusion of inclusion bodies from nucleus during chelation
therapy.

were similar to those seen in experimental animals and were related to length of exposure and presumably dose or body burden.

Wedeen, et al. [19], studied eight workers with exposure to lead. Reduced glomerular filtration was found in four of the workers. One had asymptomatic renal failure. Renal biopsy showed features of chronic lead nephropathy including glomerular sclerosis, periglomerular and interstitial fibrosis and degenerative changes in epithelial cells. No inclusion bodies were present. A second renal biopsy after chelation therapy showed improvement of the epithelial cell changes but persistence of interstitial fibrosis confirming again that this feature of chronic lead nephropathy is not reversible.

Renal biopsies were also obtained from two of three other workers with reduced glomerular filtration rate and no other functional changes. The renal biopsies were normal including glomerular morphology. Blood lead levels were below 80 μg/100 ml in all but one of the workers. Nevertheless, each worker had three or more years of lead exposure and without a more complete record of blood lead levels it is not possible to relate renal effects with a particular level of blood level.

The large study by Lilis and coworkers of two groups totaling two hundred and sixty-nine secondary smelter workers correlated blood lead, blood urea nitrogen and creatinine and zinc protoporphyrin [20]. Blood urea nitrogen was corrected for age. They found a prevalence of workers with increased blood urea nitrogen and creatinine among those workers with a long history of lead exposure. They also found a highly significant correlation of blood urea nitrogen and creatinine and duration of lead exposure. Both of these parameters correlated with blood zinc-protoporphyrin but not with blood lead. This suggests that blood levels of zinc-protoporphyrin reflect lead content of a diffusible compartment of bone lead. The relationship or common link between zinc-protoporphyrin and lead nephropathy must be total body burden of lead. Although the results of this study suggest this relationship may be a useful index of lead nephropathy, it may not be very helpful as a predictor in a specific case. There was no apparent relationship in the few cases reported by Wedeen.

In a second study by Wedeen and coworkers [21], they found reduced glomerular filtration rates in 21 of 57 lead workers in whom excessive body lead burdens had been shown by the urinary excretion of more than 1000 μg of lead per day during an edentate disodium calcium lead-immobilization test. Renal biopsies excluded other causes of renal disease in twelve patients suggesting the diagnosis of occupational lead nephropathy. Morphological confirmation of this diagnosis, however, was lacking in that none had nuclear inclusion bodies and eight had glomerular and tubular immunoglobulin deposits. This is a new finding in lead nephropathy and has not been reported in previous renal biopsies of persons exposed to lead or in experimental studies. However, gold and mercury, two other toxic metals that cause nephropathy, provoke antitubular basement membranes and immune complex disease [22, 23].

And, finally, the study by Hong, et al., measured glomerular filtration rates in six workmen with periods of lead exposure ranging from three months to six years [24]. All had normal serum urea nitrogen and creatinine. In four workers with decrease in inulin clearance, tubular functional changes were correlated with changes in glomerular filtration rate to see if any measure of tubular dysfunction was disproportionately greater than change in glomerular filtration rate. Of the tests for tubular function that were performed, the tubular reabsorptive capacity for glucose was significantly depressed but the secretory capacity for PAH and hydrogen ion were unchanged. This would appear to be the most sensitive functional indicator of lead nephropathy. However, these studies were only performed on workers with decreased glomerular filtration rates. Renal biopsies of workers with asymptomatic renal failure (azotemia) do show glomerular sclerosis and periglomerular fibrosis and in the light of Wedeen's recent study [21] glomeruli may also contain immune deposits.

GOUT AND LEAD NEPHROPATHY

A century ago it was commonly believed that chronic lead nephropathy and gout were somehow associated. Garrod, who first recognized elevated blood uric acid levels as the etiology of gout, cited lead poisoning as a cause of gout. However, this relationship was questioned by Aub [2], and the problem received little further attention and evidence accumulated that hyperuricemia itself did not appear to produce renal disease [25]. However, a number of studies appeared in the nineteen sixties again noting the relationship between lead nephropathy and gout [26, 27, 28]. Persons with lead nephropathy often have increased blood uric acid levels perhaps related to reduced renal excretion of urate [29]. A recent study of twenty-two patients with renal disease compared lead excretion following EDTA mobilization with lead excretion in patients with hyperuricemia and no renal disease [30]. Lead excretion was more than two times greater in those persons with renal disease and suggested that lead nephropathy may indeed be related to gout. The excessive mobilizable lead in the patients with gout could not be attributable to renal failure itself, since patients with renal disease, no gout, and no history of lead exposure did not have an increase in mobilizable lead.

LEAD AND RENAL ADENOCARCINOMA

The role of lead in renal carcinogenesis has received attention because life-time feeding of high doses of lead to rats results in renal adenoma and adenocarcinoma [31]. This experimental finding is species specific in that renal tumors cannot be induced in hamsters and rabbits and have not been noted to occur more often than expected in persons with occupational exposure to lead. Lead is not a mutagen [32]. Hyperplasia of renal tubular epithelial cells is prominent in both animal models and in lead nephropathy in humans but the role of lead in the progression of these lesions to neoplasia is not known. However, addition of lead acetate to the diet of rats exposed to N-(4-fluorobiphenyly)4-acetamide, a known carcinogen, increases renal tumor incidence to 100 percent suggesting that lead may be a promotor [33].

Choie and Richter noted that a single dose of lead can greatly stimulate proliferation of renal tubular epithelium in rats. Also, injection of lead acetate to mice greatly stimulated uptake of ^{3}H-thymidine in renal tubular epithelium. The increase in DNA replication is followed by increases in RNA and protein synthesis [34].

SUMMARY

Pathologic changes of lead nephropathy in man are similar to findings in experimental models. Effects on proximal epithelial cells occur in the early or acute phase and are reversible but interstitial fibrosis in the chronic phase is not reversible.

Present evidence suggests that asymptomatic renal failure (azotemia and reduced glomerular filtration rate) is associated with interstitial fibrosis. In workers without azotemia but decreased inulin clearance, there is decreased maximum reabsorption of glucose. Presumably interstitial fibrosis and irreversible renal effects are present at this stage of lead nephropathy.

There is no correlation of blood lead and renal effects but there is positive correlation of elevated blood urea and creatinine with duration of lead exposure.

Finally, there is still need for tests of renal function that can recognize lead nephropathy prior to onset of interstitial fibrosis, that is, during the stage that lead effects are still reversible. The role of immunologic mechanisms in the pathogenesis of lead nephropathy must be studied further experimentally and in persons with known excess exposure to lead.

REFERENCES

1. Tanqueral des Planches L. Lead Diseases: A Treatise, Translated from the French by Dana, SL, Daniel Bixby and Co, Lowell Massachusetts, 1848, pp.12-13, pp. 90 and 117.
2. Aub JC et al. Medicine 4:1-225, 1925.
3. Oliver T. Lead Poisoning, Lewis, London, 1914.
4. Vostal J and Heller J. Environ Res 2:1-10, 1968.
5. Goyer RA et al. Arch Environ Hlth 20:705-711, 1970.
6. Schumann GB, et al. Am Soc Clin Path 74:192-196, 1980.
7. Barry PSI. In Lead in the Environment, (P Hepple, ed.) Appl Sci Publ, Essex England, 1972, pp.79.
8. Victery, et al. Am J Physiol 237:F408-F414, 1979.
9. Goyer RA. Curr Top Pathol 55:147-176, 1971.
10. Goyer RA, et al. Lab Invest 22:245-251, 1970.
11. Moore JF, et al. Lab Invest 29:488-496, 1973.
12. Cramer, et al. Brit J Ind Med 31:113-127, 1974.
13. Goyer, et al. Lab Invest 19:78-85, 1968.
14. Goyer RA and Rhyne BC. Int Rev Exp Pathol 12:1-77, 1973.
15. Sandstead HH, et al. Arch Intern Med 123:632-635, 1969.
16. Goyer RA. Am J Path 64:167-182, 1971.
17. Goyer RA, et al. Lab Invest 32:149-156, 1975.
18. McLachlin JR, et al. Tox Appl Pharmacol 56:418-431, 1980.
19. Wedeen RP, et al. Am J Med 139:53-57, 1975.
20. Lilis et al. J Environ Pathol Toxicol 2:1447-1474, 1979.
21. Wedeen RP, et al. Arch Intern Med 139:53-57, 1979.
22. Ainsworth, SR, et al. Arch Path Lab Med 105:373-377, 1981.
23. Kelchner J, et al. Experientia 32:1204-1208, 1976.
24. Hong CD, et al. Kid Int 18:489-494, 1980.
25. Reif MC, et al. N Engl J Med 304:535-536, 1981.
26. Morgan JM, et al. Arch Int Med 118:17-29, 1966.
27. Emmerson BT. Arthritis Rheum 11:623-634, 1968.
28. Ball GV and Sorensen LB. N Engl J Med 280:1199-1202, 1969.

29. Klinenberg JF. N Engl J Med 280:1238-1239, 1969.
30. Bautman V, et al. N Engl J Med 304:520-522, 1981.
31. Moore MR and Meredith PA. Arch Toxicol 42:87-94, 1979.
32. Rosenkrantz HS and Poirier LA. J Nat'l Cancer Inst 62:873-892,
       1979.
33. Hinton DE, et al. Bull Environm Contam Toxicol 23:464-469, 1979.
34. Choie P and Richter G. In Lead Toxicity (R L Singhal and JA Thomas,
       eds), Urban and Schwarzenberg, Baltimore, 1980, pp.187-212.

GOLD RELATED NEPHROPATHY

O. Duke, M. Richter and G.S. Panayi

Department of Medicine, Guy's Hospital, London Bridge, London SE1 9RT, UK

ABSTRACT

The use of gold salts in the treatment of Rheumatoid Arthritis is now well established and a recognised complication of such therapy is the development of a membranous glomerulonephropathy. This paper considers the pharmacology of gold salts in relation to this complication, the clinical presentation and incidence of gold related nephropathy, the histopathological features, and the possible aetiopathogenic mechanisms which may be operating. In particular, the idea that gold-related nephropathy is caused through the interaction of a genetically determined inability to clear immune complexes satisfactorily from the circulation with the further depression of reticuloendothelial clearance caused by gold salts is considered.

KEYWORDS

gold salts
Glomerulonephritis
HLA-DR3
Immune Complexes
Reticuloendothelial system

INTRODUCTION

The application of gold salts in medicine began shortly after World War I when they were used in the treatment of pulmonary

tuberculosis. Although in this capacity they gradually fell into
disrepute, their application by Forestier in Rheumatoid Arthritis
(R.A.) in the late 1920s and early 1930s with beneficial effects
resulted in wider use in this condition (1).

It was noted during these early studies that the incidence of
side effects was considerable and so it was not until the double
blind, controlled, studies of Fraser (2) in 1945 and the Empire
Rheumatism Council in 1960(1) which confirmed their beneficial
effects that the use of gold salts became established. They are
now widely used as a second line drug in the treatment of RA although
the incidence of side effects is such that careful monitoring
of the patient is required.

Amongst the more serious of these side effects is the development of a gold related nephropathy (GRN) which usually manifests
itself as asymptomatic proteinuria or the development of the
nephrotic syndrome. This particular complication of gold therapy
has been extensively studied recently in both man and animal models
so that a wealth of clinical, pathological and immunological information is now available which allows us to speculate on the
mechanism of its pathogenesis and raises the important possibility
of being able to predict which patients might be at risk from this
complication.

PHARMACOLOGY

The commonly used gold preparations in man are water soluble
salts in which gold is attached to sulphur. The structural
formulae are shown in Fig. 1. The dosage and administration are
variable being adjusted to suit the individual case but usually
consists of a test dose of 5 - 10mg of the salt after which the
dose is increased to 50mg/week. This dose is continued until the
patient has received a total dose of 1G or until the disease shows
signs of remission when the dose is reduced in frequency to once
monthly.

The pharmacokinetics of gold salts are poorly understood in man
(4,5,6). Of particular interest is their localisation in relatively
large amounts in the kidney, reticuloendothelial system, and the
observation by several workers that the toxic effects of gold are
unrelated to plasma or urine levels in man, and this seems to be
particularly true of GRN (3).

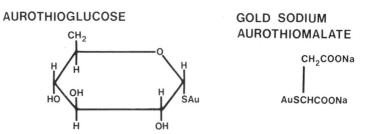

FIGURE 1. The structural formula of the commonly used gold salts,
           aurothioglucose and gold sodium aurothiomalate.

CLINICAL PRESENTATION AND INCIDENCE

There are now many case reports and small series reported of GRN and the usual forms of presentation are asymptomatic proteinuria, microscopic haematuria and the nephrotic syndrome. The clinical presentation may be accompanied by varying degrees of renal failure.

The exact incidence of this complication of gold therapy is difficult to ascertain (1,3,7,8,9). The incidence of proteinuria varies from 1% to 16%, whereas the incidence of frank nephrotic syndrome is less varying from 0 - 5% of patients receiving gold salts. The study by Kean et al (9) also noted the highest incidence of GRN in the first 6 months of therapy and this is in accord with other studies. It is important to note, however, that some patients with RA not taking gold salts may have renal abnormalities. These could, of course, be due to coincidental renal disease but there still remains a small population of patients with RA in the literature who have never had gold or penicillamine therapy that develop a nephropathy(10,11). This has raised the question as to whether or not the kidney is involved in RA and a large number of studies devoted to this end have been carried out. The consensus of opinion is that there are no really characteristic features of renal disease in RA (12,13) although there are a few patients reported who show some of the histological and immunofluorescent findings typical of gold salt nephropathy although they have never received the drug.

HISTOPATHOLOGICAL FEATURES OF GRN

The usual lesion found in patients with GRN is that of a membranous glomerulonephritis (5,10,14,15,16), the characteristic feature of which is the presence of electron dense deposits on the epithelial side of the glomerular capillary basement membrane. These so called subepithelial deposits are thought to be consistent with the deposition of immune complexes (17) and this is confirmed by immunofluorescent studies.

PATHOGENESIS

A number of possible explanations have been advanced to explain this appearance in man but first it is worth reviewing briefly the findings in GRN in animals (18,19). Payne and Saunders (18) describe a characteristic heavy metal nephropathy which occurs on administering gold to rats. Acute tubular necrosis similar to that obtained by Nagi et al (19) was seen but this type of lesion does not occur in man possibly because a not large enough dose is administered. The subacute and chronic lesions they describe also have no counterpart in man. Nagi et al (19) have, however, succeeded in producing a similar histological lesion to that seen in man using low doses of gold, and have invoked an immunological mechanism similar to autologous immune complex nephropathy in man (vide infra). It seems, therefore, that gold may cause renal damage either by direct toxic damage to the renal tubular epithelium if it is given in high enough dosages or if given in low doses gives rise to an immune complex type of glomerulonephritis. This latter mechanism seems to be the predominant one in man and possible explanations for this will now be considered.

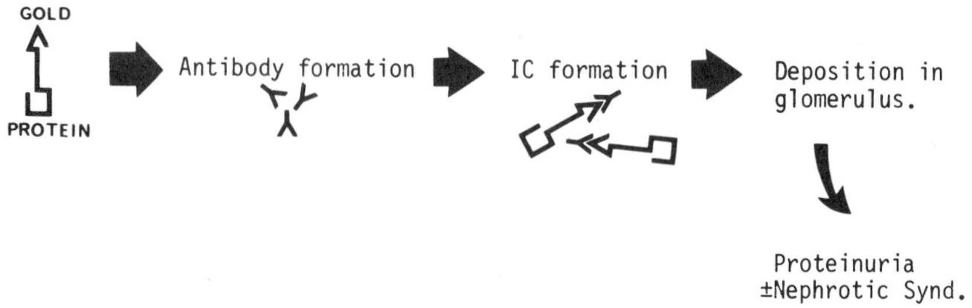

IC= immune complex.

FIGURE 2.   The hapten theory for the pathogenesis of gold-induced glomerulonephritis.

1.   The Hapten Theory

This theory supposes that gold which is heavily protein bound in plasma may initiate an immune response with the development of antibodies which then combine with the Gold-Protein complex to form immune complexes which are subsequently deposited in the glomerulus (Figure 2). The idea has some support from the work of Denman et al (20) who demonstrated lymphocyte transformation in response to Myocrisin in some patients with toxic side effects to gold therapy. However, although it has been shown that gold may cross the capillary wall, electron microprobe analysis has failed to reveal gold in the sub-epithelial deposits of patients with GRN (21) making this mechanism unlikely.

2.   Autologous Immune Complex Disease (Heymann autoimmune Nephritis)

In this model rats are immunised with repeated injections of rat kidney homogenate and Freund's complete adjuvant (22). The animal produces antibodies to renal tubular antigens (RTA) which lead to further destruction of renal tubular epithelium and the formation of antigen-antibody complexes which are deposited in the glomerulus. In the case of GRN the toxic effects of gold on the proximal renal tubular epithelium are thought to release RTA which then elicit an immune response (23). There are, however, a number of features of gold nephropathy which do not fit in with this concept.

Firstly, Heymann nephritis, once initiated, is a self perpetuating process and continues *ad infinitum* whereas GRN will cease on or shortly after gold therapy is stopped. Secondly, if this mechanism were true one would expect to find immune complexes containing RTA both in the circulation as well as in the glomerulus. These questions have not been answered for gold induced membranous nephropathy (MN) although these antigens have been looked for in other forms of MN with variable results. Naruse et al (24) found RTA deposited in the glomerular capillary walls of 3 out of the 7 patients with idiopathic MN that they looked at, but they were unable to demonstrate circulating antigen-antibody complexes in these 3 patients. A study of 74 patients with MN by Whitworth et al (25), which included one patient whose disease was gold

Autologous rat
kidney homogenate.

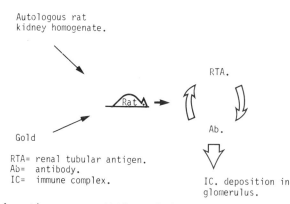

RTA= renal tubular antigen.
Ab= antibody.
IC= immune complex.

IC. deposition in
glomerulus.

FIGURE 3.   Schematic representation of the pathogenesis of autologous
immune complex disease (Heymann nephritis).

induced, failed to identify RTA in the glomerular deposits of
of any of the patients. The evidence, therefore, for such an
hypothesis in MN is scant whilst it is at the moment more or
less non existent in the gold related form of the disease and
further studies are required.

3.   Modulation of Immunological Mechanisms
An alternative hypothesis and one which is gaining support
is that the administration of gold compounds to a genetically
susceptible individual may result in an alteration of the
immunological *status quo*. It is now established by the work
of Wooley, Panayi and co-workers (26) that the development of
GRN is closely linked to the possession of the HLA antigen
DRW-3. In their study, in which they looked at the HLA-DR types
of patients having toxic reactions on gold therapy, they found
that the relative risk of developing GRN, if one possessed the
DRW-3 antigen, was increased 32 fold. The possession of the
DRW3/B8 haplotype is seen in many autoimmune conditions
characterised by the production of antibodies (e.g. myasthenia
gravis, systemic lupus erythematosus and nephritis, etc.) and
in RA it is associated with higher titres of rheumatoid factor than
in those patients without DRW3 (27). It is currently believed
that this association of DRW3 with certain autoimmune diseases
is not a direct association but by virtue of a closely related
immune response gene. This gene would be in close proximity
to the HLA-DR locus on the short arm of Chromosome 6 and in
some way controls the immune response in these DRW3 patients
such that they tend to produce large titres of autoantibody.
Furthermore, it has recently been reported by Lawley
and co-workers [28] that the HLA B8/DRW3 haplotype is associated
with defective Fc-receptor function and as the Fc-receptor
function of macrophages is thought to be important in the
clearance of immune complexes from the circulation it may be
that patients who are DRW3 positive and develop GRN, by
analogy with Lawley's work, are only poorly able to clear
immune complexes from the circulation. It is of interest in
this respect that membranous glomerulonephritis is independently
associated with the HLA-DRW3 antigen [29].

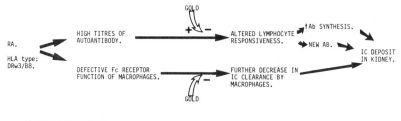

RA= RHEUMATOID ARTHRITIS.
HLA= HUMAN LEUCOCYTE ANTIGEN.
Ab= ANTIBODY.
IC= IMMUNE COMPLEX.

FIGURE 4.   Production of glomerulonephritis mediated by the immuno-
            modulating properties of gold salts.

In addition to this, patients with RA have been shown to
have poor reticuloendothelial clearance mechanisms (30) and
this may well be aggravated by the effect of gold which has
been shown to reduce the phagocytic ability of macrophages
in vitro and *in vivo* (31,32). Thus, we have now the basis of
the hypothesis shown in Figure 4. This portrays GRN as resulting from the inability to clear circulating immune complexes
efficiently and these may as a result become deposited in the
glomerulus. In addition, it is possible that gold may actually
initiate the formation of new autoantibodies thereby compound-
ing the situation. The evidence for any of these hypothetical
mechanisms is wanting, the only thing that seems certain is that
patients who continue to receive gold for their RA will continue
on occasion to develop GRN.

REFERENCES

1.   The Research Sub-committee of the Empire Rheumatism Council.
          Ann Rheum Dis 16: 95 - 116, 1960
2.   Fraser TN, Ann Rheum Dis 4: 71 - 75, 1945
3.   Silverberg DS et al, Arthritis Rheum 13: 812 - 825, 1970
4.   Smith RT et al, JAMA 161: 1197, 1958
5.   Brun C et al, Nephron 1: 265 - 276, 1964
6.   Gottlieb NL et al, Arthritis Rheum 15: 582 - 592, 1972
7.   Hartfall SJ et al, Lancet 2: 838 - 842, 1937
8.   The Co-operating Clinics Committee of the American Rheumatism
          Association, Arthritis Rheum 16: 353 - 358, 1973
9.   Kean WF and Anastassiades TP. Arthritis Rheum 22: 495 - 501,
          1979
10.   Samuels B et al, Medicine 57: 319 - 327, 1977
11.   Skrifvas B, Scand J Rheumatology 8: 242 - 247, 1979
12.   Salomon MI et al, Nephron 12: 297 - 310, 1974
13.   Pollak VE et al, Arthritis Rheum 5: 1 - 8, 1962
14.   Davies DJ et al, Pathology 9: 281 - 8, 1977
15.   Vaamonde CA and Hunt FR. Arthritis Rheum 13: 826 - 834, 1970
16.   Skrifvars BV et al, Ann Rheum Dis 36: 549 - 556, 1977
17.   Spargo BH and Seymour AE. In Renal Disease 3rd Edition (Black
          D Ed) Blackwell, Oxford 1973 pp 160 - 169
18.   Payne BJ and Saunders LZ, Vet Path 15 (suppl 5) : 51 - 87, 1978

19.   Nagi AH et al, Exp Molec Path 15: 354 - 362, 1971
20.   Denman EJ and Denman AM, Ann Rheum Dis 27: 582 - 588, 1968
21.   Strunk WS and Ziff M. Arthritis Rheum 13: 39 - 52, 1970
22.   Heymann W et al, Proc Soc Exptl Biol Med 100: 660 - 664, 1959
23.   Skrifvars B. Scand J Rheumatology 8: 113 - 118, 1979
24.   Naruse T et al, J Immunol 110: 1163 - 1166, 1973
25.   Whitworth JA et al, Clin Nephrol 5: 159, 1976
26.   Wooley PH et al, NEJM 303: 300 - 302, 1980
27.   Panayi GS et al, BMJ 2: 1326 - 1328, 1978
28.   Lawley TJ et al, NEJM 304: 185 - 192, 1981
29.   Klouda P et al, Lancet 2: 770 - 771, 1979
30.   Williams BD et al, Lancet 1: 1311 - 1314, 1979
31.   Davis P et al, J Rheumatol 6 (Suppl 5): 98 - 102
32.   Jessop JD et al, Ann Rheum Dis 32: 294 - 300, 1973

ACKNOWLEDGEMENTS

Part of the work described was financed by a grant from the Arthritis and Rheumatism Council of Great Britain.

CISPLATIN (*CIS* DICHLORODIAMMINE PLATINUM II) NEPHROTOXICITY

Peter T. Daley-Yates and David C. H. McBrien

Biochemistry Department, School of Biological Sciences, Brunel University, Uxbridge, Middlesex, UK

ABSTRACT

Cisplatin, a newly introduced antitumour drug, has nephrotoxic side effects. In a study of microscopic morphological changes induced by cisplatin in the rat kidney the collecting ducts and the pars recta of the proximal tubule were found to exhibit the earliest signs of damage. Vacuolation of the mitochondria is seen in these regions before major changes in the nuclei. There is no evidence, from x-ray microprobe analysis, for the accumulation of platinum deposits in the damaged kidneys. The effects of probenecid and furosemide upon the clearance of platinum through isolated perfused rat kidneys indicate that platinum enters the urine both by glomerular filtration and by active tubular secretion and that there is normally also a reabsorption of platinum from the urine which can be inhibited by probenecid. The Na^+/K^+-ATPase and Mg^{2+} - ATPase of rat kidney are equally sensitive to inhibition by cisplatin *in vitro* and the extent of inhibition and the time taken for it to develop are not affected by chloride ion concentration in the range 0 - 150 mM. These results are discussed in the light of a current model for the mechanism of platinum nephrotoxicity and a modified model is proposed.

(Keywords: Cisplatin, Furosemide, Probenecid, ATPase, Mitochondria, Platinum)

INTRODUCTION

Some metals have been known for many years to be nephrotoxic in experimental animals and in humans [1]. The recent introduction of platinum anti-tumour drugs has added a new dimension to clinical interest in metal-induced nephrotoxicity. Rosenberg [2] in 1965 first reported that certain platinum co-ordination compounds inhibited cell division in bacteria. The observation was the somewhat fortuitous outcome of experiments designed to investigate the effect of electric currents

upon cell growth. In 1969 Rosenberg's group [3] reported the potent
anti-tumour properties of some of the platinum complexes when tested in
mice. Of the compounds tested the most potent was cis- dichlorodiammine
platinum II (cisplatin). Following extensive toxicological evaluation
in animals   4   this was introduced into clinical trials. It was
found to have good activity against testicular and ovarian tumours but,
as with most cytotoxic drugs, its toxicity is a major complication in
its use. Amongst several reported side-effects [5] the dose-limiting
factor is nephrotoxicity, which is dose-dependent and cumulative. Cisplatin received approval for clinical use in the U.K. in March 1979.

Tissue distribution studies with radiolabelled cisplatin [6] have
shown in a variety of animal species that the kidney accumulates the
highest concentration of platinum, up to four times more than is found
in the liver for example. Hepatotoxicity has not been observed with
cisplatin [7]. Following intravenous injection of cisplatin between 70
and 90% of the dose is excreted during the first 15 minutes [6]. The
resultant high concentration of platinum in the urine is probably a significant factor in the development of kidney damage. The remaining
fraction of the dose is excreted over a period of several weeks and
patients are reported as having platinum in their urine one month after
the last dose [8]. Cisplatin binds extensively to blood cells and
plasma proteins [9] and this is the reason for the very slow loss of that
proportion of the original dose which is retained 24h after dosing. The
clinical features of platinum nephrotoxicity are uraemia, glucosuria,
proteinuria, the appearance of kidney enzymes in the urine and electrolyte imbalance [5]. In experimental animals the increase in blood urea,
glucosuria and proteinuria reach peak values approximately 4d after injection of cisplatin at 7.6 mg/kg [10].

After injection cisplatin undoubtedly undergoes a number of trans-
formations, chemical reactions with biological molecules and also
possibly metabolic alterations, but the nature of these biotransformations is not fully understood. The chemistry of platinum co-ordination
compounds is complicated [11] . It is a widely held view that cisplatin
loses its chloride ligands in aqueous media by replacement with water
molecules or hydroxyl ions and these more reactive hydrolysis products
are responsible for biological activity and toxicity [11-14]. We
present here the results of an investigation into the nature and the
mechanism of platinum nephrotoxicity.

MORPHOLOGICAL STUDIES

Information about the nature of the pathological changes in the kidney
caused by cisplatin has come from both animal and human studies.
Patients receiving cisplatin chemotherapy have had kidney structure examined at autopsy or by biopsy. These investigations have not led to
general agreement about the nature of the nephrotoxic lesion in man.
Different treatment regimens and patient histories make the interpretation of results difficult. Hardaker *et al* [15] described focal areas of
interstitial infiltrates, tubular destruction, periglomerular fibrosis,
and occasional sclerotic glomeruli in biopsy specimens from one patient
who was hypertensive and receiving other drugs. Piel *et al* [16] reported acute proximal tubular necrosis in biopsy specimens from patients
treated with cyclophosphamide and cisplatin. Gonzalez-Vitale *et al* [17]
presented detailed autopsy data from many patients treated with different dose schedules of cisplatin and mannitol. They concluded that the

primary nephrotoxic lesion was in the distal tubules and the collecting
ducts; the proximal tubules were affected but to a much lesser degree
and the glomeruli were reported as being unaffected. In patients the
dose varies between 1 and 3 mg/kg for single intravenous administrations
or approximately 0.5 mg/kg for repeated doses [18] Early animal studies
have tended to concentrate on the proximal tubule. In the first such
report Leonard *et al* [4] described swelling of the mitochondria in the
proximal tubules of rats 46h after injection of cisplatin at 10.0 mg/kg.
Elements of the brush border were reported as lost by 72h following injection. Ward and Fauvie [10] reported necrosis of the outer stripe of
the medulla 3d after rats had received 7.6 mg/kg cisplatin. Dobyan
and co-workers [19] used a dose of 6 mg/kg cisplatin in rats and described the major lesion as necrosis of the third segment of the proximal
tubule 3 to 5d after treatment.

We have extended these early studies by examining in detail, using
light and electron microscopy, all parts of the rat nephron at various
times after dosing, and have observed changes starting as early as 25h
following single intraperitoneal injections of 10 mg/kg cisplatin. Our
results [20] are summarised as follows :

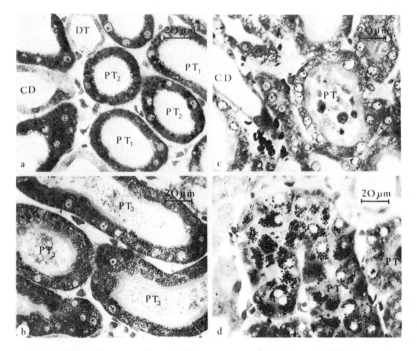

Figure 1. Light micrographs of the rat renal cortex. Kidneys were
taken from animals previously treated with cisplatin (10 mg/kg i.p.).
(a) 25h after treatment the pars convoluta (PT_1,PT_2) is normal (b) 25h
after treatment the pars recta (PT_3) has undergone cloudy swelling (c)
39h after treatment the pars recta (PT_3) has highly swollen nuclei loss
of the brush border and disrupted organelles fill the lumen (d) 70h
after treatment the proximal tubule (PT) has collapsed and contains
necrotic cells.

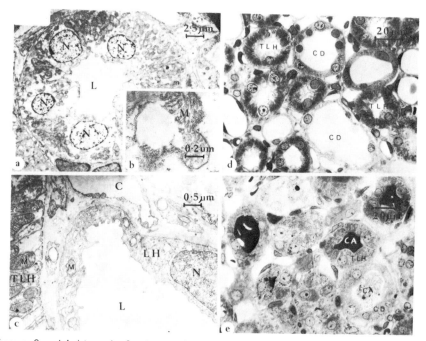

Figure 2. Light and electron micrographs of the rat renal medulla.
Kidneys were from animals previously treated with cisplatin (10 mg/kg
i.p.). (a) thick loop of Henle (TLH) 25h after treatment, mitochondrial
swelling is evident (b) shows detail of mitochondria (M) at 25h (c) thin
loop of Henle (LH) 25h after treatment, swollen mitochondria (M) and
nuclei (N) with lost heterochromatin can be seen (d) 39h after dosing
nuclei of the collecting ducts (CD) and thick loops of Henle (TLH) have
condensed chromatin and some collecting ducts are necrotic. (e) 70h
after treatment casts (CA) are found in the thick loop of Henle (TLH)
and collecting ducts (CD), most nuclei show loss of heterochromatin.

The collecting ducts. When observed with the light microscope the
dark cells of the medullary collecting ducts stain very darkly with toluidine blue 25h after treatment with cisplatin. Examined by electron
microscopy these cells exhibit dense cytoplasm, shrunken nuclei and
numerous apical vacuoles. Thirty-nine hours after treatment degradation
and dilation of the cortical collecting ducts can be seen (Fig.1c) and
the medullary collecting ducts have necrotic cells, possibly the dark
cells as these are no longer distinguishable (Fig.2d). Seventy hours
following treatment medullary collecting ducts have casts in their lumens
and the nuclei are pale and have lost chromatin (Fig.2c). The intense
staining of the collecting duct dark-cells at 25h may be due to mineral
deposition in these cells. The precise function of these cells is not
known. However, they do increase in number in hypokalemia and large numbers of apical vacuoles are seen in disorders of potassium reabsorption
[21]. These observations may be related to a deficiency of cation reabsorption in the proximal tubules. Patients receiving cisplatin do
suffer from cation imbalance [5] and cases of renal magnesium wasting
have been reported [22]. In magnesium deficiency calcium is deposited

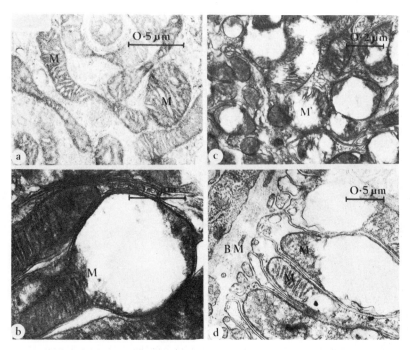

Figure 3. Mitochondrial lesions in the rat kidney. Kidneys were from animals treated with cisplatin (10 mg/kg i.p.). (a) mitochondria of the pars convoluta 39h after dosing (b) mitochondria of the thick loop of Henle 70h after dosing (c) mitochondria of the pars recta 25h after dosing (d) mitochondria at the base of a distal tubule cell showing the basement membrane (BM) 25h after treatment.

in the nephron [23] . This could be a result of impairment of transport ATPase (see later). The first portion of the collecting ducts has a con-siderable capacity for glucose reabsorption [24] . Extensive damage can therefore be caused to the proximal tubule without glucosuria becoming apparent [25] . Even at low doses cisplatin causes glucosuria [26] and so it is possible that the early damage caused to the collecting ducts is of more importance in the development of cisplatin nephrotoxicity than has previously been recognised.

The loop of Henle and distal tubules. The thick loops of Henle and distal tubules 25h after cisplatin treatment contain swollen and vacuo-lated mitochondria (Fig.2a,2b,3d). The nuclei of the cells appear normal at this stage (Fig.2a) although small casts may be seen in the lumen of some of the thick loops of Henle. Figure 2c shows the thick loop of Henle at this stage with mitochondrial swelling and loss of heterochromatin in the nuclei. Thirty nine hours after treatment the thick loops of Henle have nuclei with condensed chromatin (Fig.2d). Seventy hours after treatment many thick and thin loops of Henle contain darkly staining casts occluding their lumens and the nuclei are pale and swollen. Some cells are necrotic with cell debris filling the lumen (Fig.2c).

The glomeruli. The glomeruli are largely unaffected by cisplatin. Seventy hours after treatment there is loss of heterochromatin in some podocyte nuclei and some swelling and vacuolation of the cytoplasm of some podocytes. There is no detectable fusion of the foot processes or thickening of the filtration membrane. Aggarwal *et al* [12] reported electron dense deposits on the filtration membrane and the epithelium of Bowman's capsule but we were unable to confirm these observations (also see later). The absence of high molecular weight proteins in the urine of animals with cisplatin induced proteinuria suggests an absence of severe glomerular damage [12].

The proximal tubules. The pars convoluta shows no evidence of damage 25h after treatment with cisplatin (Fig.1a). However, cells of the pars recta (Fig.1b) have undergone cloudy swelling, nuclei have swollen and lost heterochromatin and mitochondria are swollen and vacuolated (Fig.3c). The lumen of the pars recta is filled with disrupted organelles (Fig.1b). Thirty nine hours after treatment the pars recta is extensively damaged, nuclei are highly swollen and there is an almost total absence of heterochromatin. Cell fragments fill the lumen and there is some loss of the brush border elements (Fig.1c). Swollen mitochondria can be found in the pars convoluta (Fig.3a). After 70h necrotic proximal tubules in the outer medulla are abundant (Fig.1d). Many cytoplasmic bodies (type II) are found in the pars convoluta. These bodies have crystalline inclusions and at the cell apices numerous vesicles with electron dense deposits are found [20]. By 90h after treatment many areas of the outer medulla are necrotic.

It is difficult to interpret these morphological changes in terms of the biochemical events which lead to cell death or   reversible cell damage. Many other metals which are nephrotoxic accumulate as intra-cellular deposits in the kidney cells [27] and the role of lysosomes and mitochondria in these processes have been discussed elsewhere [28] and in this symposium. Such deposition does not appear to be a feature of cisplatin nephrotoxicity (see below). The antitumour action of cis-platin is thought to be brought about by binding to DNA [29]. However, the nuclear changes which we have seen seem to be secondary to and gen-erally occur later than changes in the mitochondria. The swelling of the mitochondria might be brought about by osmotic forces caused by the cation imbalance which results when transport ATPases are inhibited (see later). We have investigated the effects of cisplatin on the mito-chondrial enzyme pyruvate dehydrogenase [30] which is sensitive to in-hibition by many metals but our results do not indicate an involvement of this enzyme in the mechanism of platinum nephrotoxicity.

SUBCELLULAR LOCALISATION OF PLATINUM

Many metals are known to form metallic deposits in the cells of kidneys of exposed individuals [27]. Aggarwal *et al* [12] reported the occurrence of electron dense deposits in the kidneys of rats "due to cisplatin". We have examined kidneys from our own experiments but have been unable to detect any electron dense regions containing platinum. For this search we used x-ray microprobe analysis using a Link Systems energy dispersive x-ray detector attached to a Jeol 100C electron micro-scope. We examined kidneys from rats treated with up to 50 mg/kg cis-platin for periods between 0.5 and 24h prior to sacrifice. The high

toxicity of cisplatin (LD_{50} = 7.7 mg/kg in the rat) and the fact
that platinum thionine complexes do not form *in vivo* (M. Webb personal
communication) means that kidneys do not accumulate platinum to
levels exceeding the detection limits of the technique (approx. 0.01%
of the sample dry weight) before death. However, if a kidney with an
average platinum content below this level has a heterogeneous platinum
distribution with some areas of high concentration these might still be
detectable with this technique. No such areas were found in any of the
kidneys which we examined. Isolated cells in tissue culture have been
used to investigate the sub-cellular distribution of platinum by x-ray
microprobe analysis. Khan and Sadler [41] detected platinum in HeLa
cells treated with cisplatin and found platinum only in electron dense
regions within the nucleus. They incubated their cells in Eagle's
minimal medium containing 200 µM cisplatin for 4h prior to fixation.
Their stock solution of cisplatin had been prepared with dimethyl-
sulphoxide (DMSO) as a solvent and consequently there was approximately
1.0 mM DMSO in their incubation mixture. We repeated and extended their
experiments by using both HeLa and Chinese Hamster Ovary (CHO) tissue
culture cells and by incubating the cells with cisplatin both with and
without DMSO. We were also able to detect platinum in cells using x-ray
microprobe analysis but only in cells treated with cisplatin and DMSO
together. Figure 4 shows data from a single CHO cell incubated for 4h
with 200 µM cisplatin and approx. 1 mM DMSO. X-ray spectra were obtained from a region in the nucleus and a region in the cytoplasm. Platinum
could be detected in both regions but was present to the highest concentration in the nucleus. The picture of the cell shown in Fig.4 lacks
detail because a thick section (200-300 nm) was used to increase the
chance of detecting low concentrations of platinum. However, the
sectioned cell has a damaged cell membrane and this was probably caused
by the DMSO. The reason for cells exposed to cisplatin absorbing more

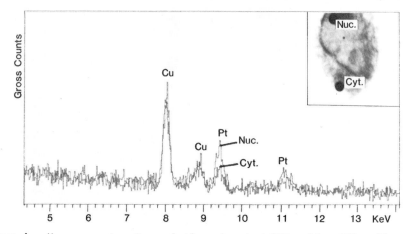

Figure 4.   X-ray spectra from platinum treated CHO cell.   CHO cells were
exposed to 200µM cisplatin and 1 mM DMSO for 4h at 37°C.   The inset shows
the cell from which the spectra were recorded.   The electron beam was
focussed upon a spot in the nucleus (Nuc) and in the cytoplasm (Cyt).
The spectra are shown superimposed and it can be seen that there is more
platinum (Pt) present in the nucleus than in the cytoplasm.   The copper
(Cu) peaks are from the specimen holder.

of it in the presence of DMSO is probably due to the increased permeability of such cells compared to those incubated without DMSO. Certainly such sub-cellular concentrations of cisplatin are not attained in the kidneys of animals treated with cisplatin *in vivo*.

RENAL CLEARANCE OF PLATINUM

The nephrotoxicity of cisplatin is controlled clinically by maintaining patients in extensive diuresis, using either hydration and mannitol [31,32] or furosemide [33]. We have investigated the clearance of platinum by the isolated perfused rat kidney and the effects upon this clearance of furosemide and of probenecid, drugs reported to ameliorate the nephrotoxicity of cisplatin in the rat [34,35].

Kidneys of male rats were perfused using the method of Bowman [36] and with a perfusate containing *inter alia* glucose, several amino acids and, when required 5% bovine serum albumin. Each kidney was perfused with 40-50 ml perfusate for approx. 1h. The urine produced was returned to the perfusate except for three periods of urine collection each lasting 2-10 min depending on the rate of urine flow and starting 20, 40 and 60 min after beginning perfusion. Samples of the perfusate were taken at the midpoint of each period of urine collection. When required cisplatin, furosemide and probenecid were added to the perfusate 3-4h before the start of perfusion. The glomerular filtration rate (GFR) was determined by measurement of the clearance of inulin. Further details of the methods and results will be published elsewhere [20].

Platinum binds to albumin and other blood proteins and approximately 47% is bound 4h after addition of cisplatin (30μM) to 50ml of perfusate. Only free (unbound) platinum is filtered at the glomerulus and the amount

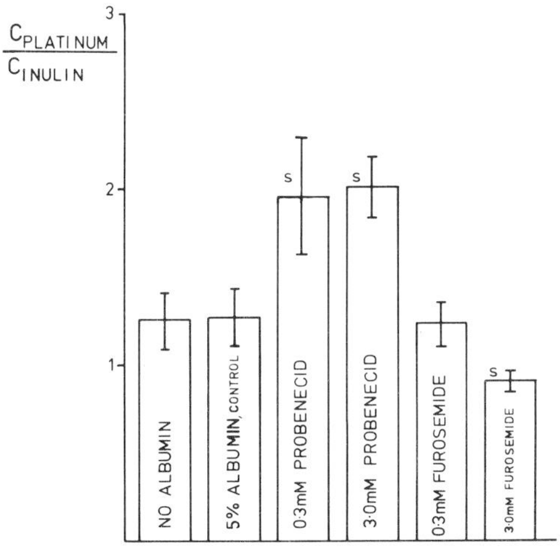

Figure 5. Ratios of the clearance of platinum to the clearance of inulin in the isolated perfused rat kidney. Clearance was measured with cisplatin (30μM) added to the perfusate and in the presence of probenecid and furosemide (see text). Each histogram represents the mean of nine clearance measurements ± standard deviation. Where indicated (S) the mean is significantly different from the control (p <0.01).

of free platinum in the perfusate for each period of urine collection was
determined by measuring platinum in the filtrate obtained after passage
of the perfusate sample through an Amicon CF25 ultrafilter. When albumin
is omitted from the perfusate all the platinum added to the perfusate is
recovered in the filtrate. The clearance of platinum from perfusates
containing 30μM cisplatin was determined with or without the presence of
furosemide or probenecid (Fig.5). The clearance of platinum was calculated from the concentration of free platinum in the perfusate. This
procedure is justifiable on the basis of the experimental evidence since
the clearance of platinum was found to be 125% of the GFR whether or not
albumin was included in the perfusate (Fig.5). This value also indicates
that there is a component of renal tubular transport in the excretion of
platinum. It can be seen that probenecid (at both 0.3 and 3.0 mM) increases the clearance of platinum to approximately twice the GFR.
Probenecid has been reported to prevent the development of platinum
nephrotoxicity in rats [35] . Clinically the drug is used principally
in the treatment of gout since it prevents renal tubular reabsorption of
uric acid. However, the renal transport of other organic acids is also
blocked [38]. Ross and Gale [35] proposed that cisplatin *in vivo* might
undergo ligand exchange for example with amino acids, to form new complexes with free carboxylate groups and that the renal transport of these
compounds might be inhibited by probenecid. If these compounds were
responsible for the kidney damage this hypothesis could account for the
amelioration of cisplatin nephrotoxicity brought about by probenecid.
The perfusate used in our experiments contains several amino-acids and we
have shown (unpublished results) that of these arginine is particularly
likely to give rise to the formation of new complexes with free carboxylate groups. Thus our observation that probenecid increases the clearance of platinum is evidence in support of the Ross and Gale hypothesis,
and if this hypothesis is correct then one must conclude that the nephrotoxic effects of cisplatin are brought about by the new platinum complexes, formed in the blood, filtered into the urine and then reabsorbed
into the kidney tubule cells. We are currently investigating further the
nature of the metabolites of cisplatin formed in the blood. However, the
results obtained when furosemide is added to the perfusate indicate that
the simple hypothesis outlined above is insufficient to explain all the
nephrotoxic effects of platinum.
    Furosemide increases the rate of urine flow from the perfused kidney
but at 0.3mM does not affect the clearance of platinum although the concentration of platinum in the urine is lower (Fig.4). At 3.0mM there is
apparently a nett reabsorption of platinum such that only 93% of the
filtered platinum appears in the urine. This could explain why both Pera
and Harder [37] and DeSimone *et al* [34] found that rats treated with
furosemide and cisplatin had more platinum in their kidneys than animals
treated with cisplatin alone. Pera and Harder [37] concluded that
furosemide reduces cisplatin nephrotoxicity by lowering the platinum concentration in the urine. If the reabsorbed platinum species are responsible for kidney damage it is a surprising observation that furosemide
does not prevent reabsorption and may even stimulate it. Moreover, probenecid and furosemide are both actively transported into the urine and
probenecid can compete with furosemide for the same transport mechanism
[39] . Passive reabsorption of compounds from urine [40] is dependent
upon the urine flow rate and is readily inhibited by diuretics such as
furosemide but, from our results, passive reabsorption of platinum does
not occur since the omission of albumin from the perfusate results in a

more rapid rate of urine flow (up to 0.8 ml/min compared with 0.2 ml/min) but does not affect the clearance of platinum. If it is not yet possible to draw detailed conclusions about mechanisms of platinum nephrotoxicity one thing is clear from these results. Platinum enters the urine via both glomerular filtration and active tubular secretion and can leave it by at least one route of tubular reabsorption.

THE EFFECTS OF PLATINUM UPON RENAL ATPase ACTIVITY

Renal ATPases have been shown to be the target of many nephrotoxic compounds [42] and some metal compounds have been shown to inhibit ATPase [43] . The Na^+/K^+-ATPase of isolated flounder kidney tubules has been shown to be inhibited by cisplatin [44] but only after exposure to high concentrations for prolonged periods. The inhibition of mitochondrial ATPase by cisplatin and its diaquo derivative has also been investigated [12] but in this case only the diaquo derivative was found to be inhibitory. Nevertheless, cisplatin has been shown to inhibit oxidative phosphorylation in isolated kidney mitochondria and to reduce whole kidney ATP concentrations [45] . Sodium transport in the frog skin is also inhibited by cisplatin[46].
We have investigated the sensitivity of both the Na^+/K^+- and the Mg^{2+}-ATPase in rat kidney to cisplatin, its hydrolysis products and some possible biotransformation products [47]. Our study was carried out using a whole kidney homogenate in MOPS (3-(N-morpholino)-propanesulphonic acid) buffer (pH 7.4) containing sodium deoxycholate.

Preparation of platinum compounds. Cisplatin was dissolved in distilled water and used immediately. Cisplatin hydrolysis products were prepared by allowing an aqueous solution of cisplatin to stand for 15d. Amino acid complexes of cisplatin were prepared by incubating 1:1 molar ratios of L-cysteine or L-methionine with cisplatin at 37° for 1.5h. This produced a mixture of the mono- and di-substituted platinum aminoacid complexes and their formation was confirmed by thin layer chromatography [47] .

Assay of ATPase. Platinum compounds were pre-incubated at 37°C for different times with 0.1 ml kidney homogenate (approx. 42 µg protein) in MOPS-KOH buffer (pH 7.4) containing potassium, sodium and magnesium sulphates [47] so that the mixture was essentially chloride free. For measurement of ouabain insensitive activity (*i.e.* Mg^{2+}-ATPase) 1 mM ouabain was included in the pre-incubation mixtures. To investigate the effect of varying the chloride ion concentration upon the ATPase activity choline chloride was added to the incubation mixture. The ATPase activity was measured, after pre-incubation period, by the addition of ATP and incubation at 37°C for 15 min. Further details will be published elsewhere [47].

Effects of cisplatin on ATPases. When ATPase activity was measured in the absence (Total ATPase = Na^+/K^+-ATPase + Mg^{2+}-ATPase) or presence (Mg^{2+}-ATPase) of 1 mM ouabain the concentration of cisplatin required for 25% inhibition was 360 µM for total ATPase and 340 µM for Mg^{2+}-ATPase (Fig.6). The similarity of these concentrations indicates that the two different ATPase activities are equally sensitive to cisplatin. Further experiments were therefore performed investigating the effects of cisplatin only upon total ATPase. The 15 day old solution of cis-

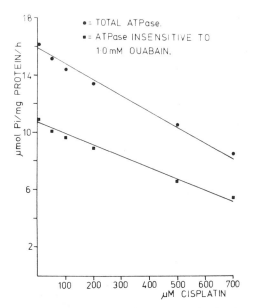

Figure 6. Inhibition of ATPase activity by cisplatin. Kidney homogenate
was pre-incubated with various concentrations of cisplatin for 1.5h at
37°C prior to assay. Assays were performed in the presence (Mg^{2+}-ATPase)
and absence (Total-ATPase) of 1.0 mM ouabain. Each point is the mean of
four determinations.

platin (cisplatin hydrolysis products) was found to be a thousandfold
more inhibitory to ATPase (ID$_{50}$ = 8.0 x 10^{-7}M) than freshly made cisplatin solutions (ID$_{50}$ = 6.5 x 10^{-4}M). The cysteine/cisplatin complexes
were not inhibitory to the enzymes at any concentration we tried but the
methionine/cisplatin complexes were more inhibitory (ID$_{50}$ = 1.1 x 10^{-4})
than cisplatin alone. To further investigate the effect of the methionine complexes solutions containing methionine and cisplatin prepared as
before but in different molar ratios (cisplatin:methionine 10:1, 2:1,
1:1, 1:2, and 1:5) were tested. The 10:1 solution would be expected to
contain mostly unsubstituted cisplatin and the monosubstituted complex
and the 1:5 solution mostly the disubstituted complex. We found the 2:1
solution was the most inhibitory (72% inhibition after 90min, 500μM
platinum) and the 1:5 solution the least inhibitory (19% inhibition after
90min, 500μM platinum). The biotransformations of cisplatin are not
fully characterised but it is known that cisplatin reacts rapidly *in
vitro* with many of the small molecules found in blood. Amino acids are
particularly likely to become involved in ligand exchange reactions [11].
It is thus likely that the two sets of amino acid complexes studied
above could form *in vivo*. Methionine probably reacts with cisplatin by
displacing a chloride ligand with sulphur and the incoming atom would
have a trans-labilising effect on an ammonia group rendering the complex
more reactive than cisplatin and presumably more toxic *in vivo*. The
equivalent mono-substituted cysteine complex would not be expected to be
subject to the same trans-labilising effect because the sulphydryl group
is deprotonated on binding [11] . The negatively charged sulphur which
results is less likely to attract electrons from platinum than the

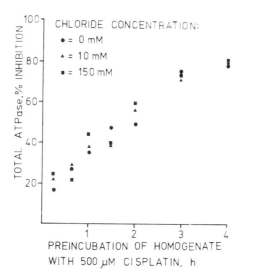

Figure 7. The effect of chloride ion concentration on the inhibition of Total-ATPase activity by cisplatin. Cisplatin (500 μM) was pre-incubated with the kidney homogenate for various times before assay, and in mixtures containing different chloride ion concentrations. Each point is the mean of four determinations.

neutral methionine sulphur atom and this would explain why the cysteine-cisplatin complexes are ineffective at inhibiting ATPase. A platinum complex of the mono-methionine type could be of importance in activating the cisplatin molecule *in vivo*.

Chloride ions and inhibition of ATPase by cisplatin. Cisplatin reacts slowly with ATPase, as shown in Fig.7 where 2h pre-incubation is required for the development of 50% inhibition. The rate of reaction is due to slow ligand exchange. Cisplatin may be reacting with a histidine imidazole group or with an amine group of arginine or lysine since these are groups in proteins with intermediate affinity for platinum. (Sulphur atoms react rapidly with platinum and if -SH or -SCH$_3$ groups were involved in inhibition of ATPase a faster reaction than that shown in Fig. 7 would be expected. Other groups, such as carboxylate and amide react much more slowly and are thus probably not involved in the observed inhibition). Rosenberg [13] and others [11,12,14] have suggested a role for hydrolysis products of cisplatin in the development of platinum toxicity. It is assumed that at chloride concentrations found in blood (approx. 103mM) cisplatin retains its chloride ligands but upon entering a cell the low cytoplasmic chloride concentration (approx. 4mM) allows hydrolysis to occur leading to the formation of more reactive and more toxic products. Water and hydroxyl ions are more effective leaving groups than chloride. Our results show that hydrolysis products of cisplatin are more effective inhibitors of ATPase activity than cisplatin *in vitro* (see above). We have investigated the effect of chloride ion concentration (0-150 mM) on the rate of development of inhibition of ATPase caused by 500μM cisplatin (Fig.7). It can be seen that the chloride ion concentration affected neither the extent of inhibition

nor the time taken to reach it. This suggests either that hydrolysis is
not affected by chloride concentration or that hydrolysis products are
not involved in the observed inhibition. The latter is more likely
since it has been calculated that in aqueous solution cisplatin undergoes hydrolysis with a half-time of about 7h [14] but at a chloride concentration of 100mM hydrolysis is arrested. This demonstration that cisplatin can directly inhibit enzyme activity raises the question of
whether the 'hydrolysis hypothesis' of platinum toxicity is valid. In a
biological environment there are so many potential ligands for platinum
of high affinity that it seems improbable that aquated derivatives of
cisplatin would form preferentially even though water is generally present at such a high concentration.

A MODEL FOR PLATINUM NEPHROTOXICITY ?

An understanding of the complicated chemistry of platinum co-ordination complexes and of the ligand exchange reactions which occur between
cisplatin and the components of a biological environment must be the
basis for an understanding of the mechanisms of toxicity and biological
activity of cisplatin. Because of this complexity the suggestions which
we make are necessarily tentative.

Many of the reactions which occur between cisplatin and biological
molecules, giving rise to new platinum compounds, will result in reduced
toxicity. The interaction with blood proteins [9] and, as we have shown,
with cysteine are examples of this. The apparent lack of reactivity of
cisplatin and the potent reactivity of cisplatin hydrolysis products[12]
has led many workers to propose the removal of the chloride ions and
their replacement by water or by hydroxyl ions as a method of activation of cisplatin *in vivo* [11-14] . The dependence of the reaction
upon chloride ion concentration has been discussed [11,14] and although
on theoretical grounds the cytoplasm has a low enough chloride concentration for hydrolysis to occur we suggest (see preceding section) that
this is unlikely to be a significant process. However, cisplatin does
react rapidly with amino-acids such as methionine under conditions found
in vivo, and we have shown that the products of this reaction are more
reactive than cisplatin itself. These complexes, once formed, would be
available for excretion. We have shown that excreted platinum compounds
may be reabsorbed in the kidney. This could possibly be via a mechanism
that normally reabsorbs amino acids. Once inside the kidney cells such
complexes could break-down either by simple chemical substitutions, by
reaction with nucleophilic atoms or even by enzymic attack upon ligands.
The nature of the targets in the cell for platinum toxicity is difficult
to determine. In tumour cells the antitumour effects of cisplatin involve the inhibition of cell division and it is generally accepted that
this requires the binding of platinum to nucleic acids, especially DNA
[29] . Kidney damage occurs in what is normally a non-proliferating
tissue, results in general necrosis and probably occurs via a different
mechanism. In the experiments on subcellular location of platinum using
tissue culture cells (see above) the concentration of platinum does
appear to be higher in the nucleus than elsewhere in the cell, but these
cells were treated with very high concentrations of cisplatin in the
presence of a powerful solvent and the results may therefore not be
typical of cells exposed to cisplatin *in vivo*. The changes in kidney
morphology caused by cisplatin indicate that mitochondria may be the
most sensitive parts of the cell to platinum toxicity but the patho-

logical changes observed may be indirect. Inhibition of ATPase has been
demonstrated and is probably a contributory factor to the loss of renal
function. It is likely that, once inside a cell, platinum may interact
in a relatively non-specific way with a variety of enzyme proteins resulting in necrosis. If the reabsorption of platinum species from the
urine is the key event in development of kidney damage it is difficult
to explain why furosemide can ameliorate such damage and more work is
required before the mechanism of platinum induced nephropathy is fully
elucidated.

ACKNOWLEDGEMENT

One of us (P.T.D-Y) gratefully acknowledges receipt of an S.E.R.C.
CASE research studentship with the co-operation and financial support of
Johnson-Matthey Research.

REFERENCES

1.   Zbinden G, in The Kidney (C Rouiller and AF Muller,eds.) Academic
      Press, New York,1969,pp.417-425.
2.   Rosenberg B,et al. Nature(London) 205:698-699,1965.
3.   Rosenberg B,et al. Nature(London) 222:385-387,1969.
4.   Leonard BJ, et al. Nature(London) 234:43-45,1971.
5.   Williams CJ and Whitehouse JMA, Br Med J 1689-1691,1979.
6.   Taylor DM, Biochimie 60:949-956,1978.
7.   Slater TF,et al. J Clin Hematol Oncol 7:534-546,1977.
8.   Williams CJ,et al. Cancer Treat Rep. 63:1745-1747,1979.
9.   Manaka RC and Wolf W, Chem Biol Interact 22:353-358,1978.
10. Ward JM and Fauvie KA, Toxicol Appl Pharmacol 38:535-547,1976.
11. Howe-Grant ME and Lippard SJ, in Metal Ions in Biological Systems,
      Vol 11 (H Sigel,ed.). Dekker,New York,1980.
12. Aggarwal SK,et al. in Cisplatin,Current Status and New Developments
      (AW Prestayko,ST Crooke and SK Carter,eds.).Academic Press,New
      York,1980.
13. Rosenberg B, Biochimie 60:859-867,1978.
14. Lim MC and Martin RB, J Inorg Nucl Chem 38:1911-1914,1976.
15. Hardaker WT,et al. Cancer 34:1030-1032,1974.
16. Piel IJ and Perlia CP, Cancer Chemother Rep 58:995-999,1975.
17. Gonzalez-Vitale JC,et al. Cancer 39:1362-1371,1977.
18. Ash CD, J Clin Hematol Oncol 10:55-62,1980.
19. Dobyan DC,et al. J Pharmacol Exp Ther 213:551-556,1980.
20. Daley-Yates PT and McBrien DCH, in preparation.
21. MacDonald MK,et al. Q J Exp Physiol 47:262-272,1962.
22. Schilsky RL and Anderson T, Ann Intern Med 90:929-931, 1979.
23. Battiflora H,et al. Am J Pathol 48:421-438,1966.
24. Frohnert PP,et al. Pfluegers Arch 66:1315-1318,1970.
25. Wen SF,Clin Res 22:550-555,1974.
26. Madias NE and Harrington JT,Am J Med 65:307-314,1978.
27. Chandler JA,in Electron Microprobe Analysis in Biology (DA Erasmus,
      ed.). Chapman-Hall,London,1978.
28. Galle P, J Microsc (Paris) 19:17-24,1974.
29. Roberts JJ and Thomson AJ,in Progress in Nucleic Acid Research and
      Molecular Biology (WE Cohn, ed.).Academic Press, New York,1978.

30. Daley-Yates PT and McBrien DCH, J Appl Toxicol Vol 1 (4) V-XXV, 1981.
31. Cvitkovic E, et al. Cancer 39:1357-1361,1977.
32. Hayes DM,et al. Cancer 39:1372-1381,1977.
33. Merrin C, Proc Am Assoc Cancer Res 18:100,1977.
34. DeSimone PA,et al. Cancer Treat Rep 63:951-960,1979.
35. Ross DA and Gale GR, Cancer Treat Rep 63:781-787,1979.
36. Bowman RH,in Methods in Pharmacology,Vol 4B (M Martinez-Moldanado, ed.). Plenum,New York,1978.
37. Pera MF and Harder HC,Proc Am Assoc Cancer Res 19:100,1978.
38. Pharmaceutical Codex,11th Ed.,Pharmaceutical Press,London,1979,p738.
39. Bowman RH, Am J Physiol 229:93-98,1975.
40. Torretti J and Weiner IM,in Methods in Pharmacology,Vol 4A, (M Martinez-Moldanado ed.).Plenum,New York,1976.
41. Khan MUA and Sadler PJ,Chem Biol Interact 21:227-232,1978.
42. Stekhoven FS and Bonting SL,Physiol Rev 16:1-77,1981.
43. Neckay BR and Saunders JP,J Environ Path Toxicol 2:283-290,1978.
44. Guarino AM,et al. in Cisplatin,Current Status and New Developments (AW Prestayko,ST Crooke and SK Carter,eds.).Academic Press,New York, 1980.
45. Simmons CF and Humes HD,Kidney Int 16:862-871,1979.
46. Van der Berg EK, Kidney Int 19:8,-981.
47. Daley-Yates PT and McBrien DCH,submitted to Chem-Biol Interact.

DIAGNOSIS OF METAL-INDUCED NEPHROPATHY IN HUMANS

R. R. Lauwerys and A. Bernard*

Unite de Toxicologie Industrielle et Médicale, Faculté de Médecine, Université Catholique de Louvain, 30.54 Clos Chapelle-aux-Champs, 1200 Bruxelles, Belgium

ABSTRACT

Several screening tests can be considered for the biological surveillance of persons chronically exposed to nephrotoxic metals; in urine : reagent strips for protein and glucose, quantitative determination of total and specific proteins, electrophoretic characterization of the proteinuria, microscopic examination of the sediment, aminoaciduria, enzymuria; in blood : BUN, creatinine, β_2-microglobulin, uric acid, immunological analyses.

The most common sign of chronic renal damage induced by metals is an increased excretion of proteins. However, in early stages of metal-induced renal dysfunction, it is usual to detect a significant increased urinary excretion of specific proteins before a significant increase of total proteinuria. Increased BUN seems also to be an early sign of chronic excessive exposure to lead.

Therefore, the following tests are proposed as screening tools for the early detection of metal-induced nephropathy : examination of urine for the presence of glucose and protein with reagent strips, immunochemical quantitation of at least two proteins one of low molecular weight such as retinol binding protein, or β_2-microglobulin and one of high molecular weight such as albumin. The determination of β_2-microglobulin in serum is also recommended. BUN determination should be made when there is exposure to lead.

Functional tests are performed when the repeated finding of abnormal screening tests suggests the presence of renal dysfunction.

Keywords : metal exposure, nephrotoxicity, early detection, cadmium mercury, lead.

* Charge de recherches du Fonds National Belge de la Recherche Scientifique

INTRODUCTION

This paper deals with the biological tests which can be used for the early detection of kidney dysfunction in workers exposed to metals. Acute excessive exposure to nephrotoxic metals usually results in tubular necrosis. These intoxications are either accidental or iatrogenic and rarely occupational; they will not be considered in this paper. Several tests have been proposed for the detection of the chronic nephrotoxic effects of metals. They can be divided in two groups.
1. The screening tests, suitable for the periodic medical surveillance in industry.
2. The functional tests which usually are only applied when the screening tests are abnormal or when the symptoms are already suggestive of renal diseases.

1. SCREENING TESTS

They are applied in urine or in blood. It should be stressed that for any of these tests, one single determination may be misleading. Repeated determinations are necessary to confirm the presence of a renal functional change.

1.1 Urine analyses. Preferably the urine analyses should be carried out on a 24 hour-urine sample but unfortunately a complete 24 hour-urine collection is extremely difficult to obtain. Even the analysis of a morning specimen is not always feasible and frequently in occupational medical practice, the analyses must be performed on spot specimens. It is therefore important to evaluate the degree of urine dilution (specific gravity, creatinine concentration, osmolality) because analyses performed on very dilute urine specimens are not reliable (false negative results).

1.1.1 Appearance of urine. Direct examination of urine (colour, cloudiness...) provides very limited information but since it is so simple to perform, it should never be neglected. No specific change in urine aspect is likely to be present at the early stage of metal induced nephrotoxicity.

1.1.2 Reagent strips for protein and glucose. Glucosuria may be detected in metal induced tubular dysfunction. An early sign of renal damage (glomerular or tubular) induced by nephrotoxic metals is an increased urinary excretion of proteins. Normally the amount of proteins excreted in urine does not exceed 200 mg per day. These proteins originate from the uro-genital tract (approximately 50%) and from the plasma.
Proteins cross the glomerular filter in proportion to their molecular dimension. The filtration of proteins through the glomerulus depends on the relationship between the electrostatic and steric properties of the protein and that of the pores of the glomerular membrane as well as on the absolute value of the glomerular filtration rate [1].
Proteins with molecular weight below 40000 pass easily through the glomerular filter, whereas proteins with MW above 40000 are more effectively retained in plasma. The filtered proteins are reabsorbed

by the proximal tubular cells of the kidney. The absorption process is energy dependent and characterized by a very high capacity, relatively low threshold and a constant fractional absorption rate over a wide range of plasma concentration of the protein. The reabsorbed proteins are catabolized within the tubular cells and the degradation products (aminoacids, polypeptides) are then returned to the circulation. In glomerular damage, the glomerular permeability is usually increased and therefore larger quantities of high molecular weight proteins enter the glomerular filtrate and ultimately appear in the urine. The urinary concentration of low molecular weight proteins is not increased since the reabsorption process in the tubule is normal. When proteinuria is a consequence of tubular dysfunction, the amount of protein filtered through the glomeruli is not increased, but the low and the high molecular weight proteins which are normally filtered appear in larger quantities in the final urine, because the tubular reabsorption is incomplete. However, the urinary concentration of low molecular weight proteins is proportionally more increased than that of high molecular weight proteins. In tubular proteinuria, the amount of protein lost is usually less than 2 g/24 h. When both sites - the glomeruli and the tubules - are damaged the proteinuria consists of a mixture of low and high molecular weight proteins [2].

It is important to realize that the reagent strip for proteins (Albustix) is more sensitive to albumin than to globulin and an increased urinary excretion of low molecular weight proteins is not detected with this qualitative test. The reagent strip is sensitive to albumin concentration ranging from 50 to 300 mg/l. False positive results can be obtained with alkaline urine and quaternary ammonium compounds. For detecting minimal proteinuria (< 0.5 g/day) as found in the early stage of renal tubular dysfunction or in the relatively inactive phases of glomerular diseases, screening tests based on reagent strips are too coarse and more sensitive, quantitative methods should be used.

1.1.3 Quantitative determination of total protein in urine. The detection of a slight increased total proteinuria (< 0.5 g/24 h) requires the use of a quantitative method (e.g. Biuret). To be of significance this test should be carried out on urine collected during a well defined time interval (24 hour or less) and the result should be confirmed on repeated measurements. However, in the early stage of metal induced renal dysfunction, it is usual to detect a significant increased urinary excretion of specific proteins (e.g. retinol binding protein or β_2-microglobulin in cadmium workers) without significant change of total protein excretion.

1.1.4 Quantitative determination of specific proteins in urine. Sensitive immunochemical methods are presently available for the quantitative analysis of specific proteins in urine. The determination of at least one low molecular weight protein (e.g. retinol binding protein, β_2-microglobulin) and one high molecular weight protein (e.g. albumin) should be included in the surveillance programme of workers exposed to heavy metals. For some proteins (e.g. β_2-microglobulin) control of the urinary pH is important.

1.1.5 Electrophoretic characterization of proteinuria. The electrophoretic or immunoelectrophoretic separation of urinary

proteins has been used for years to classify the proteinuria in
glomerular, tubular or mixed type proteinuria. However, in
practice, this method is of a limited usefulness. Because of its
low sensitivity, it requires a concentration of the urine sample.
Furthermore, the differentiation of glomerular and tubular proteinuria can be realized on the basis of more quantitative and sensitive
criterions by the simultaneous determination in urine of albumin and
β_2-microglobulin (or retinol binding protein) [3]

1.1.6 Examination of the urine sediment. Although this analysis
is useful to diagnose renal parenchymal damage (e.g. presence of
cell cylinders), it is not sensitive enough for the early detection
of renal damage induced by metals.

1.1.7 Aminoaciduria. The tubular deficit induced by some metals
(e.g. Cd) may result in aminoaciduria. Usually, all aminoacids
appear in the urine in increased amounts. In the normal adult,
urinary excretion of aminoacids does not exceed 200 mg of αamino-
nitrogen excreted in a 24 hour-period.

1.1.8 Enzymuria. The determination of several enzymes in urines
has been considered to detect toxic kidney injury. Under normal
conditions, the enzymes present in urine may originate from 4 sources :
a) serum : low molecular weight enzymes (MW < 40000) can pass into
   the glomerular filtrate and since they are not totally reabsorbed
   by the tubules, they will be found in small quantities in urine
   (e.g. lysozyme, ribonuclease).
b) epithelial cells of the urogenital tract : the desquamation of
   epithelial cells may yield the appearance of their enzyme content
   in urine. This source of urinary enzyme activities is generally
   regarded as insignificant.
c) glandular secretion of the urogenital tract : the secretion of
   the urogenital tract glands are rich in various enzymes. The
   contribution of these secretions to urinary enzyme activities is
   more important in males than in females. Acid phosphatase
   activity of urine is twice as great in males as in females.
d) kidney : kidney is also a rich source of various enzymes. For
   example, tubular cells contain a high concentration of alkaline
   phosphatase, leucine aminopeptidase, γ-glutamyl transpeptidase,
   lactate dehydrogenase and alanine aminopeptidase. The latter
   enzyme is a marker of the brush border membrane. Acid phosphatase and glucose-6-phosphate dehydrogenase are particularly active
   in the glomeruli.
When kidney is damaged, cellular enzymes are released into the
tubular lumen and their determination in urine may provide an index
of kidney disturbance. It has been suggested that even subtle changes
of the renal tubular cells provoke significant alterations of
urinary enzymatic activities. It is well known that acute toxic
tubular necrosis is associated with a marked increase of the activities of several urinary enzymes. In workers chronically exposed to
mercury vapour and cadmium, we have also found an increased activity
of some enzymes in urine.
However, we are of the opinion that on an individual basis, the
usefulness of urinary enzyme determination for the early detection
of the kidney injury following long term occupational exposure to
nephrotoxic metals is rather limited for the following reasons :

a) the inter- and intraindividual variability is very high;
b) it should be stressed that what is measured is the activity of an enzyme and not necessarily its concentration in urine. The activity may be influenced by various factors (inhibitors, activitors). A change in activity may not necessarily be a direct reflection of the amount of enzyme molecules present in urine;
c) storage conditions (t°, pH, bacterial growth...) will modify the enzyme activities.

Some of the difficulties encountered with the measurement of the activity of enzymes released in urine may be overcome by using immunochemical methods with specific anti-enzyme antibodies. This approach has already been applied with success for the determination of the concentrations of alanine aminopeptidase and carbonic anhydrase in urine. This immunochemical approach is in fact valid for the detection in urine of any antigen released by damaged kidney cells.

1.2 Blood analyses.

1.2.1 Blood urea nitrogen, creatinine, β_2-microglobulin. Although BUN is usually considered less useful than plasma creatinine to detect an impairment of glomerular filtration rate (GRF), it has frequently been observed that an early sign of lead induced nephro-toxicity is an increased BUN without change in other renal parameters. However, no single determination of BUN would serve adequate warning of impending renal disease since substantial reduction in GFR can occur in lead workers whose BUNs are in the normal range. It should therefore be determined at frequent intervals in all lead workers. In this manner upward trends within the normal range could be detected. [4].

In the absence of malignant diseases, β_2-microglobulin in serum is a very sensitive index of impaired GFR. Several studies have demonstrated the existence of a close inverse relationship between plasma β_2-microglobulin and inulin clearance [5,6]. Furthermore, contrary to plasma creatinine, the level of β_2-microglobulin in serum is not affected by the muscular mass and the diet and its immuno-chemical determination is highly specific. When a creatinine clearance study cannot be performed, and since a single determination of plasma creatinine may be misleading, the analysis of β_2-microglo-bulin in serum represents a reliable alternative to evaluate the GFR.

1.2.2 Uric acid. Increased plasma urate is usually a late manifestation of excessive exposure to lead [4].

1.2.3 Immunological analyses. Immunological mechanisms have been implicated in the pathogenesis of some metals (e.g. Hg, Pb, Au) nephrotoxicity. It might therefore be indicated to search for the presence of circulating immune complexes or anti-glomerular basement antibodies in workers chronically exposed to heavy metals. Further clinical investigations are however required to test the practical usefulness of such investigations.

The application of all the tests cited above does not cause any inconvenience for the workers; these tests can also be performed by the majority of clinical laboratories. It is clear, however, that for the routine screening of workers chronically exposed to metals a selection must be made among these analyses.

For the early detection of metal induced nephropathy, we think
that the following combination of tests is the most valid : examination of urine with reagent strips for the presence of glucosuria
and proteinuria, quantitative determination in urine of at least two
proteins : one of low molecular weight such as β_2-microglobulin or
retinol binding protein and one of high molecular weight such as
albumin. The determination of β_2-microglobulin in serum is also
recommended to check that the increased urinary excretion of
β_2-microglobulin does not result from a reduced GRF (values of β_2-
microglobulin in serum exceeding the Tm). β_2-Microglobulin level
in serum is also a sensitive index of the GFR. BUN determination
should also be made when there is exposure to lead. As already
stressed above, only serial measurements during the course of
occupational exposure to metals is of value.

2. FUNCTIONAL TESTS

These tests are only performed when the screening tests suggest
the presence of renal dysfunction. They explore the glomerular
permeability (glomerular filtration rate), the renal plasma flow,
the proximal (e.g. Tm glucose, Tm bicarbonate, phosphate reabsorption, 24 hour-calciuria) and distal (e.g. acidification test) tubular
function. They will not be commented upon in this paper.

However, the short creatinine clearance (urine collected for 1 or
2 hours) deserves a special mention. Serial measurements in the
workers in whom some screening tests are abnormal may provide an
indication of the direction of the changes in renal function. The
advantage of the short creatinine clearance is that the study can
be performed under good technical control and that a complete urine
collection can be successfully obtained over a short period of time
[7]. Renal biopsy with light, electron microscopic and immunological
studies of the specimens and radiographic examination of the kidney
are reserved for frank pathological cases.

3. APPLICATION TO WORKERS EXPOSED TO HEAVY METALS

We have recently applied some of the fore-mentioned screening
tests (enzymuria, total proteinuria, aminoaciduria, increased
excretion of specific proteins in urine) to detect signs of kidney
dysfunction in workers occupationally exposed to cadmium (n = 148),
to mercury vapour (n = 63) or to inorganic lead (n = 25). A group
of workers non occupationally exposed to heavy metals (n   88)
served as control [8]. We have shown that excessive exposure to
cadmium increases the urinary excretion of both low and high molecular weight proteins and of tubular enzymes. These changes are
mainly observed in workers excreting more than 10 μg Cd/g creatinine
or with a cadmium level in blood above 1 μg Cd/100 ml whole blood.

In the workers exposed to lead for 3 to 30 years, we have not
found any increased prevalence of signs of kidney dysfunction. But
it should be stressed that the lead group included only 25 workers,
all with Pb level in blood below 62 μg/100 ml. Recently, we have
also examined a group of workers simultaneously exposed to lead and
to cadmium. The results suggest that the degree of renal dysfunction
is more related to the intensity of exposure to cadmium than to lead

[9]. Occupational exposure to mercury vapour seems to induce mild glomerular dysfunction as evidenced by an increased urinary excretion of high molecular weight proteins and a slight increased prevalence of higher β_2-microglobulin concentration in plasma without concomitant change in urinary β_2-microglobulin concentration. β-Galactosidase activity in blood and in urine was also increased. The likelihood of these findings is greater in workers with Hg levels in blood and in urine exceeding 3 μg/100 ml whole blood and 50 μg/g urinary creatinine respectively.

REFERENCES

1. Heinemann HO, Am J Med 56:71-82, 1974.
2. Alt JM, et al. Contr Nephrol 24:115-121, 1981.
3. Peterson PA, et al. J Clin Invest 48:1189-1198, 1969.
4. Hammond PB, et al. J Occup Med 22:475-484, 1980.
5. Wibell L, et al. Nephron 10:320-331, 1973.
6. Bailey RR and Pearson S, New Zealand Med J 87:168-170, 1978.
7. Duarte CG, et al. Renal function tests. Clinical Laboratory procedures and diagnosis. Little, Brown and Company, Boston, 1980.
8. Buchet JP et al. J Occup Med 22:741-750, 1980.
9. Buchet JP et al. J Occup Med 23:348-352, 1981.

THE NEPHROTOXICITY OF MYCOTOXINS AND BOTANICALS

William O. Berndt

Department of Pharmacology and Toxicology, University of Mississippi Medical Center, Jackson, Mississippi 39216, USA

ABSTRACT

A variety of substances present in nature can affect renal function adversely. Various constituents, or their metabolites, of *Amanita phalloides* (phallotoxins, amatoxins) have been observed by electron microscopy to produce tubular necrosis. Underlying mechanisms, however, are not well understood. A number of higher plants contain several alkaloids with poisonous potential. For example, pyrrolizidine alkaloids can produce dramatic effects on liver, lung and/or kidney, depending on dose of alkaloid and species of animal under study. It may be that the major toxicity is to the small blood vessels and this in turn leads to the various necroses. Fungal toxins are well documented to affect a number of organ systems, including kidney. Citrinin (*Penicillium citrinum*) and ochratoxin A (*Aspergillus ochraceus*) both alter renal function in the rat. Proximal tubular necrosis produced by citrinin is associated with "high output" renal failure and the inability of several renal transport systems to function. Although the mechanism of mycotoxin-induced nephropathy is not certain, an active metabolite may be involved. Since all of these toxins occur in nature, the possibility exists that they may have an important role in human renal disease.

mycotoxins
citrinin
ochratoxin A
pyrrolizidine alkaloids
monocrotaline
amatoxins

MUSHROOM TOXINS

Poisoning from toxic mushrooms (so-called toadstools) has been do-cumented in almost every area of the world. Mycetism or mycetismus (mushroom poisoning) takes many forms and all too frequently results from individuals collecting and eating wild mushrooms without proper identification of the mushroom species. The genus *Amanita* contains al-most every toxic substance associated with mushrooms and is a very com-mon cause of poisoning in North America. Other toxic components do exist, for example, helvellic acid in *Gyromitra esculenta* and psilocybin in some species of *Psilocybe*. Consumption of some species of *Coprinus* or *Boletus* have been reported to lead to a disulfiram-reaction to alcohol [1].

Several common species of the toxic Amanita exist, e.g., A. *muscaria* and A. *phalloides*. It is suggested that in western Europe and North America almost all fatal mushroom poisonings occur with this latter species of mushroom. There also seem to be other species of *Amanita* that are nearly identical to A. *phalloides*, particularly in terms of toxicity and presumably by virtue of the toxins present in the fungi: A. *verna*, A. *virosa*, A. *tenuifolia*, etc.

Mushroom poisoning has been described by authorities in terms of the latency of the toxic response [2]. Both the short and long latency toxicity will be described briefly, although only the delayed onset toxicity appears to involve the kidney.

The rapid-onset toxicity is usually associated with the ingestion of the *muscaria* group of mushrooms, or other groups with a marked ability to mimic stimulation of the parasympathetic nervous system, or with ingestion of the psilocybin-containing mushrooms or other hallucinogenic species. The parasympathetic response elicited by ingestion of A. *muscaria* and other mushrooms may or may not be caused by muscarine itself, but the symptoms are unmistakable and in general, the prognosis for the patient is good. CNS effects also are observed including hallu-cinations and frequently, increased motor activity, tremors, etc. Studies defining the various causative agents which might be responsible for each of these responses have not been accomplished [2].

The delayed-onset toxicity is observed after the ingestion of A. *phalloides* and various related species or subspecies. After several hours (at least 5, as many as 20) severe gastroenteritis will be observed with vomiting, severe abdominal pain, watery diarrhea, etc. Such a syndrome may be followed by cardiovascular collapse if the fluid loss has been severe enough. After this initial illness, the patient frequently will exhibit nearly normal behavior that may last for several days. After this normal period the severe, often life threatening toxicity will develop, which is first observed with jaundice and other signs of hepatic cell necrosis. Severe damage may also arise in the renal tubular epithelium as well as in other tissues. There are no spe-cific antidotal procedures for *phalloides* poisoning and as many as half of such cases may be fatal [3].

At least two groups of orally active toxic substances are known to exist in A. *phalloides* and probably in other related subspecies of fungi. The so-called phallotoxins are cyclic heptapeptides. Phalloidin is the most commonly recognized member of this group, although at least five other chemically distinct toxins have been identified. Phalloidin has been suggested to cause the initial gastroenteritis produced by ingestion of these mushrooms, but it is also thought to be involved in the production of the severe liver lesion seen several days after ingestion [4]. Studies on mechanisms underlying the action of the phallotoxins are few. It is not even clear whether it is the parent compound or a metabolite that is active. Some have suggested that phalloidin may act without being metabolically activated [5], at least as far as the liver damage is concerned. Frimmer and Schischke [6] have obtained contrary data which suggest that phalloidin must be altered chemically in the liver before it can produce injury to that organ.

The other group of toxins, the so-called amatoxins, are cyclic octapeptides. Overall, the amatoxins are more toxic to man than the phallotoxins and it is generally agreed that most of the symptoms associated with ingestion of A. *phalloides* are attributable to these compounds [2, 3]. Not uncommonly, a single specimen of A. *phalloides* could contain enough α-amanitin to kill a man. The LD_{50} of α-amanitin has been reported to be as little as 0.1 mg/kg in some species.

Renal damage produced by these toxic fungi has been reported in the literature, although detailed studies of mechanisms have been lacking. Several reports of acute renal failure in humans are available, for example, Myler *et al.*, [7]. Electron microscopic studies of biopsy samples indicated that both proximal and distal tubular cells were affected, although clear evidence of direct necrosis was absent. No glomerular lesions were observed. The pathogenesis of the renal tubular changes was not known. Although intermittent peritoneal dialysis was used sucessfully in the treatment of some poisonings, i.e. renal function returned to normal, some evidence of permanent diffuse interstitial fibrosis was observed.

An early experimental study in the mouse by Fiume *et al.*, [8] demonstrated the sensitivity of this species to α-amanitin. Damage was restricted to the proximal convoluted tubule. In related studies on the rat no evidence of renal damage was observed by electron microscopy. The lack of toxicity in the rat was suggested to be attributable to the inability of that species to reabsorb (secrete?) the toxin so that it did not achieve significant concentrations within the proximal tubular cells. If the toxin was coupled with albumin, which permitted the toxin to be taken intracellularly by pinocytosis, renal damage was observed in the rat. With respect to hepatic damage, the same degree of toxicity was observed whether or not the toxin was attached to albumin. Nonetheless, greater penetration of hepatocytes occurred with the albumin conjugate [10]. Unfortunately all of these studies have been done only with morphological observations. The alterations in physiological behavior of the kidneys were not characterized for α-amanitin toxicity.

Because the earliest morphological changes observed are in the nuclei of the proximal tubule cells, Fiume and colleagues have examined α-amanitin effects on nucleic acids. For example, Stirpe and Fiume [11] found α-amanitin to inhibit the activity of RNA polymerase activated by Mn^{++}. From these and related studies, these investigators have suggested that alterations in nucleic acid metabolism may underlie the renal failure syndrome. However, the exact relationship between nucleic acid metabolism and renal function is somewhat obscure.

Human consumption of *Cortinarius speciosissimus* has led to acute renal damage. Nieminen and colleagues [12, 13, 14] have examined the effects of this mushroom in rats with morphological techniques. Necrotic lesions were observed in both male and female rats by 2 to 4 days after administration of *Cortinarius* extract (250 mg mushroom per Kg). In the female rats, the necrotic lesions were most marked in the inner cortex.

HIGHER PLANT TOXINS

A large number of species of plants have been reported to be poisonous to man and other animals [15]. Apparently there are representatives of poisonous species at almost every level of the plant kingdom. Furthermore, the organ systems on which these plants and their constiuents exert their effects are as varied as the number of poisonous plants themselves. There are suggestions of renal damage produced by plants, although these are not as common as actions on other organ systems. Consumption of plants containing oxalates may lead to crystallization of those oxalates in kidney tubules resulting in a quite predictable type of renal insufficiency. Events of this sort also are known to occur with other toxins.

The pyrrolizidine alkaloids are an interesting group of esters of amino-alcohols derived from the heterocylic pyrrolizidine nucleus. These compounds appear distributed throughout the plant kingdom without any obvious rationale for that distribution. In general there have been few suggestions concerning the function of these compounds in the overall economy of the plants which manufacture them. The most common suggestion has been that because of their bitter taste they serve as a protective mechanism for the plants, but based on the occurrences of poisonings in grazing animals, it is not so clear that this is a tenable hypothesis. Although poisoning by plants such as *Senecio jacoboea* is not a common occurrence when pastureland is plentiful, when the pastures become restricted cattle do graze on the ragwort and poisoning is noted. Other genera which produce these alkaloids are *Crotalaria*, *Echium*, *Heliotropium*, etc. Monocrotaline produced by *Crotalaria spectabilis* and several of the *Senecio* alkaloids (e.g. senecionine, seneciphylline) have been studied most commonly.

Apparently three organs are affected primarily by the pyrrolizidine alkaloids: liver, lung, kidney. Which organ is attacked seems to depend to some extent on which species of animal is being studied [16, 17]. In any event, hepatic damage is a common report and this is usually expressed as a severe necrotic syndrome [18]. Lungs of rodents fed plant seeds showed enlarged cells in the bronchial epithelium, large alveolar cells, large macrophages with cytoplasmic invagination as well as certain vascular disorders [18]. The vascular effects observed in lungs also are noted in liver and kidney and may underlie much of the toxicity. The so-called venous occlusive disease produced by pyrrolizidine alkaloids suggests a direct effect of some of these compounds or their metabolites on capillary endothelia. The nature of the toxic event is not known, however, although similarities in action are observed in all of the organs where toxicity is found.

Renal damage produced by the pyrrolizidine alkaloids varies tremendously with species [19, 20, 21]. The rat seems relatively insensitive to renal damage compared to other animals [22], while the mouse [18] and the pig [23] seem to be relatively sensitive. Megalocytosis is reported commonly with significant nuclear as well as cytoplasmic enlargements in the epithelial cells. These changes are seen in proximal tubules as well as in the glomeruli. The degenerative changes in the capillary of the glomeruli also are reported commonly. The cytoplasmic swelling in the glomeruli may lead to occlusion of the capillary lumina with various dense deposits noted in those lumina, possibly proteins. If damage is severe, clear detachment of endothelial cells is observed and marked areas of hemorrhage are seen.

Unfortunately, very few attempts have been made to study the changes in renal physiological events which result from pyrrolizidine poisoning. The morphological changes suggest the occurrence of a "nephrosis", but exactly how fluid and electrolyte balance is or is not maintained has not been commented upon.

Although evidence is far from clearcut, it is likely that all of the toxicities are produced through the same mechanisms. Pyrrolizidine alkaloids are metabolized to pyrrole derivatives as well as to N-oxides. The weight of evidence [16, 19, 22] suggests that the pyrrole derivatives are the toxic compounds. These substances probably act as alkylating agents and as such can produce damage to intracellular as well as membrane structures leading to mitochondrial dysfunction and other metabolic abnormalities. Part of the support for that position comes from the studies of Chesney and Allen [24] designed to examine the relative resistance of the guinea pig to pyrrolizidine alkaloid toxicity. In these studies with monocrotaline, it was found that the pyrrole derivatives were formed much more readily in the rat than the guinea pig, while both species produced N-oxide derivatives with about equal efficiency. Administration of monocrotaline pyrroles directly to the guinea pig did produce toxicity suggesting that the absence of the synthetic pathway, or its activity at a reduced level, was responsible for the relative resistance of that species. Interestingly, the resistance of the rabbit to *Senecio* alkaloids administered in the diet does not seem to relate to metabolism [25]. Apparently this species is resistant because of poor GI absorption of the alkaloids. Hence, if the purified alkaloids are administered intravenously, toxicity develops. Furthermore, the rabbit liver has a high rate of pyrrole production. Finally, several studies have shown that certain substances can afford protection against pyrrolizidine alkaloid toxicity. Recent studies from Buhler's laboratory [26] indicate that butylated hydroxyanisole (BHA) will protect against the acute toxicity of monocrotaline. BHA reduced the level of pyrrole metabolism in the liver as well as increased the concentrations of liver sulfhydryl groups. Hence, the protective effects of BHA stem from the reduction in the available pyrrole metabolites produced by the liver of the mouse. Studies have not been done on the intrarenal metabolism of pyrrolizidine alkaloids, the effects of pyrroles on renal function, etc., but it is likely that these reactive alkylating agents would have detrimental effects on kidney and lung much like those on liver.

An extensive study of the possible protective role of sulfhydryl containing compounds was undertaken by Buckmaster *et al.*, [27]. These authors suggested that, for example, cysteine might be expected to react with electrophilic pyrrole metabolites preventing their attack on cellular components. Although crude plant fractions were added to the diet of rats, chemical analyses of the dried, powdered plants were performed. Overall, cysteine afforded better protection than did methionine.

Pyrrolizidine alkaloid toxicity may be a serious problem for man as well as for animals. Cattle which feed on plants containing these alkaloids may well transfer those substances in their active form in the milk. In a study by Dickenson *et al.*, [28] cows were fed dried tansy ragwort for two weeks. Five alkaloids were isolated from the dried plant material and one of these, jacoline, was isolated from the milk. In addition, Deinzer *et al.*, [29] has demonstrated the occurrence of some of the pyrrolizidine alkaloids from the ragwort in honey. This is thought to occur since the bees that collect the pollen do so from the ragwort as well as other plants and the alkaloids are present in the pollen. Hence, either through milk, honey, or perhaps other sources it is possible for man to become contaminated with pyrrolizidine alkaloids. The extent of toxicity so produced is not known and the exact role of such events in the production of human renal or liver disease is similarly unknown.

MYCOTOXINS

A large variety of molds produce secondary metabolites. These compounds of widely varied chemical structures have been observed to produce many different effects in farm and test animals [30]. The diversity of mold from which the compounds are produced is matched only by the diversity of chemical structure of the compounds themselves. Within a given class of mold, however, one might anticipate the production of compounds of similar structure. Hence with related species of mold, similar types of effects should be observed.

There is a long documented history of the effects of fungal toxins in man and other animals [31]. The ergotism observed and reported in the Dark Ages was an example of the consequences of consumption of mold contaminated rye. The active ergot alkaloids produced by *Claviceps purpurea* led to the toxicity. In more recent times (early 1930's), *Fusarium* toxicity in pigs was noted and expressed as digestive illnesses. In the 1940's, *Fusarium* was again implicated in the production of toxic alimentary aleukia in the U.S.S.R. The products of *Aspergillus flavus*, the aflatoxins, were suggested as causative agents in outbreaks of "Turkey X disease" in the 1960's. Both hepatotoxic and carcinogenic effects of aflatoxins have been documented. Aflatoxicoses in farm animals have been well documented. It also is clear that man is susceptible to such contamination [31]. Documentation of this latter situation, has come mainly from epidemiological data collected from various areas of the world. In these studies a close correlation was demonstrated between the consumption of certain contaminated foodstuffs and the incidence of an unusually rare hepatocarcinoma. Although reported from many countries, clear documentation was obtained first in a study in Uganda in the mid-1960's. A highly significant correlation was found between the occurence of hepatoma and the presence of aflatoxins in the human food supply in those areas of Uganda where the hepatomas occurred. Where the incidence of hepatomas was low, aflatoxins were not found in the food. Similar correlative, epidemiological studies were conducted in Swaziland, Thailand, Kenya, etc. Many of these data have been summarized by Hayes [32].

The rubratoxins, and in particular, rubratoxin B, have been demonstrated to have hepatotoxic effects in several experimental animals. Similarly, feeding of rubratoxin B producing molds results in the same hepatoxic syndromes [33]. Penicillic acid, produced by a variety of molds, produces lesions in the liver. Although several suggestions have been made that penicillic acid has adverse effects on several organ systems, the severe hepatic necrosis is most striking. In addition, a number of these substances (e.g., patulin, penicillic acid) have affects on specific enzymes such as the ATPases.

Obviously, concern needs to be expressed about the carcinogenic, teratogenic, and mutagenic potentials of mycotoxins. In addition specific organ toxicity has been observed and reported with fungal toxins. All of this is to indicate that these toxic fungal metabolites are not

only of varied chemical structures, but also of varied biological actions. Specific effects on the kidney will be examined in detail.

Studies on and the documentation of the occurrence of a mycotoxin-induced nephropathy have come from several sources. Larsen in 1928
reported on the occurrence of abnormal appearing kidneys in pigs brought
to slaughter [34]. Subsequently, with isolation and purification of
citrinin from P. *Citrinum* [35], it was possible to demonstrate that this
substance could produce a syndrome which resulted in the same gross
morphological changes as those observed by Larsen [36, 37, 38]. Similar
alterations in renal physiology as well as morphology could be produced
by the feeding of purified ochratoxin A, feeding of mold which produced
this compound, or the feeding of grain contaminated with ochratoxin
A-producing mold [39, 40, 41]. Although many studies were directed at
an examination of porcine nephropathy, various studies suggested that
other species were as susceptible as the pig to the effects of citrinin
and/or ochratoxin A. For example, Berndt and Hayes [42] found rats to
be susceptible to citrinin, and Elling *et al.*, [43] were able to associate a poultry nephropathy with ochratoxin A. The association of mycotoxin-induced nephropathy with citrinin and/or ochratoxin A has been
demonstrated both with field (correlative in nature) and laboratory
studies.

Although relatively strong epidemiology data indicate the involvement
of humans with aflatoxicosis, similar evidence for a mycotoxin-induced
renal disease in humans is not yet available. The suggestion has been
made, however, that the endemic Balkan nephropathy may be such a disease
[44]. Although at the time the suggestion was made, it was based
largely on the elimination of other causes for the disease and an
abundance of circumstantial evidence rather than direct evidence, this
suggestion seems to be standing the test of time and is gaining support
[45]. Although there is some debate as to the role of glomerular
dysfunction in the endemic Balkan disease relative to that in porcine
nephropathy, all and all the descriptions of renal behavior in the
endemic Balkan disease are not dissimilar from those seen in the
citrinin- or ochratoxin A-induced disease in laboratory or farm animals.
In all instances, proximal tubular necrosis is observed, associated with
proteinuria, glucosuria, etc. In addition, a high incidence of renal or
bladder cancers have been observed in patients with the Balkan disease,
and this correlates nicely with suggestions that citrinin or ochratoxin
A may have a role in the production of renal carcinomas in rats [46].
Finally, ochratoxin A has been demonstrated in the home-made foodstuffs
in areas of Yugoslavia where the incidence of the disease is high [47].
This suggests the possibility of greater exposure of certain families to
ochratoxin A, an event which might be associated with the renal disease.
This observation also would be consistent with the original comments of
Barnes [44] concerning the relatively high humidity in some of the
valley bottoms and the possibility that families or groups of families
might store their own grain before food preparation.

Of course, the studies of Krogh *et al.* [47] did not demonstrate the
presence of fungal toxin in every patient with the disease nor were all
affected households equally exposed to ochratoxin. Nonetheless, these
human, epidemiological-like studies offer a strong suggestion that
mycotoxin induced nephropathy may be an underlying explanation for the
endemic Balkan disease.

Whatever the role of fungal toxins in endemic Balkan nephropathy
there is no doubt that both citrinin and ochratoxin A (Fig. 1) can
significantly alter renal function, e.g. see Berndt *et al.* [48]. Both

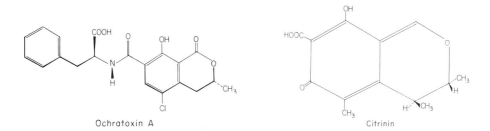

Ochratoxin A   Citrinin

Figure 1.   Structures of ochratoxin A and citrinin

compounds are produced by commonly occurring molds and at least some
molds produce both substances. Hence, not uncommonly when one compound
is found in contaminated grain, so is the other. Porcine nephropathy
was first documented to be produced by citrinin, although subsequently
Krogh and colleagues demonstrated that ochratoxin A was equally
effective [39, 40, 41]. Indeed, the effects of ochratoxin A are seen at
lower doses than with citrinin. Although veridicatum toxin may also be
a likely candidate for the production of renal disease, both citrinin
and ochratoxin A presently are the leading candidates. Because of the
potential for the production of renal damage and the relative ready
availability of the toxins a better understanding of this phenomenon
seems essential.

Laboratory model for mycotoxin-induced nephropathy.   Barnes and colleagues [49] and Berndt, Hayes, and colleagues [42, 50-54] have demonstrated the utility of the laboratory rat as model for mycotoxin-induced
nephropathy. In the Barnes' study rats were fed fungal toxins chronically in an effort to examine changes in renal morphology. Studies from
Berndt's laboratory have emphasized the monitoring of physiological
parameters.
     Studies with unanesthetized rats have demonstrated that citrinin can
produce renal dysfunction after the intraperitoneal administration of a

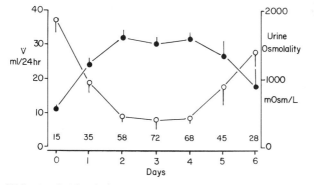

Figure 2.   Effect of citrinin on renal function in the rat. One con-
     trol urine sample was collected (C) before injection of one dose of
     citrinin (55 mg/kg, i.p.). The days are the days after the in-
     jection. The numbers at the bottom of the graph are typical BUN
     values. For urinary values, N = 4.

single dose of the toxin. Depending on dose, the animals may exhibit
either a high-output (non-oliguric) renal failure or the more classical,
oliguric or anuric renal disease. The typical pattern of non-oliguric
renal failure is given in Fig. 2. The animals that excrete large
volumes of urine (often 2-4 x normal) also excrete large quantities of
glucose and protein. In addition, citrinin causes the formation of
hypo-osmolar urine (250-300 mOsm/L), which appears to be the earliest
change in renal function observed. All of these effects are sustained
throughout the period of nephrotoxicity. Again, depending on dose, the
renal dysfunction may be self-limiting and completely reversible.
Animals which survive a moderate to large dose of citrinin will show
nearly normal renal function by 7-9 days after administration of the
toxin.   Electron   microscopic   studies   confirmed   these   temporal
relationships with maximal necrosis seen at days 2-4 with complete
recovery by days 7-9.
       The effects produced with ochratoxin A were somewhat different,
although alterations in renal function in the rat were clear [50]. It
was not possible to find a single dose of ochratoxin A which would
produce renal dysfunction without other consequences. Doses large
enough to produce measurable effects on urine flow, osmolality, etc.
usually resulted in severe diarrhea and/or death. Only after the
administration of small doses of ochratoxin A on a repeated daily basis
was it possible to see a syndrome somewhat like that observed with
citrinin. After 4 or 5 days of treatment, the rats began to produce a
hypo-osmotic urine of enhanced volume containing large quantities of
glucose and protein. This syndrome was complicated with ochratoxin A
because the animals lost a large amount of body weight (as much as 15 to
20% over 7 to 10 days) and this excessive weight loss alone will have
some effects on renal function. Nonetheless, it would appear that both
ochratoxin A and citrinin can produce a qualitatively similar renal
dysfunction in the rat. Furthermore, this response is not unlike that
reported with porcine nephropathy and may serve as a reasonable model
for the human disease, endemic Balkan nephropathy.

Table 1. Citrinin Effects on Renal Function

Measurements were done 120 minutes after anesthesia and start of PAH
and inulin infusions. For acute citrinin experiments, citrinin was
administered at zero time.

	% of Control	
	Citrinin 50 mg/kg acute	Citrinin, 50 mg/kg 24 hours before experiment
Urine flow, ml/min	89	22^a
GFR, ml/min	65^a	8^a
Na$^+$ excretion, µEq/min	81	2^a
K$^+$ excretion, µEq/min	24^a	15^a
% Δ in filtered K$^+$	35^a	-80^a

[a]Significantly different from control, P < .05

The temporal differences between ochratoxin A and citrinin are marked. For example, the effects produced by citrinin can be seen very early after administration of the compound if given under the correct circumstances in sufficient dose (Table 1). Anesthesized rats prepared for clearance experiments permit demonstration of an effect of nephrotoxic dose of citrinin in as little as 20 minutes after its administration [54]. Although the daily, 24-hour urine output in the unanesthesized rat exceeded by 2 to 3 times the urine output of a normal animal 24 hours after citrinin administration, the anesthesized rat had very low urine flow. Dramatic effects also were seen on glomerular filtration rate and electrolyte excretion. Early effects (i.e., 2 hours) on sodium excretion were not seen after an acute dose of citrinin. However, potassium reabsorption was reduced by 75%. Indeed, with a sufficiently large dose of citrinin net potassium secretion occurred. It is not clear whether the relatively large amount of potassium added to the urine came from the extracellular space or directly from to the kidney tissue as a result of tissue damage. In the latter situation the increased urinary potassium would reflect loss of renal intracellular potassium stores. Also acute citrinin administration significantly reduced glomerular filtration rate. The effects of citrinin in both the anesthetized and unanesthesized rats are summarized in Table 1.

The rat model also has proven useful for the assessment of the pharmacokinetic characteristics of citrinin. The availability of a specific analytical method for citrinin [52] as well as ^{14}C-labeled compound permitted these studies from which certain predictions were possible concerning the effects of citrinin in both the experimental and field situation.

The radioactivity from a non-nephrotoxic dose of ^{14}C-citrinin was eliminated from the plasma very rapidly. The kinetics of elimination suggested a two compartment process with half-lives of 2.5 and 15 hours. Over 24 to 48 hours, nearly all of a single dose of citrinin was accounted for in the urine and feces of normal animals, with the largest fraction of the label in the urine (75-85%). If the tracer dose of citrinin was administered to an animal with citrinin-induced nephrotoxicity (50 mg/kg, 72 hours before tracer), a different kinetic pattern was observed. The plasma disappearance curve for the labeled compound still resolved into two compartments, but only one of these compartments appeared to be the same as in the control ($t\frac{1}{2}$ = 15 hr). The kinetic parameters are summarized in Table 2.

Table 2. Pharmacokinetic Parameters for the Plasma Disappearance of ^{14}C after Administration of ^{14}C-Citrinin

For controls, 5 mg ^{14}C-citrinin per Kg was given i.v. For the experiments with "nephrotoxic animals", 55 mg citrinin per Kg was administered i.p. 3 days before the i.v. injection of 5 mg ^{14}C-citrinin per Kg.

Controls: $(Cp)_t = 10.5\ e^{(-0.27)t} + 0.54\ e^{(-0.046)t}$

"Nephrotoxic
    Animals": $(Cp)_t = 29.4\ e^{(-1.18)t} + 11.4\ e^{(-0.049)t}$

The short half-life compartment in control animals was replaced by a compartment with an even shorter half-life ($t_{1/2}$ = .59 hr), probably associated with redistribution of the compound in the animal. It may be concluded that the compartment with the 2.5 hr half-life was associated with renal elimination. This supposition is substantiated by balance studies wherein it was observed that only approximately 35% of a given dose of labeled citrinin was accounted for in the urine of an animal with mycotoxin-induced nephropathy compared to 75-85% in the urine of healthy animals.

This observation is consistent with the fact that the renal tissue of a nephrotoxic animal contained less citrinin than the renal tissue of a normal, healthy animal. In addition, clearance experiments in anesthesized rats suggested that citrinin could be secreted as a component of the elimination process. When corrected for protein binding, citrinin:inulin clearance ratios were about three. In rats that had been pretreated with citrinin before the administration of the tracer compound, citrinin:inulin clearance ratios were approximately one.

The relatively rapid elimination of citrinin after the administration of a single dose would support the prediction that cumulative effects of citrinin might not be expected. Indeed, in preliminary experiments in our laboratory it has not been possible to demonstrate renal dysfunction in rats receiving single daily doses of 10 or 15 mg/kg of citrinin for 13 days or approximately 10 mg/kg of citrinin per day in the diet for a matter of 20 to 30 days. Obviously over these time periods no accumulation of citrinin was seen (as judged by lack of toxicity) probably because of the rapid urinary elimination.

In addition to alterations in standard renal function parameters in intact animals, citrinin and ochratoxin A also altered specific renal transport processes. Pretreatment of rats either with a single dose of citrinin or with repeated doses of ochratoxin A resulted in a reduction of renal transport of organic anions and organic cations. Similar effects were seen when citrinin or ochratoxin A were added directly to renal slices prepared from non-pretreated rats. Although one might speculate that citrinin and ochratoxin A, both organic anions, might alter PAH transport by a competitive mechanism, this is not a likely explanation for the inhibition of TEA transport. The effects of these compounds on divergent transport systems in the pretreatment experiments may well reflect the general demise of the renal cortex, i.e., the acute tubular necrosis with acute renal failure. Such an explanation, however, is not likely for those experiments where the fungal toxins were added directly to fresh renal cortex slices. Renal necrosis has not occurred in these slices and the actions of the fungal toxins probably reflect a direct action of the compounds on the membrane transport processes, energy supply mechanisms, or some other central event important in the renal transport of the organic ions. That is to say, both the *in vivo* and *in vitro* studies would indicate that citrinin and ochratoxin A produce a very early event capable of disrupting some renal function parameters promptly, but more importantly leading to the subsequent development of renal tubular necrosis and acute renal failure several days after the administration. Hence, although one can assess the renal dysfunction two or three days after administration of a single dose of citrinin, for example, studies related to the mechanism of toxicity would appear to require an examination of events in the tissue occurring within 30 to 60 minutes of the administration of the citrinin. Examination of subcellular events at two or three days when the renal dysfunction is maximal might or might not be useful for understanding

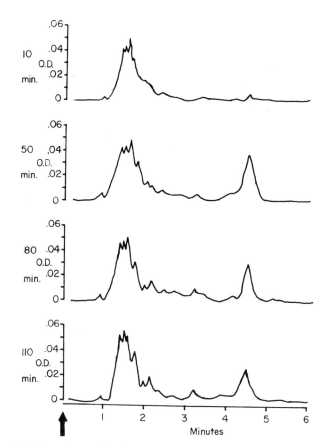

Figure 3. HPLC tracings showing presence of citrinin metabolites and citrinin. Bile from isolated perfused liver collected at various times after start of perfusion was injected on a Waters C-18 μBonda-pak reverse phase column using the method developed for citrinin [52]. Citrinin (5 x 10^{-5}M) was added to liver perfusate. The large peak at 4.3 minutes was authentic citrinin; peaks at 130 and 190 seconds were citrinin metabolites.

mechanisms. Examination of subcellular events within 30 to 60 minutes after administration of citrinin might yield changes in important processes which could be correlated with the subsequent development of toxicity.

Possible mechanisms of toxicity. In the pharmacokinetic studies it was demonstrated that citrinin metabolism occurred. At least two metabolites were formed and appeared in the urine of animals treated with a nephrotoxic dose of citrinin. Quantitatively, these metabolites accounted for no more than 10 to 15% of a dose of citrinin, but their possible role or roles in the production of toxicity could not be overlooked. To date the metabolites have not been identified. It is known, however, that these compounds are not glucuronides or sulfates based on glucuronidase and sulfatase incubation experiments. Both metabolites are more polar than the parent compound which suggests that they are either oxidation products or mercapturic acid derivatives of citrinin, or mercapturic acid derivatives of citrinin metabolites. Studies with the isolated perfused liver preparation indicate that the liver can form these metabolites (Fig. 3). In the bile from an isolated perfused liver preparation, a progressive increase in the quantity of metabolites was observed. These metabolites had the same retention times on HPLC analysis as the metabolites found in the urine of intact animals. If one is to project metabolism as important in the production of nephrotoxicity, one might anticipate finding a metabolite formed in the target organ itself. Studies with the isolated perfused rat kidney preparation do not indicate renal metabolism of citrinin. Metabolites were not found in either the urine or perfusate over ninety minutes of perfusion. These data suggest that either the parent compound is nephrotoxic or if a metabolite is involved in the toxicity that a critical metabolic step occurs in the liver.

The possible role of metabolism is emphasized by SKF-525A pretreatment experiments. Renal slice transport was protected from the effects of citrinin by pretreatment with SKF-525A (Table 3).

When renal slice transport was examined three days after the administration of the citrinin in SKF-525A pretreated rats, renal slice transport of PAH and TEA were significantly protected compared to transport by kidney slices from animals treated with citrinin alone. Protection was not complete, but less inhibition of transport was observed after SKF than in its absence. Because of the known effects of SKF-525A, these data suggest a role of metabolism in the citrinin-induced nephrotoxicity.

Although the nature of the "reactive" metabolite is not known, it has been demonstrated that covalent binding of carbon-14 to renal tissue can occur after the administration of the carbon-14 labeled compound.

Table 3.   Effect of SKF-525A Pretreatment
on Citrinin-Induced Nephrotoxicity

SKF-525A was administered in a dose of 30 mg/kg, i.p., 30 minutes before citrinin and 3.5 hours after. Citrinin was given i.p. in a dose of 55 mg/kg. Renal slice experiments were performed 72 hours after citrinin administration. N = 4.

	PAH	PAH with lactate	TEA
		S/M ratios (% of control)	
Control	3.7 ± 0.2	9.3 ± 0.4	10.2 ± 0.3
Citrinin	1.0 ± 0.2 (27)	1.1 ± 0.2 (12)	3.5 ± 0.3 (34)
Citrinin + SKF	3.5 ± 0.3 (95)	5.0 ± 0.2 (54)	7.5 ± 0.5 (74)

Covalent binding is defined as that radioactivity remaining in a TCA precipitable material after repeated extraction of that precipitate with organic solvents selected because of their ability to dissolve authentic citrinin. The covalent binding is organ specific in that approximately three times more binding occurs in renal cortex than in liver. This differential exists at all doses studied except low doses which are not nephrotoxic. Consistent with the covalent binding argument is the fact that citrinin can reduce significantly renal and hepatic glutathione. The reduction of renal glutathione is to approximately 60% of normal and the reduction in the liver to about one-half of normal. Although neither depletion is of the same magnitude as that observed with other nephrotoxic compounds thought to act through "reactive intermediates", the glutathione depletion is a consistent finding [48].

Because the glutathione depletion is not as great as might be anticipated, and because covalent binding persists at a significant level for only 24 hours, it was necessary to examine the role of the unmetabolized citrinin in the nephrotoxic response as well. As with certain antibiotics such as the cephalosporins [55], it is possible that citrinin itself in the kidney tissue is responsible for the nephrotoxicity. This possibility would be supported greatly if a strong correlation could be found between accumulation of the parent compound in the kidney and the development of toxicity. The availability of a specific analysis for citrinin facilitated this study.

It has already been suggested above that citrinin is actively secreted by renal transport mechanisms and, since this compound is an organic anion, it is likely that secretion by the PAH mechanism is the important one [54]. Hence, the next set of experiments was designed to examine the effects of probenecid on citrinin lethality, citrinin-induced renal dysfunction, and the accumulation of citrinin by renal tissue.

Citrinin toxicity is reduced significantly by pretreatment with probenecid before the administration of citrinin. In a 72 hour mortality study with several doses of probenecid (30-120 mg/kg) it was possible to demonstrate significant protection against citrinin-induced death. Citrinin was given at 55 mg/kg, approximately the LD_{50}.

Renal slice transport of PAH and TEA was monitored as an indicator of renal function. Renal slices prepared from animals pretreated with

Table 4. Effect of Probenecid on Citrinin-Induced
Inhibition of Renal Transport

Pretreatment with probenecid was 30 minutes before citrinin (55 mg/kg). Experiments were performed 72 hours after citrinin administration.

Probenecid	PAH	% of Control	TEA
		PAH with lactate	
0	32	17	55
30	80	53	88
60	95	71	89
120	122	80	87

Table 5.   Effect of Probenecid on Tissue Accumulation of ^{14}C-Citrinin

Probenecid (120 mg/kg, s.c.) was injected 30 minutes before citrinin. Measurements were made 1 hour after injection of 55 mg/kg ^{14}C-citrinin i.p. Values are means ± SE for N = 4.

	CPM/ml homogenate		% of Control	P
	Control	Probenecid		
Kidney	3448 ± 319	1094 ± 396	32	<.05
Liver	3215 ± 179	2713 ± 541	82	NS

probenecid 30 minutes before the administration of citrinin showed a significantly greater degree of transport of these test compounds 72 hours after citrinin administration than did tissue from animals not pretreated with probenecid. The data in Table 4 were obtained with various doses of probenecid given prior to citrinin. Even with a dose of probenecid as low as 30 mg/kg a significant protection was observed, although somewhat greater protection was afforded at 120 mg/kg.

The ability of probenecid to protect against lethality and to promote renal transport is correlated well with the ability of probenecid to prevent entry of citrinin into the renal tissue. The data in Table 5 indicate a significant reduction in tissue citrinin content 1 hour after the administration of citrinin in those animals pretreated with probenecid compared to controls.

This appears to be an organ specific effect since no reduction in liver citrinin uptake was observed in the same experimental animals. Probenecid also reduced the covalent binding observed in kidney tissue after the administration of labeled citrinin, but did not produce a similar effect in liver tissue. These data suggest that citrinin itself may be involved in the renal covalent binding process or probenecid blocks the entry into renal tissue of a liver-produced citrinin metabolite. If probenecid can interfere with renal transport of a citrinin metabolite, it is not possible to determine from these studies whether the parent citrinin or a liver-produced metabolite is responsible for the nephrotoxicity. It is possible to determine, however, that renal transport of either citrinin or a metabolite is essential for the production of a nephrotoxicity since probenecid, a known blocker of active tubular secretion, does protect against renal dysfunction and death.

Whatever the mechanism of transport and whether or not metabolism is important in the production of nephrotoxicity, there is still little direct information concerning the event or events which might initiate the nephrotoxic response. Trump and others sometime ago suggested that alterations in calcium binding, transport, etc. might mediate necrotic processes.

The effects of citrinin on calcium-45 accumulation have been studied in fresh renal cortex slices [56]. It can be seen from Figure 4 that both citrinin and ochratoxin A enhanced the accumulation of the labeled calcium by renal cortex slices. The enhanced uptake of the label is a precise reflection of the accumulation of total tissue calcium as determined by atomic absorption spectrometry. That is, citrinin or ochratoxin A caused a net uptake of calcium by fresh rat renal cortex

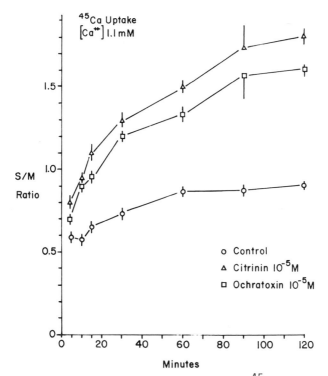

Figure 4. Effect of citrinin or ochratoxin A on ^{45}Ca uptake by fresh
rat renal cortex slices. Each point is mean ± SE for N = 4.

slices. Possibly the accumulation of large quantities of calcium
intracellularly might interfere with mitochondrial function (energy
generation?) or specific transport functions and lead to the subsequent
development of the nephrotoxic syndrome.

Finally, whatever the mechanism of the nephrotoxicity produced by the
fungal toxins, it should be noted that this problem is a potentially
important one. Although mycotoxin contamination of food supplies is not
a major problem in those areas of the world where food processing and
storage are at a high level of sophistication, fungal contamination of
food supplies is a common occurrence where care is not taken in food
processing or storage. The fungal toxins discussed here have a remark-
able propensity for producing disruption of renal function in
experimental animals and may do likewise in man. In addition, these
substances may interact with other pollutants in the environment which
might lead to an enhanced toxicity. How many of the various human
diseases are produced by fungal toxins is unknown, as is the role of
fungal toxins or other environmental contaminants in human kidney
disease. However, it is possibly noteworthy that such events could
occur and this will continue as an important area of investigation for
the future.

REFERENCES

1. Tyler VE Jr, Prog. Chem. Toxicol. 1:339-389,
    1963.
2. Lampe KF, Ann. Rev. Pharmacol. Toxicol. 19:85-104, 1979.
3. Gosselin RE, Hodge HC, Smith RP and Gleason MN, Clinical Toxicology
    of Commercial Products, The Williams and Wilkins Co., Baltimore,
    1976, pp. 10-16.
4. Weiland T, Science 159:946-952, 1968.
5. Floersheim GL, Bioch. Pharmacol. 15:1589-1593, 1966.
6. Frimmer M and Schischke B, Naunyn Schmiedebergs Arch. Pharmakol. 272:44
    449, 1972.
7. Myler RK, Lee JC and Hopper J, Arch. intern. Med. 114:196-204, 1964.
8. Fiume L, Marinozzi V and Nardi F, Br. J. Exp. Pathol. 50:270-276, 1969.
9. Bonetti E, Derenzini M and Fiumi L, Arch. Virchows B 16:71-78, 1974.
10. Bonetti E, Derenzini M and Fiumi L, Arch. Toxicol. 35:69-73, 1976.
11. Stirpe F and Fiumi L, Biochem J. 105:779-782, 1967.
12. Nieminen L, Mottonen M, Tirri R and Ikonen S, Exp. Pathol. 11:239-
    246, 1975.
13. Nieminen L and Pyg K, Acta Pathol. Microbiol. Scand. Sect A 84:222-224,
    1976.
14. Mottonen M, Nieminen L and Heikkila H, Z. Naturforsch. 300:668-
    671, 1975.
15. Kingsburg JM, In Toxicology, The Basic Science of Poisons, Doull J
    Klaassen CD and Amdur MO, (eds), MacMillan Publishing Co. Inc.,
    New York, 1980, pp. 578-590.
16. McLean EK, Pharmacol. Rev. 22:429-483, 1970.
17. Peckham JC, Sangster LT and Jones OH Jr, J. Amer. Vet. Med. Assoc.
    165: 633-638, 1974
18. Hooper PT, J. Pathol. 113:227-230, 1974.
19. Cooper P, Fd. Cosmet. Toxicol. 17:547-549, 1979.
20. Hooper PT, In Effects of Poisonous Plants on Livestock, Keeler RF,
    van Kamper KR and James LF, (eds.) Academic Press Inc., NY, 1978,
    pp. 161-176.
21. Culvenor CCJ, In Effects of Poisonous Plants on Livestock, Keeler
    RF van Kamper KR and James LF (eds.) Academic Press Inc., NY 1978,
    pp. 189-200.
22. Miranda CL, Cheeke PR, Schmitz JA and Buhler DR, Toxicol. Appl.
    Pharmacol. 56:432-442, 1980.
23. McGrath JPM, Duncan JR and Munnell JF, J. Comp. Path. 85:185-194,
    1975.
24. Chesney, CF and Allen JR, Tox. Appl. Pharmacol. 26:385-392, 1973.
25. Pierson ML, Cheeke PR and Dickinson EO, Res. Comm. Chem. Path. and
    Pharmacol. 16:561-567, 1977.
26. Miranda CL, Reed RL, Cheeke PR and Buhler DR, Toxicol. Appl.
    Pharmacol. 59:424-430, 1981.
27. Buckmaster GW, Cheeke PR and Shull LR, J Animal Science 43:464-473,
    1926.
28. Dickinson JO, Cooke MP, King RR and Mohamed PA, J. Am. Vet. Med.
    Assoc. 169:1192-1196, 1976.
29. Deinzer ML, Thomson PA, Bargett DM and Isaacson DL, Science 195:
    497-499, 1977.
30. Wyllie TD and Morehouse LG (eds.), Mycotoxic Fungi, Mycotoxins,
    Mycotoxicoses, vol. 1, Marcel Dekker, Inc., New York, 1978, pp.
    1-15. ISBN 0-8247-6552-4

31. Shank RC, In Mycotoxic Fungi, Mycotoxins, Mycotoxicoses, vol. 3, Wyllie TD and Morehouse TG (eds), Marcel Dekker, Inc., NY, 1978, pp. 1-15. ISBN 0-8247-6552-4
32. Hayes AW, Mycopathologia 65:29-51, 1979.
33. Hayes AW, In Mycotoxins in Human and Animal Health, Rodricks JV, Hesseltine CW and Mehlman MA (eds), Pathotox Publishers, Park Forest, IL, 1977, pp. 507-524.
34. Larsen S., Maanedsskr Dyrl 40:259-284, 289-300, 1928.
35. Hetherington AC and Raistrick H, Trans. Royal Soc. (London) B 220: 269-296, 1931.
36. Ambrose AM and DeEds F, Proc. Soc. Exp. Biol. Med. 59:289-291, 1945.
37. Carleton WW, Sansing G and Szczech GM, Fd. Cosmet. Toxicol. 12:479-490, 1974.
38. Ames DD, Wyatt RD, Macks HL and Washburn KW, Poultry Sci. 55:1294-1301, 1976.
39. Krogh P, Hasselager E and Friis P, Acta Pathol. Microbiol. Scand. 78:401-413, 1970.
40. Krogh P, Hold B and Pedersen EJ, Acta Pathol. Microbiol. Scand 81: 689-695, 1973.
41. Krogh P, Oxelsen NH, Elling F, Gyrd-Hansen N, *et al.*, Acta Pathol. Microbiol. Scand. Sec. A Suppl. 246, 1974.
42. Berndt WO and Hayes AW, J. Environ. Path. Tox. 1: 93-103, 1977.
43. Elling F, Hold, Jackobsen C and Krogh P, Acta Pathol. Microbiol. Scand. 83: 739-741, 1975.
44. Barnes JM, In Ciba Foundation Study Group, Wolstenholme GEW and Knight J (eds.), Little, Brown and Co., Boston, 1967, pp. 110-120.
45. Krogh P. Proc. 2nd Int. Symp. on Endemic Nephropathy, Sofia, Bulgaria, 1972, pp. 266-270.
46. Shinohara Y, Arai, M, Hirao K, Sugihara S, Nakanishi K, Tsunoda H and Ito N, Gann 67:147-155, 1976.
47. Krogh P, Hold B, Plestina R and Ceovic S, Acta Pathol. Microbiol. Scand. Section B 85:238-240, 1977.
48. Berndt WO, Hayes AW and Phillips RD, Kidney Intern. 18:656-664, 1980.
49. Barnes JM, Carter RL, Peristianis CTC, Austwick PKC, Flynn FV and Aldridge WN, Lancet 1:671-675, 1977.
50. Berndt, WO and Hayes AW, Toxicology 12:5-17, 1979a
51. Phillips RD, Berndt WO and Hayes AW, Toxicology 12:285-298, 1979.
52. Phillips RD, Hayes AW and Berndt WO, J. Chromatog. 190:419-427, 1980.
53. Lockard VG, Phillips RD, Hayes AW, Berndt WO and O'Neal RM, Exper. Molec. Path. 32:226-240, 1980.
54. Phillips RD, Hayes AW, Berndt WO and Williams WL, Toxicology 16: 123-137, 1980.
55. Tune BM and Fravert D, Kidney Intern. 18:591-600, 1980.
56. Berndt WO and Hayes AW, The Toxicologist 1:9, 1981.

RENAL NECROSIS PRODUCED BY HALOGENATED CHEMICALS

Edward A. Lock

Imperial Chemical Industries PLC, Biochemical Toxicology Section, Central Toxicology Laboratory, Alderley Park, Nr Macclesfield, Cheshire SK10 4TJ, UK

ABSTRACT

Several halogenated chemicals of industrial, agricultural and medicinal importance have been shown to be nephrotoxic in man or experimental animals. In this article the known nephrotoxic action of three chemicals, chloroform, tris(2,3-dibromopropyl)phosphate and S-(1,2-dichlorovinyl)-L-cysteine has been reviewed. Although chloroform produces hepatic necrosis in several species, the mouse appears unusually susceptible to chloroform-induced renal necrosis and displays a marked age, sex and strain difference in nephrotoxicity. This hormonal and genetic influence on chloroform-induced nephrotoxicity may be a reflection of a requirement for metabolism of chloroform to a reactive intermediate, possibly phosgene, which can bind covalently to critical sites in the kidney to produce necrosis. Tris(2,3-dibromopropyl)phosphate produces acute renal tubular necrosis in rodents with minimal hepatic injury. This compound undergoes metabolism in the rat to produce reactive metabolite(s) which become covalently bound to cellular macromolecules in the kidney. This binding may be related to the onset of renal necrosis and to the production of renal tumours which are observed following chronic administration of tris(2,3-dibromopropyl)phosphate. S-(1,2-dichloro-vinyl)-L-cysteine (DCVC) produces acute renal tubular necrosis in all species tested. Metabolism of DCVC to a reactive intermediate appears to be necessary to produce its toxic action. This metabolic activation does not involve a cytochrome P-450 system but requires the presence of a C-S lyase enzyme located in the kidney which produces a reactive alkylating moiety containing the thiovinyl group. This reactive intermediate inhibits the *in vitro* oxidation of 2-oxoacids by mitochondria probably by inhibition of the enzyme lipoyl dehydrogenase. Another nephrotoxic halogenated chemical hexachloro-1:3-butadiene, causes depletion of hepatic but not renal glutathione. It is suggested that the HCBD-glutathione conjugate formed in the liver is transported to the kidney where it is degraded to the HCBD-cysteine conjugate and that this latter conjugate (like

DCVC) is a substrate for the C-S lyase enzyme. Further work is
needed, at the molecular level, to understand the mechanism(s) of
nephrotoxicity of halogenated chemicals.

Keywords: Renal necrosis, chloroform, tris(2,3-dibromopropyl)
phosphate, S-(1,2-dichlorovinyl)-L-cysteine, hexachloro-1:3-butadiene,
chlorotrifluoroethylene.

INTRODUCTION

There are many halogenated chemicals of industrial, agricultural
and medicinal importance which have been shown to be nephrotoxic in
man or experimental animals [for recent review articles see references
1-3]. Three such chemicals have been selected and the likely
mechanism whereby they produce their nephrotoxic action will be
discussed. As will become apparent there is a paucity of information
in certain areas. It is hoped that by highlighting these areas,
further work will be stimulated. The three chemicals are chloroform,
tris(2,3-dibromopropyl)phosphate (Tris-BP) and S-(1,2-dichlorovinyl)-
L-cysteine (DCVC).

CHLOROFORM

The main use today of chloroform is as a solvent and chemical
intermediate mainly in the manufacture of fluorocarbon compounds.
However, it was once used as a general anaesthetic for man. For a
recent review of the biochemical toxicology of chloroform see Pohl [4].
The major target organs for chloroform toxicity are the liver and
kidney; liver necrosis being produced in both rats and mice whereas
renal necrosis is only readily produced in mice. Thus the bulk of
work on chloroform-induced nephrotoxicity has been carried out in the
mouse.

Sex and strain differences. Eschenbrenner [5] first described the
marked sex difference in chloroform-induced renal tubular necrosis
showing that male mice had extensive renal necrosis after oral
administration whereas no necrosis was found in female mice of the
same strain which were similarly treated. Eschenbrenner and Miller
[6] later reported that castration of male mice abolished their
susceptibility to renal necrosis following the administration of
chloroform but that treatment of the castrated animals with testosterone could restore their susceptibility. These original observations have been confirmed and extended [7,8], and for a summary see
Table 1.
Recently Clemens and co-workers [9] have reported that testosterone
sensitisation of female mice to chloroform-induced nephrotoxicity can
be blocked by treatment with the antiandrogenic compound flutamide.
They also reported that the Tfm/Y strain of mice which lack androgen
receptors were not responsive to chloroform-induced renal damage even
if androgen treated. These findings suggest that the androgen
induced renal susceptibility to chloroform toxicity is mediated via
the androgen receptor, which is located in the proximal convoluted
tubular cells.
Sex differences in the morphology of the mouse kidney have been
reported [10]. In female mice the parietal layer of most of the
Bowman's capsules are composed entirely of squamous cells while in

TABLE 1 The influence of hormonal status on the susceptibility to chloroform-induced renal necrosis in mice

Sex	Hormonal status/or treatment	Susceptibility to renal necrosis
Male	<27 days of age	-
"	>30 days of age	+
"	<15 days of age + testosterone	-
"	15-30 days of age + testosterone	+
"	Castrated	±
"	Castrated + adrenalectomised	-
"	Castrated + testosterone	+
"	Castrated + corticosteroids	+
"	Oestrogen	±
Female	Mature	-
"	Testosterone	+
"	Testosterone + flutamide	-
Male/female	No androgen receptor	-
"	No androgen receptor + testosterone	-

+ Completely susceptible, ± partially susceptible, - not susceptible. Data from references [7,9].

male mice they are composed partly or entirely of cuboidal cells similar to those of the proximal tubule. Subsequent work by Crabtree [11,12] showed that the percentage of capsules having cuboidal cells did not reach a high value in male mice until sexual maturity, and that in castrated mice this value remained low and was similar to that of normal female mice. Chloroform primarily causes necrosis of the proximal tubule, the parietal layer of Bowman's capsule being undamaged. Eschenbrenner and Miller [6] reported that kidneys with a high percentage of cuboidal cells (60-70%) lining the Bowman's capsule (i.e. kidneys from adult males or castrated males treated with testosterone) were susceptible to chloroform-induced damage whereas kidneys with a low percentage of cuboidal cells (20-30%) (i.e. kidneys from females or castrated males) were resistant to chloroform induced renal damage. Thus both the differentiation of parietal cells of the Bowman's capsule and the ability of chloroform to produce renal tubular necrosis appear to be under androgenic control in the mouse kidney.

Several cases of accidental exposure of mouse colonies to small concentrations of chloroform vapour have been reported [13-17]. In every case a high proportion of males either died with renal damage or sustained gross renal damage, whereas females exposed did not exhibit renal damage. Taylor and co-workers [18] using three different strains of mice found that more radioactivity from radio-labelled chloroform was present in male kidneys than in female kidneys 5 h after a single oral dose. Radiolabelled chloroform bound to renal protein was also higher in male than female mice indicating greater metabolite formation in the male kidney. Unweaned male mice exposed to chloroform are also resistant to renal damage [7,14,15] indicating that there is not only a marked sex difference but that there is also an age-dependence for the onset of necrosis.

In addition to chloroform toxicity being dependent on the sex and age of the mouse, it is also dependent on the strain of mouse used [13-17, 19,20]. The LD50 of chloroform to male C57Bl/6j mice was found to be four times higher than in male DBA/2j mice and that about twice as much radioactivity from radiolabelled chloroform was present in the kidneys of the sensitive strain as compared with the resistant strain. The first generation male offspring were intermediate between the parental strains for both toxicity and the presence of radioactivity in the kidney, suggesting a genetic control of chloroform-induced toxicity and renal damage [9,21].

Metabolism of Chloroform. The major metabolite of chloroform is carbon dioxide, accounting for 50% of an administered dose in man [22] and about 60% in rats and 80% in mice [23]. Studies *in vitro* have established that both rat liver and kidney slices can convert chloroform to carbon dioxide [24]. However the carbon dioxide generated does not appear to be of toxicological importance, suggesting that an intermediate in the metabolism of chloroform to carbon dioxide may be responsible for the toxicity. Phosgene has been identified as a metabolite of chloroform in rat liver preparations from both *in vitro* and *in vivo* studies [25-27] A possible mechanism of chloroform toxicity, therefore, is the alkylation of critical cellular macromolecules by phosgene leading to cell necrosis.

Ilett and co-workers [28] reported the generation of a chemically reactive metabolite of chloroform which became covalently bound to hepatic and renal proteins in mice. This binding to renal protein was greater in male than in female mice. Autoradiographic studies showed accumulation of radioactivity in proximal convoluted tubular cells, which is the site of the necrosis, strongly suggesting that the binding and necrosis were related events [28]. The activation of chloroform to a reactive intermediate by liver microsomes appears to be cytochrome P-450 dependent as the covalent binding to microsomal protein (a) requires NADPH and (b) can be inhibited by carbon monoxide and SKF525A [28,29]. However, in contrast to the results with liver, the covalent binding of chloroform metabolites to renal protein was (a) only minimally affected by the omission of NADPH and was (b) not altered by incubation under carbon monoxide or nitrogen. These observations indicate that the pathway of chloroform metabolism leading to covalent binding in kidney microsomes may be different from that in liver microsomes.

Indirect evidence that a metabolite of chloroform is probably involved comes from studies using modifiers of drug metabolism: piperonyl butoxide protects [28,30] whilst polybrominated biphenyls potentiate the renal necrosis [31]. However, treatment with other inducers e.g. 3-methylcholanthrene, 2,3,7,8-tetrachlorodibenzo-p-dioxin or polychlorinated biphenyls reduces renal toxicity, whilst phenobarbitone treatment has no effect [32]. Based on these latter findings Kluwe and co-workers [32] suggested that the reactive metabolite(s) of chloroform responsible for the renal necrosis are probably generated in the kidney (as opposed to being transported from the liver) as a compound like phosgene would be expected to alkylate macromolecules very readily or rapidly be metabolised to carbon dioxide.

Chloroform depletes both liver and kidney glutathione in the mouse [30] whereas in the rat it only depletes liver glutathione [33-35].

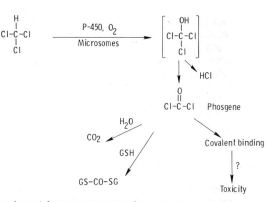

Figure 1   A schematic representation of the proposed metabolism of chloroform by mouse kidney.

One of the physiological functions of glutathione and the glutathione transferase enzymes is to scavenge electrophilic compounds, which can react with tissue macromolecules to cause tissue damage [36,37]. Thus glutathione may protect the mouse kidney from the deleterious effects of chloroform. Docks and Krishna [35] reported that at least three non-volatile metabolites of radiolabelled chloroform were excreted in the bile after administration to rats pretreated with phenobarbitone. The amounts of these non-volatile metabolites corresponded approximately to the molar equivalents of glutathione depleted [38]. Recently the depletion of hepatic glutathione has been shown to correlate with an increased secretion of the glutathione conjugate of phosgene (GS-CO-SG) in the bile of rats [39]. For a schematic representation of chloroform metabolism see Figure 1.
    Thus, although we can readily produce renal necrosis with chloro-form in the mouse, we do not know the mechanism by which it occurs. Is chloroform metabolised to phosgene in the mouse kidney? If so, is the generation of this metabolite under hormonal control and by what mechanism? What are the critical site(s) to which the reactive metabolite(s) of chloroform bind, and what is the sequence of biochemical events leading to the tubular necrosis? Why does pre-treatment of mice with polybrominated biphenyls enhance chloroform-induced renal necrosis and yet pretreatment with polychlorinated biphenyls reduces the necrosis? Many questions remain unanswered.

TRIS(2,3-DIBROMOPROPYL)PHOSPHATE

    Tris(2,3-dibromopropyl)phosphate (Tris-BP) was extensively used in synthetic fibres, polyurethane foams and plastics as a flame retardant. Initially it was thought to have low toxicity and would not represent a health hazard for use in fabrics for human wear e.g. children's sleepwear: its LD50 in the rat being about 5 g/kg [40]. However, studies by several workers [41-44] using the Salmonella mutagenicity assay showed that Tris-BP was a potent mutagen. These findings led to the discontinuation of the use of Tris-BP in fabrics. Subsequently, it was demonstrated that feeding Tris-BP to rats and mice led to renal tubular adenomas and carcinomas that were assumed to originate from the epithelia of the proximal convoluted tubule [45,46]. Renal

changes were observed following dermal application of Tris-BP for 90
days to rabbits [47] and following subchronic oral administration to
rats [48].

Soderlund and co-workers [49] carried out a detailed study of the
acute organ damage produced by Tris-BP in the rat. A single ip
injection of Tris-BP at 250 mg/kg or above produced observable renal
necrosis by 24 h. Histological examination of the damaged kidneys
showed that at the lower doses the lesion was confined to the straight
portion of the proximal tubule (pars recta) whereas at higher doses,
in addition to the straight portion, there was evidence of necrosis
in parts of the proximal convoluted and distal convoluted tubules.
At doses which produced very marked renal necrosis (i.e. 250 mg/kg)
there was no histological evidence of liver damage. No increase in
liver to body weight ratio was observed and only at very high doses
(750 mg/kg) was there evidence of some centrilobular necrosis. Thus,
in the rat Tris-BP appears to produce renal necrosis with little
involvement of the liver.

The metabolic fate of Tris-BP in the rat is not fully understood.
Radiolabelled Tris-BP, when administered orally, is rapidly absorbed
and 50-75% of the radiolabel appears in the urine within 24 h. The
kidneys and liver are the organs containing the highest concentration
of radioactivity [50]. Tris-BP is metabolised by dealkylation at the
phosphate group, and most of the halogenated alkyl group formed is
thought to be subsequently metabolised to carbon dioxide. However
2,3-dibromopropanol has been detected in the urine after absorption
of Tris-BP through the skin [51,52] and the diester metabolite
bis(2,3-dibromopropyl)phosphate has been identified [53] as a minor
component in rat urine after iv administration. Recently several
metabolites have been isolated from urine, bile and faeces, and it
has been demonstrated *in vitro* that liver enzymes can degrade Tris-BP
to the same polar metabolites identified from urine and bile [54].
The enzymes responsible for the activation and metabolism of Tris-BP
are concentrated in the microsomal and soluble portions of the rat
liver. The mutagenicity of Tris-BP to Salmonella typhimurium TA100
requires the presence of microsomes, NADPH and oxygen. Inhibitors of
cytochrome P-450 reduced the mutagenicity as did the addition of
reduced glutathione (GSH) [44], leading these authors to suggest that
Tris-BP is oxidised to a reactive electrophile, possibly the 2-keto
derivative, which could react with DNA and produce the mutagenic
event. Both bromines in the 2,3-dibromopropyl moieties of Tris-BP
have been shown to be essential for the mutagenic effects of Tris-BP
in vitro [43,44]. Similarly, the monobrominated analogues of
Tris-BP are much less active than Tris-BP itself in causing renal
damage and the hydrolysis product of Tris-BP (2,3-dibromopropanol)
does not appear to produce renal damage [49].

Incubation of radiolabelled Tris-BP with rat liver microsomes
in vitro generated a metabolite which became covalently bound to the
microsomal protein [55]. This binding was NADPH and oxygen dependent
and the binding was markedly reduced by carbon monoxide, by the
cytochrome P-450 inhibitors metyrapone and SKF525A and by the addition
of GSH. The *in vitro* binding of radiolabelled Tris-BP to rat kidney
microsomes was only 7% of that produced by liver microsomes. However,
administration of radiolabelled Tris-BP to rats leads to covalent
binding to renal protein and DNA, the binding (per mg of protein or
DNA) in the kidney being 4-5 times that found in the liver [55,56].
This indicates that the binding to macromolecules *in vivo* may be
relevant to the renal necrosis and carcinogenesis.

In vivo, Tris-BP administration to rats causes a marked depletion of both hepatic and renal glutathione content [49], the glutathione conjugate being excreted in the bile [54]. Pretreatment of rats with either diethylmaleate or with the cytochrome P-450 inducers pheno-barbitone or polychlorinated biphenyl, had no effect on the renal necrosis.

Thus, in the rat, Tris-BP appears to be significantly metabolised by the liver and yet it produces no damage to that organ. The role of hepatic cytochrome P-450 dependent metabolism *in vivo* is not clear. Toxicity is not produced by modifiers of this system and little covalent binding occurs. However, conjugation via a glutathione-S-transferase presumably occurs to a significant extent. The basis for the renal lesion is not understood; the metabolic pathway(s) responsible for generating the toxic metabolite (P-450 dependent?) may only be a minor pathway in the liver but a major pathway in the kidney. If the toxic metabolite is generated in the kidney by cytochrome P-450 dependent enzymes, this may explain the site specificity of the lesion as cytochrome P-450 dependent enzymes are thought to be concentrated in the pars recta of the proximal tubule [57-59]. An alternative explanation is that the liver may metabolise Tris-BP to a non-toxic metabolite(s) e.g. a glutathione conjugate, which may be transported to the kidney where it could undergo further metabolism to a 'toxic' metabolite. The ability of the kidneys to concentrate urine (containing metabolites) to a high concentration in the pars recta, and the location of the organic anion transport system in that part of the nephron, may facilitate the entry of high concentrations of metabolites into those renal cells. Further work is needed to identify the toxic metabolites of Tris-BP and to establish the relative roles of the liver and kidney in their generation.

S-(1,2-DICHLOROVINYL)-L-CYSTEINE

S-(1,2-dichlorovinyl)-L-cysteine (DCVC) was tentatively identified as the toxic agent responsible for the outbreaks of aplastic anaemia in cattle fed soya bean meal which had been extracted with trichloro-ethylene. DCVC was therefore synthesised from trichloroethylene and L-cysteine [60] and administered to calves where it was shown to produce similar symptoms to those produced by feeding soya bean meal extract.

In the rat (and several other laboratory species), only renal tubular necrosis was found [61,62] whereas in the case of the calf, recovery from the renal lesion is followed by the onset of aplastic anaemia [63]. Histological examination of the rat kidney, 24 h after a single ip dose (100 mg/kg) of DCVC, showed a distinct band of damage to the pars recta of the proximal tubules [65]. Histological examination of the mouse kidney showed tubular necrosis comparable to the rat except that necrotic tubules were frequently found in the pars convoluta in addition to the pars recta [62]. Treatment of mice with large doses of trichloroethylene produces liver necrosis with little evidence of renal impairment [64,65], thus any formation of DCVC *in vivo* either does not occur or not to a significant extent to produce renal damage.

Studies of the metabolic fate of DCVC in the calf [66] have shown that it is very different from that in the rat [67]; the ability of

the rat but not the calf to N-acetylate DCVC may partially explain
the different toxicological response of these two species. Cleavage
of DCVC at the C-S bond has been shown to occur enzymatically in
bovine liver and kidney extracts [68,69] in rat liver mitochondrial
and cytosolic fractions [70,71] and also non-enzymically [72]. The
products identified from this cleavage reaction were pyruvic acid,
ammonia and a fragment of unknown structure containing the thiovinyl
moiety of DCVC. The enzyme responsible for the C-S cleavage of DCVC
is a β-lyase and it has been isolated and purified from bovine liver
and kidney [68,69] and is probably the same enzyme recently isolated
and characterised from rat liver cytosol by Tateishi and co-workers
[73]. The thiovinyl moiety generated *in vitro* from the cleavage of
DCVC has been shown to be a very reactive alkylating fragment which
can combine with a variety of acceptors including proteins,
glutathione [72] and DNA [74].
     Biochemical studies have shown that DCVC inhibits uncoupler-
stimulated respiration of isolated rat liver and kidney mitochondria
in vitro, whilst mitochondria isolated from rat kidneys 2-4 h after
ip administration of DCVC also had impaired respiration [75]. DCVC
produces a delayed inhibition of respiration and a delayed stimulation
of ATP hydrolysis by rat liver mitochondria *in vitro* [76] and this
delay is thought to be related to the generation of a reactive
metabolite by this fraction. The site of action within the mitochondria is thought to be lipoyl dehydrogenase, an enzyme present in
both of the 2-oxoacid dehydrogenase complexes [71,76], whilst in the
cytosolic fraction the activity of glutathione reductase is inhibited
in vitro [71]. The active site of glutathione reductase and lipoyl
dehydrogenase are thought to be similar, both containing a disulphide
bond and requiring FAD as a prosthetic group.   See Figure 2 for a
schematic representation of the proposed action of DCVC on renal
metabolism.

OTHER HALOGENATED COMPOUNDS WHICH MAY PRODUCE RENAL DAMAGE VIA CYSTEINE
CONJUGATES

     Several unsaturated halogenated compounds have been reported to
produce marked renal tubular necrosis, with minimal liver involvement
following inhalation exposure e.g. Chlorotrifluoroethylene (CTFE)
[78-80], hexafluoropropene (HFP) [79,80], hexachlorobutadiene (HCBD)
[81], difluorodichloroethylene (CDFE) [82].
     Inhalation of 0.3% CTFE for 4 h produces marked renal tubular
necrosis in mice by 24-48 h, enzyme histochemistry showing defects in
kidney mitochondria within 30 min of exposure [78]. Similarly,
inhalation exposure of rats to a range of concentrations of CTFE or
HFP for 4 h produces, by 24 h, impairment of renal function;
histological examination of the kidneys shows necrosis localised in
the pars recta of the proximal tubules after CTFE exposure and
in the pars recta and pars convoluta after HFP exposure [80].
These authors also reported an increased urinary excretion of fluoride
ions 24 h after exposure, however, the amount of fluoride ion
liberated from either CTFE or HFP was not considered to be enough to
account for renal toxicity.
     Recently Gandolfi and co-workers [83] have reported that halogenated
cysteine conjugates prepared from CTFE or CDFE produce renal tubular
necrosis of the pars recta of mice three days after a 5-10 mg/kg
dose. *In vitro* the vinyl cysteine conjugate of CTFE undergoes rapid

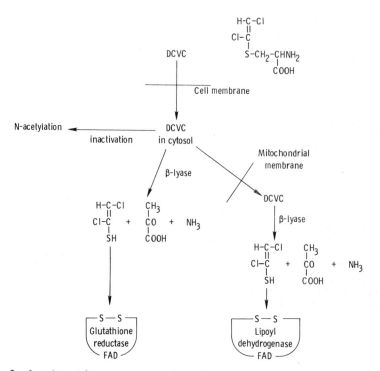

Figure 2 A schematic representation of the proposed action of DCVC in rat kidney adapted from reference [77].

degradation by enzymes present in rabbit renal tubules to produce pyruvate [84] and presumably generates a reactive thiovinyl moiety which can react with glutathione in an analogous manner to that reported for DCVC. Thus the organ specific nephrotoxicity of CTFE, CDFE and perhaps HFP could be explained by the formation of a vinyl cysteine complex *in vivo* which in the kidney is activated by a β-lyase enzyme, to form a reactive fragment capable of producing tubular necrosis analogous to DCVC (see Figure 3). However, to date, these conjugates have not been shown to occur *in vivo*. The double bond in the molecule appears to be required to produce necrosis as S(chloroethyl)- or S(hydroxyethyl)cysteine were non-nephrotoxic to mice at doses up to 20 mg/kg [83].

HCBD produces renal tubular necrosis in several species and by a variety of routes of administration [85-89] with minimal liver injury. In the rat a single ip injection of 200 or 300 mg/kg produces a distinct band of necrosis located in the pars recta of the proximal tubules [88,90] whereas in the mouse, a single ip injection of 50 mg/kg produces a lesion in the pars recta and pars convoluta [91].

The metabolic fate of HCBD in the rat is not known. Following ip administration of a nephrotoxic dose of radiolabelled HCBD, radio-activity appears mainly in the faeces (being eliminated via the bile) with about 10% appearing in urine. The tissues containing the highest concentration of radioactivity are the kidneys, fat and liver [92]. HCBD appears to undergo extensive metabolism, several water

soluble metabolites being found in bile and urine [92,93]. In the
male rat, HCBD administration causes a marked depletion of hepatic,
but not renal glutathione content [94]. Evidence from our laboratory
has shown that incubation of HCBD with rat liver microsomes and
glutathione causes a loss of glutathione which can be accounted for
by the formation of a glutathione conjugate. The formation of the
conjugate appears to be catalysed by a glutathione transferase enzyme
present in the microsomal and cytosolic fraction [95]. A component
with chromatographic characteristics similar to the glutathione
conjugate of HCBD has been observed in rat bile [93]. Pretreatment
of rats with diethylmaleate markedly increased the HCBD-induced
impairment of renal function [96], whereas pretreatment with
glutathione [89] or cysteine [97] was without effect. Treatment of
rats *in vivo* with a variety of inhibitors or inducers of both hepatic
and renal mixed function oxidases was without effect on HCBD-induced
renal necrosis [94-96] indicating that cytochrome P-450 monooxygenase
reactions do not appear to play a major role in this type of toxicity.

Thus, in the rat, HCBD appears to be metabolised to a significant
extent by the liver, where it forms a glutathione-conjugate. The
glutathione conjugate of HCBD is then presumably transported to the
kidney (via the bile) for excretion. Glutathione-conjugates are
converted to their cysteine conjugates in the kidney by the enzymes
γ-glutamyl transferase and cysteinyl glycinase. These enzymes are
concentrated to a significant extent in the pars recta of the proximal
tubules [98]. The cysteine conjugate is then thought to enter the

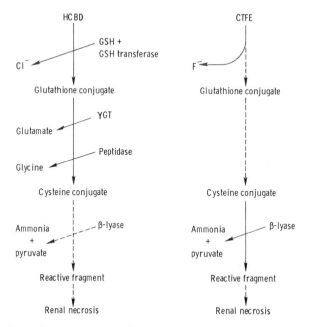

Figure 3 A schematic representation of the proposed nephrotoxic
action of hexachloro-1:3-butadiene and chlorotrifluoroethylene in the
rat, based on both *in vitro* and *in vivo* data. Established pathways
are shown in solid lines whilst broken lines represent postulated
pathways.

renal tubular cells to undergo acetylation [98]. Thus analogous to
DCVC the HCBD cysteine conjugate could be activated by a β-lyase
enzyme (presumed to be located in that part of the nephron) to generate
a reactive thio-chlorobutadiene moiety which could be toxic by virtue
of its alkylating potential. This may, therefore, be an interesting
example of lethal synthesis, where the liver converts HCBD to a
glutathione conjugate which is then transported to the kidney where
it undergoes further metabolism to a toxic product responsible for
the tubular necrosis. Figure 3 summarises our current proposed
mechanism whereby certain halogenated alkenes cause toxicity.
Further work is needed in this area to establish whether cysteine
conjugates of some of these compounds are formed *in vivo*, and if so,
whether they are activated via the β-lyase enzyme.

In summary, further work is needed, at the molecular level, to try
and understand the mechanism whereby halogenated chemicals produce
their nephrotoxicity. In particular, it is important (i) to
understand the metabolism of the chemical in the target organ and the
role, if any, of other organs in the biotransformation process, (ii)
to identify the critical site(s), (e.g. enzymes) to which reactive
metabolites, if formed, bind and the cascade of biochemical events
which leads to tubular necrosis. Only by understanding these
processes will we be in a better position to explain the marked sex,
age, strain and species differences in nephrotoxicity produced by
some halogenated chemicals.

ACKNOWLEDGEMENTS

The author wishes to acknowledge valuable discussions with Dr's J
Ishmael, M D Stonard, T Green and R C Wolf; whilst preparing the
manuscript.

REFERENCES

1.   Hook JB et al in Reviews in Biochemical Toxicology (E Hodgson,
       JR Bend and RM Philpot, eds). Elsevier, New York 1979 1:53-78.
       ISBN 0-444-00317-7.
2.   Kluwe WM, in Toxicology of the Kidney (JB Hook, ed.) Raven
       Press, New York 1981 172-226. ISBN-0-89004-475-9.
3.   Mazze RI, in Toxicology of the Kidney (JB Hook, ed.) Raven
       Press, New York 1981 135-150. ISBN-0-89004-475-9.
4.   Pohl LR, in Reviews in Biochemical Toxicology (E Hodgson, JR
       Bend and RM Philpot, eds) Elsevier, New York 1979 1:79-108.
       ISBN 0-444-00317-7.
5.   Eschenbrenner AB, J Natl Cancer Inst 5:251-255 1945.
6.   Eschenbrenner AB and Miller E, Science 102:302-303 1945.
7.   Culliford D and Hewitt HB, J Endocrinol 14:381-393 1957.
8.   Krus S et al. Nephron 12:275-280 1974.
9.   Clemens TL et al. Toxicol Appl Pharmacol 48:117-130 1979.
10. Crabtree C. Science 91:299 1940.
11. Crabtree C. Anat Rec 79:395-413 1941.
12. Crabtree C. Endocrinology 29:197-203 1941.
13. Shubik P and Ritchie AC. Science 117:285 1953.
14. Deringer MK et al. Proc Soc Exp Biol Med 83:474-479 1953.
15. Hewitt HB. Brit J Exp Pathol 37:32-39 1956.
16. Christensen LR et al. Z Versuchstienkd 2:135-140 1963.
17. Jacobsen L et al. Acta Pathol Microbiol Scand 61:503-573 1964.

18. Taylor DC et al. Xenobiotica 4:165-174 1974.
19. Bennet RA and Whigman A. Nature 204:1328 1964.
20. Zaleska-Rutczynska and Krus S. Patol Pol 23:185-188 1972.
21. Hill RN et al. Science 190:159-161 1975.
22. Fry BJ et al. Arch Int Pharmacodyn Ther 196:98-111 1972.
23. Brown BM et al. Xenobiotica 4:151-163 1974.
24. Paul BB and Rubinstein D. J Pharmacol Exp Ther 141:141-148 1963.
25. Mansuy D et al. Biochem Biophys Res Commun 79:513-517 1977.
26. Pohl LR et al. Biochem Biophys Res Commun 79:684-91 1977.
27. Pohl LR et al. Toxicol Appl Pharmacol 48:A110 1979.
28. Ilett KF et al. Exp Mol Pathol 19:215-229 1973.
29. Sipes IG et al. Life Sci 20:1541-1548 1977.
30. Kluwe WM and Hook JB. Toxicol Appl Pharmacol 59:457-466 1981.
31. Kluwe WM et al. J Pharmacol Exp Ther 207:566-573 1978.
32. Kluwe WM and Hook JB. Toxicol Appl Pharmacol 45:861-869 1978.
33. Johnson MK. Biochem Pharmacol 14:1383-1385 1965.
34. Brown BR et al. Anesthesiology 41:554-561 1974.
35. Docks EL and Krishna G. Exp Mol Pathol 24:13-22 1976.
36. Mitchell JR et al. In Glutathione Metabolism and Function (IM
    Arias, WB Jakoby, eds). Raven Press, New York 1976 357.
37. Jakoby WB and Keen JH. Trends Biochem Sci 2:229 1977.
38. Docks EL et al. Pharmacologist 16:239 1974.
39. Branchflower RV et al. Toxicologist 1:98 1981.
40. Kerst AF. J Fire Flammability/Fire Retardant Chem 1:205-215 1974.
41. Prival MJ et al. Science 195:76-78 1977.
42. Blum A and Ames BN. Science 195:17-23 1977.
43. Nakamura A et al. Mutat Res 66:373-380 1979.
44. Soderlund GJ et al. Acta Pharmacol Toxicol (kbh) 45:112-121 1979.
45. Reznik G et al. J Natl Cancer Inst 63:205-212 1979.
46. Reznik G et al. Lab Invest 44:74-83 1981.
47. Osterberg RE et al. J Toxicol Environ Health 3:979-987 1977.
48. Osterberg RE et al. Toxicol Appl Pharmacol 45:254-255 1978.
49. Soderlund E et al. Toxicol Appl Pharmacol 56:171-181 1980.
50. Ulsamer AG et al. Toxicol Appl Pharmacol 45: 251-252 1978.
51. StJohn LE Jr et al. Bull Environ Contam Toxicol 15:192-197 1976.
52. Blum A et al. Science 201:1020-1023 1978.
53. Lynn RK et al. Res Commun Chem Pathol Pharmacol 28:351-360 1980.
54. Matthews HB and Nomeir AA. Toxicologist 1:35 1981.
55. Dybing E et al in Mechanisms of Toxicity and Hazard Evaluation
    (B Holmsted et al, eds.) Biomedical Press, Elsevier, North
    Holland 1980, 265-268.
56. Morales NM and Matthews HB. Bull Environ Contam Toxicol 25:34-38
    1980.
57. Wattenberg LW and Leong JL. J Histochem Cytochem 10:412-420 1962.
58. Fowler BA et al. J Pharmacol Exp Ther 203:712-721 1977.
59. Wolf CR et al. J Appl Toxicol 1:xxii 1981.
60. McKinney LL et al. J Am Chem Soc 79:3932-3 1957.
61. Schultze MO et al. Proc Soc Exp Biol Med 111:499-502 1962.
62. Terracini B and Parker VH. Food Cosmet Toxicol 3:67-74 1965.
63. Schultze MO et al. Blood 14:1015-1025 1959.
64. Plaa GL and Larson RE. Toxicol Appl Pharmacol 7:37-44 1965.
65. Klaassen CD and Plaa GL. Toxicol Appl Pharmacol 9:139-151 1966.
66. Derr RF et al. Biochem Pharmacol 12:475-488 1963.
67. Derr RF and Schultze MO. Biochem Pharmacol 12: 465-474 1963.
68. Anderson PM and Schultze MO. Arch Biochem Biophys 111:593-602
    1965.

69. Bhattacharya RK and Schultze MO. Comp Biochem Physiol 22:723-735 1967.
70. Stonard MD and Parker VH. Biochem Phrmacol 20:2429-2437 1971.
71. Stonard MD. Biochem Pharmacol 22:1329-1335 1973.
72. Anderson PM and Schultze MO. Arch Biochem Biophys 109:615-621 1965.
73. Tateishi M et al. J Biol Chem 253:8854-8859 1978.
74. Bhattacharya RK and Schultze MO. Arch Biochem Biophys 153:105-115 1972.
75. Parker VH. Food Cosmet Toxicol 3:75-84 1965.
76. Stonard MD and Parker VH. Biochem Pharmacol 20:2417-2427 1971.
77. Stonard MD. PhD Thesis, University of London 1971.
78. Walther H et al. Acta Biol Med Ger 23:685-706 1969.
79. Clayton JW. Environ Health Perspect 21:255-267 1977.
80. Potter C et al. Toxicol Appl Pharmacol 59:431-440 1981.
81. Gage JC. Brit J Ind Med 27:1-18 1970.
82. Sakharova LN and Tolgskoya MS. Gig Tr Prog Sabol 5:36-42 1977.
83. Gandolfi AJ et al. Fed Proc 39:546 1980.
84. Bonhaus DW and Gandolfi AJ. Toxicologist 1:100 1981.
85. Gradiski D et al. Eur J Toxicol 8:180-187 1975.
86. Kociba RJ et al. Environ Health Perspect 21:49-53 1977.
87. Duprat P and Gradiski D. Acta Pharmacol Toxicol (kbh) 43:346-353 1978.
88. Lock EA and Ishmael J. Arch Toxicol 43:47-57 1979.
89. Berndt WO and Mehendale HM. Toxicology 14:55-65 1979.
90. Ishmael J et al. J Pathol in press.
91. Lock EA and Ishmael J. Unpublished observation.
92. Davies ME et al. Toxicology 16:179-191 1980.
93. Nash J et al. Unpublished observation.
94. Lock EA and Ishmael J. Toxicol Appl Pharmacol 7:79-87 1981.
95. Wolf CR et al. Unpublished observation.
96. Lock EA and Ishmael J in Adv Pharmacology and Therapeutics II vol 5 Toxicology and Experimental Models. Pergamon Press, Oxford, in press.
97. Davis ME et al. Toxicologist 1:9 1981.
98. Curthoys NP and Hughey RP. Enzyme 24:383-403 1979.

ACUTE AND CHRONIC NEPHROTOXICITY OF DICHLOROACETYLENE IN MICE AND RATS

D. Reichert, U. Spengler, W. Romen* and D. Henschler

*Institute of Pharmacology and Toxicology and *Institute of Pathology of the University, Versbacher Strasse 9, D-8700 Würzburg, Federal Republic of Germany*

INTRODUCTION

Dichloroacetylene (DCA) is a by-product of the synthesis of certain chlorinated aliphatic hydrocarbons. In particular, the synthesis of vinylidene chloride is accompanied by DCA formation. DCA also occurs as a decomposition product of trichloroethylene and acetylene. DCA is highly reactive, and in the presence of air oxygen it decomposes into various hydrocarbons (mostly perchlorinated), which have been identified in earlier studies [1]. For experimental applications, DCA must be stabilized to avoid decomposition. Severe nephrotoxic properties have been established in DCA inhalation experiments with several animal species [2,3].

We report here on further studies of the acute and chronic nephrotoxic activity of DCA; these studies have been designed to clarify the influence of different stabilizers on the acute toxicity and to evaluate the toxic risk of DCA exposure.

MATERIALS AND METHODS

Chemicals. DCA was freshly synthesized from trichloroethylene and anhydrous potassium hydroxide in steady state concentration in nitrogen as described previously [2].

Animals. NMRI mice and Wistar rats (Zentralinstitut für Versuchstiere, D-3000 Hannover, FRG) were used throughout the experiments. Animals were kept in an air-conditioned room with an artificial 12h day/night rhythm. Food (Altromin[R]) and tap water were freely available. For the duration of the exposures, animals had no access to food and water.

Exposure system. During the exposure the bodies of the animals were kept in place in tubular, transparent plexiglass casings [2,3]. The

exposure time in the acute toxicity study was 1h; in the chronic inhalation experiments of 12- and 18-months duration the exposures were
as follows: mice: 9ppm 6h/day, 1day/week; rats: 14ppm 6h/day, 2days/
week.

Synthesized DCA was analytically controlled continuously in an
infrared spectrometer at 990 cm^{-1}. DCA has a pronounced characteristic
band at this wave length. In the exposure mixture DCA was selectively
and quantitatively determined by a Hall electrolytic conductivity
detector. This detector is specific for halogen-containing molecules
and allows rapid, sensitive and reproducible control of the exposure
mixture. DCA decomposition into toxic products, e.g. phosgene, hexachlorobutadiene and chloroform, was therefore immediately recognized
[4].

Histological examination. Deceased animals were autopsied, organs
were weighed and tissue sections were fixed in 10% formalin prior to
being embedded in Paraplast. Hematoxylin-eosin staining was used
routinely, but other stains were employed if needed.

RESULTS AND DISCUSSION

Acute nephrotoxicity. To ascertain whether different stabilizers
influence the acute toxicity of DCA (e.g. by intermolecular reactions,
adduct formation and rearrangement), the LD$_{50}$s of DCA mixed with different potent stabilizers were determined with mice in 1h inhalation
experiments. For each DCA concentration, 10 mice were exposed. The
regression of the dose-effect lines failed to show significant differences in slope when 1,2-dichloroethylene (1:4, v:v), acetylene (1:1,
v:v), and trichloroethylene (1:2, v:v) were admixed as stabilizers.
Under the assumption of parallelism, the acute toxicity of DCA is not
influenced by the stabilizers. These data are supported by the fact
that the IR-spectra reveal no further bonding in the DCA mixtures;
such bonding would probably influence the biological activity of DCA.

In the kidneys of spontaneously deceased animals, extensive tubular
necrosis and focal necrosis of the collecting tubuli were observed.
There was a significant increase in cytoplasmic basophilia in many
preserved tubuli together with impaired tubular regenerations and formation of strikingly large nuclei. Acute kidney damage was the cause
of death in all cases.

Chronic nephrotoxicity. Acetylene was used as the stabilizer in the
chronic toxicity study. In comparison to the controls after 4 months,
increased polyuria and glucosuria were observed, indicating an early
manifestation of nephrotoxicity. Blood glucose remained at normal
levels. The survival time for both exposed animal species was significantly reduced in comparison with control animals. Mean survival times
in weeks were as follows (controls in parentheses): male mice 54.8$\pm$3.0
(100.4$\pm$5.6), female mice 70.9$\pm$2.6 (88.5$\pm$4.6); male rats 113.2$\pm$5.6
(136.4$\pm$5.5), female rats 104.9$\pm$5.3 (136.0$\pm$5.5). The markedly reduced
life expectancies of exposed male mice are consistent with the general
observation that male mice inhale a considerably larger dose due to
their substantially higher respiratory rate as compared to female mice.

TABLE 1. TUMORS OBSERVED IN MICE AND RATS AFTER DCA EXPOSURE

| | MICE | | | | RATS | | | |
| | MALE | | FEMALE | | MALE | | FEMALE | |
ORGAN TUMOR	9 PPM	CONTROLS	9 PPM	CONTROLS	14 PPM	CONTROLS	14 PPM	CONTROLS
NO. OF AUTOPSIED ANIMALS	30	30	30	29	30	24	29	25
KIDNEY CYSTADENOMA	23	8	15	0	6	0	2	0
ONCOCYTOMA	0	0	0	0	0	6	0	2
ADENOCARCINOMA	4	0	0	0	1	0	0	0
NEPHROBLASTOMA	0	0	0	0	0	0	0	1
TRANSITIONAL CELL PAPILLOMA	0	0	0	0	0	1	1	0
TRANSITIONAL CELL CARCINOMA	0	0	0	0	0	2	0	0
LIVER CHOLANGIOMA	0	0	0	0	6	0	11	2
HEPATOCELL. ADENOMA	0	0	0	0	2	0	2	0
HEPATOCELL. CARCINOMA	0	0	0	0	0	1	0	0
TUMORS (TOTAL) BENIGN	30	21	26	7	20	14	18	13
MALIGN (LYMPHOMAS IN PARENTHESES)	5(1)	14(14)	5(2)	22(17)	12(6)	12(3)	16(11)	16(4)
NOT DETERMINED	0	3	0	1	1	1	2	2

The above described damage due to the acute toxic kidney lesion persists later on in the form of atypical cells and poorly differentiated tubular epithelia. It is suggested that this damage leads to disturbed reabsorption and subsequently to nephrohydrosis and cystic degeneration. After 1 year of exposure, almost all test animals developed cysts of the kidney cortex (i.e., in part, cysts of the glomeruli, along with cystic dilations of the proximal tubuli with atrophic epithelia and a thickened, split-up basal membrane).

The tumor rates in kidney and liver, from the nearly completed experiment, are given in Table 1. The most important result is a striking increase in the formation of cystadenomas of the proximal tubuli in male and female mice as well as in male rats. Cystic adenocarcinomas were found in four male mice and in one male rat. Besides the onset of renal cystadenomas in rats, we found a highly significant increase in DCA related cholangiomas of the liver (Table 1). No liver tumors were found in mice.

The toxicological risk in handling chlorinated aliphatic hydrocarbons is essentially increased by the decomposition product DCA. The results confirm DCA as a substance with pronounced organotropic properties. The main tissue target in acute as well as in chronic inhalation studies is the kidney. The extreme toxic effects are unique among other chlorinated hydrocarbons in both severity and organ specificity. In part, the effects are comparable with those of hexachlorobutadiene. This fact is interesting, because this compound is one of the main degradation products of DCA [1]. In future studies, it should be determined if the similar toxic effects of hexachlorobutadiene and DCA are based upon common molecular mechanisms of biotransformation.

REFERENCES

1. Reichert D, Metzler M, Henschler D, J Environ Pathol Toxicol 4:525–532, 1980.
2. Reichert D, Ewald D, Henschler D, Food Cosmet Toxicol 13:511–515, 1975.
3. Reichert D, Henschler D, Bannasch P, Food Cosmet Toxicol 16:227–235, 1978.
4. Reichert D, Spengler U, Henschler D, J Chromatogr 179:181–183, 1979.

ANTIBIOTIC NEPHROTOXICITY

J. P. Fillastre, D. Kleinknecht, M. Godin, G. Viotte, B. Olier and J. P. Morin

Groupe de Physiopathologie de Rouen, Hôpital de Montreuil, France

ABSTRACT

Antibiotics are the principal cause of drug-associated nephropathy. They are responsible for acute interstitial nephropathy (AIN) or acute tubulo-interstitial nephropathy (ATIN) due to two different pathophysiologic mechanisms.

1. AIN of immunologic origin. These are rare and are induced either by β-lactamines or by rifampicin. Among the β-lactamines, it is reported most frequently with methicillin, less often with penicillin and ampicillin and only rarely following carbenicillin, oxacillin, nafcillin, cephalothin or cephalexin. Macroscopic hematuria occurring 10 to 15 days after initiation of treatment usually reveals renal involvement. It is associated with or preceded by fever, skin eruptions and blood eosinophilia. Renal insufficiency (RI) is not severe and rarely requires hemodialysis (HD). The course is usually favourable. Rifampicin-induced AIN is observed in two circumstances, either during intermittent treatment or when previous treatment is resumed. Macroscopic hematuria is rare and RI often severe. Anti-rifampicin anti-bodies are usually found.

2. ATIN due to direct toxicity. Several classes of antibiotics may be responsible : cephalosporins, polymyxins or cyclins, but it is usually observed with aminoglycosides (AG). The incidence of renal involvement due to the latter group is estimated to be 4 to 10%. Nephrotoxicity is initially reflected by polyuria, tubular proteinuria and increased enzymuria, followed by cylinduria and reduced glomerular filtration. HD is rarely required. The proximal tubule is predominantly affected; pathological findings are disappearance of the brush border and tubular necrosis. Electron microscopy shows lysosomal alterations with numerous myelinic bodies. Tubular regeneration occurs within 15 to 30 days. These mechanisms have been well studied. AG accumulate in the renal cortex, where concentrations can attain 20 times that of the serum concentration peak.
Cortical elimination is slow, taking weeks. All AG's are not equally nephrotoxic, with varying accumulation and alteration of subcellular components. Several therapeutic or clinical factors may favour their toxic effect. Short-term treatment and monitoring of

concentrations should avoid excessive renal accumulation. Certain
factors such as age, pre-existing renal disease and water and salt
depletion (furosemide), as well as certain therapeutical associations
(dextran, iodized products) favour this toxicity and call for
modification of dosage and increased monitoring.

Keywords : antibiotics, immunology, toxicity, lysosomes, enzymology.

INTRODUCTION

     Since the beginning of the chemotherapeutic era, nephrotoxicity has
been recognized as a complication of antibiotic therapy. The risk of
kidney damage was great with agents such as sulfonamides, bacitracin
and neomycin. With new antibacterial agents the problem of
nephrotoxicity has persisted. Antibiotics are the principal cause of
drug-associated nephropathies. They are responsible for acute
interstitial nephropathy (AIN) or acute tubulo-interstitial nephropathy
(ATIN) due to two different pathophysiologic mechanisms: a drug-
induced immunologic process and direct action due to drug accumulation.
The kidneys are particularly susceptible to toxicity because they have
- a large blood supply relative to their weight, thus delivering a
large drug dose to the kidneys - a large endothelial surface where
antigen-antibody complexes can localize - a high concentraion of
excretory products on the tubular luminal surfaces - tubular cells with
high metabolic rates which are susceptible to poisoning by drugs
located on their surfaces or within the cells as a result of the
reabsorption secretory processes.

IMMUNOLOGICALLY-MEDIATED ACUTE INTERSTITIAL NEPHRITIS

     The possibility that drug-induced immunologically mediated renal
damage might occur in man is now widely accepted.

     β-lactam agents. A list of offending β-lactam agents has been
recently reported (1). Methicillin is the prime offender implicated in
about 100 cases. The clinical picture is often characteristic.
Patients were treated with normal doses of methicillin over 10 or 20
days of therapy. The daily dose received was quite variable and ranged
from 4 to 18 grams per day. The interval between the beginning of
treatment and drug reactions ranged from 5 to 60 days. Presenting
symptoms included fever, skin rash, macroscopic hematuria and marked
eosinophilia (10-40%). Appel and Neu noted that despite the common
occurrence of features of hypersensitivity only 31% of patients had the
complete hypersensitivity triad of rash, fever, eosinophilia. Thus,
one must not wait for the appearance of the classic picture in making a
presumptive diagnosis of β-lactam related acute interstitial nephritis.
Some degree of proteinuria was commonly found usually quantitated 1 +
to 3 +. Hematuria remains the cardinal urinary finding, it was noted
in 91% of the cases and seen macroscopically in a third of the cases.
Eosinophils in urine sediment were detected by Wright stain in 15 out
of 18 cases examined. Since this technique has only recently become
popular, it is likely that is will become a common finding in drug

induced acute interstitial nephritis. Non-oliguric acute renal failure developed in only some of these patients and renal recovery was usual after discontinuation of therapy, though permanent renal damage has been observed (2). It is noteworthy that symptoms may recur when patients are given another penicillin derivative or even cephalosporin (3). Renal biopsy was performed in approximately half of the patients. The renal lesion is generally formed by patchy tubular cell damage, interstitial edema and leucocyte infiltration with mononuclear phagocytes, lymphocytes, plasma cells and often eosinophils. Epithelioid cell granuloma with giant cells were observed. Glomerular and vascular lesions are rarely found.

The pathogenesis of this hypersensitivity reaction is unclear. In some patients, a dimethoxyphenyl penicilloyl (DPO) hapten and IgG deposits were detected in a linear pattern along the tubular basement membrane (TBM). Linear deposits of C_3, IgG and DPO deposits along the glomerular basement membrane (GBM) were found in only one case. The initial step may be binding of penicillin hapten to structural protein of the renal interstitium and for tubular basement membranes leading to the formation of a stable hapten-protein conjugate. Subsequently, either humoral or cell mediated mechanisms or renal damage may predominate. A humoral mechanism is supported by the presence of circulating antibodies reactive against the TBM's, the presence of linear TBM deposits and a decreased serum complement level. Many cases however have not shown evidence of circulating anti TBM or anti-interstitial antibodies or of linear deposits. It has been suggested that anti TBM antibodies are an epiphenomenon - a result of an association with a primary cell mediated form of renal damage (4,5). There is some evidence for cell mediated tubulo-interstitial nephritis in experimental animal models (6). Thus, both humoral and cell mediated mechanisms appear to play a role in these β-lactam related AIN (7).

Penicillin is widely used and 30 years after the introduction of penicillin G, only occasional cases of AIN have been described (3). The clinical symptoms and the pathological picture were similar to those of methicillin-induced AIN. A typical biphasic temperature response occurred with subsidence of fever due to the underlying infection for which the antibiotic was prescribed followed by a recurrence of fever 8-44 days later and accompanied by skin rash, eosinophilia, proteinuria, macroscopic hematuria and renal insufficiency. An interstitial mononuclear infiltration and eosinophils were observed. The glomeruli appeared normal and no vasculitis was found (6). Immunofluorescence studies were performed in a few reports. Traces of IgG in the renal interstitium and rare granular C_3 deposits near the tubules were noted (5). A rabbit antiserum to penicillin G bound diffusely to the interstitium, TBM and GBM, it bound equally well to the autopsy tissue of several patients with normal kidneys who had received penicillin shortly before death (5).

AIN has also been noted in association with treatment with ampicillin (8-10), carbenicillin (1), oxacillin (1,11), nafcillin (12) and amoxicillin (13). AIN can also certainly occur with cephalosporin therapy, cephalothin however usually produces acute tubular damage, clinical and pathological findings suggested interstitial nephritis (11, 14,15).

The optimal therapy for drug induced AIN is still uncertain. Discontinuation of the offending agent is necessary. The use of corticosteroids or immunosuppressive agents remains controversial.

Some authors have indicated a beneficial and occasionally striking improvement with corticosteroid therapy. There are equally clear reports of no apparent beneficial results from such therapy (16). Kleinknecht et al (3) think that a different penicillin derivative or even a cephalosporin are to be avoided in patients with histories of antibiotic-induced AIN.

Rifampicin. About 60 cases of acute renal failure (ARF) due to rifampicin have been reported (17). The reason for rifampicin treatment was always tuberculosis. Patients receiving rifampicin on an intermittent basis have a much higher incidence of renal disease. In these cases it was noted that intermittent treatment, once or twice weekly for 1-6 months led to ARF of short duration whereas discontinuous treatment - eg continuous treatment for 3-12 months, interrupted for 4 days to 9 months and then followed by resumption of rifampicin; led to severe ARF occurring shortly after intake of a single dose of rifampicin. The interval between the last dose and reactions to drug ranged from a few hours to 10 days. Dizziness, chills, fever, lumbar pain and myalgia appeared. Skin rash and dark urine were also noted. Eosinophilia was uncommon. Thrombocytopenia and hemolysis were present in a very few cases. The urine contained proteins, numerous red cells and urinary casts; macroscopic hematuria was exceptional. Severe oliguric ARF, requiring hemodialysis or peritoneal dialysis, was more frequently observed than non-oliguric ARF. Full renal recovery was usual but permanent renal damage has been occasionally reported (8). It is not clearly stated whether prednisone therapy may be beneficial. Renal biopsy was performed in approximately half of the patients. Interstitial edema and mononuclear cell infiltration without eosinophils were prominent. Diffuse or focal necrosis or degeneration of the proximal tubular cells were also frequent. Immunofluorescence was negative in most cases. Kleinknecht (3) noted, in their review, focal C_3 and C_4 deposits along the TBM in only four cases. C_3 and immunoglobulin deposits were exceptionally found in the glomerular mesangium or within some arteriolar walls.

Rifampicin-dependent antibodies were found in at least 13 patients (3). The antibody titers declined within months to undetectable values. The anti-rifamcipin antibodies are of the IgG and/or IgM type, reacting in the presence of the drug. Patients receiving rifampicin on an intermittent basis have a much higher incidence of rifampicin-dependent antibodies than those receiving the daily therapy. In addition, the incidence of adverse reactions is higher in patients with such antibodies than in patients without them. Therefore, it has been postulated that daily administration of rifampicin may result in formation of antigen-antibody complexes, preventing antibody excess and thereby the adverse reactions that occur with high levels of free antibody (18). From a practical point of view, avoiding an intermittent rifampicin regimen is mandatory. Determination of the serum anti-rifampicin titre may be useful when rifampicin is to be started again within weeks or months after continuous treatment has been stopped (3).

DRUG-INDUCED NEPHROTOXICITY

Cephalosporin nephrotoxicity is reviewed by Balazs (this volume).
We will discuss only tetracycline, vancomycin, polymyxin and
aminoglycoside nephrotoxicities.

Tetracycline. Administration of tetracycline to patients with pre-
existing renal disease can worsen uremia. For the most part this is
not due to a toxic effect of tetracycline on the kidney but rather to
the increased load of urea which results from the anti-anabolic effect
of tetracycline on protein synthesis. In certain circumstances,
however tetracycline can be nephrotoxic. The use of outdated
tetracycline has been associated with a reversible Fanconi syndrome,
characterized by a proximal tubular defect leading to proteinuria,
glycosuria, aminoaciduria, hypercalciuria, hyperphosphaturia and
uricosuria (19).
The impairment in concentrating ability was slowly reversible after
cessation of the drug. These effects are related to the degradation
products of tetracycline (epitetracycline, epianhydrotetracycline and
anhydrotetracycline) that are apt to occur when the outdated product is
exposed to acid and heat (20,21). Citric acid is now no longer used as
a preservative for tetracycline capsules and this precaution has
prevented recurrences of Fanconi syndrome.
Demethylchlortetracycline administration has been associated with
vasopressin resistant nephrogenic diabetes insipidus. Polyuria and
polydipsia develop a variable time after the ingestion of the drug and
is reversible with cessation of therapy (8,22). Demethylchlortetracycline has been used to treat the syndrome of inappropriate
antidiuretic-hormone secretion.
Because uremia can be exacerbated by the tetracyclines they should
not be given to patients with renal failure - nevertheless doxycycline
does not accumulate in renal failure and can be prescribed.

Vancomycin. Nephrotoxicity of vancomycin has not been clearly
established in man. Vancomycin has been incriminated in the renal
injury of several patients treated for severe staphylococcal
infections. Proteinuria, hematuria, increased BUN were noted (9). In
many other cases, vancomycin has been administered without renal damage
(23). It was suggested that reports of vancomycin nephrotoxicity may
have been related to impurities in the drug (24). Thus, whether
vancomycin itself is nephrotoxic is debatable but it should be used
cautiously in patients with prior renal disease since ototoxicity is
more frequent in these patients.

Polymyxin. Nephrotoxicity is a well recognized side effect of
polymyxin B and polymyxin E (colistimethate). These antibiotics are
not so frequently used as in the past. Observations of nephrotoxic
effects of polymyxin are now very rare. Nephrotoxicity of polymyxin B
is characterized by proteinuria, cylinduria, leucocyturia. At doses of
3mg/kg/day nitrogen retention and a decreased glomerular filtration
rate occur in patients with previously normal renal function. In the
presence of prior renal dysfunction, lower doses cause renal damage
(1). Renal alterations are usually reversible but renal function may
be permanently impaired (25). Colistimethate can also produce renal
damage with proteinuria, casts, blood urea nitrogen and creatinine
increasing. This appears more likely to occur in patients with pre-

existent renal damage. The renal dysfunction is reversible with cessation of therapy. Accidents due to massive doses of colistin given to patients with previously normal renal function have been observed on many occasions (26,27). Acute renal failure with preserved diuresis, accompanied with psychiatric symptoms could appear. Renal biopsies have shown proximal tubular damage and acute tubular necrosis. Renal function returned slowly to normal when colistimethate was withdrawn. In a review by Koch-Weser et al (28) on the adverse effects of colistin methane sulfonate during 317 courses of therapy in a variety of severe infection states, it was noted that adverse renal effects occurred in 20.2% of the patients. The antibacterial effect of polymyxins derives from a surfactant disorganization of the bacterial cell membrane. Essential to this action is the presence of free terminal amino groups. Colistimethate, with one less free amino group than polymyxin B could be less nephrotoxic. In fact, if the surface active amino groups are covered by methane sulfonation, diminution of antibacterial activity results and it is necessary to administer a higher dose of the antibiotic and nephrotoxicity could be the same. Nephrotoxicity may be mediated through the drug's action as a surfactant on renal tubular cells. Thus, polymyxins should be used only when other, less toxic antibiotics, are not available.

Aminoglycosides. Nephrotoxicity has been recognized as a major complication of aminoglycoside antibiotics for many years. The incidence is between 10 to 20% of treated patients. Aminoglycoside nephrotoxicity is characterized by a wide range of nephron disturbances (29-31). Polyuria due to a decrease in urine concentrating capacity is one of the earliest abnormalities of renal function. Low level tubular proteinuria, increased urinary β_2-microglobulin, increased urinary excretion or lysosomal enzymes as well as membrane bound enzymes derived from proximal tubular cells are early indicators of tubular changes and this occurred with all aminoglycosides. Depression of glomerular filtration rate is a later manifestation of aminoglycoside nephrotoxicity. Aminoaciduria or glycosuria are less frequent. Acute renal failure was rarely noted. Aminoglycosides induce tubular cell necrosis which is confined almost exclusively to the pars convoluta and pars recta of proximal tubules. Aminoglycosides are concentrated within the renal cortex in animals and humans. Microinjection studies demonstrated net absorption of ^{3}H gentamicin in the proximal tubule without transtubular secretion (32). Just and Haberman (33) and Silverblatt and Kuehn (34) by elegant radioautographic techniques demonstrated apical transfer of aminoglycosides by pinocytosis with lysosomal sequestration. This uptake can be inhibited by anoxia, metabolic inhibitors, cationic amino acids and other aminoglycosides (35). Using a technique of micro-dissection of rabbit kidney nephron, we have been able to examine the distribution of gentamicin along a single nephron from the glomerulus to the collecting duct. No detectable amount of labelled product was found within the glomeruli, the descending and ascending loop of Henle and the distal tubular cells. Large amounts of silver grain were seen within the proximal tubular cells. The gentamicin distribution was not homogenous all along the proximal tubular cells: an increasing gradient of intra cellular gentamicin concentraion was recorded from the initial portion of the proximal tubule (36). Subcellular localization of gentamicin was studied after centrifugation of kidney cortex homogenates in a linear sucrose gradient. The distribution pattern of gentamicin resembles closely those of two marker enzymes of lysosomes: N-acetyl-β-D-glucosaminidase and cathepsin B (36). We have measured free and total activity ratios of lysosomal enzymes on a fraction enriched in lysosomes in the presence of increasing doses of aminoglycosides. All aminoglycosides labilize the lysosomes of rat kidney *in vitro* at concentrations ranging from 5 to 50μg/ml of standard lysosmal suspension. It was thus possible to classify the aminoglycosides in terms of decreasing intensity of their labilizing effect: sisomicin, tobramycin, gentamicin, neomycin, lividomicin, kanamycin, amikacin, netilmicin, streptomycin, paromomycin and kasugamycin (36). This labilizing effect of lysosomes was also observed *in vivo* after an 8 day treatment with gentamicin 10mg/kg/day. Lysosomes show prominent alterations after treatment with aminoglycosides. The earliest identifiable lesion seen by electron microscopy in animals and man is an increase in the number and size of the secondary lysosomes which contain myeloid bodies. The myeloid bodies are an electron dense lamellar structure suggestive of concentric and densely packed membranes. These lesions resemble those induced by treatment with amphiphillic cationic drugs. Subsequently, other changes became evident including a decrease in the number and height of microvillae of brush border membrane, swelling of mitochondria, cytoplasmic vacuolization and dilation of the cisternae of rough endoplasmic reticulum. The changes progress to total disorganization and disruption of cellular organelles with frank cellular necrosis. The activity of lysosomal enzymes has been studied in kidney cortices of rats treated with 10, 20, 50 and 100mg/kg of gentamicin, tobramycin, amikacin, netilmicin for 2 to 24 days. Most of the enzymes including glycosidases, proteases, hydrolases showed no significant changes in their specific activity. We have noted a striking decrease in sphingomyelinase and alanine aminopeptidase. This decrease in sphingomyelinase activity had to be paralleled to the phospholipidosis demonstrated recently in the renal cortex (36).

Aminoglycoside nephrotoxicity has attracted the attention and interest of a number of investigators. The exact mechanism of renal failure is still unknown. Several factors contribute to nephrotoxicity. 1) High concentration of aminoglycoside in the renal cortex. For a given aminoglycoside, the risk of nephrotoxicity increases as the renal concentration of drugs increases. This concentration is a function of dose, frequency of drug, administration and duration of drug treatment until a plateau is reached that reflects saturation of the transport process. In fact, this accumulation is not the only factor or the predominant one to explain the nephrotoxicity of aminoglycosides. These antibiotics exhibit different nephrotoxicity potential and these do not correlate with the degree to which these drugs are concentrated in renal cortex. Neomycin is concentrated in renal cortex at a relatively low rate, yet this drug had the highest nephrotoxicity potential. Netilmicin is accumulated to approximately the same extent as gentamicin. Yet netilmicin's nephrotoxicity seems to be significantly less than that of gentamicin (31). 2) The intrinsic toxicity of these aminoglycosides is reflected by the effect of these molecules on structural latency of the lysosomal membranes (36). 3) The extent to which the drug affects the lysosomal catabolism of phospholipids resulting in a renal phospholipidosis. It should be metioned that the formation of myeloid bodies per se does not explain why the epithelial cells undergo necrosis since amphiphillic drugs may produce a still more pronounced lipid storage in tubular cells without induction of necrosis. The disturbance of the lipid metabolism within the lysosomes increases the concentration of certain

reactive intermediates which by themselves damage the lysosomal
membrane. 4) Exposure of other intracellular structures to the
contents of altered lysosomes could perhaps result in cell injury or
death. We have noted that *in vitro* exposure of mitochondria from
hepatic and renal tubular cells to aminoglycosides has shown impairment
of state 3 respiration and stimulation of state 4. The effect is
dependant on the Na, K, Ca and Mg content in the incubation medium.
The relative potency of various aminoglycosides in producing effects on
mitochondrial respiration correlates with the number of free amino
groups on the molecule (37). 5) It is known that the acidic
phospholipids are linked to the functional properties of the cell
membrane via their capacity to bind calcium and magnesium. Competition
of aminoglycosides with divalent cations Ca and Mg have been described
in a number of systems. Thus, the initial binding of aminoglycosides
to plasma membrane phospholipids may be important in the pathogenesis
of aminoglycoside-induced acute renal failure via alterations in both
membrane structure and function.

CONCLUSION

    Although animal experimentation contributes to the understanding of
the basic mechanism of antibiotic nephrotoxicity the extrapolation of
these data to the human remains premature. The compilation of the
available clinical studies are not always easy to interpret. The
definition of adverse effects on kidney function is not uniform. In
many observations, it is noted "probable" or "possible" nephrotoxic
effect but it is really completely artificial. A multiple cause
etiology could not be ruled out. It is really difficult to separate
the antibiotic-induced nephrotoxic element from adverse effects of
underlying disease. Severe infections, sepsis, shock, dehydration
especially in elderly patients, affect the kidney function by lowering
the glomerular filtration rate. Thus, it is necessary to follow up
prospective studies in man with the control of many parameters to know
in the future the safer antibiotics to use.

REFERENCES

1.   Appel GB and Neu HC, New Engl J Med 296:663, 1977.
2.   Mayaud C, et al, New Engl J Med 292:1132-1133, 1975.
3.   Kleinknecht D, et al, Contr Nephrol 10:42-52, 1978.
4.   Baldwin DS, et al, New Engl J Med 279:1245-1252, 1968.
5.   Colvin RB, et al, Ann Intern Med 81:404-405, 1974.
6.   Heptinstall RH, Amer J Path 83:214-222, 1976.
7.   Appel GB, Clin Nephrol 13:151-154, 1980.
8.   Maxon MR, and Rursky EA, Millit Med 138:500-501, 1973.
9.   Ruley EJ and Lisi LM, J Pediat 84:878-881, 1974.
10. Tannenberg AM, et al, J Amer Med Ass 218:449, 1971.
11. Burton JR, et al, Johns Hopk Med J 134:59-62, 1974.
12. Parry MF, et al, J Amer Med Ass 225:178-181, 1973.
13. Appel GB, et al, Arch Intern Med 138:1265-1268, 1978.
14. Engle J E, et al, Ann Intern Med 83:232-233, 1975.
15. Harrington JP and McCluskey RT, New Engl J Med 293:1308-1316,
     1975.

16. Border WA, et al, New Engl J Med 291:381-384, 1974.
17. Kleinknecht D, et al, Med Mal Infect 7:117-121, 1977.
18. Kleinknecht D et al, Lancet 1:1238-1239, 1972.
19. Gross JM, Ann Intern Med 58:523-528, 1963.
20. Benitz KF and Dierneier HF, Proc Soc Exp Biol 115:930-935, 1964.
21. Frimpter GW, et al, J Amer Med Ass 184:111-113, 1963.
22. Singer I and Rotenberg D, Ann Intern Med 79:679-683, 1973.
23. Waisbren BA, et al, Arch Intern Med 106:179-193, 1960.
24. Kirby WMM and Divelbiss CI, Antibiot Ann 4:107-117, 1956.
25. Jawetz E, Pediat Clin N Amer 8:1057-1071, 1961.
26. Lissac J, et al, J Urol Nephrol 70:789-793, 1964.
27. Rapin M, et al, Press Med 73:1529-1531, 1965.
28. Koch-Weser J, et al, Ann Intern Med 72:857-862, 1970.
29. Fabre J, Nephrologie 1:37-43, 1980.
30. Fillastre JP, et al, Néphrologie 1:145-152, 1980.
31. Kaloyanides GJ and Pastoriza-Munoz E, Kidney Int 18:571-582, 1980.
32. Pastoriza-Munoz E, et al, Kidney Int 16:440-450, 1979.
33. Just M and Haberman E, Naunyn-Schmiedeberg's Arch Exp Path Pharmak 30:67-76, 1977.
34. Silverblatt FJ and Kuehn C, Kidney Int 15:335-345, 1979.
35. Porter GA and Bennett WM, Amer J Physiol 10:F1-F13, 1981.
36. Morin JP, et al, Kidney Int 18:583-590, 1980.
37. Weinberg JM and Humes HD, Arch Biochem 205:222-231, 1980.

NEPHROPATHIES ASSOCIATED WITH THE USE OF ANESTHETICS

Richard I. Mazze

Department of Anesthesia, Stanford University School of Medicine, Stanford, California 94305, USA and Veterans Administration Medical Center, Palo Alto, California 94304, USA

Anesthetic nephrotoxicity is due to biotransformation of the fluorinated hydrocarbon inhalation agent to inorganic fluoride. This is a clinically significant problem only with methoxyflurane. The predominant factor in the production of methoxyflurane nephrotoxicity appears to be anesthetic dosage. Possible secondary factors include: 1) a high rate of methoxyflurane metabolism and sensitivity of the kidney to inorganic fluoride toxicity; 2) concurrent treatment with other nephrotoxic drugs; 3) pre-existing renal disease; 4) surgery of the urogenital tract, aorta or renal vasculature; 5) repeat administration of methoxyflurane leading to accumulation of inorganic fluoride; and 6) concurrent treatment with enzyme inducing drugs, such as, phenobarbital.

Isoflurane and halothane are not metabolized to a sufficient extent to cause inorganic fluoride nephropathy under any circumstance. Enflurane administration will not result in clinically significant renal impairment although it can cause a detectable decrease in concentrating ability. (Key Words: Nephrotoxicity; Inorganic fluoride; Methoxyflurane; Enflurane; Isoflurane; Halothane.)

Specific anesthetic induced nephrotoxicity was first reported by Crandell et al. [1] in 13 of 41 patients anesthetized with methoxyflurane (Penthrane; $CH_3-O-CF_2-CHCl_2$) for abdominal surgical procedures. They noted polyuria with a negative fluid balance; elevation of serum sodium, osmolality, and urea nitrogen levels; and fixed urinary osmolality, close to that of serum. Patients were unable to concentrate urine despite fluid deprivation and vasopressin administration, suggesting that the difficulty was of renal origin and was not due to antidiuretic hormone (ADH) deficiency. Impairment persisted for 10 to 20 days in most patients, but in three, abnormalities still were present after more than one year. In 1971, Mazze et al. [2,3] confirmed these findings. They reported a controlled, randomized, prospective clinical evaluation of renal function following methoxyflurane anesthesia in which abnormalities were found in all cases. Patients exhibited polyuria unresponsive to ADH administration, marked weight loss, delayed return of normal urinary concentrating ability, hypernatremia, serum hyperosmolality,

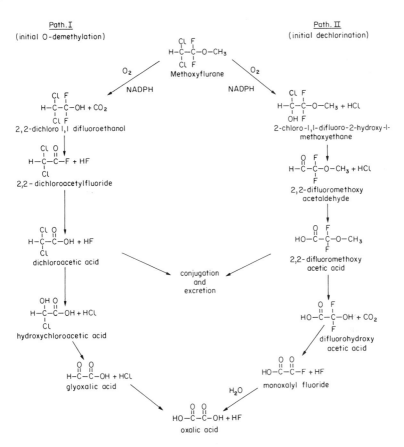

FIGURE 1.   Metabolic pathways for the metabolism of methoxyflurane.
In pathway I, methoxyflurane is O-demethylated in the liver, producing 2,2-dichloroacetyl fluoride and a molecule of hydrogen
fluoride.   Dichloroacetyl fluoride is further hydrolyzed to
dichloroacetic acid, liberating another molecule of hydrogen
fluoride.   A portion of the dichloroacetic acid is excreted in the
urine while a second part is oxidatively dechlorinated to glyoxalic
acid.   The latter is enzymatically oxidized to oxalic acid.   In
pathway II, methoxyflurane is enzymatically dechlorinated to 2,2-
difluoromethoxyacetic acid.   A portion is excreted in the urine and
a second part is O-demethylated in the liver.   Subsequent
dehydrofluorination and hydrolysis result in oxalic acid formation.   From Mazze et al. [3], reproduced with permission of
Anesthesiology.

elevated BUN and serum creatinine, increased serum uric acid and a
decrease in uric acid clearance. Of particular interest, all patients
demonstrated increased serum and urinary concentrations of two
nephrotoxins, inorganic fluoride and oxalic acid, with the highest
levels found in individuals with the greatest impairment of renal function. To explain the increased levels of inorganic fluoride and oxalic

Serum Fluoride

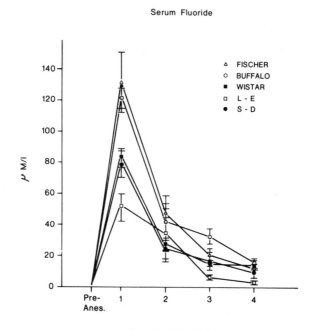

FIGURE 2. Daily serum inorganic fluoride activity (mean ± S.E.) before anesthesia and after 3 hr of 0.5% methoxyflurane anesthesia. Fischer 344 and Buffalo rats had significantly greater increases than rats of the other three strains. n = 6, each group. Abreviations: (L-E) Long-Evans rats; (S-D) Sprague-Dawley rats. From Mazze et al. [8], reproduced with permission from the Journal of Pharmacology and Experimental Therapeutics.

acid following methoxyflurane anesthesia, two complementary metabolic routes for biotransformation of methoxyflurane were proposed (Fig. 1).

EVIDENCE OF METHOXYFLURANE NEPHROTOXICITY IN AN ANIMAL MODEL

In spite of the clinical evidence [1-5], a cause-effect relationship between methoxyflurane administration and renal dysfunction was not clearly defined until a series of animal studies by Mazze and associates [6-9]. In one experiment they administered methoxyflurane to rats of five different strains and found that Fischer 344 and Buffalo rats metabolized methoxyflurane to a greater extent than did Sprague-Dawley, Wistar or Long-Evans rats, as evidenced by higher serum fluoride levels (Fig. 2). However, only Fischer 344 rats developed functional (Fig. 3) and morphological evidence of a renal lesion [8]. Also, when Fischer 344 rats were injected with inorganic fluoride (NaF), they developed a much greater degree of renal insufficiency than did identically treated Buffalo rats. From these data it was concluded that there were strain differences among rats in the rate of metabolism of methoxyflurane to inorganic fluoride and in the susceptibility to the nephrotoxic effects

Urine Volume

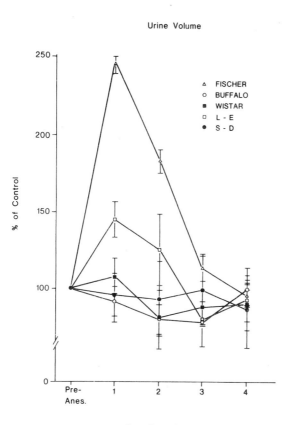

FIGURE 3.   Daily 24-hr urine volume (mean ± S.E.) before and after 3
hr of 0.5% methoxyflurane anesthesia.   Significant postanesthetic
increases occurred only in Fischer 344 rats. From Mazze et al. [8],
reproduced with permission of the Journal of Pharmacology and
Experimental Therapeutics.

of inorganic fluoride. A high rate of methoxyflurane defluorination and
increased sensitivity to inorganic fluoride results in polyuric renal
insufficiency in Fischer 344 rats.

In another study inorganic fluoride rather then oxalic acid was
implicated as the primary nephrotoxic metabolite. Sodium fluoride injection resulted in dose-related polyuric renal insufficiency and
morphological abnormalities similar to those found after methoxyflurane
anesthesia [9].   Injection of oxalic acid did not cause these changes
(Fig. 4). Clinical observations support these conclusions: acute
oxalic acid intoxication results in classical anuric renal failure
whereas chronic oxaluria is associated with kidney stone formation but
not polyuria [10,11]. Also, inorganic fluoride has a potent inhibitory
effect on many enzyme systems including those thought to be involved in
solute transport [12], a property not shared by oxalic acid. Other
studies in Fischer 344 rats showed that renal functional and morpho-

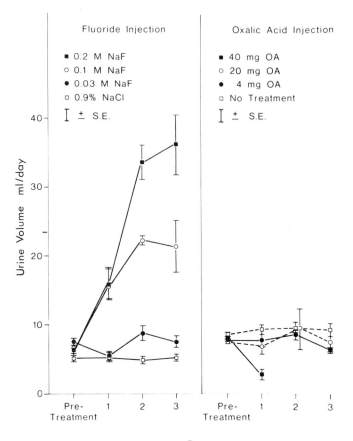

FIGURE 4.   Daily urine volume (mean ± S.E.) before and after treatment
with oxalic acid (OA) and sodium fluoride (NaF).   Dose-related
polyuria occurred after NaF injection but not after OA.   Treatment
with 444 μmole of oxalic acid resulted in oliguria. From Cousins et
al. [9], reproduced with permission of the Journal of Pharmacology
and Experimental Therapeutics.

logical changes were proportional to the dose of methoxyflurane and that
polyuria, whether resulting from methoxyflurane anesthesia or from
direct injection of NaF, was ADH-resistant (Figs. 5 and 6) [6-8].
Later, it was established that biotransformed methoxyflurane rather than
the unmetabolized, molecular form of the anesthetic was the cause of
nephrotoxicity [9]; induction of the hepatic mixed function oxidase
system by phenobarbital treatment resulted in increased defluorination
and nephrotoxicity (Fig. 7) whereas enzyme inhibition with SKF 525A
resulted in decreased defluorination and an attenuated renal lesion
(Fig. 8).
    Previous animal studies with methoxyflurane [13,14] had not been of
value in detecting the renal lesion for several reasons. Urinary output

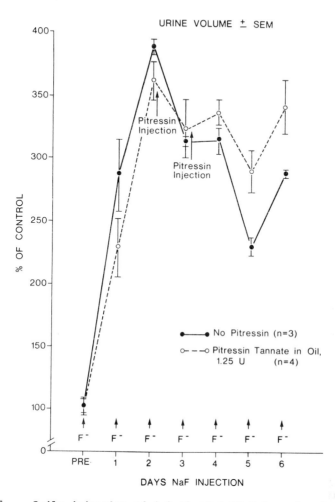

FIGURE 5.   Daily injection of 1.0 ml of 0.1M NaF produced a sustained
  increase in 24-hr urine volume which was not affected by pitressin
  (ADH) administration.   F⁻ denotes inorganic fluoride injection.
  From   Mazze,   et   al   [22],   reproduced   with   permission   of
  Anesthesiology.

had not been monitored, methoxyflurane dosage was too low and the
species tested (dogs and monkeys) were relatively insensitive to the
nephrotoxic effects of inorganic fluoride.

SITE AND MECHANISM OF THE ACUTE RENAL LESION

    Because polyuria following methoxyflurane anesthesia was ADH-resis-
tant, it was originally postulated [3] that high levels of inorganic
fluoride caused nephrotoxicity by interfering with the action of ADH in
the distal convoluted tubule and collecting duct.   However, in animal

URINE VOLUME ± SEM

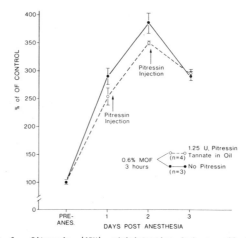

FIGURE 6.   Pitressin (ADH) administration had no effect on the
increase in 24-hr urine volume following administration of 0.6%
methoxyflurane for 3 hr. SEM=standard error of mean. From Mazze, et
al. [22], reproduced with permission of Anesthesiology.

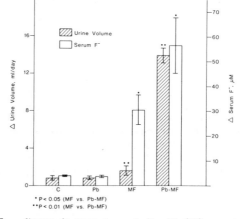

FIGURE 7.   Changes in serum inorganic fluoride (F⁻) concentration and
urine volume for the first 2 days after anesthesia (day 15): (C)
control group I; (Pb) phenobarbital, 25 mg/kg, b.i.d., days 11 to
14, group II; (MF) methoxyflurane, 0.25% for 1.5 hr, day 15, group
III; (Pb-MF) phenobarbital preceding methoxyflurane, group IV. Δ =
days 7 to 10 minus days 16 to 17, mean ± S.E. From Cousins et al.
[9], reproduced with permission of Journal of Pharmacology and
Experimental Therapeutics.

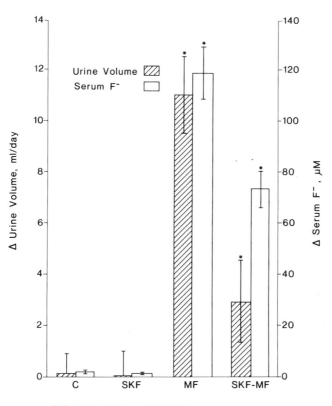

* P < 0.01 (MF vs. SKF-MF)

FIGURE 8.   Changes in serum inorganic fluoride (F⁻) concentration and
      urine volume for the first 2 days after anesthesia (day 11): (C)
      control, group I; (SKF) SKF 525-A, 50 mg/kg, group II; (MF) methoxy-
      flurane, 0.5% for 3 hr, group II; (SKF-MF) SKF 525-A followed by
      methoxyflurane, group IV.   Δ = days 7 to 10 minus days 12 to 13,
      mean ± S.E. From Cousins et al. [9], reproduced with permission of
      the Journal of Pharmacology and Experimental Therapeutics.

[6-9] and human [4,15,16] studies, the majority of structural changes
have been in the proximal convoluted tubule with damage ranging from
mitochondrial swelling to necrosis of epithelial cells. Proximal tubular dilatation and oxalate crystal deposition also have been described.
Few abnormalities have been noted in the distal nephron. Currently it
is thought that inorganic fluoride acts by a number of mechanisms: 1)
by interfering with iso-osmotic reabsorption of proximal tubular fluid.
This would place an excessive load on the more distal nephron, particularly the ascending limb of the loop of Henle, and would lead to reduced
renal medullary osmolality and decreased reabsorption of water from the
collecting ducts. Large volumes of dilute urine would then be formed in
spite of the presence of ADH; 2) by inhibiting enzyme systems necessary
for ion transport in the ascending limb of the loop of Henle. This
would result in decreased renal medullary osmolality and in polyuria;

and 3) by damaging the collecting ducts thereby rendering them insensitive to ADH.   The morphological components of the lesions suggested in
2) and 3) may be to subtle to be detected by available histological
techniques.

STUDIES IN MAN

After animal studies appeared conclusive, a randomized, prospective
study was undertaken in surgical patients in which methoxyflurane dosage
was precisely documented and the renal functional changes that occurred
at each dosage level were carefully determined [17].   The results of
that study clearly established that methoxyflurane was a dose-related
nephrotoxin in man.   A positive correlation was observed among the
following variables: degree of nephrotoxicity; methoxyflurane dosage
expressed in MAC-hours; and serum inorganic fluoride concentration.
(MAC is the minimum alveolar concentration of anesthetic necessary to
prevent movement in respone to surgical incision in 50% of patients.
MAC-hours is determined by multiplying alveolar anesthetic concentration
by the duration of administration of anesthetic.) Patients exposed to
methoxyflurane for 2.0 MAC-hours or less had peak serum inorganic
fluoride concentrations below 40 µM; this was not associated with
nephrotoxicity (Fig. 9). The threshold of subclinical toxicity occurred
at an exposure of 2.5-3 MAC-hours, corresponding to peak serum inorganic
fluoride levels of 50-80 µM.   These patients had a delayed return to

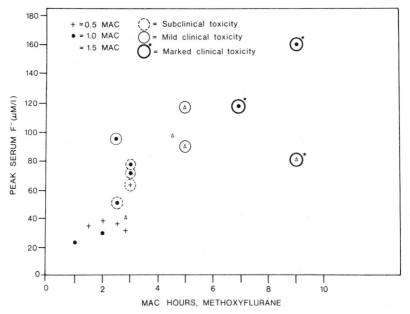

FIGURE 9.   Peak serum inorganic fluoride concentration (F⁻) and degree
of nephrotoxicity are shown at increasing doses of methoxyflurane.
Methoxyflurane dose correlated with both peak serum inorganic
fluoride concentration and degree of nephrotoxicity.   From Cousins
and Mazze [17], reproduced with permission of the Journal of the
American Medical Association.

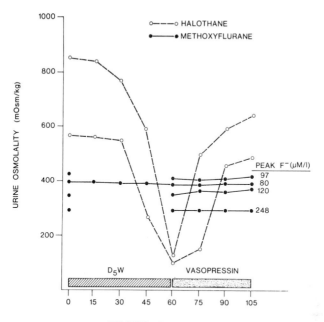

FIGURE 10. Vasopressin (ADH) infusion test in four patients with
polyuric renal dysfunction following methoxyflurane anesthesia.
Control infusions are shown for two patients following halothane
anesthesia. Patients anesthetized with methoxyflurane were unable
to decrease urine osmolality in response to a one liter fluid load
of 5% dextrose in water or increase urine osmolality after ADH
infusion. From Cousins and Mazze [17], reproduced with permission
of the Journal of the American Medical Association.

maximum preoperative urine osmolality, unresponsiveness to ADH
administration and elevated serum uric acid concentration. Mild
clinical toxicity occurred at an exposure of 5 MAC-hours (serum
inorganic fluoride concentration, 90-120 μM). In addition to the
abnormalities noted above, serum hyperosmolality, hypernatremia,
polyuria, and low urinary osmolality were present. Clinical toxicity
occurred in all three patients exposed to methoxyflurane for more than 7
MAC-hours (peak serum inorganic fluoride levels, 80-175 μM). Abnormalities in serum and urinary variables were even more pronounced than
at lower methoxyflurane dosages and polyuria in all patients was
resistant to ADH (Figure 10).

A significant permanent reduction in creatinine clearance was seen in
only one patient who was exposed to 9 MAC-hours of methoxyflurane and
required a course of gentamicin for a postoperative *Pseudomonas* wound
infection. His creatinine clearance was reduced from 107 ml/min prior
to gentamicin treatment to 40 ml/min after four days of antibiotic therapy [18]. It is likely that initially he had an inorganic fluoride
induced renal lesion which was aggravated by gentamicin treatment. The
additive nephrotoxicity of methoxyflurane and gentamicin have subsequently been demonstrated in Fischer 344 rats [19].

From these studies we can conclude that the Fischer 344 rat is an appropriate model for studying methoxyflurane (inorganic fluoride) nephrotoxicity in man because: 1) both species metabolize methoxyflurane to inorganic fluoride and oxalic acid; 2) both species develop polyuria after methoxyflurane anesthesia which is proportional to the serum inorganic fluoride level and is pitressin-resistant; 3) both species develop other similar renal functional abnormalities (hypernatremia, elevated BUN, hyperuricemia) after methoxyflurane; and 4) both species develop similar renal morphological lesions.

RENAL EFFECTS OF OTHER FLUORINATED INHALATIONAL ANESTHETICS

Enflurane (CHC1F-CF$_2$-OCHF$_2$; Ethrane).   In a study in which Fischer 344 rats were exposed to enflurane for 6 to 10 hours, vasopressin-resis-

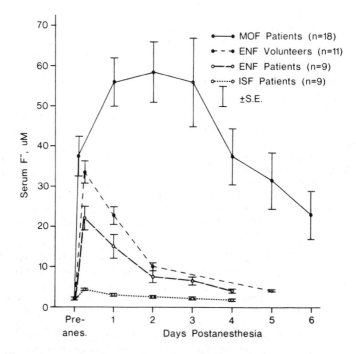

FIGURE 11.   Serum inorganic fluoride (F$^-$) concentrations prior to and following enflurane, isoflurane and methoxyflurane anesthesia. There was a significant increase in F$^-$ concentrations immediately following enflurane anesthesia reaching a mean peak value of 22.2 ± 2.8 µM, 4 hours after anesthesia was terminated; mean duration of anesthesia was 2.7 ± 0.3 MAC hours [21]. F$^-$ levels in volunteers receiving enflurane anesthesia peaked at 33.6 ± 2.8 µM [22]; mean duration of exposure was 9.6 ± 0.1 MAC hours. Following 2-3 MAC hours of methoxyflurane [17], mean peak serum F$^-$ concentration was higher, 61 ± 8 µM, and declined more slowly than after enflurane. There was almost no increase in F$^-$ following isoflurane administration [27].

tant polyuria resulted; as with methoxyflurane this occurred when serum inorganic fluoride concentration was approximately 50 µM [20]. The latter findings suggest that there may be a potential for enflurane nephrotoxicity in man. However, studies in patients and volunteers without renal disease have not supported this suggestion [21,22]. Following enflurane exposure of surgical patients averaging 2.7 ± 0.3 MAC-hours, peak serum inorganic fluoride concentrations in the nephrotoxic range generally did not occur. Exceptions were noted in two patients: one obese patient had a peak serum inorganic fluoride level of 51 µM following a dose of 4.2 MAC hours of enflurane; another patient exposed to isoniazid, a compound which can induce enflurane defluorination, had a peak serum inorganic fluoride level of 106 µM following an enflurane exposure of 3.8 MAC-hours. However, in all patients anesthetized with enflurane, including the two mentioned above, serum inorganic fluoride peaked earlier and at a lower level, and fell much more rapidly than after methoxyflurane anesthesia, as noted in a comparable group of patients from a previous study (Fig. 11) [17]. It is the peak serum inorganic fluoride level and the duration this level is maintained which primarily determines whether nephrotoxicity will occur. Results of renal function studies support the conclusions that may be inferred from these metabolism data. The absence of postoperative hypernatremia, serum hyperosmolality, increased serum creatinine and BUN and the normal response to vasopressin is conclusive evidence that postoperative renal function was normal.

In the study of volunteers exposed to enflurane for an average of 9.6 MAC-hours [22], a clinically insignificant concentrating defect was observed. Mean maximum urinary osmolality before enflurane anesthesia was transiently reduced from approximately 1030 ± 50 mOsm/kg to 770 ± 50 mOsm/kg the day after anesthesia. Values had returned to normal by the next time they were tested on day 5 after anesthesia. These findings are in agreement with the results of previous studies in surgical patients without kidney disease. There was no increase in BUN or serum creatinine in surgical patients studied by Dobkin, et al. [23], and Graves and Downs [24] have made a similar observation.

Isoflurane (CHF_2-O-$CHClCF_3$; Forane). Isoflurane, like enflurane is a pentafluorinated methylethyl ether. It is metabolized to inorganic fluoride in man and animals [25,26], but to a much lesser extent than methoxyflurane. Animal studies with isoflurane have failed to demonstrate any evidence of nephrotoxicity [26]. Its renal effects and metabolism were studied in nine surgical patients; six control patients received halothane [27]. Isoflurane was metabolized to a slight extent with a mean peak serum inorganic fluoride concentration of 4.4 ± 0.4 µM, measured six hours postanesthesia. Postanesthetic renal function including the response to vasopressin was normal in both groups. It appears that the metabolism of isoflurane to inorganic fluoride is of insufficient magnitude to cause renal dysfunction.

Halothane ($CF_3CClBrH$; Fluothane). Halothane, although biotransformed to a greater extent than isoflurane or enflurane is not defluorinated under normal conditions of clinical administration. Thus, it has no potential for causing inorganic fluoride nephrotoxicity [3,17,22,26,27,].

TABLE 1. Nephrotoxic potential of fluorinated anesthetic agents.[*]

Agent	nmol F$^-$/ 30 min/ mg Protein	Oil:Gas X λ	Defluorination = Index	Nephrotoxic Potential
MOF	2.00	930	1860	1.00
DOC	1.41	275	387	0.23
ENF	1.31	99	129	0.07
SEVO	1.82	56	101	0.05
ISO	0.51	94	48	0.03
HAL	0	230	0	0.00

[*] Modified from Mazze, et al. [28].

ABBREVIATIONS: MOF, Methoxyflurane; DOC, Dioxychlorane; ENF, Enflurane;
SEVO, Sevoflurane; ISO, Isoflurane; HAL, Halothane.

IN VITRO STUDIES

   While *in vivo* studies with Fischer 344 rats may be the most unequivocal approach outside of human investigations for examining anesthetic
induced nephropathy, compared with *in vitro* studies they are costly and
time consuming. Since the inhalational anesthetics are nephrotoxic only
as a consequence of their defluorination, a more convenient method of
screening for nephrotoxic potential might be simply to measure *in vitro*
inorganic fluoride formation.   However, this would give us only one
dimension of a two dimensional variable, as the length of time the serum
inorganic fluoride level remains elevated after anesthesia, not just the
peak value, is related to the development of nephrotoxicity. Assuming,
then, that anesthetic exposure is the same, the area under the serum
inorganic fluoride curve reflects both the biological stability of the
anesthetic agent and the availability of the drug for postoperative
metabolism.   Solubility of the drug in body tissues, particularly fat,
is the best index of the latter property of anesthetic agents. Thus, we
have formulated a defluorination index which is the product of *in vitro*
inorganic fluoride formation and the oil:gas partition coefficient of
the anesthetic agent (Table 1) [28].
   To determine inorganic fluoride production, hepatic microsomes from
untreated Fischer 344 rats are prepared in the usual fashion [28] and
then reacted with the inhalational anesthetic agents.   Nanomoles of
inorganic fluoride liberated in 30 minutes per mg of microsomal protein
are then determined.   The corn oil:gas partition coefficient is used to
approximate anesthetic solubility in body fat. The defluorination index
for methoxyflurane, 1860, has been assigned a nephrotoxic potential of
one.   Other drugs have been given proportional values based on their
defluorination index. The derived values correlate well with the demonstrated nephrotoxicity of the fluorinated inhalational agents tested to
date.   Enflurane has a nephrotoxic potential of 0.07; a clinically
insignificant, inorganic fluoride induced, urinary concentrating defect
has been observed after prolonged enflurane exposure of volunteers
[22]. Fischer 344 rats also demonstrate minimal polyuria and vasopressin resistance after 6-10 hours of enflurane administration [20].   Of

the other clinically available agents listed in Table 1, halothane has a nephrotoxic potential of 0.00 and its administration has not been associated with a concentrating defect in humans [17] or in the animal model [7,9]. Isoflurane has a very low nephrotoxic potential, 0.03 and also is devoid of adverse renal effects in patients [27] and in Fischer 344 rats [26]. Another investigational agent, sevoflurane [C(CF$_3$)$_2$H-O-CH$_2$F] is also free of adverse renal effects in Fischer 344 rats [29]; its nephrotoxic potential is quite low, 0.05. The effect of sevofluorane on urinary concentrating ability has not been determined in man.

The index of nephrotoxic potential also may have predictive value for new agents. We recently tested dioxychlorane (C$_3$H$_2$Cl$_2$F$_2$O$_2$), an experimental inhalational anesthetic agent of dioxolane ring structure in our hepatic microsomal preparation. Inorganic fluoride production was 1.41 nmol/30 min/mg protein. The oil:gas partition coefficient of dioxychlorane is 275 (Table 1). These data yield a defluorination index of 387 and a nephrotoxic potential of 0.23, a value more than three times higher than that calculated for enflurane, an agent which causes a sub-clinical concentrating defect. Because of this, dioxychlorane was not synthesized commercially.

REFERENCES

 1. Crandell WB, Pappas SG, Macdonald A, Anesthesiology 27:591-607, 1966.
 2. Mazze RI, Shue GL, Jackson SH, J Amer Med Assoc 216:278-288, 1971.
 3. Mazze RI, Trudell JR, Cousins MJ, Anesthesiology 35:247-252, 1971.
 4. Taves DR, Fry BW, Freeman RB, J Amer Med Assoc 214:91-95, 1970.
 5. Frascino JA, Vanamee P, Rose PP, N Engl J Med 283:676-679, 1970.
 6. Kosek JC, Mazze RI, Cousins MJ, Lab Invest 27:575-580, 1972.
 7. Mazze RI, Cousins MJ, Kosek JC, Anesthesiology 36:571-587, 1972.
 8. Mazze RI, Cousins MJ, Kosek JC, J Pharmacol Exp Ther 184:481-488, 1973.
 9. Cousins MJ, Mazze RI, Kosek JC, Hitt BA, Love FV, J Pharmacol Exp Ther 190:530-541, 1974.
10. Hockaday TDR, Clayton JE, Frederick EW, Smith Jr., LH, Medicine 43:315-345, 1964.
11. Jegher J, Murphy R, N Engl J Med 233:208-215, 1945.
12. Wiseman A, Handbook of Experimental Pharmacology, Pharmacology of Fluorides, F.A. Smith, Ed., Springer-Verlag, New York, 1970, pp 48-93.
13. Byles PH, Dobkin AB, Jones DB, Can Anaesth Soc J 18:397-407, 1971.
14. Cale JO, Orarjs CR, Jenkins MT, Anesthesiology 23:248-250, 1967.
15. Aufderheide AC, Arch Pathol 92:162-166, 1971.
16. Halpren BA, Kempson PL, Coplon NS, J Amer Med Assoc 223:1239-1242, 1973.
17. Cousins MJ, Mazze RI, J Amer Med Assoc 225:1611-1616, 1973.
18. Mazze RI, Cousins MJ, Brit J Anesth 45:394-398, 1973.
19. Barr GA, Mazze RI, Cousins MJ, Kosek JC, Brit J Anesth 45:306-312, 1973.
20. Barr GS, Cousins MJ, Mazze RI, Hitt BA, Kosek JC, J Pharmacol Exp Ther 188:257-264, 1974.
21. Cousins MJ, Greenstein LR, Hitt BA, Mazze RI, Anesthesiology 44:44-53, 1976.

22. Mazze RI, Calverley RK, Smith NT, Anesthesiology 46:265-271,
    1977.
23. Dobkin AB, Kim D, Choi JK, et al., Can Anaesth Soc J 20:494-498,
    1973.
24. Graves CL, Downs NH, Anesth Analg (Cleve) 53:898-903, 1974.
25. Hitt BA, Mazze RI, Cousin MJ, et al., Anesthesiology 40:536-542,
    1974.
26. Cousins MJ, Mazze RI, Barr GA, Kosek JC, Anesthesiology
    38:557-563, 1973.
27. Mazze RI, Cousins MJ, Barr GA, Anesthesiology 40:536-542, 1974.
28. Mazze RI, Beppu WJ, Hitt BA, Br J Anaesth 51:839-844, 1979.
29. Cook TL, Beppu WJ, Hitt BA, Kosek JC, Mazze RI, Anesthesiology
    43:70-77, 1975.

CHEMICAL ASSOCIATED RENAL PAPILLARY NECROSIS

Peter H. Bach and James W. Bridges

Robens Institute for Industrial and Environmental Health and Safety, and the Department of Biochemistry, University of Surrey, Guildford, Surrey GU2 5XH, UK

ABSTRACT

Renal papillary necrosis in man has been associated most often with an inappropriate chronic intake of analgesic or, more recently, non-steroidal anti-inflammatory drugs. Histologically similar lesions can be induced chronically or acutely by the administration of several groups of chemicals.

Previously attempts to define the molecular pathogenesis of the lesion have suggested:-

i) counter-current concentration, ii) ischaemic injury, iii) inhibition of prostaglandin synthesis, iv) the generation of biologically reactive intermediates, v) perturbed intermediate metabolism or vi) an immunological response. None of these proposed mechanisms have, however, provided a unifying hypothesis by which to explain the lesion and its secondary consequences.

Recent data have shown that disruption of the medullary glycosaminoglycan matrix is the earliest histochemically discernable change, which precedes an acutely induced "model" lesion. Perturbation of the ground substances has also been confirmed biochemically. Loss of the ground substance could lead to the subsequent disruption of the nephron (and its associated vascularity) in the medulla. There is also a secondary loss of the unique urinary Tamm-Horsfall glycoprotein from the distal nephrons of the kidney, aggregates of which lodge in the residual collecting ducts of necrosed papilla.

A similar sequence of events may underly both the chronically induced lesions in animals and the pathological course seen in man, although a different molecular pathogenesis could be responsible. Perturbation of the medullary matrix is common to several types of papillary necrosis, irrespective of aetiology. Analgesics and non-steroidal anti-inflammatories depress glycosaminoglycan synthesis, an effect which would be most marked in the kidney by virtue of the pharmacokinetics of these compounds.

Altered medullary glycosaminoglycans and glycoproteins would also explain the loss of urine concentrating ability and could contribute to

the common clinical features of secondary renal degeneration, recurrent
urinary tract infection and renal stone formation.

Key Words: Renal papillary necrosis, Analgesic, Non-steroidal anti-
inflammatory, Proteoglycan - Glycosaminoglycan, Tamm-Horsfall
Glycoprotein.

INTRODUCTION

Renal papillary necrosis (RPN) was first recognised as an iatrogenic
disease when Spuhler and Zollinger (1) drew attention to the apparent
increase in the incidence of "chronic interstitial nephritis" and
highlighted the association between this condition and an abusive intake
of analgesics. The mixed analgesics preparations consumed by these
patients all contained phenacetin, which was assumed to be the solitary
aetiological common denominator. Current evidence favours the idea that
most, if not all, analgesics and anti-inflammatory drugs have the
potential to give rise to the lesion. Several other classes of widely
used industrial chemicals and environmental contaminants also cause a
similar lesion experimentally, a potential toxicological problem which
has not been fully evaluated.

RPN has many possible underlying causes (Table 1). The lesion is most
difficult to diagnose (except at autopsy, and even here it can easily be
overlooked), thus the true incidence of drug-induced papillary
necrosis in man can only be a poor estimate. The low reported incidence
in the USA (0.2%) may be under-diagnosis (2) and Cove-Smith (3) has
reported a probable 30% underestimation in the prevalence of this lesion
in the UK. The literature relating to the topic of analgesic associated
renal papillary necrosis is extensive (2-11) and up to 1973 over 3200
confirmed cases had been reported (4).

DIAGNOSIS OF RPN IN MAN

The clinical symptoms now known to be caused by the early development
of analgesic associated renal papillary necrosis (Table 2), are unlikely
to draw attention to themselves. It is only the observed presence of a

Table 1. Factors associated with the development of renal papillary
necrosis.

FREQUENTLY REPORTED FACTORS:-
Diabetes Mellitus   Analgesic Abuse
High Dose Non-steroidal Anti-inflammatory Drug Treatment
Upper Urinary Tract Obstructive Uropathy (consequence?)
Recurrent Urinary Tract Infection (consequence?)
Sickle Cell Haemoglobinopathy
Acute Pyelonephritis (superimposed?)
Dehydrated Newborn Infants (frequently jaundiced)

LESS FREQUENTLY REPORTED FACTORS:-
Renal Vein Thromboses   Glomerulonephritis
Chronic Alcoholism   Renal Transplant
Severe Jaundice   Systematic Candidosis
Calycael Artheritis   Prolonged Hypotension
Dehydration in Children   Trauma

Table 2.   Clinical features associated with renal papillary necrosis.

PATIENT GROUP
 Females predominate 3:1 to 8:1
 Most commonly 40 to 60 year age group

EARLY SYMPTOMS
 Psychiatric abnormalities:- dependence, anxiety, neurosis, headaches.
 Upper gastrointestinal disease:- peptic and duodenal ulcers*.
 Haematology:- anaemia (due to gastric bleeding*), cyanosis*.

INTERMEDIATE SYMPTOMS
 Urinary tract disease:- bacteriuria, sterile pyuria, nocturia, dysuria,
   microscopic haematuria, ureteral colic, lower back pain.
 Renal function:- defective concentrating capacity and acidification,
   proteinuria, azotemia.

LATE SYMPTOMS
 Hypertension
 Cardiovascular malfunction
 Renal calculi
 Renal malfunction (increase in BUN)
 Urothelial carcinoma
 Acute renal failure

* Direct consequence of high dose analgesic intake.
Data from (4-11,90).

papilla in the urine, a rare and oft overlooked occurrence (7), that is likely to pinpoint the lesion. The progression of renal damage is insidious and as much as 60 to 85% of renal function may be compromised before symptoms become obvious. These will not, however, in themselves, be indicative of the underlying cause.

Radiological examination may not identify papillary necrosis, if the necrosed papilla remains in situ,(12) and even when loss of the papilla is obvious the only available criteria for confirming the underlying cause of a diagnosed papillary lesion as excessive analgesic intake is:-
i) the absence of other possible clinical causes,
ii) the identification of abnormally high plasma or urine levels of these compounds (or their metabolites) over long periods, and/or
iii) a history of high dose, long term analgesic usage (13). Patient histories are, however, notoriously unreliable, especially if, as is the case, there is a social stigma associated with abusive drug consumption. Further, the question of what quantity, and which analgesic(s) has been abused have been obscured by failure to identify the causative agents and hence the lack of a definition of what constitutes "an abusive consumption".

The reasons underlying excessive use have been evaluated by many research reports (2-4) and include such factors as the mood altering effects of constituents such as codeine, caffeine and other sedatives or stimulants; attempts to "overcome" caffeine withdrawal headaches; personality traits or an accepted social custom.

The criteria for abuse of "analgesics" is poorly defined, and covers the broad range of 2 to 35kg (of phenacetin) over 3 to 45 years. Other reports suggest an accumulative estimate of each of the separate analgesic intakes, or the total mixed analgesic consumption (3,14), which are probably a more valid measure of abuse.

The Epidemiology, Geographical Distribution and Incidence of RPN in Man. A number of reports (6,8,13) have highlighted the cause and effect relationship between analgesics and RPN. There is an increased incidence of lesions in these patients, a proportionality relationship between the estimated amount of analgesic (phenacetin) consumed and the extent of renal damage, and the renal function stabilises (or improves) in patients who ceased to abuse analgesics, while those who continued to consume excessive amounts showed a steady deterioration in renal function.

Much of the early data supported the theory that phenacetin was the solitary underlying cause of RPN. Gilman (15), however, questioned the validity of this theory, and suggested that each or all of the constituents in mixed analgesics may have contributed. The question has still not been resolved, but most analgesic and nonsteroidal anti-inflammatory drugs (NSAID) have been shown to induce the lesion experimentally, if not in humans. There have been no reports of the development of papillary necrosis in patients who took only phenacetin, but the prescribing of phenacetin on its own has always been uncommon. Recently there has been some evidence to support the view that salicylates can cause RPN in rheumatic patients, but has this been questioned and refuted (3,6,16).

The dangers of "therapeutically induced" papillary damage from mixed analgesics has been highlighted by Cove-Smith (3) who reported that 42% of patients who were taking prescribed high dose, longterm mixed analgesic therapies for either rheumatoid arthritis or osteoarthritis developed "analgesic nephropathy", and 88% of these patients died from chronic or acute renal failure. The analgesics taken were either aspirin-phenacetin or aspirin-paracetamol mixtures.

Recently, a number of reports have suggested that the "second generation" NSAID may induce papillary necrosis on man at commonly prescribed doses. The NSAID so far linked to this lesion include propoxyphene (2), fenoprofen, naproxen, phenylbutazone, indomethacin, ibuprofen and alclofenac (17). One unsubstantiated report suggests that therapeutic doses of dapsone have induced RPN (18).

Over the last few years increasing attention has been focussed on the possible importance of paracetamol (acetaminophen) in the underlying aetiology of analgesic associated renal disease. The attempts to link paracetamol and RPN have been speculative, especially those that draw inferences on the chronic nephrotoxicity of paracetamol from its acute effects. Rosner (4), is of the opinion that the initial "link" between papillary necrosis and paracetamol was forged by the observations that paracetamol (a major metabolite of phenacetin) was concentrated across the medulla, but that phenacetin was not. This tenuous association has most probably been strengthened by the uncompromised view that phenacetin was the original and only cause of papillary necrosis, and failure to decrease the frequency of analgesic nephropathy when phenacetin was replaced by paracetamol in mixed analgesics. Mitchell et al. (19) have described a mechanism to explain the acute hepatic necrosis that develops as a consequence of high doses of paracetamol. This mechanism has been transposed to "fit" chronically induced renal papillary necrosis. Recently, Duggin's group (20) have shown that paracetamol undergoes co-oxygenation with arachidonic acid to form a reactive intermediate, the formation and covalent binding of which was most pronounced in the medulla.

Dubach has reported a prospective study where urinary paracetamol was used as the distinguishing criterion of patient analgesic abuse (13). However, these investigations fail to differentiate between patients who took analgesic mixtures which contain paracetamol as opposed to those containing phenacetin, nor did it define the actual analgesic mixtures.

One of the other puzzling features underlying the aetiology of RPN is the varying incidence between countries and especially within countries (2,4-8,14). Some of these variations may relate to a lack of awareness, and consequently failure to diagnose the condition, but it is equally possible that the extent of abuse and the nature of the offending chemicals varies both between and within countries. The per-capita consumption of phenacetin (still assumed by many to be representative of total analgesic intake) has been used to support this hypothesis (14). A number of workers have questioned the origins of these figures, the validity of the assumptions underlying the calculations (2,4) and the fact that "consumptions" are similar in Canada, South Africa, the United Kingdom and the USA, but there are markedly different incidences of analgesic associated nephropathies.

THE PATHOLOGICAL COURSE OF RPN IN MAN

The evolution of papillary necrosis shows that the lesion is primarily one of the apex of the papilla and this then progresses slowly to include secondary cortical changes (7). Burry (7,21) has defined the lesion in terms of early, intermediate and total necrosis.

Early papillary necrosis. The earliest reported changes related to papillary necrosis include necrosis of the limbs of Henle, the capillaries and interstitial cells (with or without calcification) and PAS staining shows a thickening of the basement membrane. Burry et al., (7,21) report a more intense staining of mucopolysaccharide, but Gloor (22) suggested loss of this ground substance from the interstitial matrix. Cryostat sections showed an accumulation of lipid material deposited in the necrosed tissue, which constitute columns progressing up the medulla, but leaving the vasa recta, some limbs of Henle and the collecting ducts intact. Needle shaped crystals have been noted in lipid-rich necrosed areas. These were reported to be cholesterol esters and possibly arachidonic acid (21).

Intermediate papillary necrosis. Those anatomical elements in the medulla which were previously unaffected, with the exception of collecting ducts and occasional vasa recta, are necrosed. Calcium deposits are more extensive in the necrosed area and the outer medulla may show atrophy and sclerosis, and varying degrees of fibrosis and inflammatory response. Bone formation may also occur in the necrosed papilla.

The necrosed papilla ghost may remain attached or separate from the medulla. The separated papilla may remain in situ, or it may leave the minor calyces either whole or fragmented. The medulla above the line of sequestration is never histologically normal, but, nevertheless, is coated by transitional epithelium. Bacterial infection may be superimposed upon these changes (7,21,22).

Total papillary necrosis. Total papillary necrosis develops from the progressive destruction of the inner medulla, following either a crescent or a central course.

Cortical   changes   associated   with   papillary   necrosis.
Microscopically the cortex appears normal until the papilla which
"functionally underlies it" is totally necrosed. The form of cortical
changes then depend on the degree of sclerosis at the line of
sequestration (if the papilla is cast off).   The cortical changes are
essentially characterised as "chronic interstitial nephritis", and
include   tubular   atrophy,   interstitial   fibrosis,   inflammatory
infiltration, glomerular changes, hyalinization within collecting ducts
and destruction of vascularity.

Changes in the pelvis, ureter and bladder associated with papillary
necrosis. An association between analgesic abuse and carcinoma of the
pelvis, ureter and bladder transitional epithelia has been clearly
established (21-23).   The underlying pathogenesis is not clear, but it
has been suggested to be induced via biologically reactive intermediates
formed from phenacetin.   There appears to be little experimental work
published in this area, but recent studies on cyclo-oxygenase mediated
xenobiotic metabolism suggest this may be a key factor. (See Rush and
Hook, this volume).

In addition, non-malignant histopathological changes in the pelvis,
ureter and bladder (such as thickening of capillary walls, sclerosis of
lamina propria, and changed fat and collagen deposition) have been
reported (21,22).

The Prognosis for Patients Suffering from Papillary Necrosis.   The
prognosis for patients with RPN depends on an early diagnosis. If the
patient stops abusing the offending compounds the kidney function may
either improve dramatically or it may stabilise. If, however, (as more
often seems to be the case) large doses of the drugs are still consumed
the kidney function will deteriorate and eventually the patient will
develop renal failure.

Even if patients are part of a sophisticated dialysis or transplant
programme their prognosis is poor Kingsley et al. (24) have reported a
51% death rate in a 5 year period, while Cove-Smith (3) reported a mean
survival of 31.3 months from the time when patients were diagnosed to be
suffering from RPN.

EXPERIMENTALLY INDUCED RPN

Investigations into the pathogenesis of experimentally induced
nephrotoxicity is hampered by species and sex variation in renal
morphology, the complexities of renal function and the inherent
limitations of the available means of assessing renal malfunction.
These difficulties are further compounded by the many and varied
degenerative changes that are often encountered in untreated control
animals over long periods.   These are either genetically linked
spontaneous lesions, or they occur with increasing frequency in aging
animals.

Murine strains and hybrids develop an age related RPN that occurs with
increasing frequency and severity after 12 months.   The necrosis was
preceded by amyloid infiltration of the interstitium at the papillary
apex and extended to other functional areas, but was limited to the
medulla. The changes in the cortex were secondary to papillary necrosis
and included amyloid deposits and cystic dilatation (25).

Papillary necrosis has also been reported to occur in adult homogenous Gunn rats (26) where the necrotic lesion developed from the papilla tip and was always associated with a deposit of bilirubin-like crystals in the interstitial matrix.

NON-CHEMICALLY INDUCED RENAL PAPILLARY NECROSIS.
    Dietary induced RPN. Renal papillary necrosis can be induced by maintaining rats on a fat-free diet for a long period (27); see also Molland this volume. The molecular pathogenesis has generally been explained on the basis of an essential fatty acid deficiency limiting the availability of prostaglandin precursors, but several other possible mechanisms will be discussed below.

    Renal papillary necrosis induced by "manipulating" renal haemodynamics. Ligating the ureter caused both hydronephrosis and papillary necrosis in 64% of dogs (28), and in uninephrectomized rabbits (29), but not rats (30). The induction of necrosis was explained on the basis of an increased intra-pelvic pressure altering renal haemodynamics (28,29).
    Occluding the major renal blood vessels may also cause papillary necrosis. Total renal vein occlusion caused a complete medullary necrosis, with some cortical lesions (31) and chronic partial renal vein occlusion caused necrosis (of varying complexity) in the medulla, but occluding the renal artery caused necrosis of the cortex with only minimal changes in the medulla (29,32-34).

    Heterologous serum-induced renal papillary necrosis. RPN develops in rats within 72h of injecting human serum iv (35). The incubation of this heterologous serum with rat erythrocytes resulted in haemolysis and agglutination, but the papillotoxic potential of the incubated serum was lost.
    It seems likely that agglutinated rat erythrocytes could disrupt medullary blood flow, but Patrick et al (35) also suggested a direct antigenic effect of human serum components on the rat kidney. This may be supported by the tremendously violent and rapid (within 30s) fixation of human antibodies, and of complement, when the rabbit kidney is xenoperfused with fresh human blood (36), Recently, Rudofsky et al (37) reported (without comment) that SJL mice were found to have papillary necrosis 56 days after immunization with rabbit tubular basement membrane. The possibility that this was a spontaneous lesion (vide supra) cannot, however, be excluded until similar nephroimmune responses have been induced in other species.

CHEMICALLY-INDUCED RENAL PAPILLARY NECROSIS.

    A diverse array of chemicals are now known to have papillotoxic potential. However, the induction of renal papillary necrosis is disturbingly irreproducible for many of these agents (4), presumably because of unrecognised and uncontrolled variables. A detailed review of the extensive literature on the topic is, however, beyond the scope of this chapter (see 4-8, 17 and 38 for reviews).
    The pathological course and possible molecular pathogenesis of the experimentally induced lesions are considered below. Several important points must, however, be highlighted. The diagnosis of chemically-induced papillary necrosis is not easy. The behaviour and appearance of test and control animals are normal and weight gains are similar (38).

Changes in blood biochemistry have been described, but they are either transitory and non-specific, or they reflect secondary cortical changes (39-41). Intravenous urograms apear normal in rats with an acutely induced total papillary necrosis (42) and conventional urine analysis fails to give a clear cut diagnosis of papillary necrosis, although it may demonstrate renal malfunction. The exfoilation of renal tubular cells follows the administration of many analgesics (see 5), but it is not indicative of an acutely induced papillary necrosis per se (43) and most likely reflects a response to an irritant compound. The pattern of enzymuria is not specific for papillary lesions (40,41) and, in common with proteinuria, may reflect cortical changes. Decreased urinary osmolality (due to the destruction of the anatomical elements responsible for concentration), lack of concentrating capacity and failure to acidify the urine after oral ammonium ion loading are the only features ascribed to papillary necrosis, but these may be transitory (11,9,41) and a number of other chemicals have been described which produce the same responses where the papilla appears to be morphologically normal (see Hansen this volume). Thus none of these functional changes are specific indications of papillary necrosis, and there are circumstances where apparently normal renal function is recognised in the presence of marked histological changes (39), although it is likely that the renal functional reserve capacity would fail under stress such as infection or dehydration.

The presence of RPN can only be established histopathologically, but the papilla tip may be missed unless painstakingly careful sectioning is undertaken. This difficulty is compounded by the re-epithelialisation of the truncated medulla when the necrosed area sloughs off. Thus a section of the medulla that appears to be cut obliquely may, in fact, be adjacent to the remnants of a necrosed area (39).

The papillotoxicity of analgesic and non-steroidal anti-inflammatory compounds and their structural analogues. Much of the published data is conflicting, often experimental details have been omitted (such as strain, sex, age, weight, dose regimens, routes of dosing, etc.) many of the findings are irreproducible (sometimes even in the same laboratory) and only a proportion of test animals ever suffer from the lesion after a protracted period of dosing (4). Within these constraints it has not been possible to establish the likely papillotoxic potential of each of the analgesic-NSAID group of medications, nor to delineate the molecular pathogenesis which underlies the development of RPN. A number of hypotheses have, however, been proposed and each will be considered below.

The papillotoxicity of non-analgesic compounds. A number of non-analgesic compounds have been shown to cause RPN. Two of these, ethylenimine (EI, 44) and 2-bromoethanamine (BEA) hydrobromide (45) were shown to cause an acutely developing lesion well over 50 years ago. BEA undergoes spontaneous cyclization to form EI, under aqueous alkaline conditions (46), which is commonly assumed to be the proximate papillotoxin which causes this lesion (47) for both compounds, but this has never been proved.

Experimentally, the most important features of the BEA- or EI-induced lesion include:-
i) the extent of the lesion is dose related, from a threshold value
(which causes an apex limited lesion) to a plateau level, where the
tissue is necrosed up to, but never beyond the corticomedullary
junction (48,49),

Table 3. Comparison of pathological changes in experimentally induced renal papillary necrosis and the lesions found in man.

Morphological and functional Changes	Type of renal papillary necrosis		
	Acutely induced (BEA and EI)	Chronically induced (Analgesic and fat-free diet)	Analgesic associated (Man)
Early:-			
Papilla apex primary site of lesion	Yes	Yes	Yes
Extends to include medulla but not beyond corticomedullary junction	Yes	Yes	Yes
Loss of thin loop of Henle and interstitial cells	Yes	Yes	Yes
Loss of vasa recta	Yes	Yes	Yes
Microvascular occlusion	No	Yes	Yes
Intermediate:-			
Loss of collecting ducts and covering epithelia	Yes	Yes	Yes
Changed staining of MPS matrix	increase then loss	loss	increase or loss
Epithelial hyperplasia	Yes	Yes	Yes
Inflammatory response	No	Yes	Yes
Regeneration and re-epithelialisation	Yes	Yes	Yes
Fatty changes	No	Yes	Yes
Calcification	Yes	Yes	Yes
Renal and bladder calculi	?	?	Yes
Urinary tract infection	Yes	Yes	Yes
Hyperplasia of transitional urothelia of pelvis, ureter and bladder	Yes	Yes	Yes
Late:-			
Secondary cortical changes overlying necrosed papilla	Yes	Yes	Yes
Cystic dilatation	Yes	Yes	Yes
Hypertension	After salt loading	Yes	Common
Fatty changes in papilla	No	Yes	Yes
Carcinoma of transitional urothelia of pelvis, ureter and bladder	No	No	Commonly associated with analgesic abuse

ii)   the extent of damage is reproducible within a particular dose
      range (48,49), particularly after BEA administration (48),

iii) the lesion develops in all animals given an effective dose, within
      48h (48,50,51).

iv)   the secondary consequences of RPN are indistinguishable from those
      associated with a chronically induced lesion (52).
      A major disadvantage of using EI is that it is chemically unstable,
explosive (46) and an established mutagen (53): BEA does not, however,
suffer from these particular limitations.

THE MOLECULAR PATHOGENESIS OF RENAL PAPILLARY NECROSIS.

     Surprisingly, there are many similarities between the pathological
course of the acutely and chronically induced lesions in animal model
systems, and those changes reported in humans. Table 3 compares these
pathological changes, although they develop on a different time scale.
     A number of theories have been postulated to explain the sequence of
events which precedes papillary necrosis in man and the experimentally
induced lesions in animals, but several different molecular events may
give rise to the same end effect. Thus mechanistic differences may exist
between the acutely (EI and BEA) and chronically (analgesic) precipated
lesions, despite the striking similarities in the pathological course of
the lesion.   In discussing the possible molecular pathogenesis it has
been convenient to establish artificial boundaries between what may be
similar or inter-related mechanisms.

     The Counter-current Concentration Mechanisms.   One of the most oft
cited mechanisms to explain papillary necrosis is based on the
supposition that a concentration gradient of the offending compound
(increasing from the cortex to the papilla) develops as a consequence of
the counter-current concentration mechanism.   This concentration
gradient is assumed to be high enough to exert a "direct" (although never
defined) toxic effect.
     The data is conflicting, whereas concentration gradients of
paracetamol (of 10 to 1 for conjugated molecule and 19 to 1 for free
compound) have been found in dehydrated dogs, there were no gradients for
phenacetin or aspirin (54-56).   Gault (57, 58) found only modest
increases in the medullary concentrations of phenacetin, aspirin and
paracetamol.   More recently, Molland (38) showed the distribution of
aspirin (assessed by autoradiography at the light microscopic level) was
greater in the medulla, where it was confined largely to the epithelium
of the proximal tubule, principally near the pars recta.
     These discrepancies may relate to the state of hydration of test
animals, species differences, or the methods used (chemical assay versus
radiolabel distribution, respectively), but all are of questionable
relevance because they were single dose studies. The autoradiographic
distribution of aspirin described by Molland (38) is also inconsistent
with the degenerative changes seen in the medullary interstitial cells
after chronic dosing.   More meaningful results may be derived from
autoradiographic studies during the course of chronic dosing.
     The counter-current concentration hypothesis also fails to take into
account the fact that both EI and BEA (48) induce a marked, almost
immediate diuresis.   Furthermore, there is a loss of concentrating
ability shortly after rats are given larger doses of analgesics

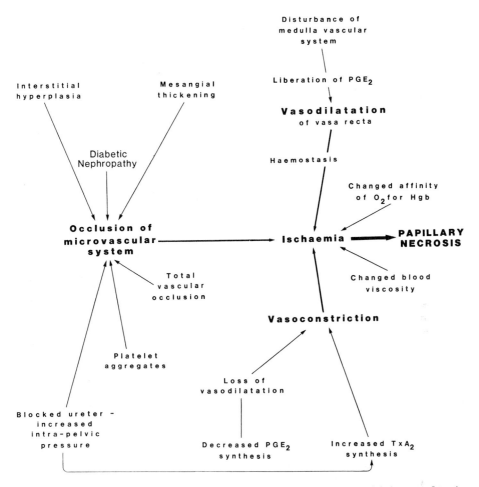

Figure 1. The possible pathophysiological changes which result in medullary ischaemic injury, from data of Shelley (8).

analogues (39) and one of the earliest "preclinical" symptoms of analgesic abuse in man (11) is similarly a nephrogenic-based failure to produce a urine of high osmolality.

Antipyrine has been shown to produce RPN (59), but this compound is apparently present in higher concentrations in the cortex than in the medulla, although the data needs to be confirmed by autoradiographic techniques, and after chronic dosing.

The fact that dehydration favours the exerimental induction of the lesion together with the suggested contribution of "hot climates" to human papillary necrosis (4-8) is thought to strengthen the importance of this mechanism. Dehydration would, however, put an added stress factor on the kidney. This mechanism does not alone explain the molecular pathogenesis underlying the lesion, but favours the concept that factors which lead to active water counter-current concentration may make the papilla more sensitive to toxic insult.

Medullary Ischaemia. The medulla is poorly perfused (compared to the cortex) and functions with a relatively low oxygen tension. This is assumed to predispose the papilla to "anoxic injury" and several possible mechanisms have been proposed by which a localised ishaemic injury might be induced chemically (Fig 1).

The induction of medullary lesions by vascular occlusion is assumed to support this concept, but stopping the blood supply to an organ for several hours will cause profound changes, especially so in the kidney where vascular flow is the quintescence of renal function.

Attempts to resolve the contribution of microvascular changes to papillary necrosis have given conflicting data. There is ample evidence (47,48,51,60,61) to show that micro-vascular change parallels or lags behind cell necrosis in the acutely induced models of RPN. Thus vasoconstriction does not appear to be a prerequisite to the development of the lesion. It is possible, however, that vasodilation of the vasa recta could cause haemostasis and lead to ischaemic injury.

Extensive vascular changes have been described for both the chronically-induced lesions in animals and for human kidneys (7,8,38,62,63), but it is impossible to be certain if these were the primary cause, parallel changes, a secondary effect or unrelated to the aetiology.

Alternatively, the whole concept of medullary anoxic injury may be a total misnomer. It is widely agreed that the medulla receives only about 10% of the renal blood flow, but it is generally overlooked that the kidneys process 25% of the resting cardiac output. The actual amount of blood which therefore perfuses the medulla is substantial, and has been estimated to be of the same order of flow as that perfusing the brain and 15 times that of muscle (64). Recently, Cohen (65) has highlighted the fact that the medulla cells have an extensive aerobic metabolism, although they possess the ability for anaerobic glycolysis. The difficulty in defining the metabolic nature of this tissue may rest in the heterogeneous nature of the cell population (See Bonner et al, this volume).

The Role of Renal Prostaglandins (PG) in Papillary Necrosis. Attention has been focussed on the fact that most analgesic and NSAID (and their analogues) inhibit PG synthesis by blocking the enzyme cyclo-oxygenase. It has been argued:-

a) that perturbation of PG synthesis might cause a reduced synthesis of PGE_2, or an increased synthesis of TXA_2, and either or both effects might cause vaso-constriction and hence local ischaemic injury (Fig. 1),

b) The analgesic compounds may cause profound changes in renal haemodynamics and induce ischaemic injury, and

c) Perturbation of prostaglandin synthesis might alter the trans renal osmotic compartments (see 8 and 11).

One of the theories offered to explain the papillary necrosis that develops after prolonged fat-free diet (38) is that the limited ingestion of arachidonic acid or its precursors might lead to the depletion of prostaglandin precursors. The role of altered prostaglandin metabolism in the pathogenesis of renal papillary necrosis is difficult, if not impossible, to assess on present evidence. The function of each prostaglandin in the normal kidney is far from clear, prostaglandins are rapidly metabolised, chemically unstable and most difficult to assay with qualitative and quantitative certainty. Furthermore, those substances which do inhibit "prostaglandin synthetase" may also cause several different effects on prostaglandin metabolism and many other

Table 4. The in vivo papillotoxic potential of biphenyl analogues, analgesics and NSAID compared to their inhibition of PG synthesis.

TEST COMPOUND	RPN INDUCED	INHIBITION OF PGE
Diphenylamine	++++	++++
Flufenamic acid	++++	
Indomethacin	+++	
Aspirin	+++	
N-Phenylanthranilic acid	+++	++
Diphenyl ether	-	
Diphenyl	+	
Diphenyl methyl alcohol	+++	+
Amidopyrine	++	
Diphenyl-2-carboxylic acid	-	-

From Hardy TL, Unpublished data.

effects which are totally unrelated to the prostaglandin system. Thus despite the relationship between the papillotoxic potential of various analgesics, NSAID and biphenyls and their inhibition of PGE synthesis (Table 4) this does not establish a cause and effect relationship. Similarly, the decreased levels of prostaglandin E_2 in the renal vein of rats treated with analgesics (11) may not establish any more than an already proven relationship between analgesics and the inhibition of PG synthesis.

Biologically reactive intermediates. The concept of metabolically generated electrophilic molecules disrupting cellular function by binding to "essential" macro- or micro-molecules has served to explain many toxicological enigmas. This approach has clarified much of the genesis of paracetamol-induced acute hepatic necrosis, and recently a similar mechanism was proposed to help explain a chronically induced lesion in the medulla (19). Mudge et al. (66), have since reported a marked depletion of renal glutathione and extensive covalently binding in both the cortex and the papilla after a single high dose of paracetamol. The papilla had lower endogenous glutathione concentrations, and a slower turnover of covalently bound radiolabelled paracetamol than the cortex.

The true significance of this covalent binding to the medulla must remain a matter for speculation, because a single high dose of paracetamol cause a proximal tubular lesion, and its only under very special conditions that chronic dosing with paracetamol causes papillary necrosis (63). Similarly, the significance of paracetamol co-oxygenation with arachidonic acid to form an active intermediate, most prominently in the medulla (20), still has to be related to the chronic nature of the lesion and other papillotoxic molecules.

The view that active metabolites contribute to renal papillary necrosis may be given some support by the fact that aspirin provides the acetyl group for which transacetylates macromolecules, most notably prostaglandin cyclo-oxygenase (67); that BEA may cyclize to ethylenimine (46) a potent alkylating agent (53) and that cyclophosphamide has been reported to cause papillary necrosis (68).

The generation of a reactive intermediate and its covalent binding to macromolecules does not, in itself, predestine cell necrosis. Nor does covalent binding related necrosis explain the molecular pathogenesis per se: it only suggests that some essential function is altered.

Chemically Induced Changes in Intermediate Metabolism as the Underlying Cause of Papillary Necrosis. A number of workers have probed the possibility that the increased concentration of papillotoxins (due to counter-current activity) could accentuate the inhibition of normal medullary metabolic functions. Davidson et al. (69,70) showed that paracetamol failed to alter the de novo synthesis of protein, but it did exacerbate the inhibitory effects of salicylic acid.

Goldberg et al. (71) reported that high concentrations of salicylate inhibited the pentose phosphate shunt, decreasing cellular concentrations of reduced glutathione, which might predispose to the covalent binding of electrophilic molecules. The effects of various compounds on key aspects of anaerobic glucose metabolism have given conflicting data (see ref 8) probably because some studies were on medulla tissue and others on outer medulla and cortex tubules. Thus the observations of Dawson, (72,73) and Szinicz et al., (74) are probably inapplicable to the medulla because in the former case medullary cells were absent from the in vitro preparations and in the latter mixed medulla and cortex cell types were used. Even the use of medulla slices or cell suspensions might not be appropriate to differentiate between the metabolic effects on different cell types unless additional techniques are applied to solve the problem of heterogeniety.

The Contribution of Immunological Changes to the Pathogenesis of Papillary Necrosis. A number of workers have speculated on the contribution of immunological changes to the chronically induced RPN, but evidence is conflicting. Hook et al. (75) raised the possibility that the development of RPN in only some of the human analgesic abusers might indicate an immunological basis for the disease. The possible contributions of the immunogenicity of salicylate and several phenacetin metabolites (e.g. phenetidine) has been discussed (4,13), but no immunodeposits in the medulla or cortex of patients with early analgesic nephropathy have been found (76). Similarly, there were no immunopathological changes in the medulla which might have suggested that an immune response had a part in the pathogenesis of the BEA-induced lesion (77).

Functional Changes in the Cortex as an Underlying Cause of Renal Papillary Necrosis. It is commonly assumed that papillary necrosis is caused primarily by a direct effect on one or more of the elements of the medulla. The nephron is, however, a highly structured and ordered array of cell types, each of which shows inter-dependance on the functioning of other cell types. It is thus possible that an altered function (without pathophysiological consequences) in one cell type of the nephron could have profound secondary effects on a more distal cell population, which could manifest as a pathological lesion.

The concept would be most difficult to probe, but such a mechanism might explain many of the anomalies associated with this lesion. A precedent for this concept has been set by the continuing failure to recognise that an important underlying cause of diphenylamine-induced cystic kidney (78) is, in fact, papillary necrosis (79).

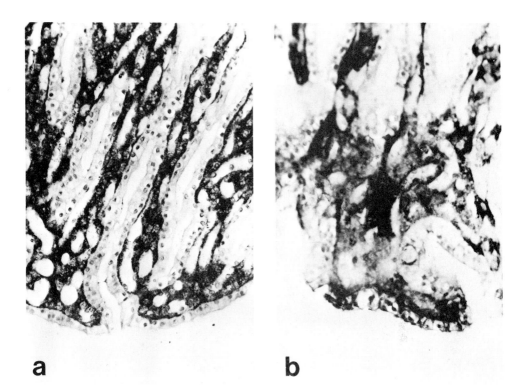

a   b

Figure 2. The histochemical changes in the medullary glycosaminoglycan ground substance of the rat papilla following the administration of BEA (50mg/kg,ip), a) Control and b) 18h after BEA. Hale's colloidal iron, counter stained with neutral red. X 3300

THE MEDULLARY GROUND SUBSTANCE AND RENAL PAPILLARY NECROSIS

It is widely appreciated that the medulla, particularly the papilla, is rich in extra cellular matrix material. This is made up of proteoglycans (POG) and their composite glycosaminoglycans (GAG). (These molecules have, in the past, been known as acidic or sulphated mucopolysaccharides). Very little attention has, however, been accorded the possible significance of this macromolecular ground substance in either the pathogenesis or the sequelae of papillary necrosis.

Whereas Burry (7,21) reported an increased intensity in the histochemical staining of the medullary matrix of human analgesic abusers, Gloor (22) reported that staining was much reduced. By contrast rats with a renal papillary necrosis which had been induced chronically with fat-free diet or with aspirin (38), or induced acutely with BEA (80) showed a lack of POG-GAG histochemical staining.

We have recently re-evaluated the time course changes in the medullary POG-GAG matrix during the course of BEA-induced RPN (48). Within an hour of BEA dosing the staining intensity of the medullary matrix increased dramatically. This changed to a granular appearance between 4 and 8h and a diffusive loss of histochemical staining of the medulla matrix paralleled, and was confined to those areas where necrotic change was taking place between 12 and 24h (Fig 2 a and b).

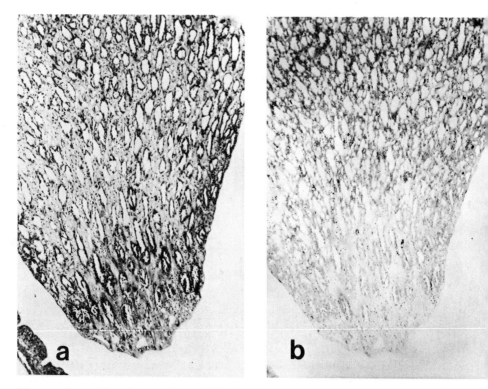

Figure 3.   The loss of medullary glycosamonoglycans 24h after BEA treament; a)H and E, and b) Hale's colloidal iron, counter stained with neutral red.   X 830

Between 24 and 48h (when the necrotic change had run its course and cellular repair processes were active) POG-GAG staining was lost almost totally from the necrosed areas,(Fig 3) but was apparently normal in the unaffected adjacent areas (48).   Preliminary data (81) confirms the perturbation of the matrix material during the development, and as a consequence, of the lesion. The urinary profile of different molecular weight fractions containing uronic acid (as a means of monitoring POG-GAG) have been measured using the method of White and Kennedy (82).   The polydispersion of uronic acid containing material (Fig. 4) showed marked changes over the first 48h, and there was a 50% loss of ^{35}S from the medulla after BEA treatment, but very little difference in other areas of the kidney or extra-renal tissue (Table 5).

It seems unlikely that the early increase in the staining intensity of the ground substance represented a quantitative increase (48).   These changes are more likely to have represented conformational changes which have made more binding sites available, a hypothesis which has been substantiated by the massive increase in free solute (as opposed to that bound to the polyanionic matrix) within the kidney (81).   It remains uncertain, at this stage, if the loss of staining later in the course of the development of the lesion was a result of loss of anionic binding groups (as shown by loss of ^{35}S) or total disruption of the protein and/or polysaccharide back-bone as well.   Irrespective of the nature of

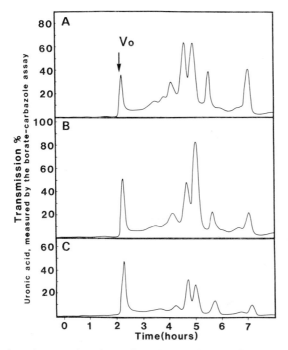

Figure 4. The changes in the molecular weight polydispersion of urinary uronic acid (as a marker of glycosaminoglycans and their degraded products) in response to BEA treatment (50mg/kg, ip).
A) 24h before BEA   B) 0 to 24h after BEA, and   C)24 to 48h after BEA.

Table 5   The residual radiolabel sulphur contents of different tissue following BEA treatment.

TYPE OF TISSUE	^{35}S DPM PER 100 mg TISSUE	
	Controls*	BEA-treated*
Medulla	36852	19558
Corticomedulla	9937	9432
Cortex	5174	5352
Liver	2198	1869
Lung	9679	10106
Muscle	2678	2142
Heart	2612	3147
Spleen	2655	2871

* Rats were given 300 μCi of ^{35}SO$_4$ ip, and after 5 days 2 rats were given 50 mg/kg BEA ip and 2 rats left as control. The rats were killed 72h later and duplicate samples of the different tissues digested and counted. Colour quenching was corrected by the use of internal standards.

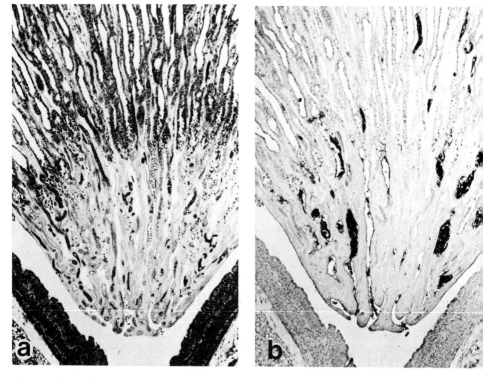

Figure 5.   Aggregates of immunohistochemically positive Tamm-Horsfall glycoprotein in the medullary collecting ducts 7 days after BEA treatment (100 mg/kg, ip), a) Masson's trichrome and b)immunoperoxidase. X 830

the molecular change the necrosed medulla was not subsequently repopulated by interstitial cells (although it may be re-epithelialised) and the ground substance was not re-deposited (48,80,81).

TAMM-HORSFALL GLYCOPROTEIN, PAPILLARY NECROSIS AND CYSTIC TUBULAR DILATATION

The normal role of Tamm-Horsfall glycoprotein (THG) includes "water proofing" the distal nephron, although its other possible functions in health and disease remain poorly defined (83). This unique molecule, may play an important role in the development of the secondary degenerative cortical changes which follow RPN. We have recently shown that massive amounts of THG were deposited within the collecting ducts following the administration of BEA, almost exclusively in those which had been necrosed Fig. 5. Time course studies have shown that the deposition of this material only began to take place after the loss of POG-GAG ground substance had occurred (81). Much of the THG positive staining material was lost from the distal tubule, but if animals had been treated with low doses of aspirin before BEA (84) there was a total absence of distal tubule staining, the collecting duct deposits of THG were most marked and there was extensive dilation of the cortical nephrons. THG immuno-

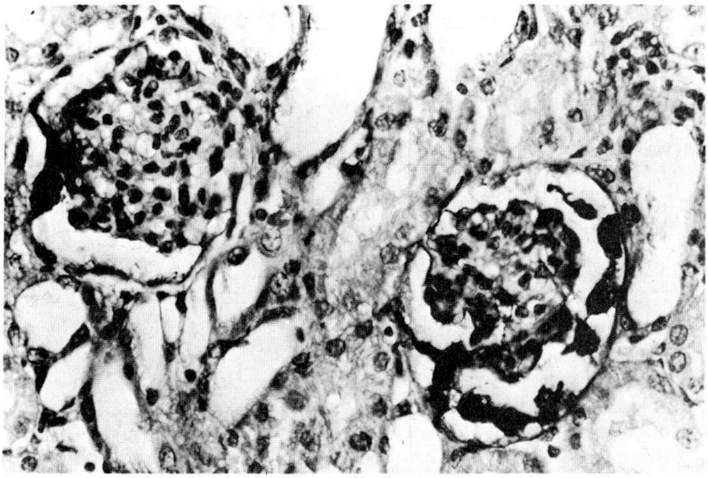

Figure 6. Aggregates of immunohistochemically positive Tamm-Horsefall glycoprotein within the Bowman's Capsule of the superficial nephrons of rats treated with Aspirin (0.1 mmol/kg,po per day for 2 days) and then given BEA (35mg/kg,ip). X 5280

histochemical staining also occurred within the Bowman's capsule of the superficial, but never the juxtamedullary nephrons (Fig. 6). The route by which the THG reaches the Bowman's capsule remains enigmatic, but more importantly its subsequent effects on nephron function might be expected to be profound if it exerts its waterproofing effects.

The exact significance of these findings, together with their consequences to renal function need to be carefully assessed. It is, however, tempting to speculate that:-

i) THG forms the major constituent of the eosinophilic cast material in the necrosed medulla,

ii) loss of THG from the distal nephron contributes to the urinary concentrating defect,

iii) blocking of the collecting duct or nephron with precipitated deposits of THG plays a role in secondary cystic dilation and the subsequent development of cortical damage.

PROTEOGLYCANS, GLYCOPROTEINS AND THE ACUTELY INDUCED RENAL PAPILLARY NECROSIS.

The molecular pathogenesis which underlies BEA-induced RPN is still uncertain, although our own data suggests that neither the counter-current mechanism, microvascular constriction, the conversion of BEA to E1 (the proximate reactive intermediate) nor an immune response play any part in its development (48,81,85).

Perturbation of the medullary ground substance has not previously been associated with the development of RPN. The pathogenesis which underlies the BEA-induced changes in the medullary matrix are uncertain and may be mediated via damage to the interstitial cells or by direct or indirect action on the ground substance itself. The consequences, however, might include and explain the urine concentrating defect that accompanies the development of the lesion, the loss of microvascalature, interstitial and other cell types and the substantial electrolyte wastage (86). The massive release of electrolyte from the disrupted matrix and the urinary acidosis (81) would favour the precipitation and aggregation of THG (83) and the absence of the polyanionic matrix from the necrosed papilla could be decisive in the lodging of negatively changed aggregates of THG in the collecting ducts.

Chronically Induced Renal Papillary Necrosis. No attempt will be made to extrapolate this data from an acutely induced model chemical system in animals to human analgesic abusers, but certain parallel changes do occur.

Most analgesics depress POG-GAG synthesis (87,88) and by virtue of their physicochemical characteristics (and by that of their metabolites) these compounds are excreted via the kidney (89,90). Thus the potential of these molecules to depress medullary matrix and other POG-GAG synthesis will therefore be quite substantial and might explain the urinary concentrating defect which develops in human analgesic abusers (11).

The POG-GAG which is excreted into the urine, that which covers the urothelia and makes up the medullary matrix has an important role in preventing bacterial colonisation (91). Thus depressing its synthesis may predispose to recurrent urinary tract infection (92) and retrograde bacterial pyelonephritis, both of which are commonly associated with RPN in human analgesic abusers (2,3,5,6-11,13,14).

The excretion of POG-GAG in the urine is commonly thought to bind cations and thus prevent or limit the supersaturation and crystallisation of calcium, magnesium and other complexes, which would otherwise exceed their solubility product. The formation of these microcrystals may provide the niduses from which calculi subsequently develop (93). The depression of urinary POG-GAG synthesis may, therefore, also have a direct consequence of favouring a higher frequency of nephrolithiases in those patients who consume large quantities of analgesics (94).

There is also evidence which suggests that THG may be perturbed in human analgesic abusers. Hyaline casts are frequently encountered and Burry has described hyalinised glomeruli in patients with RPN (7, 21). Altered THG deposits could also contribute to:-
  i)   the loss of urine concentrating capacity (11) because of loss of the effective "waterproofing" of the distal nephron (83).
  ii)   the high incidence of recurrent urinary tract infection, because THG is normally thought to entangle bacterial fimbrae and preventtheir attachment to the urothelial wall and subsequent colonisation (95), and finally
  iii) THG forms aggregates in the urine which could provide an important binding material on which microcrystalline deposits would gather and form nuclei for the growth of calculi, but this area remains most controversial however (96,97).

CONCLUSION

The pathogenesis which underlies RPN, and its secondary consequences, are most likely multi-factorial. This is particularly so in man where the early changes in response to an ill defined chronic chemical insult could predispose to factors such as bacterial infection or nephrolithiases, both of which would exacerbate renal degenerative changes on route to chronic renal failure.

In addition to analgesics and non-steroidal anti-inflammatory drugs there are a diffuse array of chemicals, with industrial uses that contaminate our ecosystem, which are known to cause renal papillary necrosis. There is an important need to assess the clinical risks associated with exposure to these and as yet unidentified compounds which may cause RPN or predispose to the development of the lesion.

There has, however, been almost no progress in terms of real patient care in attempts to establish a reliable means of diagnosing the early changes which precede papillary necrosis. This is also a problem which plagues the Toxicologist, who has only recourse to the arduous task of histopathology in order to establish the existence of this lesion. The most immediate need, therefore, is to produce a specific and sensitive means of identifying those early renal changes which subsequently progress to RPN. This will allow the Toxicologist to define the full spectrum of compounds which predispose to or cause the lesion, as well as other contributing factors (such as diet, concomitant disease etc). Most importantly this would provide the experimental basis for an essential advance in preventive medicine.

REFERENCES

1. Spuhler O and Zollinger HN, Z Klin Med 151:1-50, 1953.
2. Murray TG and Goldberg M, Kidney Int 13:64-71 1978.
3. Cove-Smith JR, J Clin Pathol 34:1255-1260, 1981.
4. Rosner I, CRC Crit Rev Toxicol 4:331-352, 1976.
5. Shelley JH, Clin Pharmacol Ther 8:427-471, 1967.
6. Duggin GG, Aust J Pharmaceut Sci 6:44-48, 1977.
7. Burry AF et al, Pathol Ann 12:1-31, 1977.
8. Shelley JH, Kidney Int 13:15-26, 1978.
9. Kincaid-Smith P, Contr Nephrol 16:57-64, 1979.
10. Duggin GG, Kidney Int 18:553-561, 1980.
11. Nanra RS, Brit J Clin Pharmacol 10:359S-368S, 1980.
12. Lindvall N, Kidney Int 13:93-106, 1978.
13. Dubach UC, Contr Nephrol 10:75-83, 1978.
14. Gault MH et al, Ann Intern Med 68:906-925, 1968.
15. Gilman A, Amer J Med 36:167-173, 1964.
16. Kincaid-Smith P, Kidney Int 17:250-260, 1980.
17. Prescott LF, Brit J Clin Pharmacol 7:453-462, 1979.
18. Hoffbrand BI, Brit Med J 1:78, 1978.
19. Mitchell JR et al, Amer J Med 62:518-526, 1977.
20. Mohandas J. et al, Res Commun Chem Pathol Pharmacol 34:69-80, 1981.
21. Burry AF, Kidney Int 13:34-40, 1978.
22. Gloor FJ, Kidney Int 13:27-33, 1978.
23. Lomax-Smith JD and Seymour AE, Amer J Surg Pathol 4:565-572, 1980.
24. Kingsley DPE et al, Brit Med J 4:656-659, 1972.
25. Cornelius EA, Amer J Pathol 59:317-323, 1970.
26. Axelsen RA, Pathology 5:43-50, 1973.
27. Borland VG and Jackson CM, Arch Pathol 11:687-708, 1931.
28. Muirhead EE et al, J Amer Med Assoc 142:627-631, 1950.
29. Sheehan HL and Davis JC, Arch Pathol 68:185-225, 1959.

30. Edmonson HA et al, Arch Intern Med 79:148-175, 1947.
31. Beswick IP and Schatzki PF, Arch Pathol 69:733-739, 1960.
32. Sheehan HL and Davis JC, J Pathol Bactiol 78:351-377, 1959.
33. Baum M et al, Brit Med J 2:229-231, 1969.
34. Davies DJ, MD Thesis, University of Liverpool, 1967.
35. Patrick RL et al, Arch Pathol 78:108-113, 1964.
36. Rossmann P and Matousovic K, Virchow Arch A382:95-111, 1979.
37. Rudofsky UH et al, Lab Invest 43:463-470, 1980.
38. Molland EA, Kidney Int 13:5-14, 1978.
39. Hardy TL, Brit J Exp Pathol 51:348-355, 1970.
40. Ellis BG et al, Chem-Biol Interact 7:131-142, 1973.
41. Ellis BG and Price RG, Chem-Biol Interact 11:473-482, 1975.
42. Sherwood T et al, Invest Radiol 6:239-244, 1971.
43. Davies DJ et al, Ann Rheum Dis 27:130-136, 1968.
44. Levaditi C, Arch Int Pharcodyn Therap 8:45-63, 1901.
45. Oka A, Virchows Arch 214:149-160, 1913.
46. Dermer OC and Ham GE, in Ethylenimine and Other Aziridines,
          Academic Press, New York, 1969.
47. Murray G et al , Amer J Pathol 67:285-302, 1972.
48. Bach PH et al, Toxicol Appl Pharm (Submitted).
49. Axelson RA, Virchow Arch A 301:79-84, 1978.
50. Fuwa M and Waugh D Arch Pathol 85;404-409, 1968.
51. Ham KN and Tange JD, Aust Ann Med 18:199-208, 1969.
52. Axelson RA, Virchow Arch A Path Anat Histol 381:63-77, 1978.
53. Ninan T and Wilson GB, Genetica 40:103-119, 1969.
54. Bluemle LW and Goldberg M, J Clin Invest 47:2507-2514, 1968.
55. Duggin GG, Brit J Pharmacol 54:359-366, 1975.
56. Duggin GG and Mudge GH, J Pharmacol Exp Ther 199:10-16, 1976.
57. Gault MH, Proc Amer Soc Nephrol, 4th Meeting: 28, 1970.
58. Gault MH, Clin Res 19:808, 1971.
59. Brown DM and Hardy TL, Brit J Pharmacol Chemother 32:17-24, 1968.
60. Hil GS et al, Amer J Pathol 68:213-234, 1972.
61. Vanholder R et al, Archiv Internat Physiol Biochim 89:63-73, 1981.
62. Zollinger HU et al, Schweiz Med Wschr 110:106-107 1980.
63. Furman KI et al, Clin Nephrol 16:271-275, 1981.
64. Thurau K, Amer J Med 36:698-719, 1964.
65. Cohen JJ, Amer J Physiol 236:F423-F433, 1979.
66. Mudge GH et al, J Pharmacol Exp Ther 206:218-226, 1978.
67. Caterson RJ et al, Brit J Pharmacol 207:584-593, 1978.
68. Solez et al, Amer J Pathol 76:521-528, 1974.
69. Davidson W et al, Clin Res 21:227
70. Davidson W et al, Clin Res 21:683, 1973.
71. Goldberg M et al, J Clin Invest 50:37a, 1971.
72. Dawson AG, Biochem J 130:525-530, 1972.
73. Dawson AG, Biochem Pharmacol 24:1407-1411, 1975.
74. Szinicz L et al, Arch Toxicol 42:63-73, 1979.
75. Hook JB et al, Rev Biochem Toxicol 1:53-78, 1979.
76. Gault MH et al, Amer J Med 151:740-756, 1971.
77. Murray G and Van Stowasser V, Brit J Exp Pathol 57:23-29, 1976.
78. McCormack KM et al, in Toxicology of the Kidney (JB Hook ed) Raven
          Press, New York, 1981, pp 227-250.
79. Hardy TL, Proc Europ Soc Study Drug Toxicity 15:337-344, 1974.
80. Shimamura T and Bonk K, Invest Urol 14:111-114, 1976.
81. Bach PH et al, Unpublish data.
82. White CA and Kennedy JF, Clin Chim Acta 95:369-380, 1979.
83. Hoyer JR and Seiler MW, Kidney Int 16:279-289, 1979.

84. Wirdnam PK et al, J Appl Toxicol 1:xxii, 1981.
85. Bach PH and Bridges JW, in Mechanisms of Toxicity and Hazard Evaluation
    (B Holmstedt, R Lauwerys, M Mercier, M Roberfroid, eds.) Elsevier-
    North Holland, Amsterdam, 1980, pp 533-536.
86. Sabatini S et al, Amer J Physiol 241:F14-F22, 1981.
87. Palmoski MJ and Brandt KD, Arthritis Rheum 23:1010-1020, 1980.
88. Dekel S et al, Prostaglandins Medicine 4:133-140, 1980.
89. Ransford KD et al, Arch Int Pharmacodyn 250:180-194, 1981.
90. Prescott LF, Drugs 23:75-149, 1982.
91. Parsons CL et al, Science 208:605-607, 1980.
92. Waters WE et al, Lancet 1: 341-344, 1973.
93. Nordin BEC et al, in Nephrology (J Hamburger, J Crosnier & J-P Grunfeld,
    eds.). Wiley-Flammarion, New York-Paris, 1979, pp 1091-1128.
94. Blackman JE et al, Brit Med J 2:800-802, 1967.
95. Orskov I et al, Lancet 1:887, 1980.
96. Wenk RE et al, Pathobiol Ann 11:229-257, 1981.
97. Bichler KH et al, Brit J Urol 47:733-738, 1976.

NEPHROTOXICITY ASSOCIATED WITH THE USE OF RADIOLOGICAL CONTRAST DRUGS

Gilbert H. Mudge

Departments of Pharmacology and Toxicology and of Medicine, Dartmouth Medical School, Hanover, New Hampshire 03755, USA

ABSTRACT

Our knowledge of this type of nephrotoxicity depends almost completely on clinical reports, owing to the absence of relevant animal models. The literature from '55 to the present is reviewed. Two types of drugs should be clearly distinguished. First, the urographic or angiographic drugs. These are lipid insoluble and are excreted in the urine without being metabolized. Second, the cholecystographic agents. These are lipid soluble and are excreted principally in the bile as glucuronide conjugates.

Approximately 300 cases of acute renal failure have been reported after urographic drugs. Reduction in filtration rate is frequently, but not always, accompanied by oliguria. Sensitivity-like reactions are extremely rare. Incidence seems unrelated to dose of contrast drug. Prognosis is reasonably good in absence of diabetes or cardiac disease; prognosis is worst with concomitant multiple myeloma. Of proposed mechanisms, acute tubular obstruction appears the most probable.

About 50 cases have been reported after oral cholecystographic drugs, frequently with co-existent liver disease or jaundice. Most cases have followed large doses. Prognosis appears less good than with urographic drugs.

The most urgent unanswered question involves incidence. Alleged rates vary enormously and appear higher in American series than European. However all incidence rates are of doubtful validity due to methods of case selection, absence of statistical evaluation, etc. With increased use of urographic drugs anticipated in conjunction with CAT scans, a large but simple prospective study is urged. As a minimum this would involve daily determinations of plasma creatinine for 3 days. This period of observation is recommended on the basis of the patterns observed in the published case reports.

Key Words. Radiocontrast drugs, obstructive nephropathy, uricosuria, Tamm-Horsfall protein, proteinuria.

INTRODUCTION

By most criteria the radiocontrast drugs are so pharmacologically inert that they are often referred to as dyes, agents or materials. Within recent years there has been an increasing interest in toxic reactions and their underlying mechanisms. It is of some historical interest that there have appeared several recent surveys of toxic reactions conducted by radiologists in which the subject of nephrotoxicity was not even mentioned. This is understandable since attention was directed to the immediate reactions that occur during the course of the radiological examination itself. Minor reactions such as transient nausea are quite common. For understandable reasons the reaction which is of greatest concern to the radiologist is that of anaphylactoid shock. This is life threatening and fortunately very rare. It appears to be a hypersensitivity type of reaction but is not well understood. However, as the literature has grown, it is now apparent that nephrotoxicity is one of the most common of the major reactions. Except for one or two case reports there is no evidence that nephrotoxicity results from hypersensitivity.

Our knowledge of nephrotoxic reactions depends almost completely on clinical case reports. In essence the diagnosis has been based on the occurrence of renal failure following the administration of a radiocontrast drug in a situation in which other known causes can be excluded. Although a cause and effect relationship has been challenged in the past, with the publication of a large number of clinical reports and the establishment of readily recognized clinical pattern, there can be little doubt but that radiocontrast drugs can cause renal failure in man. Despite considerable effort useful animal models are not available. Several laboratories are making use of the high risk factors that occur in man, such as diabetes mellitus, but results are not yet available.

A word on the case report may be appropriate. This is an important part of the medical literature but one which apparently does not receive high editorial priority. In the field of nephrotoxicity of radiocontrast drugs, I am astounded at the number of reports which are accepted for publication in which the descriptive material is limited to the nature of the radiological procedure and in which no mention is made of the name of the drug, or its dose, or its exact formulation. This is essential information and because of its absence many cases are worthless for critical analysis. Such information should be included in any report in which drug toxicity is the point of principal interest. In this respect radiocontrast drugs are no different from any other drug.

In a few papers all radiocontrast drugs have been considered together as a single group. This is an unfortunate oversimplification. Two general classes of drugs should clearly be recognized, first the urographic radiocontrast drugs (Uro-RCD) and second the oral cholecystographic drugs (Chole-RCD). Although there are also a few reports which suggest that the intravenous cholangiographic drugs may produce renal failure, the number of cases is too small to warrant further analysis. Historically, the Uro-RCD were introduced in order to diagnose disorders of the urinary tract. The technique of the intravenous pyelogram (IVP) was developed with the early agents such as iodopyracet (Diodrast). By the 1950's these were largely replaced by the better tolerated tri-iodinated derivatives of benzoic acid, such as diatrizoate or iothalamate. (For convenience, the tri-iodinated derivatives of benzoic acid will be referred to as the modern Uro-RCD). These are relatively strong acids and are administered as the sodium or meglumine salt, or a combination of the two. Within recent years non-ionic Uro-RCD have been synthesized

in order to decrease the osmolality which must necessarily result from
the dissociation of the parent compound into cationic and anionic particles
Within the past several decades the clinical use of the Uro-RCD has
expanded enormously with the development of angiography and computerized
axial tomography. The use of Uro-RCD for the latter two purposes far
exceeds the urographic use in most hospitals. The Uro-RCD are lipid
insoluble and diffuse poorly across epithelial barriers. Hence they
are poorly absorbed across the gastrointestinal tract and do not undergo
reabsorption across the renal tubule. They are not bound to plasma
protein and are thus freely filtered at the glomerulus. In general,
their distribution is limited to the extracellular space. They are
excreted almost completely in the urine and as the parent compound without metabolic alteration.

In comparison, the Chole-RCD are iodinated organic acids which
are lipid soluble. Although they exist principally in their anionic
form at the pH of the body fluids, the concentration of undissociated
acid is sufficiently high to allow its ready diffusion across the lipid
like cell membranes. Thus, following oral administration these drugs
are absorbed across the gastrointestinal tract. They gain ready access
to the drug-metabolizing enzymes of the endoplasmic reticulum of the
liver and are more or less completely converted to glucuronide conjugates. These in turn are readily excreted into the bile by the organic
acid transport system of the liver. Their high concentration in the
bile makes them useful for the visualization of the gall bladder. The
parent compounds are strongly bound to plasma protein and hence are
filtered in only insignificant amounts at the glomerulus. The small
amount that is filtered is also subject to tubular reabsorption so that
urinary excretion is normally very small. It is thought that the glucuronides are actively secreted by the organic acid transport system
of the proximal tubule. Under some circumstances these may also be
reabsorbed. Normally the total amount of drug excreted into the urine
is only a small fraction of that excreted into the bile.

NEPHROTOXICITY OF CHOLE-RCD

Within the past two decades at least 53 cases of acute renal failure
attributeable to oral Chole-RCD have appeared in the literature. The
summary of Table 1 includes 5 additional cases of the author. The
percentage classified as "unfavorable outcome" appears higher than with
the Uro-RCD. Jaundice and/or liver disease are unequivocal risk factors.
A small number of patients have had diabetes or cardiac disease but the
role of these disorders is difficult to evaluate since in half of them
there has been coexistent hepatic disease. There appears to be a definite
relationship of dosage to nephrotoxicity. Of the 58 cases in only one
instance was a single standard dose of Chole-RCD given. In all others
the dose was either doubled or repeated one or more times, or in a few
instances a clearly excessive dose was given at a single time. At least
four different compounds have been involved.

There has been a recent proliferation of the case reports of renal
failure due to the urographic agents. This has not been the case for
the cholecystographic drugs. The reasons are not completely certain.
One probable factor has been the realization that nephrotoxicity is
dose related. In those patients in whom the gall bladder has failed
to visualize on the first examination, at one time it was common practice to repeat the examination with a double dose. This is no longer
the recommended procedure. Secondly, other diagnostic techniques such

as ultra-sound have probably decreased the use of Chole-RCD, particularly
in ill patients who are at high risk. This is opposite to the trend
that appears to be occurring with Uro-RCD, for which the introduction
of one new diagnostic technique, namely computerized axial tomography,
has increased the use of the contrast drug.

Table 1. Summary of nephrotoxic reactions reported in literature.

		Total Cases	Unfavorable Outcome	
		Number	Number	Percent
Uro-RCD	--Total	270	48	18
	--Mult. Myeloma	9	8	89
	--Cardiac &/or Diabetic	141	33	23
Chole-RCD	--Total	58	23	40
	--Jaundice &/or Liver dis.	34	19	56
	--Cardiac &/or Diabetic	12	7	58

Cases of Uro-RCD are limited to "modern drugs", see text. Unfavorable
outcome is defined as death in uremia or as renal failure of sufficient
magnitude to require chronic dialysis. Data include previously unreported
cases of the author -- 17 for Uro-RCD and 5 for Chole-RCD. For primary
references for Uro-RCD, see [5].

Competition for Biliary and Urinary Excretion. Because of the clinical
association of kidney damage with pre-existing hepatic disease it has
frequently been postulated that nephrotoxicity results from decreased
excretion of the contrast drug by the liver which thus increases the
load to the kidney. The quantitative implications of excretion by two
routes should be recognized. In most species, including man, under normal conditions approximately 5% of an ingested dose of Chole-RCD is
excreted in the urine and the remaining 95% in the bile. The mechanisms
of biliary excretion are complex and involve several inter-related steps:
Hepatic uptake, storage and metabolism (principally glucuronidation),
transport of the conjugate from hepatocyte to bile, and also transport
from either the hepatocyte or the bile into the blood. A number of
factors determine the rate of bile flow and secondarily the concentration
of contrast drug within it. These include the endogenous bile acids as
well as other drugs which may be excreted into the bile. In addition
the radiocontrast drugs themselves have a variable action on the rate
of bile production [1]. It would not be surprising therefore if the
rates of biliary excretion of Chole-RCD were to fluctuate considerably,
both in normal subjects as well as those with various diseases. For
the present argument, assume that biliary excretion decreases from 95
to 90% of the ingested dose. While this represents only a negligible
change in elimination by that route, if the alternate route were to be
considered one would calculate that excretion into the urine would increase from 5 to 10%, a two fold change.
    In studies on iopanioc acid in the dog the rate of bile flow was
inversely related to the amount of glucuronide eliminated by the urine
[2]. This relationship varies with species and with different radiopaque
compounds. There are no direct measurements on how the two excretory

routes are effected by hepatic disease in man. The problem has been studied with several different types of experimental liver injury in the rat [3]. The amount of iopanoic acid excreted by the alternate urinary route depends on the type of hepatic injury. Possibly of most immediate relevance to the clinical problem is that the highest rate of urinary excretion was produced by chronic surgically induced stasis of the biliary tree.

Tissue drug levels should theoretically correlate with toxicity. In the case of the kidney such levels are compounded by the heterogeneous nature of the organ, which involves not only an additional tissue compartment, the tubular fluid, but also the gradients from cortex to papilla established within that compartment as well as within the interstitium. In the case of Chole-RCD there is an additional complication imposed by distinguishing analytically between the highly lipid soluble parent compound and the relatively lipid insoluble conjugates. It might be anticipated that these have different nephrotoxic potencies, but no data are available. In isolated cell systems the cholecystographic drugs, represented by iopanoic acid, are far more cytotoxic than the urographic drugs [4]. Such studies may eventually elucidate mechanisms of nephrotoxicity.

It has been repeatedly asserted that pre-existing kidney disease is a risk factor for the nephrotoxicity produced by Chole-RCD. This concept finds little support from the published cases. Of the 58 patients (Table 1) the levels of plasma creatinine or blood urea nitrogen (BUN) were determined in 47 prior to the radiological examination. Of these 43 were within normal limits; 4 patients had a slight elevation of BUN with an average value of 33 mg/dl. Several patients with an unfavorable outcome had proteinuria, but the available data are insufficient to evaluate.

NEPHROTOXOCITY OF URO-RCD

In a recent review an extensive bibliography was published to which the reader is referred [5]. The present summary focusses on the nature of the clinical picture and its relationship to some of the proposed mechanisms of toxicity.

Clinical Syndrome. From the 270 cases summarized from the literature the acute renal failure caused by Uro-RCD is a relatively benign disorder with an "unfavorable outcome" in only 17% (Table 1). This is less than with many other etiologies. Of the patients who recovered, renal function returned completely to normal in 83%. Other signs of drug toxicity such as acute hypotension or hypersensitivity are so rare that they be discounted as playing a role. The onset of the renal injury as judged by the appearance of oliguria may occur within hours after the radiological procedure. However, it is of considerable interest that a number of cases have been observed in which the IVP was normal and the patient then went on to develop acute renal failure. Since a normal IVP depends on normal excretory function, it follows that in these patients the Uro-RCD had no immediate effect on renal function at a time when the blood levels of Uro-RCD were at their highest. (With normal renal function the plasma half-life of Uro-RCD is 2-3 hours in man). In the cases that were first reported anuria was so prominent that it was considered to be an essential feature. However, in subsequent reports renal failure (i.e. a sudden rise in plasma creatinine or blood urea) has occurred without oliguria in about 15%.

In patients who eventually recover the peak plasma creatinine varies from 1 to 10 mg/dl above control levels; most cases are in the range from 2-4 mg/dl. This implies that the renal injury can vary in its intensity.

As to the radiological procedure, the IVP and most angiographic procedures produce the same pattern of nephrotoxicity. This does not include renal arteriography in which a high concentration of contrast drug is injected directly into the renal artery. However, case reports with this procedure are too few to be evaluated further. There is an enormous variation in the dose of Uro-RCD which appears to be nephrotoxic. However, it is clear that many cases of nephrotoxicity result from "standard" IVP doses. Whether there is a higher true incidence with larger doses is not known.

In patients who recover, the time at which the plasma creatinine reaches its peak value varies from the first to tenth day after the radiological procedure. This raises the possibility that renal injury might be an on-going or progressive process and not necessarily limited to the period immediately after drug administration. In this connection, although it is clear that the onset of oliguria may occur within the first 24 hours, it is not known whether or not in some patients the on-set might be later. This has important implications both for surveillance and for mechanisms of toxicity.

The role of associated diseases has been controversial. In the early papers multiple myeloma was frequently reported as a risk factor (Table 1). There is no doubt that these patients have had the least favorable prognosis. However, in several series the incidence of nephrotoxicity in well hydrated myeloma patients is said to be no higher than in controls. Within the past decade diabetes and cardiac disease have been recognized as risk factors. The significance of pre-existing renal disease remains controversial. This appears to add an additional risk in the presence of concomitant diabetes and cardiac disease, but not in their absence.

Hyperosmolarity. There are few aspects of renal physiology in which greater confusion has been generated than the relationship of osmotic diuresis to hyperosmolarility. It has also been claimed that hyperosmolarity per se is an important factor leading to nephrotoxicity. Since this is at best only a partial truth, it may be useful to examine the basic concepts of osmolarity and their diverse relationships to renal function.

By definition, an osmotic diuretic is a substance which is filtered at the glomerulus and to which the tubular epithelium is essentially impermeable. Therefore the amount that is eventually excreted in the voided urine is the same as the amount that is filtered. Usually such compounds are otherwise pharmacologically inert. Most are lipid insoluble. It is for this reason that they do not back diffuse across the renal tubule and for the same reason that they are excluded from most cells. As a result they do not gain access to drug metabolizing enzymes and do not undergo metabolic transformation. Mannitol is generally considered the prototype and has various non-radiological applications. However by many criteria the modern Uro-RCD are virtually indistinguishable from mannitol.

As a matter of pharmaceutical convenience most osmotic diuretics are dispensed as hyper-osmotic solutions. However, their action as diuretics

is unrelated to hyper-osmolarity itself. Consider as an example the
effect of injecting 500 ml of 5% mannitol (isosmotic, 278 mOsmole/kg)
and compare this to the effect of 100 ml of 25% mannitol (hyperosmotic,
1390 mOsmole/kg). Assume that the extracellular fluid volume is 15,000
ml and, for present purposes, also assume that renal excretion is negligible
prior to the time at which extracellular distribution reaches equilibrium.
The dose of mannitol, 139 mOsmole, is the same in both instances. In the
first example the mannitol is diluted into 15,000 plus 500 ml to a final
concentration of 8.97 mOsmole/liter. In the second example the mannitol
becomes diluted into 15,000 plus 100 plus 200 ml. The final term is the
result of water diffusion from intracellular to extracellular fluid.
Thus the injected mannitol is diluted in 15,300 ml for a final concentratic
of 9.09 mOsmole/liter. This is barely different from the isosmotic injection. The magnitude of diuresis depends on the amount of the osmotic
agent filtered at the glomerulus which is the product of the glomerular
filtration rate (GFR) and the plasma concentration. Both solutions will
be almost identically active as osmotic diuretics.

As suggested above, hyperosmotic solutions of Uro-RCD (which are dis-
trubuted extracellularly) are diluted within the body by two mechanisms.
Consider sodium diatrizoate as an example and at an injected dose of 50
ml with an initial osmolality of 1490 mOsmole/kg. As this dose equilibrate
within the extracellular space it is diluted by a volume of 15 liters with
an initial osmolality of 280 mOsmole/kg. Simply by this dilution the
final osmolality at equilibrium would be 284 mOsmole/kg. When the diffusion of water from the intracellular space is taken into account, extracellular volume would increase by an additional 120 ml to make the final
equilibrium value 282 mOsmole/kg.

If an angiographic injection is given directly into an occluded branch
of the renal artery, the transient osmolality will be the same as that of
the pharmaceutical preparation. If the injection is at a distance from
the kidney the contrast agent will be diluted by blood and perhaps other
tissue fluids prior to its arrival at the kidney. We took samples of
femoral blood at 5 second intervals in the dog following the injection
of sodium diatrizoate at a concentration in the syringe of 1490 mOsmole/
kg. With an initial plasma osmolality of 280 mOsmole/kg the peak initial
concentration to reach the kidney was calculated as 422 mOsmole/kg when
the injection mimicked aortography of the thoracic aorta, and 317 mOsmole/
kg when it mimicked an intravenous pyelogram with a bolus into the brachial
vein. In both instances the hyperosmolality was rapidly dissipated. In
the dog at a dose of diatrizoate of 900 mg Iodine/kg, which is slightly
higher than the most frequent clinical dose, the increase in the
osmolality of femoral artery plasma was 18, 12, and 8 mOsmole/kg
at 2,6 and 12 minutes, respectively, after intravenous dosing [6].

It is extremely unlikely that the increase in the osmolality of
the renal blood is of sufficient magnitude to be incriminated in acute
renal failure following intravenous pyelography. As an isolated factor
the higher degree of transient hyperosmolality following arteriography
is difficult to evaluate. In both instances the diuretic action of the
Uro-RCD lowers urine osmolality to less than control periods. In the
clinical syndromes of hyperosmolality damage to the central nervous
system is the most prominent feature [7]. This has not been reported
in Uro-RCD induced nephrotoxicity. Microscopic lesions of the tubular
epithelium have been experimentally produced at plasma osmolalities
of 430 mOsmole/kg sustained for several hours. Because of the severity
of the conditions the findings may have little relevance for the present

problem. However, the possibility can not be excluded that transient
severe hyperosmolality of the renal blood might be a factor in renal
angiography.

   Renal Response to Acute Osmotic Diuresis. The basic feature of
osmotic diuresis involves the filtration by the glomeruli of an
osmotically significant amount of non-reabsorbable solute. This
obligates an increase in intraluminal volume because of the limitations
of the dital nephron in modifying the osmolality of the tubular fluid
at high rates of solute and water exretion. In most radiological
procedures the urographic agents are injected rapidly as a bolus.
As a result the status of the kidney is rapidly changed from anti-
diuresis to diuresis. This transformation has been studied in the
vasopressin infused dog with the following findings [8,9]: 1) as
urine flow increases urine osmolality decreases towards isosmotic
levels; 2) there is a sudden brief increase in negative free-water
formation resulting from the increased volume of tubular fluid
delivered to the hypertonic papilla; 3) the high concentrations
of urea in the papilla are dissipated by the diffusion of urea in
a secretory direction into the tubular fluid; 4) changes in the
excretion rates of other solutes are variable; and 5) there is a
sudden reduction in both GFR and renal blood flow which recovers toward normal within 10 to 15 minutes.
   Of the above changes, the latter is most relevant to the present
problem. In terms of hydrodynamics the path of least resistance for
the disposition of the fluid filtered at the glomerulus is that it be
largely (about 99%) reabsorbed by the tubular epithelium and gain egress
from the kidney by way of the renal vein. When water reabsorption is
blocked by osmotic diuretics there is an increase in the volume and
pressure of the intraluminal fluid. The increased pressure acts as a
counterforce to filtration pressure and thereby reduces GFR. The
intraluminal pressure also dilates the lumen of the distal nephron thus
decreasing resistance to intraluminal flow and eventually permitting
intraluminal pressure to be reduced. Besides the direct measurements
of intraluminal pressure [10] this mechanism is supported by studies
on Uro-RCD. As an intravenous bolus meglumine diatrizoate reduced GFR
to a nadir of 45% of controls; following a slow infusion of the same
dose GFR fell to only 78% of controls; and when the bolus was superimposed on a pre-exisiting mild diuresis the GFR fell to 77% of controls
[8].
   The above results were observed after intravenous administration
and were determined by the clearance technique. When renal blood flow
is monitored directly by a flowmeter and when the contrast drugs are
administered in a manner to mimic renal arteriography, a biphasic response is observed [11]. As in other vascular beds, in response to acute
hypertonicity blood flow increases for almost one minute; however, unlike
other organs, blood flow in the kidney then falls below normal for an
equally brief time. The initial response of hyperemia can not be studied
by clearance methods because of wash-out artifacts as a result of diuresis.
The fall in the GFR measured by clearances persists longer than the fall
in renal blood flow measured by flowmeter, but both may reflect the
changes in intrarenal pressure induced by the osmotic diuretic. It has
also been proposed that angiotensin may be involved [11].

Despite repeated statements to the contrary there is little evidence that Uro-RCD are nephrotoxic by means of an anoxic mechanism. Under the most extreme circumstances of antidiuresis GFR and renal blood flow are reduced by only about 50%, and this only for a period of 5-20 minutes. It should be recalled that above the basal oxygen requirements the renal oxygen consumption is proportional both to the GFR and to the amount of sodium reabsorbed [12]. Thus a modest hemodynamic change resulting from acute osmotic diuresis reduces both oxygen demand and oxygen supply and does not produce tissue anoxia in the usual sense. Futhermore, in vascular surgery it is the generally accepted practice to cross-clamp the aorta above the renal arteries for as long as 20 minutes under normothermic conditions. This degree of anoxia does not produce renal failure. It exceeds by many fold the anoxia resulting from the administration of Uro-RCD.

It is not known whether an acute rise in intraluminal pressure or a sudden dilatation of the tubular lumen may themselves be injurious to the tubular epithelium.

Uricosuria. The moderate uricosuric action of both Chole-RCD and Uro-RCD is of undoubted importance in the evaluation of resultant hypouricemia. It has also been proposed that uricosura might be a factor contributing to nephrotoxicity [13] but subsequent experience makes this hypothesis unlikely. As indicated in Table 2, the urate/creatinine excretion ratio is approximately doubled by Uro-RCD, Chole-RCD and iodipamide, the intravenous cholangiographic agent. In the case of Chole-RCD the action is sufficiently prolonged to be detectable for 24 hours, but for Uro-RCD the action is largely over within 2 hours. Acture urate nephropathy has been attributed to a uric acid concentration in the urine which exceeds solubility and hence produces crystalluria and obstructive nephropathy. As seen in Table 2, the urinary concentration of uric acid increased after Chole-RCD and i.v. cholangiography, but not after Uro-RCD. In no instance did the degree of uricosuria meet the requirements of acute urate nephropathy described for other causes of uricosuria [14]. Likewise there is no correlation between nephrotoxicity and hyperuricemia in 78 cases after Uro-RCD [5]. Of 58 cases of Chole-RCD related renal failure, plasma urate was determined in only five and was normal except for one of which was slightly elevated. Nevertheless it would be prudent when dealing with patients with severe hyperuricemia to bear the uricosuric action of the contrast agents in mind and to embark on radiological studies only after appropriate deliberation.

Tubular Permeability to Uro-RCD. The early drugs such as iodopyracet undergo tubular secretion and hence traverse the renal tubular epithelium. At a constant dose the concentration achieved within the kidney varies from one compound to another [15]. Although there is substantial evidence for man and the dog that the renal tubule is impermeable to the modern Uro-RCD such as diatrizoate, there is considerable species variation and diatrizoate itself is secreted in the rat and rabbit [16]. Other modern Uro-RCD may also be secreted in man to a slight extent [17]. In the rat, increased intrarenal pressure makes the tubule permeable to iothalamate [18]. Whether reabsorption occurs by a transcellular or intercellular route is not known. As a factor in the pathogenesis of nephrotoxicity, tubular permeability to Uro-RCD can not be excluded. If this were to occur at a site in the lower nephron at which high concentrations of Uro-RCD had been established

within the tubular fluid, the reabsorption of a small absolute amount
of Uro-RCD might give rise to high intracellular concentrations. The
toxicological consequences might well be different from those for
high extracellular concentrations. Following *in vivo* injection of
radioactive Uro-RCD, small amounts of radioactivity were found in
the nuclear, mitochondrial and microsomal sub-cellular fractions of
kidney homogenates [19]. Whether the radioactivity gained access to
the organelles before or after homogenization is not know, and the
implications for nephrotoxicity mechanisms are uncertain.

Table 2. Effect of radiocontrast drugs on urinary excretion of uric
          acid in man.

	Minutes of Observation mean	Urine conc. Uric acid ug/ml		Urine Urate/Creatinine Ratio
		Before	After	After/Before
IVP, Uro-RCD (11)	47	482 ± 72	436 ± 69	1.96 ± 0.16
(5)	1440	413 ± 112	291 ± 71	1.15 ± 0.11
Chole-RCD (9)	1440	527 ± 108	720 ± 145	1.71 ± 0.23
Iodipamide (4)	211	616 ± 308	1152 ± 210	1.69 ± 0.07

All IVP's were with diatrizoate either as sodium or meglumine salt. For
Chole-RCD iopanoic acid was used for 8, ipodate for 1, all in single
standard doses. Iodipamide was administered for i.v. cholangiography.
All values are means + SE. Minutes of observation refers to time after
administration of radiocontrast drug. Number of cases examined are in
parenthesis.

Tubular Obstruction. Since the time of the first descriptions of
acute renal failure following intravenous pyelography in patients with
multiple myeloma [20] there has been good evidence for an obstructive
uropathy. This mechanism was extended to other patients [21,22] with
the demonstration that Uro-RCD form insoluble precipitates with Tamm-
Horsfall protein (T-H). At the present time a number of points are well
established [5]. T-H is a muco-protein that is synthesized by the kidney
and is the major constituent of urinary casts. It is a normal component
of the urine and is detectable in the tubular cells, the tubular fluid
and sometimes in the interstitium. The formation of insoluble gels
of T-H is facilitated by serum albumin, Bence-Jones protein and Uro-
RCD. The recovery from the oliguric renal failure induced by Uro-RCD
is accompanied by an increased excretion of T-H and urinary casts.
These findings have led to the proposal that renal failure results
from the interaction of T-H and Uro-RCD within the tubular fluid and
that this leads to precipitation and intrarenal obstruction. To this
mechanism should be added the more recent observation that in a rare
patient Uro-RCD may produce massive proteinuria [23] and that this
might also enhance precipitation of T-H. There is also suggestive
evidence that myoglobin may react with Uro-RCD [24].
        When considered in relation to the clinical picture the hypothesis
of intratubular obstruction has many attractive features. It would
explain both oliguric and non-oliguric renal failure by similar mechanisms
since the latter might represent the obstruction of a small fraction of
the nephrons. It might also explain the variability in the clinical
picture both in relation to the range of peak plasma creatinine concentrations and to the time span over which they are observed. Although

detailed observations are not available it may be presumed that the
formation of precipitates would require a finite amount of time and
also that the process would be dependent on the local concentrations
of the reactants. Such a mechanism would also be consistent with
the normal excretory pyelogram observed in patients who then later go
on to develop renal failure. In addition, it would be consistent with
the late appearance of a nephrogram following renal impairment [25].
It has recently been demonstrated that there is a low urinary concentration of sodium in patients with renal failure induced by Uro-RCD
[26]. This is more consistent with an obstructive lesion than with
primary cell damage or necrosis. As to associated risk factors, in
multiple myeloma the excretion of Bence-Jones protein is well known.
To our knowledge the excretion of T-H protein has not been quantified
for either diabetes or cardiac disease. In both instances underlying
vascular disease might also enhance the proteinuria induced by Uro-RCD.
    In considering intraluminal obstruction, the interaction between two
or more substances which leads to precipitation should depend directly
on their concentrations within the tubular fluid rather than on their
rates of excretion. Micropuncture studies of tubular fluid are not
available. However, from analysis of the voided urine the composition
of the tubular fluid can be evaluated with reasonable certainty. An
additional cascade effect may also be operative [21]. Assume for the
sake of illustration that the concentrations of T-H and Uro-RCD have
reached critical levels within the tubular fluid so that precipitation
occurs and the lumen is blocked. Filtration to this nephron decreases
but does not cease and there is continued reabsorption upstream to the
point of blockade. This increases the concentrations of the reactants
within the tubular fluid and accelerates the process of precipitation.
Although this mechanism is difficult to document directly it has considerable theoretical merit. It may be of major importance in obstructive nephropathy.

    Urinary Composition after Intravenous Pyelography. Most of the
studies on the renal excretion of Uro-RCD are limited to the one or two
hours after dosing and focus on the factors underlying uroradiological
procedures. With a primary interest in nephrotoxicity we have conducted
preliminary studies on the composition of the urine for up to 24 hours
after intravenous urography in a small number of patients. Each subject received 60 ml of 60% meglumine diatrizoate (Renograffin). All
major or relevant urinary solutes were monitored except for T-H which
was not measured. Several observations of interest have emerged. First,
it was found in control samples that the Lowry method gave far higher
values for urinary protein than other standard methods, and it was
then also discovered in the post-IVP specimens that this method measures
meglumine. The Coomassie Blue method for protein [27] was then explored
and the results are considered reliable. In the comparison of the final
urine voided before the IVP to the first one after it, in nine patients
the protein/creatinine ratio consistently increased. The average after/
before ratio was 1.95 ± .44 (SEM). In none of these specimens was proteinuria detectable by the usual clinical test (Bili-Labstix, Ames).
Thus intravenous pyelography produces a slight proteinuria in all patients
examined. This was detectable for up to approximately 200 minutes. A
more drastic response in an occassional patient might not be unexpected.
    Second, the urinary concentration of diatrizoate was determined in 7
patients for up to 24 hours. All subjects had normal renal function as
judged by plasma creatinine. This was confirmed by the observation that

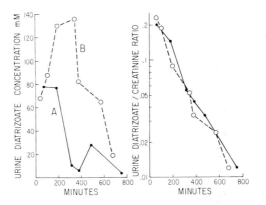

Figure 1. Patterns of urinary excretion of diatrizoate for two subjects (A and B) for 800 minutes after IVP. Time refers to interval after i.v. injection of meglumine diatrizoate. All voidings were on voluntary schedule. Diatrizoate was determined by UV spectroscopy.

in the post-IVP specimens the diatrizoate/creatinine fell as a first order reaction and with a similar slope in all subjects (Figure 1). This would be anticipated if GFR and creatinine production remained constant and if there were no interference between the mechanisms by which diatrizoate and creatinine are excreted. The linearity of the slope is also indirect evidence for the completeness of the voidings which were on a voluntary time schedule. As shown in Figure 1, two patterns were observed. For both subjects the half-times for diatrizoate excretion, as estimated by the line of best fit, were identical at 230 minutes. However, for subject A the urinary concentration of diatrizoate was maximal within the first 200 minutes and for subject B the peak occurred approximately 200 minutes later. Three subjects followed pattern A. Of the four who ressembled B the peak concentration of diatrizoate occurred at 340, 420, 440 and 530 minutes after injection. Parenthetically, most radiological examinations are completed within 30 minutes after injection of the contrast drug and many studies on actual excretion have been limited to 60-120 minutes.

The pattern of subject B (Figure 1) is contrary to the firm impression frequently held by radiologists. It has significant implications for the pathogenesis of nephropathy, patricularly for those proposed mechanisms, such as intraluminal obstruction, in which the concentration of Uro-RCD within the tubular fluid is considered critical.

The factors which determine the urinary concentration of Uro-RCD are complex and can vary independently from each other. Using diatrizoate as an example, these include the rate of diatrizoate excretion (plus its attendant cation), the rate of excretion of other solutes, and the magnitude and direction (either positive or negative) of free-water formation [8]. The latter is regulated both by the liberation of anti-diuretic hormone from the posterior pituitary and by the magnitude of total solute excretion. As shown in Figure 1, in the presence of a normal GFR the urinary concentration of diatrizoate can peak over a wide time span. In the patients studied this varied from about 30 to over 500 minutes after injection. This indicates directly that there is no necessary relationship between urinary concentration and rate of excretion and indirectly that there may be similar discrepancies between urinary concentrations and administered dose. These findings in man are similar to those previously reported for the dog [8]. It should be emphasized that we observed only a relatively narrow range of concentrations of diatrizoate in the urine. However, the same physiological factors might greatly augment these differences in an occasional patient. In the dog the highest observed concentration of diatrizoate in the urine was 425 mM, approximately one-half that of the concentration in the syringe.

Incidence and Prophylaxis. There are certainly few problems on which there is greater disagreement than the incidence of Uro-RCD induced nephrotoxicity. Estimates vary from zero to at least 12 percent depending on the radiological procedure, the criteria for nephrotoxicity, the selection of patients, the method of study and possibly the country of origin. Most reports have been retrospective and inevitably heavily weighted by patient selection. From an analysis of over 30 papers in which a numerical value for alleged incidence has been presented this author is of the opinion that a valid estimate of incidence has yet to be presented in the medical literature.

From a different point of view there is the question of the incidence of radiocontrast drugs as the cause of renal failure in a population of patients with kidney impairment. In a total of 357 cases of acute renal failure, radiocontrast drugs were implicated in 4%, but this represented 21% of the cases in which known nephrotoxic compounds or drugs were involved [28]. However, in the long run these figures may be of less importance than the actual incidence of the complication in the population at risk, i.e. the patients to whom the diagnostic drugs are administered. With the newer developments in angiography and with the introduction of computerized axial tomography, the use of urographic radiocontrast drugs is bound to increase enormously. Even though renal failure is relatively mild compared to that caused by other agents, both morbidity and mortality are far from insignificant.

Within recent years there have been several proposals to prevent renal failure by the prophylactic administration of intravenous fluids. Old and Lerner [29] have suggested 5% mannitol in 5% glucose and water; Eisenberg et al [30] have used 550 ml of normal saline plus an additional 250 ml of heparinized saline given as a flush solution during each hour of procedure time. These protocols have the merit of being clearly stated and as such stand in contrast to the often vague admonition that patients "be well hydrated". By the same token, however, they have the weakness of establishing a rigid protocol which itself may produce morbidity. Cardiac patients might well be at a double risk, particularly with large routine infusions of intravenous saline. During the period that the need for more elaborate protocols is being evaluated, simpler techniques for hydration, e.g. the oral ingestion of water, might suffice.

The incidence of nephropathy induced by urographic agents should be determined in a prospective study. As a minimum this should involve the determination of the plasma creatinine levels for the day prior to the radiological procedure and for at least three days thereafter. Cases should be categorized by radiological procedure and by dose and type of contrast drug. Intravenous pyelography should be clearly separated from intra-arterial procedures. If possible serial serum creatinine levels should be determined on disease matched controls who do not receive radiocontrast drugs. Whether a late nephrogram is a practical method of surveillance is still uncertain. Such a project might well become a major undertaking but one fully justified by the nature of the clinical problem.

Acknowledgements. The orginal investigations reported here in were supported by NIH grants AM 16960 and AM 06818.

REFERENCES

1. Barnhart JL, Berk RN and Combes B, Invest Radiol 15:S124-S131, 1980.
2. Cooke WJ and Mudge GH, Invest Radiol 10:25-34, 1975.
3. Cooke WJ, Berndt WO and Mudge GH, J Pharmacol Exp Ther 192:618-629, 1975.
4. Nelson JA, Liou I-F, Tolman KG, et al., Invest Radiol 15:S97-S101, 1980.
5. Mudge GH, Kidney Int 18:540-552, 1980.
6. Mudge GH, Berndt WO and Cooke WJ, Am J Physiol 227:369-376, 1974.
7. Rush BF jr, Finberg L, Daviglus GF, et al., Surgery 50:359-366, 1961.
8. Mudge GH, Invest Radiol 15:S67-S78, 1980.
9. Mudge GH, Cooke WJ and Berndt WO, Am J Physiol 228:1304-1312, 1975.
10. Gottschalk CW and Mylle M, Am J Physiol 189:323-328, 1957.
11. Caldicott WJH, Hollenberg NK and Abrams HL, Invest Radiol 5:539-547, 1970.
12. Valtin H, in Renal Function:Mechanisms preserving fluid and solute balance in health. Little Brown and Co., Boston, 1973, p. 92. ISBN 0-316-89555(C).
13. Mudge GH, N Engl J Med 284:929-933, 1971.
14. Kelton J, Kelley WN and Holmes EW, Arch Intern Med 138:612-615, 1978.
15. Morris SE, Lasser EC, Fisher B, et al., Radiology 77:764-775, 1961.
16. Mudge GH, Berndt WO, Saunders A and Beattie B, Nephron 8:156-172, 1971.
17. Golman K, J Belge Radiol 60:229-238, 1977.
18. Lorentz WB jr, Lassiter WE and Gottschalk CW, J Clin Invest 51:484-492, 1972.
19. Guidolet J, Barbe R, Borsson F, et al., Invest Radiol 15:S215-S219, 1980.
20. Bartels ED, Brun GC, Gammeltoft A, et al., Acta Med Scand 50:297-302, 1954.
21. Berdon WE, Schwartz RH, Becker J, et al., Radiology 92:714-722, 1969.
22. Schwartz RH, Berdon WE, Wagner J, et al., AJR 108:698-701, 1970.
23. Golman K and Holtas S, Invest Radiol 15:S61-S66, 1980.
24. Winearls CG, Ledingham JGG and Dixon AJ, Br Med J 281:1603, 1980.
25. Older RA, Karobkin M, Cleeve DM, et al., AJR 134:339-342, 1980.
26. Fang LST, Sirota RA, Ebert TH, et al., Arch Intern Med 140:531-533, 1980.
27. Bradford MM, Anal Biochem 72:248-254, 1976.
28. Bennett WM, Luft F and Porter GA, Am J Med 69:767-774, 1980.
29. Old CW and Lehrner LM, Lancet 1:885, 1980.
30. Eisenberg RL, Bank WO and Hedgock MW, AJR 136:859-861, 1981.

THE NEPHROTOXIC EFFECTS OF NEUROTROPIC DRUGS

Hans Erik Hansen

Department of Medicine C, Aarhus Kommunehospital and University of Aarhus, Denmark DK 8000

Abstract: The nephrotoxic properties of neurotropic drugs are reviewed with special reference to the lithium ion. During long-term lithium treatment a chronic interstitial nephropathy with reduced renal concentrating ability may develop. Glomerular filtration rate is normal or almost normal. This lithium-induced renal lesion is presumably a result of a direct dose related nephrotoxicity exerted by the lithium ion. The main risk to long-term lithium treated patients is not end-stage renal failure, but lithium intoxication a condition which may be life threatening if not properly treated. The most efficient treatment for lithium intoxication is haemodialysis. The lithium-induced nephrotic syndrome is a rare condition of unknown etiology. Neuroleptics combined with lithium may possibly contribute to the development of chronic renal changes. The possible nephrotoxic properties of H_1-receptor blockers are discussed. An immunologically mediated, acute interstitial nephritis may complicate treatment with hydantoin preparations, and valproic acid is suggested to affect proximal tubular renal function.

Key words: Nephrotoxicity. chronic interstitial nephropathy, acute interstitial nephritis. lithium, psychotropic drugs, antiepileptics.

INTRODUCTION.

The anatomic configuration and complexity of physiological function performed by the kidney makes it very sensitive to the action of toxic agents.

Nephrotoxic compounds can be divided into two relatively distinct categories, either direct dose-related nephrotoxins or drugs which mediate renal toxicity by a hypersensitivity mechanism. Both categories may present clinically as acute renal insufficiency. When direct toxic mechanisms are involved a slow progressing abnormality in renal function may result from long-term treatment with what are thought to be pharmacological doses of the drug concerned.

In this chapter the nephrotoxic effects of neurotropic drugs are described, with special reference to the lithium ion, the major neurotropic agent used for long-term treatment, which is proved to affect renal function in a relatively large proportion of treated patients [1]. The possible nephrotoxic properties of other psychotropic drugs, antiepileptics and drugs which affect the central nervous system will be discussed briefly.

ACUTE AND CHRONIC NEPHROTOXICITY OF THE LITHIUM ION IN MAN.

The present study deals with the following problems:-
1) An evaluation of the renal toxicity of the lithium ion during lithium intoxication as well as during long-term lithium treatment where serum lithium values are within therapeutic limits [2].
2) The mechanisms behind the slow developing lithium intoxication which occurs during long-term lithium treatment.
3) Guidelines for treating and preventing intoxication.
4) Possible measures which might delay or prevent chronic renal changes during long-term lithium treatment.

Lithium excretion. About 90% of ingested lithium is excreted in urine [2,3]. The lithium ion is freely filtered through the glomerular membrane [4] but 70 to 83% is reabsorbed, presumably in the proximal tubules [5-8]. This means that:-
1) Lithium transport in the kidneys is high. The kidneys have to handle 80 to 200 mmol of lithium per day if the daily lithium dosage is 20 to 50 mmol.
2) Lithium concentrations in the distal part of the nephron and in urine might exceed the toxic concentrations in plasma (1.5 mmol/l) [3,9].
3) If acute and chronic toxic effects of lithium occur and the toxicity is related to lithium concentration, the main target would be the kidneys especially the distal part of the nephron.

Lithium intoxication. In a study on lithium intoxicated dogs Radomski et al. [10] demonstrated that:-
1) Acute renal insufficiency might complicate lithium intoxication.
2) Sodium depletion took place and urine volumes increased.
3) Some dogs developed hypernatriemia, probably due to the diuretic effect of the lithium ion leading to a condition where water excretion exceeded sodium excretion.
4) Microscopically, lesions confined to the distal convoluted tubules and the collecting ducts were present. Later studies [11] revealed intracellular changes in tubule cells during lithium intoxication.

Studies on lithium intoxication in man [12] were based on 100 cases from the literature and 23 of our own cases. Lithium intoxication was due to reduced lithium elimination; 21 of 23 patients developed lithium intoxication on a daily dose which had been unchanged for months or years. Events which might lead to water and sodium loss had preceded lithium intoxication in a majority of these patients. A partly reversible reduction in renal function was present in a majority of patients on admission. two suffered from acute anuria and seven patients had creatinine clearance values between 10 and 20 ml/min. The patients were generally normotonic dehydrated [13]. but four patients demonstrated excessive water loss during the period of study after lithium intoxication. presenting a nephrogenic diabetes insipidus [12], and six patients studied about four weeks after intoxication (when renal function had stabilized) had reduced renal concentrating ability [13].

Lithium-induced nephropathy. The results of these studies suggested that lithium had induced a chronic renal lesion in some patients. In our first series of patients with lithium intoxication [12] seven renal biopsies were performed. Lesions evidencing acute renal failure were few and insignificant [14].

In a further study on 14 patients including quantitative studies on renal biopsy specimens [15] a combination of lithium treatment, impaired renal concentrating ability and focal interstitial nephropathy was seen in a selected group of patients in whom the only common factor was lithium treatment for extended periods of time complicated by one or more episodes of lithium intoxication. In two studies including renal biopsy specimens a relationship between tubular damage and the degree of impairment of renal concentrating ability was found [3.16].

From studies of lithium treated patients including 110 [3] and 237 patients [17]. respectively, it appeared that the main renal change was a markedly reduced renal concentrating ability in 18 of the 110 patients studied 3 which could be related to the duration of lithium treatment. In 8 patients who had been treated with lithium for a significantly longer period of time (9.3 years) serum creatinine had increased by more than 0.3 mg/100 ml (26.5 μmol/1) during the period of treatment, the maximal value being 2.0mg/100 ml (177 μmol/1). Studies on renal biopsy specimens from 14 of 18 patients [3] revealed focal interstitial fibrosis with glomerular sclerosis, tubular atrophy and microcysts. The degree of tubular damage was significantly correlated to the degree of impairment of renal concentrating ability. The studies indicated that the lithium-induced lesions were located to the distal part of the nephron where regulation of water excretion takes place. Studies on albumin and beta$_2$-microglobulin excretion have excluded any severe constant toxic action on the glomeruli and proximal tubules [18.19]. The lithium-induced renal change is of nephrogenic, not hypothalamic, origin because these patients excrete four times more arginine-vasopressin compared to other psychiatric patients [20]. This has been confirmed by studies on plasma arginine-vasopressin concentrations in lithium treated patients during water deprivation as well as during water loading [9]. The antidiuretic hormone is neither blocked nor inhibited during long-term lithium treatment. on the contrary baseline plasma arginine-vasopresin levels are increased and the hypothalamic system reacts to water deprivation as well as to water loading [9].

Renal pathology. function and concentrating ability have been evaluated in long-term lithium treated patients [3.17-29]. Renal biopsy specimens have revealed changes similar to those described previously [21.22.24.27.29]. Interstitial fibrosis has also been found in renal biopsy specimens from psychiatric patients prior to the start of lithium treatment [27], but the lithium treated patients had a significantly higher frequency of distal tubular changes (such as tubular dilatation and microcysts) compared to psychiatric patients prior to the start of lithium treatment [29].

Table 1. Results of studies on renal concentrating ability in patients on long-term lithium treatment. A = Total number of patients studied. B = Number of patients with impaired renal concentrating ability.

Reference number	Number of patients A/B	Duration of lithium treatment (months) A/B	Average maximal urine osmolal concentration mOsm/kg H_2O/number of patients included
3	110/18	43/71	496/18
17	237/39	60/71	516/39
18	30/10	39/43	718/10
20	123/30	74/-	509/10
22	68/66	74/74	540/66
23	43/-	27/-	602/43
24	46/17	73/-	-
25	50/41	70/-	725/50
26	100/56	60/-	757/100

Studies on renal function (Table 1) have shown that reduced renal concentrating ability is frequently seen in patients on long-term lithium treatment [3.9.15-18.20.22-26.29]. The highest frequency and the lowest average maximal urine osmolal concentrations have been found in those patients who have been treated for the longest periods of time. In two studies [3.25] a relationship between the duration of lithium treatment and the impairment of renal concentrating ability was present. Albrecht et al. [24] demonstrated a relationship between the product of serum lithium concentration and the duration of lithium treatment and the degree of impairment of renal concentrating ability. Glomerular filtration rate has been normal, or almost normal, in the majority of patients studied [3.9.15-18.22-26.28]. and in only a few patients, with a mean period of lithium treatment of about 10 years, a slight reduction in glomerular filtration rate has been seen [3.17]. In one study [28] a not age related. slight decrease in glomerular filtration rate has been related. to the duration of lithium treatment. In two studies [20.26] reduced renal concentrating ability was found in psychiatric patients not treated with lithium. In other studies [30.31] renal concentrating ability was found to be normal in psychiatric patients prior to the start of lithium treatment.

Few studies have been done on the reversibility of the lithium-induced impairment of renal concentrating ability. According to these studies the condition is only partly reversible [16,22,25] after cessation of lithium treatment. In a follow-up study [31] Vestergaard and Amdisen found that the impairment of renal concentrating ability had progressed in those patients who had continued lithium treatment. In the patients where lithium treatment was stopped, renal concentrating ability had improved but had not returned to normal, when compared to results obtained in psychiatric patients prior to start of lithium treatment.

Combination of lithium and other psychotropic drugs. In a number of psychiatric patients a combination of lithium and other psychotropic drugs have been used. and it has been suggested that some of these drugs, especially neuroleptics. might contribute to the impairment of renal function. Renal biopsy specimens have revealed fibrotic changes in patients prior to the start of lithium treatment [27]. Bucht et al. [22] found the most severe impairment of renal concentrating ability in patients treated with lithium and neuroleptics, but recent studies have shown [32] that these patients had received larger doses of lithium compared to those who had had no neuroleptics. In two studies [20.26] impaired renal concentrating ability was present in psychiatric patients.not lithium treated while two other groups found normal renal concentrating ability in patients prior to start of lithium treatment [30.31].

Lithium-induced changes in the rat nephron. Recent studies have shown focal interstitial changes. with fibrosis, in rats treated with lithium for 9 weeks [33]. Histochemical studies have revealed enzymic and tubular changes in the distal part of the nephron [34]. Studies in new-born rats have shown severe dilatation of the distal convoluted tubules as well as interstitial inflammation and fibrosis [35]; changes in new-born rats were more severe than those seen in adult rats.

Lithium-induced nephrotic syndrome. Proteinuria is not related to the lithium-induced renal changes described above. Long-term lithium treated patients. presenting signs of a chronic interstitial nephropathy. had normal or almost normal albumin excretions [19]. In three cases [36,37] a nephrotic syndrome has been associated with lithium treatment. This disappeared after withdrawal of lithium and recurred on reinstitution of lithium therapy. Renal biopsy specimens revealed a minimal-change nephropathy in these patients.

Conclusions from studies on lithium-induced nephropathy. Reduced renal concentrating ability of nephrogenic not (hypothalamic) origin is frequently seen in patients on long-term lithium treatment. The reduction in renal concentrating ability has been correlated with the degree of tubular damage and to the duration of lithium treatment and is only partly reversible. In the majority of patients glomerular filtration rate is normal. and in only a few patients with a mean period of treatment of about 10 years was a slight reduction in glomerular filtration rate found. Studies on renal morphology have revealed a chronic, focal interstitial nephropathy with tubular atrophy. cystic dilatation and microcysts. Similar changes have been found in rats treated solely with lithium. It cannot be ruled out that other psychotropic drugs may contribute. because fibrotic tissue has been found in psychiatric patients prior to the start of lithium treatment. In one study a combination of lithium and neuroleptics has been related to the degree of impairment of renal concentrating ability. Similar functional abnormalities. with a disproportionate reduction in renal concentrating ability in relation to glomerular filtration rate. have been reported in other renal diseases which mainly affect the medulla of the kidney (polycystic kidney disease and medullary cystic kidney disease). The well preserved glomerular filtration rate present in almost all lithium treated patients studied indicates that the risk of developing end-stage renal failure, due to long-term lithium treatment, would take decades. The main risk to these patients is lithium intoxication. a not rare condition which may be life threatening.

The lithium-induced nephrotic syndrome is a rarely seen condition of obscure aetiology. Presumably it has no relation to the lithium-induced chronic interstitial nephropathy where patients have normal or almost normal albumin excretion.

Table 2. Conditions contributing to lithium intoxication in 23 patients
  12 .

Acute overdosage:	1	Acute pyelonephritis	1
Initial dosage too high	1	Acute mania:	1
Fever associated with upper respiratory tract disease or influenza symptoms or gastroenteritis:	8	Depression	1
		Slimming diet:	1
Chlorothiazide treatment	2	Nausea vomiting and diarrhoea of unknown etiology	2
Anorexia and vomiting due to: peptic ulcer, carcinoma of the common hepatic duct:	1	Unknown:	3

Mechanisms behind the slowly developing lithium intoxication. From a
study on 100 cases from the literature and 23 of our own cases [12] it
appeared that lithium intoxication was a gradually progressing condition
which developed in patients who had been on long-term lithium treatment
for months or even years. Events which had induced a negative water and
sodium balance did often precede the slowly developing lithium
intoxication (Table 2).

Lithium intoxication could be characterized as follows:
1) This condition developed in about half of the patients given long-
term lithium treatment (68 of 123 cases).
2) Lithium intoxication was often preceded by events which might induce
water and sodium loss.
3) Intoxication developed and progressed slowly.
4) Often associated with acute reduction in renal function.
5) Patients were dehydrated on admission.
6) The patients studied about 4 weeks after intoxication had impaired
renal concentrating ability, a feature commonly seen in long-term
lithium treatment. Increased water and sodium loss or decreased water
and sodium   intake may lead to decreased lithium elimination and
increasing serum lithium concentrations. The low therapeutic index of
lithium is   exceeded   and   lithium intoxication develops.   The
pathogenesis of acute renal insufficiency during lithium intoxication is
unknown [1,12.13], and can not be explained by dehydration alone.

Guidelines for diagnosis, treatment and prevention of lithium
intoxication. Lithium intoxication is a serious condition with a
mortality rate of 9 - 25% depending on the type of intoxication [12]. In
the majority of our own patients(21 of 23) lithium intoxication developed
gradually and in 13 patients the symptoms had been present for more than
four days before treatment was initiated. Lithium intoxication cannot
be diagnosed from the symptoms alone. mainly because it is characterized
mental and neurological symptoms. Initially these were decreased
alertness or slight apathy followed by muscular rigidity and/or muscular
fasciculation with varying localization and slight ataxia. The symptoms
worsened gradually and impaired consciousness, more severe fasciculation
and coarse irregular tremor of the limbs and worsening ataxia developed.

The severest state was characterized by a stupor-like impairment of consciousness and spontaneous twitching movements of the limbs, body and head often simulating a state of agitation in some patients and epilepsia in others [12].

Symptoms often progressed in spite of cessation of lithium and decreasing serum lithium concentrations, and the patients who probably had an elevated serum lithium for the longest period of time were those who took longest to recover (2 died) and had the longest persisting electrocardiographic and electroencephalographic abnormalities. Thus promoting the early diagnosis and elimination of lithium from the body is necessary.

Different procedures have been proposed for treatment of lithium intoxication [12]. Our studies [12] revealed no specific effect of sodium chloride in enhancing lithium excretion from the body, where the effect obtained could be related to volume expansion alone. Furthermore, large volumes of sodium chloride should be avoided because of the risk of developing hypernatriemia in patients with severely impaired renal concentrating ability. Any kind of fluid therapy or forced diuresis treatment [12.13] should only be undertaken in patients with early symptoms of lithium intoxication and normal renal function. During treatment serum lithium should be monitored at short intervals to ensure that a concentration of 1.0mmol/1 is reached within 30 hours. Electrolytes should be assessed in the light of the unpredictable reduction in renal function that may occur during lithium intoxication.

In our experience haemodialysis is the most effective way to remove lithium from the body. Haemodialysis should be undertaken for long enough to ensure a serum lithium concentration of less than 1.0 mmol/1 after equilibration between intra-and extra-vascular lithium has occurred (6 to 8 hours after end of dialysis). Since our initial study [12] another 25 patients have been treated for lithium intoxication. Of the 25 patients 22 were dialysed (1 had peritoneal dialysis and 21 had haemodialysis). All 25 patients recovered from lithium intoxication. Peritoneal dialysis gives a slower reduction in serum lithium concentration than haemodialysis [12].

Lithium intoxication may be prevented if patients know that they can neither tolerate fluid deprivation or conditions which may lead to increased water and salt loss or decreased water and salt intake. The effect of fluid deprivation in a patient with severely impaired renal concentrating ability (nephrogenic diabetes insipidus) is illustrated in Figure 1. Factors other than glomerular filtration rates (see Table1) may influence renal lithium excretion, thus consecutive measurement of serum lithium concentration related to the daily dosage gives the best information about changes in renal lithium elimination, provided that the serum lithium values are comparable. Therefore serum lithium should be measured as 12h-stSLi (12h-stSL is defined as the serum lithium concentration in a morning blood sample 12 hours after the last lithium dosage given to a patient receiving more than one lithium dose per day 2). Serum creatinine should be measured once or twice per year in patients on long-term lithium treatment. There is no reason for routine measurements of renal concentrating ability, but it is important to be aware that renal concentrating ability might be reduced and the patients instructed accordingly. Treatment with diuretics may reduce renal lithium elimination [38].

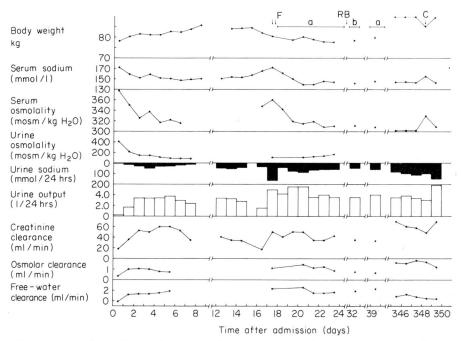

Figure 1. The clinical course in a 53-year old woman who developed polyuria during a 6-year period of lithium treatment. Lithium treatment was stopped 3 weeks before admission when an ovarian cyst had been removed. She was admitted after 24 hours of water deprivation in a state of hypertonic dehydration with renal insufficiency and improved after fluid therapy. An episode of fever from day 10 led to another episode of hypertonic dehydration. Renal biopsy taken on day 32 revealed a chronic interstitial nephropathy. During the following 11 months conditions improved. Creatinine clearance stabilized serum osmolality normalized, and osmolar clearance increased a permanent positive free water clearance being present. After treatment with diuretics a weight loss was seen and serum sodium decreased. A 26-hour renal concentration test done one year after cessation of lithium treatment revealed severely impaired renal concentrating ability with a maximal urine osmolal concentration of 317mOsm/kgH$_2$0 [15]. F: Furosemide 40 mg. a: cyclopenthiazide 0.50 mg/day. b: spironolactone 100 mg/day. R.B.: Renal biopsy. c: 26-hour renal concentration test.

Possible measures which might delay or prevent renal changes during long-term lithium treatment. As the degree of impairment of renal concentrating ability has been related to the duration of lithium treatment 3,25 or to the product of serum lithium concentration and duration of treatment [24], the lowest possible lithium dose should be used for maintenance therapy. Lithium intoxication should be prevented because of the risk of inducing acute renal insufficiency, which may be only partly reversible [12,13].

The lithium induced renal lesion affects the distal part of the nephron [3, 9-11, 33-35], thus dehydration may lead to increased lithium concentration in the distal part of the nephron. Recurrent episodes of reduced fluid intake in a patient with normal renal concentrating ability may lead to toxic lithium concentrations in the distal part of the nephron. Therefore a high fluid intake of not less than 2 to 3 litres per day should be recommended for patients starting lithium treatment.

NEPHROTOXIC EFFECTS OF OTHER PSYCHOTROPIC DRUGS.

The nephrotoxic effects of neuroleptics combined with lithium have been discussed above. The possible acute nephrotoxicity of the neuroleptic drug, chlorprothixene, has recently been studied in a patient who developed acute renal failure after an overdosage [39]. Apart from a slight dilatation of some distal tubules and a fine vacuolization of the tubular epithelium renal histology was normal, and it was concluded that there was no evidence of specific nephrotoxicity. The renal failure was thought to have resulted from ischemia during a transitory episode of hypotension. which is a well-known side-effect of chlorprothixene.

Increasing abuse of the well-known antihistamine H_1-receptor blocking agent. iphenhydramine. has been described among young people in Denmark [40]. An overdosage of diphenhydramine is associated with agitation, acute psychosis. tachycardia and eventually stupor. An association between diphenhydramine intoxication and acute renal insufficiency has not previously been described but within the last two years we have seen two males. aged 18 and 39 years respectively. develop acute renal insufficiency after an overdose of 5g of diphenhydramine. Both patients had severe psycho-social and drug abuse problems. Both had normal serum creatinine values 8 days and one year. respectively. before admission. In one of the patients renal function normalized during 6 days after a maximum serum creatinine value of 8.9mg/100 ml (787µmol/1) had been reached. The other patient was anuric and treated with peritoneal dialysis twice. and a slightly elevated serum creatinine of 1.8 mg/100 ml (160µmol/1) was present at discharge from hospital 3 weeks after admission. Renal biopsy studies including electron microscopy did not reveal any specific abnormalities in the non-dialysed patient. In the other patient changes consistent with tubulo-interstitial nephropathy were present. During the disease course both patients had stable blood pressure. neither cardiac arrthymia nor respiratory depression was present. one of the patients went into stupor; the other did not. The action of diphenhydramine on renal function is uncertain. In studies on dogs [41] a decreased glomerular filtration rate has been observed during intravenous infusion of diphenhydramine, but no decrease in glomerular filtration was seen when diphenhydramine was given to rats [42]. It is possible that hypotension had been present before admission in both patients and/or that they had withheld information concerning other drugs involved. An association between the intake of a large amount of diphenhydramine (5 g) and an acute renal insufficiency has been observed, but there is no evidence that it was a cause and effect relationship.

THE NEPHROTOXIC PROPERTIES OF ANTIEPILEPTICS

Among the reported side-effects to anticonvulsant therapy with hydantoins are generalized lymphadenopathy and nephrotic syndrome [43]. and an acute immunologically induced interstitial nephritis with acute renal failure [44]. Our patient (Fig.2). a 23 year old female. developed

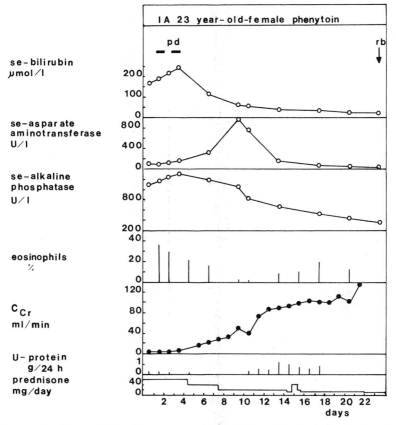

Figure 2. The clinical course of a diphenylhydantoin (phenytoin) induced allergic reaction with liver damage eosinophilia and acute renal failure in a 23-year old female. For details see text. pd: Peritoneal dialysis. rb: Renal biopsy.

generalized tonic-clonic seizures during the second month of pregnancy. there was normal blood pressure. normal renal function and no proteinuria. Neurologic investigations concluded that a cryptogenic epilepsia was present. and treatment with diphenylhydantoin (phenytoin) was started. From day 14 to day 22 after start of treatment fever. generalized exanthema. eosinophilia. liver affection and finally acute renal insufficiency developed.

Peritoneal dialysis was undertaken twice. and during prednisone treatment liver and kidney function normalized over the following 3 weeks. Renal biopsy revealed a focal interstitial nephritis with lymphocyte infiltration and granuloma with giant cells [45]. Toxic-allergic drug reactions involving the kidneys have been related to a number of drugs. Considering the number of patients treated with hydantoin preparations. related to the number of cases reported, acute toxic allergic interstitial nephritis and nephrotic syndrome are rarely seen complications.

484 H. E. HANSEN

Anticonvulsive treatment with valproic acid is associated with side-effects such as acute hepatic failure. thrombocytopenia. alopecia and anorexia [46]. In one case valproic acid has been reported to induce a proximal tubular renal dysfunction [47]. This patient developed proteinuria. reduced tubular reabsorption of glucose with glucosuria. acidosis and hypocalcemia during valproic acid treatment. after cessation of treatment immediate improvement occurred. Renal biopsy revealed giant mitochondria in the proximal tubular cells and ultrastructural studies disclosed abnormal round granular inclusions located in the cystosol of the tubular cells. A 20-year old female who had taken an overdosage of 75 g of sodium valproate with a maximal serum valproate concentration of 2100 μg/ml developed a slight and transient increase in serum creatinine from 80-141 μmol/1 during the first 24 hours after admission proteinuria was also present during the first 10 days with a maximal concentration of 2.3 g/l [48]. The renal damage could not be explained by circulatory insufficiency as the patient was admitted to the hospital 1.5 hour after intake of the overdosage and before symptoms of intoxication occurred. During the disease course she went into coma. but no episodes of hypotension or cardiac arrthymias were seen. The induction of renal insufficiency as a consequence of valproic acid intoxication removed rapidly because it was by haemodialysis treatment. followed by haemoperfusion. Within the first 30 hours after admission. however. a maximal urine valproate concentration of 400 μg/ml was measured. The present information calls for further studies on renal function during valproic acid treatment and during valproic acid intoxication.

Summary

1) Lithium concentrations in urine may exceed plasma levels by 40 to 50 times. indicating very high lithium concentrations in the distal part of the nephron.
2) Lithium may induce a chronic interstitial nephropathy with focal interstitial fibrosis. tubular atrophy and microcysts.
3) Reduced renal concentrating ability is a common finding in patients on long-term lithium treatment. The impairment of renal concentrating ability has been related to the duration of lithium treatment and to the degree of tubular damage.
4) In the majority of long-term lithium-treated patients glomerular filtration rate is normal or almost normal.
5) The major risk to long-term lithium treated patients is lithium intoxication not end-stage renal failure. Patients with reduced renal concentrating ability do not tolerate those conditions which lead to increased extrarenal water and sodium loss. or reduced fluid and salt intake. Such conditions have preceded the majority of intoxications which have developed during long-term treatment.
6) To avoid high lithium concentrations in the distal part of the nephron a fluid intake of 2 to 3 litres per day is recommended from the beginning of lithium treatment.
7) Lithium-induced nephrotic syndrome is a rarely seen condition of unknown etiology.
8) The combination of lithium treatment and treatment with neuroleptics may contribute to the development of chronic renal changes.
9) Acute renal insufficiency seen during intoxications with neuroleptics (chlorprothiene) could be related to hypotension.

10) The possible nephrotoxic properties of H_1-receptor blockers (diphenhydramine) are unsettled.
11) Hydantoin preparations may induce an immunologically mediated acute interstitial nephritis with acute renal insufficiency. but based on the number of patients reported it is a rarely seen condition.
12) Valproic acid has been suggested to affect proximal tubular renal function but the available data are too few to draw any clear-cut conclusions. and further studies on the influence of valproic acid on renal function are recommended.

References

1.   Hansen HE. Drugs. In press.
2.   Amdisen A. Clin Pharmacokinet 2:73-92.1977.
3.   Hansen HE. et al. Q J Med 48: 577-591. 1979.
4.   Foulks J, et al. Am J Psychol 168:642-649. 1952.
5.   Thomsen K and Schou A. Am J Psychol 215:823-827,1968.
6.   Steele TH. et al. Am J Med Sci 269:349-363.1975.
7.   Thomsen K. et al. Pfluegers Arch 308: 180-184. 1969.
8.   Thomsen K. Dan Med Bull 25: 106-115. 1978.
9.   Hansen HE et al. To be published.
10. Radomski JL. et al. J. Pharmacol Exp Ther 100:429-444. 1950.
11. Evan PA and Ollerich D. Am J Anat 134:97106.1972.
12. Hansen HE and Amdisen A. Q J Med 47: 123-144.1978.
13. Hansen HE. et al. Acta Med Scand 205:593-597. 1979.
14. Olsen S. Kidney Int 10 (suppl. 6):2-8.1976.
15. Hestbech J. et al. Kidney Int 12:205-213.1977.
16. Hansen HE. et al. In Proceedings of the European Dialysis and Transplant Association. Pitman Medical. London. 1977. vol. 14. p.518-527.ISBN 0-272-79501-1.
17. Vestergaard P et al. Acta Psychiatr Scand 60:504-520. 1979.
18. Donker AJM. et al. Clin Nephrol 12: 254-262, 1979.
19. Hansen HE. et al. Nephron. In print.
20. Hullin RP. et al. Br Med J 1: 1457-1459, 1979.
21. Burrows GD. et al. Lancet 1: 1310.1978.
22. Bucht G. et al. Nord Psykiatr T 32:445-456.1978.
23. Gerner RG. et al. Am J Psychiatry 137:834-837,1980.
24. Albrecht J. et al. Pharmakopsychiatr Neuropsychopharmakol 13:228-234. 1980.
25. Grof P. et al. Can J Psychiatry 25:535-544. 1980.
26. Coppen A. et al. Acta Psychiatr Scand 62:343-355.1980.
27. Davies B and Kincaid-Smith P. Neuropharmacology 18: 1001-1002.1979.
28. Depaulo JR jr. et al. Am J Psychiatry 138-324-327. 1981.
29. Kincaid-Smith PS. et al. Kidney Int 19:121.1981.
30. Walker RG and Kincaid-Smith PS. Aust NZ J Med 10:487.1980.
31. Vestergaard P and Amdisen A. Acta Psychiatr Scand. In print 1981.
32. Bucht G, et al. Acta Med Scand 208:381-385, 1980.
33. Hestbech J. et al. Acta Pathol Microbiol Scand 86: 195-197.1978.
34. Jacobsen NO. et al. In Abstracts of the 8th International Congress of Nephrology. 1981. p. 202.
35. Christensen S. et al. In Abstracts of the 8th International Congress of Nephrology. 1981. p. 194.
36.   Richman AV. et al. Ann Intern Med 92: 70-72,1980.
37. Alexander F and Martin J. Clin Nephrol 15:267-271.1981.

38. Petersen V. et al. Br Med J 3: 143-145,1974.
39. Rossen B and Steiness I. Acta Med Scand 209: 525-527,1981.
40. Staffeldt H von. et al. Ugeskr Laeger 142: 1149-1150, 1980.
41. Banks RO. et al. Am J Physiol 235: F570-F575, 1978.
42. Ichikawa J and Brenner BM. Circ Res 45:733-745,1979.
43. Snead C. et al. Paediatr 57:98;101.1976.
44. Kleinknecht D. et al. In Contributions to Nephrology vol. 10.:
     Toxic Nephropathies.S. Karger. Basel. 1977. pp42-52.
     ISBN 3-8055-2832-9.
45. Brun C and Olsen S. Atlas of Renal biopsy. Munksgaard. Copenhagen.
     W.B. Saunders Co. Philadelphia. London. Toronto 1981, p.136. ISBN
     87-16-02722-1.
46. Browne TR. N Engl J Med 302:661-665. 1980.
47. Lenoir GR. et al. J Pediatr 98:503-504. 1981.
48. Mortensen PB. et al.Clin. Pharmacol. Ther. Toxicol. in print.

NEPHROTOXICITY OF ETHYLENE GLYCOLS, CEPHALOSPORINS AND DIURETICS

Tibor Balazs, Benjamin Jackson and Mark Hite*

Food and Drug Administration, Washington, DC, USA and
*Merck Institute for Therapeutic Research, West Point, Pennsylvania, USA

ABSTRACT

Ethylene glycol and diethylene glycol have been involved in human exposures that have resulted in fatalities. Results obtained with animal models for glycol nephrotoxicity resemble the clinical events occurring in humans: necrosis or hydropic degeneration of the proximal convoluted tubules leading to anuria, uremia, and death. The lack of metabolic information on diethylene glycol and the uncertain role of crystal (oxalate) deposition in the mechanism of ethylene glycol nephrotoxicity leaves the question of mechanisms unanswered. Among the large number of cephalosporin antibiotics, cephaloridine and, to a much lesser extent, cefazolin and cephalothin are nephrotoxic. They are taken up by peritubular anionic transport into the proximal convoluted tubules, where cephaloridine reaches the highest renal-to-plasma concentration ratio. A reactive metabolic intermediate or its polymer has been postulated to have a role in the mechanism of its nephrotoxicity. Lysosomes are the primary targets, since perilysosomal lysis precedes the tubular necrosis that is dose related in each species. Diuretics have produced few nephrotoxic effects in humans. Allergic interstitial nephritis has been associated with furosemide and thiazide. These reactions have not as yet been reproduced in experimental animals and thus could not have been predicted from safety evaluation studies.

Ethylene glycol; Cephalosporins; Thiazides; Furosemide; Ethacrynic acid; Mercurials

INTRODUCTION

Chance occurrence plays no lesser role in advancing toxicological knowledge than it does in advancing knowledge of other sciences. The full safety assessment of chemicals demands an interplay between experimentation in the laboratory and experience in the clinic. Rare toxic events that have occurred in humans after exposure to drugs often could not have been foreseen by initial test results in an animal model. On the other hand, when results in animals during preclinical testing suggest a hazard, they often must await accidental findings in humans before their full significance is appreciated. The interplay between the clinic and laboratory and the resultant advances in knowledge are translated into information on safe use that is designed to prevent future accidents. This situation is illustrated by the toxic renal effects of diethylene and ethylene glycol, and of a few cephalosporin antibiotics.

The lack of premarketing toxicity studies resulted in numerous deaths due to renal failure because of the use of diethylene glycol as a solvent for sulfanilamide. This tragedy catalyzed legislation in the United States to require toxicity tests of drugs in experimental animals before their use in humans (Federal Food, Drug, and Cosmetic Act, 1938). The saga of cephalosporins is attributed to another kind of error. Although preclinical toxicity tests revealed a nephrotoxic potential of cephaloridine, results were not taken seriously, perhaps because this effect occurred at doses above those providing therapeutic blood concentrations. Nevertheless, severe nephrotoxicity developed in numerous patients, particularly when predisposing factors were present that could not be foreseen from the animal experiments.

The limitations in the state of the art of animal experiments are demonstrated by the nephrotoxicity of diuretics, the third class of compounds discussed in this review. Some of the chlorothiazide diuretics induced a renal injury that is considered to be a hypersensitivity reaction. However, an immune response-mediated effect with these agents has not been reproduced or even studied in experimental animal models. Recent advances in immunology, such as the recognition of major histocompatibility genes and immune response gene-dependent reactions to drugs, may provide impetus for studies of this nature in experimental animals.

ETHYLENE GLYCOL AND DIETHYLENE GLYCOL

Ethylene glycol and diethylene glycol are widely used as solvents in industrial processes. Both have been involved in intentional and unintentional human exposures that have resulted in fatalities. The use of ethylene glycol in antifreeze formulations has made it easily available for intentional ingestion by humans for purposes of inebriation and suicide. In 1937, a high concentration of diethylene glycol was used to prepare an elixir of sulfonamide, resulting in more than 100 human deaths.

<u>Clinical picture of acute toxicity.</u> In humans, the clinical events following ingestion of ethylene glycol can be divided into three stages [1]. The events during the first 12 hours involve the central nervous system and resemble those of ethyl alcohol intoxication; symptoms consist of vomiting, ataxia, prostration, cyanosis, convulsions, and

coma [2]. Cardiopulmonary effects may appear beyond the first 12-24 hours, and include tachypnea, cyanosis, pulmonary edema, and death in cardiac failure. The third phase, which occurs after the second day, is renal impairment, characterized by proteinuria, oliguria, anuria, and death in uremia [1]. The clinical events after ingestion of diethylene glycol resemble those of ethylene glycol except that they are somewhat slower in onset and do not include cardiopulmonary effects. Oliguria and anuria may develop after 24 hours; the patients become comatose and death in uremic coma occurs 2-7 days after the onset of anuria [3].

Rats given high doses of ethylene glycol developed ataxia, lethargy, and dyspnea within 20 minutes after treatment. Rats given comparable dosages of diethylene glycol developed a lesser degree of these effects [2].

Lethal toxicity data. Both ethylene glycol and diethylene glycol are potentially lethal in humans in amounts of about 1 ml/kg of body weight, which corresponds to a dosage of 1-2 g/kg [4]. In laboratory animals, the median lethal doses of both compounds was an order of magnitude less. Deaths from ethylene glycol in animals [4] and humans [1] usually occurred within 24-48 hours whereas deaths from diethylene glycol in humans occurred 2-7 days after the onset of anuria [3]. Toxicity was cumulative in chronic tests in rats. Blood [5] reported that survival of rats was compromised when ethylene glycol was administered in the diet for prolonged periods at levels of 1% and greater; however, female rats fed diets containing 4% survived over twice as long as males fed this diet and survival of females fed 1% in the diet was unaffected.

Nephrotoxicity. Findings of experimental nephrotoxicity in animals resemble those detected in humans exposed to lethal amounts of ethylene glycol and diethylene glycol. The deposition of oxalate crystals in the renal tubules was a constant and conspicuous feature of ethylene glycol exposure in both humans and animals [1]. Tubular epithelial changes were more variable. In humans, degeneration of tubular epithelium was observed within 72 hours after exposure to ethylene glycol [6]. Necrosis of tubular epithelium has been reported to occur in monkeys [7] and swine [8]. In studies with rats, Winek et al. [2] reported that little cellular damage was evident despite oxalate deposition when a range of doses, including a lethal dose, was used in acute tests. Crystal deposition was not a feature of diethylene glycol nephrotoxicity in either humans or animals. Renal tubular changes characterized as hydropic degeneration have been observed in humans as well as in laboratory animals [2,3,9]. Necrosis of the epithelium of proximal convoluted tubules was observed by Kesten et al. [9] after repeated exposure of rats to 3% diethylene glycol in the drinking water.

In multiple dose tests, effects on the kidneys of male and female rats were different. Deposits of calcium oxalate crystals and tubular damage were observed in renal tubules of females rats given diets containing 1 and 4% ethylene glycol but were seen in male rats only at the 0.5% concentration. Renal calculi were observed in both sexes at the high dose but not in females at the next lower dose [5].

Fitzhugh and Nelson [10] reported that marked renal and bladder changes occurred in rats fed diets containing 0.5-4% diethylene glycol for 2 years. Bladder stones and bladder tumors, in addition to kidney and liver damage, were produced by feeding diets containing 2 and 4% of the compound.

Residues of ethylene glycol have been detected in parenteral formulations of antibiotics sterilized by ethylene oxide. Similarly, residues of ethylene glycol have been found in medical devices, such as dialyzing machines for patients with kidney diseases, after sterilization with ethylene oxide.

Although it is unlikely that trace amounts of ethylene glycol would produce renal injury even after repeated exposure, there have been no reported studies of the possible role of predisposing factors encountered in its use, e.g., drug combinations or the presence of 2-chloroethanol, which is also formed from ethylene oxide and depletes glutathione, or the presence of existing renal injury.

Metabolism. In humans, ethylene glycol undergoes extensive oxidation in a manner analogous to ethanol. Glycolaldehyde, glycolic acid, and glyoxylic acid may be implicated in several biochemical reactions related to ethylene glycol toxicity [2]. The prominent cerebral symptoms that occur during the first stages of ethylene glycol toxicity coincide with the greatest amounts of aldehyde production. This metabolite may also be responsible for the cardiopulmonary symptoms. The renal damage produced by ethylene glycol ingestion is attributed to the accumulation of oxalate crystals. Support for this mechanism is supplied by the success of therapy based on prevention of the crystal formation by blocking the metabolism of ethylene glycol with ethyl alcohol.

Although both ethylene glycol and diethylene glycol produce toxic nephropathy and have somewhat similar clinical effects, there appear to be some differences between them. These include the absence of calcium oxalate crystals in kidneys after diethylene glycol exposure and the lack of necrosis of the tubular epithelium. Winek et al. [2] showed that oxalate concentrations in blood and kidneys of rats after treatment with ethylene glycol were much higher than those following diethylene glycol.

Pathogenesis of renal injury. The resemblance of the renal effects produced by ethylene glycol to those produced by oxalic acid seems to implicate the oxalate pathway in the renal injury. Roberts and Siebold [7] have questioned whether oxalate formation can account entirely for the renal injury, and Gershoff and Andrus [11] showed that morphologic tubular changes occur even when crystallization is prevented by feeding vitamin B_6. In rats, the absence of marked cytological changes in tubules containing large deposits of calcium oxalate crystals, as reported by Winek et al. [2], suggests that the deposition of oxalate crystals and tubular damage may be separate processes. On the other hand, Elferink and Riemersma [12] reported that calcium oxalate microcrystals induce cytolysis and suggest that positive charges on the crystals may play a role in the cell injury. The crystals used for their studies were less than 0.5 μm and would not likely be visible under ordinary microscopic examination.

CEPHALOSPORINS

Among the large number of cephalosporin antibiotics, cephaloridine, cefazolin, and cephalothin are nephrotoxic in both experimental animals and in humans. Cephaloridine caused renal tubular necrosis in each species tested, and the incidence and severity of the lesions were dose related. Cefazolin was nephrotoxic in rabbits, but the toxic dose was twice that of cephaloridine [13,14]. The potential nephrotoxicity of cephalothin was detected in animals and in patients with impaired renal function [15,16].

In addition to the renal injury due to direct toxic mechanisms, various types of immune system-mediated nephrotoxicity have been attributed to the use of cephalothin in humans [16].

Renal transport. The kidneys handle cephaloridine by glomerular filtration, to a lesser extent by cortical tubular transport, and to a very limited extent by reabsorption. The peritubular anionic transport is an active process, i.e., it is oxygen-dependent and is inhibited by dinitrophenol and probenecid. The nephrotoxicity of cephaloridine is related to its renal cortical accumulation; the magnitude of its cortex-to-plasma ratio correlates with the signs of nephrotoxicity. The transport pool can be estimated by the differences between the cortex-to-serum ratios of cephaloridine in control and probenecid-treated animals. An inverse relation exists between the size of the pool in the species and the nephrotoxic dose [17]. Probenecid reduced the cortex-to-serum ratios in decreasing magnitude in the rabbit, guinea pig, and rat, which can be correlated with the protective effect.

The pool size and the nephrotoxicity increased with the age of rabbits. The cortex-to-serum ratios were 1.7, 6.5, and 12.2 at 2 and 5 weeks of age and in the adult, respectively. Pretreatment at 2 weeks of age with p-aminohippurate or penicillin stimulated the uptake of cephaloridine and enhanced its nephrotoxicity [18].

Cephaloridine is removed from tubular cells by the cationic transport system, which is inhibited by cyanine 863 or mepiperphenidol. Pretreatment of rabbits with cyanine enhanced the nephrotoxicity of cephaloridine [13]. Thus this transport system may be responsible for the accumulation of cephaloridine in the tubular cell. Cefazolin and, to a lesser extent, cephalothin are secreted like p-aminohippurate in and out of the tubules. Probenecid also reduced the nephrotoxicity of cefazolin in rabbits.

The rabbit is the most sensitive laboratory animal species for investigating the nephrotoxicity of cephalosporins because of its large tubular transport pool. The blood level of cephaloridine associated with nephrotoxicity is 150 μg/ml, which can be attained by a single intramuscular dose of 200 mg/kg. Wold [13] showed that in vitro cortical slice functions declined after rabbits had been treated with a single s.c. dose of 100 mg of cephaloridine/kg and the cortical slice concentration was about 1.2 mg/g. A dosage of 200 mg/kg produced a cortical slice concentration of 4 mg/g. Subacute daily administration of 1/3 to 1/2 of an acute nephrotoxic dose did not produce nephrotoxic effects, implying that the drug was not accumulated, i.e., the healthy kidney could quantitatively excrete amounts below the nephrotoxic dose [19].

Although the nephrotoxic blood concentration of cephalothin is not much greater than that of cephaloridine, a dose about five times greater is needed to reach that level.

Pathogenesis of renal injury. Cephaloridine is similar to most direct nephrotoxins in that a single large dose can produce renal injury. Proteinuria and glucosuria developed in mice in less than 24 hours after i.p. administration of cephaloridine at 1.2 g/kg. The kidneys were enlarged and pale, and histologic examination revealed necrosis in the proximal convoluted tubules [20].

Silverblatt and associates [14] followed the time sequence of development of the lesion in rabbits treated with 200 mg cephaloridine/kg intramuscularly; by light microscopy, they detected the loss of brush borders in the mid-portion of the proximal convolution within 1 hour after treatment. The height of the epithelium was reduced and the tubular lumens were dilated 4-10 hours thereafter, and frank necrosis appeared at 10 hours. The lesion was prominent in the mid-portion of the proximal convolution, whereas a single dose of 100 mg/kg produced lesions only in a number of tubules and 50 mg/kg did not seem to cause any injury.

Watanabe [21] conducted an electron microscopic study of the cephaloridine-induced lesion in the rat. Changes in the tubular membranes that were probably related to transport of the drug were seen 30 minutes after s.c. administration of 2 g of cephaloridine/kg. These changes consisted of basal infoldings and an increase in the number and size of apical vacuoles. The vacuoles moved to the mid-region of the cell and fused with lysosomes. The membranes of some of these enlarged lysosomes ruptured and the cytoplasm around them were destroyed. Later the mitochondrial cristae became destructed. Neither lysosomal rupture nor mitochondrial changes were seen in rats treated with cephalothin, and only the membrane changes were detected.

Molecular toxicology of cephaloridine. The molecular toxicology of cephaloridine has been the subject of a number of studies. The genesis of a reactive intermediate, e.g., an electrophilic metabolite that would interact with vital macromolecules and lead to tubular necrosis, has been postulated. Pretreatment of rabbits with phenobarbital, an inducer of enzyme systems that can generate reactive metabolites, potentiated the nephrotoxicity of cephaloridine [22]. Pretreatment of rats or mice failed to potentiate the effect. These findings suggest that reactive intermediates generated in situ have a role in the pathogenesis of the lesion, since phenobarbital is known to induce the synthesis of renal enzyme systems in rabbits but not in mice or rats. Pretreatment with inhibitors of microsomal enzymes such as cobalt chloride or piperonyl butoxide inhibited development of the lesions in each of the three species [22]. This finding also supports the role of a reactive metabolite in the pathogenesis of the lesion. Nevertheless, data of a recent study of Kuo and Hook [23] favor the concept that phenobarbital-induced potentiation is attributable to enhanced transport rather than to metabolism of cephaloridine.

Another concept about the chemical mechanism of biotransformation is the polymerization of cephaloridine in the tubular cells. Commercial preparations contain the monomer, dimer, and polymer of the compound. The monomer and dimer were more nephrotoxic when given i.p. to rats than the polymer, perhaps because they are transported more readily. However, polymerization occurs in the cell and it is conceivable that this initiates the lysosomal changes described above [24].

Interaction studies. Several authors have investigated the role of various factors that may sensitize to the nephrotoxicity of cephalosporins. Linton and associates [15] treated rats with glycerol (50%, 4 ml/kg) and furosemide (50 mg/kg) concurrently with various cephalosporins. Cephaloridine and cephalothin produced tubular necrosis at serum antibiotic levels comparable to the therapeutic concentrations in humans. Cephalexin and cephapirin did not produce lesions. Glycerol alone was able to produce renal functional impairment and destruction of enlarged lysosomes in the renal epithelium.

Furosemide or ethacrynic acid alone (i.e., without glycerol) increased the nephrotoxicity of cephaloridine in mice [25]. In studies of the mechanism of the potentiating effect of furosemide, an increased resorption of the antibiotic brought about by sodium depletion was postulated.

Groups of CR/FRF2 female albino mice were treated i.p. with 20 mg of furosemide/kg 15 minutes before the i.p. administration of 600 or 1200 mg of cephaloridine/kg [20]. Other groups of mice received only cephaloridine. All animals were killed 48 hours after treatment and the kidneys were examined histologically. Furosemide pretreatment enhanced the severity of the cephaloridine-induced lesion and also significantly increased the renal cortical concentrations of antibiotics at 15, 60, and 240 minutes after their administration. The interaction of furosemide with cefazolin (6 g/kg), cephalothin (4.8 g/kg), cefamandole (4.5 g/kg), cephapirin (5 g/kg), and cephacetrile (4 g/kg) was also tested. No lesion was detected with these drugs alone or in combination.

The interaction of cephalosporin and aminoglycoside antibiotics has been investigated by several authors. Most of the aminoglycosides are themselves nephrotoxic. Data from animal experiments indicate that cephalosporins have a protective effect against the nephrotoxicity of aminoglycosides; this effect required a molar ratio of cephalothin to gentamicin of 500:1. The mechanism of the protection involved increased excretion and decreased cortical concentration of the aminoglycoside [26,27], and there may have been a specific protection on the lysosomal membrane. Clinical studies in humans failed to show protective effects with the combination of cephalothin and gentamicin. Some of the results indicated greater nephrotoxicity of this combination, particularly of gentamicin plus cephaloridine, than of gentamicin alone. The cephalosporin:aminoglycoside ratios were, however, only about 50:1 in these studies [28].

Studies in humans have demonstrated the role of pre-existing renal functional deficits related to age, e.g., decreased glomerular filtration rate or disease, as well as the role of loop inhibitor diuretics or aminoglycosides as contributory factors to the cephaloridine or cephalothin nephrotoxicity [16].

Although experimental or clinical data are not sufficient, it is possible that under certain conditions some of the newer cephalosporins will produce nephrotoxic reactions. Consequently, the dosage of these antibiotics should be modified in patients with pre-existing renal disease and renal function should be monitored throughout therapy.

DIURETICS

Diuretics produce their action on the kidney, but they have generally not caused toxicity to this organ.

Thiazides and related compounds. These drugs are sulfonamide derivatives, although not all have the benzothiadiazine nucleus. Their

mode of action is to inhibit sodium resorption in the cortical portion
of the ascending tubule and in the distal convoluted tubule, where less
than 10% of the filtered sodium is resorbed. The most noteworthy
action of the thiazides is to increase the renal excretion of sodium
and chloride with an accompanying volume of water; this effect is
virtually independent of acid-base balance. The thiazides also evoke a
significant augmentation of potassium excretion. They have a flat
dose-response curve, so that increasing the dose above the therapeutic
level yields little additional benefit and may increase the incidence
of side effects.

The most common side effects are related to electrolyte imbalance
and disturbances in blood chemistry that frequently remain undetected.
These include hypokalemia, hyponatremia, hyperuricemia, hypercalcemia,
hyperglycemia, and azotemia. Other, more rare adverse effects have
been observed; these include purpura, dermatitis, photosensitivity, and
bone marrow depression, all of which represent hypersensitivity
reactions. In animal experiments, the demonstrable toxic dose for all
thiazides is many-fold greater than that required for their
pharmacological action. For example, large acute doses can depress
central nervous system function. In addition, megadose amounts have
precipitated in the kidneys to produce mechanical injury in
experimental animals [29,30].

High-ceiling or loop diuretics. These drugs achieve a peak diuresis
far greater than that observed with other agents. They inhibit sodium
resorption in the ascending limb of Henle's loop, where approximately
20% of the filtered sodium is resorbed. Their electrolyte excretion
pattern is the same as that of thiazide diuretics, except that loop
diuretics also increase calcium excretion. These agents have an
infinite dose-response curve that makes them effective even in patients
with renal failure, but they are potentially more dangerous because the
larger the dose the greater the diuresis. The two principal members of
this class of drugs are ethacrynic acid and furosemide.

The adverse effects of loop diuretics are similar to those of the
thiazides, with only a few exceptions. Furosemide, since it is a
sulfonamide derivative, has the same potential for producing skin
rashes, photosensitivity, and bone marrow depression that the thiazides
have, and cross-hypersensitivity reactions between furosemide and the
thiazides should be anticipated in clinical use. The development of
deafness, either transient or permanent, is a serious and rare
complication of treatment with ethacrynic acid. Transient deafness
also has been reported to occur with furosemide treatment.
Drug-induced changes in the electrolyte composition of the endolymph
represent a possible mechanism. From available data, ototoxicity from
diuretics appears to be unique to this class of drugs [29,30].

Nephrotoxic effects. Acute interstitial nephritis has been noted in
rare instances with both the thiazides and furosemide diuretics
[31-36]. It is characterized by an acute onset, often with macroscopic
hematuria. On roentgenographic examination the kidneys are
symmetrically enlarged. Acute renal failure may develop insidiously.
Renal biopsy shows interstitial infiltration of mononuclear cells and
eosinophils without marked fibrosis, and tubular lesions are present
with degeneration, necrosis, and/or atrophy. When the interstitial
infiltration is only moderate, it may be difficult to distinguish acute
interstitial nephritis from acute tubular necrosis. Usually there are
no glomerular or vascular lesions [37,38].

Other associated clinical features include fever, arthralgias, skin rash, and blood eosinophilia. Moreover, the reaction is not dose related and can be elicited by a rechallenge of the patient [37]. All of these suggest an underlying immunological mechanism. This condition has not as yet been reproduced in experimental animals.

An acute renal tubular necrosis was consistently produced by furosemide after i.p. administration in male Fisher rats and male Golden Syrian hamsters, and less consistently in male Swiss mice [39]. It was suggested that metabolic activation in situ in the kidney might be responsible for drug-induced renal injury. In addition, there was a possibility that the drug-induced nephrotoxicity might be caused by selective uptake and concentration of the drugs and anoxic damage resulting from shock or respiratory depression. Altered renal blood flow with resulting hypoxia can contribute to the pathogenesis of toxic renal damage and cannot be excluded as a contributing factor [20,34,40].

Acute renal failure due to tubular urate or cast-induced obstruction in humans has been reported to be caused by tienilic acid, a uricosuric loop diuretic structurally related to ethacrynic acid [41,42].

Thiazides may occasionally cause the formation of calculi, e.g., urate stones [37]. Furosemide has also been implicated in the precipitation of renal calcifications in infants who received the drug for control of patent ductus arteriosus and later for bronchopulmonary dysplasia [43]. The calcifications were noted on radiologic examination at 1-3 months of age, and included isolated stones to nephrocalcinosis and staghorn calculi. Metabolic alkalosis was present. Amorphous crystals and calcium oxalate crystals were found in the urine. A possible mechanism for the stone formations is the hypercalcinuria and alkaline urine produced by furosemide therapy.

The syndrome of inappropriate secretion of antidiuretic hormone, as described by Curtis [37], consists of hyponatremia and reduced plasma osmolality together with a urine osmolality usually exceeding that of the plasma. Despite hyponatremia, urinary sodium excretion often exceeds 50 mEq/day. Edema and fluid depletion are absent. The condition is produced by continuous release of antidiuretic hormone in concentrations inappropriate for the plasma osmolality and it occurs in the absence of renal disease [44]. Clinically, lethargy, apathy, nausea, vomiting, headache, irritability, disorientation, increasing confusion, convulsions, and coma occur and are thought to be due to water intoxication. Mild hyperthermia may occur. Several drugs have been incriminated in this syndrome, among which are the thiazide diuretics [34,37]. The mechanism of this phenomenon has not as yet been established.

Mercurial diuretics. Before the advent of the previously described diuretics, mercurials were widely used. The classical symptoms of systemic mercury poisoning may follow the injudicious use of mercurial diuretics. Mercury has toxic effects involving numerous organ systems that have been well described [45].

Since mercury, regardless of the chemical form, is concentrated in the kidney, renal lesions may develop. These are confined largely to the tubular epithelium [37,46]. If the circulation is adequate, the first response of the kidney may be diuresis due to the suppression of tubular resorptive function. Thereafter, the renal damage becomes so extensive that oliguria and anuria result. Experimental evidence from animal studies suggests that several factors are involved in the mechanism; these include tubular obstruction, increased back-diffusion of tubular filtrate, and preglomerular vasoconstriction. The phase of polyuria is characterized by decreased renal concentrating capacity, and probably results mainly from a substantial inhibition of proximal tubular sodium resorption. In severe mercury poisoning, disturbances in tubular function may persist for several months after poisoning [45].

Chronic mercury poisoning produced by these diuretics is characterized by proteinuria [47]. If severe, the nephrotic syndrome is observed, wherein the loss of plasma protein is great enough to cause hypoproteinemia with edema of dependent parts, for example, the ankles [41]. In the mechanism of this syndrome, an immune system-mediated reaction can be postulated in view of the recent discovery of $HgCl_2$-induced autoimmune renal glomerulonephritis in rats [48].

ACKNOWLEDGMENT

The help of Dr. J.S. Wold in providing data on cephalosporins is gratefully acknowledged.

REFERENCES

1. Schreiner GE and Maher JF, Am J Med 38:409-449, 1965.
2. Winek CL, et al. Clin Toxicol 13:297-324, 1978.
3. Geiling EMK and Cannon PR, J Am Med Assoc 111:919-926, 1938.
4. Browning E, in Toxicity and Metabolism of Industrial Solvents. Elsevier, Amsterdam, London and New York, 1965, pp. 597, 627.
5. Blood FR, Food Cosmet Toxicol 3:229-234, 1965.
6. Parry MF and Wallach R, Am J Med 57:143-150, 1974.
7. Roberts JA and Seibold HR, Toxicol Appl Pharmacol 15:624-631, 1969.
8. Ostweiler GD and Eness PG, J Am Vet Med Assoc 160:746-749, 1972.
9. Kesten HD, et al. J Am Med Assoc 109:1509-1511, 1937.
10. Fitzhugh OG and Nelson AA, J Ind Hyg Toxicol 28:40-43, 1946.
11. Gershoff SN and Andrus SB, Proc Soc Exp Biol Med 109:99-102, 1962.
12. Elferink JGR and Riemersma RC, Agents Actions 10:439-444, 1980.
13. Wold JS, in Toxicology of the Kidney. (JB Hook, ed). Raven Press, New York, 1981, pp. 251-266.
14. Silverblatt F, et al. J Infect Dis 122:33-44, 1970.
15. Linton AL, et al. Can Med Assoc J 107:414-417, 1972.
16. Foord RD, J Antimicrob Chemother 1 (Suppl):119-133, 1975.
17. Tune BM, J Infect Dis 132:189-194, 1975.
18. Wold, JS, et al. J Pharmacol Exp Ther 201:778-785, 1977.
19. Atkinson KM, et al. Toxicol Appl Pharmacol 8:407-428, 1966.
20. James G, et al. Proc Soc Toxicol Annu Meeting 1975, Abstr No 194.
21. Watanabe M, Acta Pathol Jpn 28:867-889, 1978.
22. McMurty RJ and Mitchell JR, Toxicol Appl Pharmacol 42:285-300, 1977.
23. Kuo CH and Hook JB, Pharmacologist 23:190, 1981.
24. Boyd JF, et al. Int J Clin Pharmacol 7:307-315, 1973.
25. Doods MG and Foord RD, Br J Pharmacol 40:227-236, 1970.
26. Roos R and Jackson GG, Proc 10th Int Congr Chemother 2:962-964, 1978.
27. Barza M, et al. Proc 10th Int Congr Chemother 2:964-968, 1978.
28. Giamarellon H, et al. Proc 10th Int Congr Chemother 2:968-970.

29. Mudge GH, in The Pharmacological Basis of Therapeutics, 6th ed. (AG Gilman, LS Goodman and A Gilman, eds.). Macmillan, New York, 1980, pp. 892-915.
30. Gifford RW, J Am Med Assoc 235:1890-1893, 1976.
31. Lee HA, Br Med J 2:104-107, 1979.
32. Magil AB, et al. Am J Med 69:939-943, 1980.
33. Lyons H, et al. N Engl J Med 288:124-128, 1973.
34. Erickson SB, Geriatrics 35:55-63, 1980.
35. Fialk MA, et al. Ann Int Med 81:403-404, 1974.
36. Fuller TJ, et al. J Am Med Assoc 235:1998-1999, 1976.
37. Curtis JR, Drugs 18:377-391, 1979.

TESTING FOR RENAL TOLERABILITY: CEFSULODIN IN RATS AND RABBITS

E. D. Wachsmuth and P. Thomann

Research Department, Pharmaceuticals Division, Ciba-Geigy Ltd, CH-4002, Basel, Switzerland

Cefsulodin (3-(4-carbomoyl-1-pyridiniomethyl)-7β-(D-α-sulphophenyl-acetamido)-ceph-3-em-4-carboxylate monosodium salt) is a newly developed cephalosporin derivative with highly selective antibacterial activity against *Pseudomonas aeruginosa* (1). Although single i.v. injections of doses up to 1200 mg/kg (2) did not produce nephrotoxic effects in rabbits, kidney lesions were seen in rats after multiple i.m. injections (3). In view of this difference the question arose whether cefsulodin might cause lesions after administration in both species under comparable conditions. A subacute i.v. toxicity study was therefore performed in rats and rabbits. The results were compared with those obtained after injection of a nephrotoxic dose of cephaloridine, amongst the cephalosporines, the antibiotic most extensively studied in respect to nephrotoxicity and supposedly also nephrotoxic in man (4).

MATERIAL AND METHODS

ANIMALS. Male and female rabbits, Russian breed (SPF), Hoechst AG, Germany, weighing 1.5 to 2.0 kg and male rats, RAIf (SPF),Tif., weighing 200 to 300 g were used. The animals were kept singly in metabolic cages designed for the separation of urine and faeces for at least three days before treatment. Water and food were given *ad libitum* (5).

TREATMENT OF ANIMALS. Test compounds were injected i.v. once daily at around 9 a.m. in rabbits and at 2 a.m. in rats. Urine samples were collected at 24h intervals before and after injection and serum samples at the time of autopsy. The animals were sacrificed 24 hours after the last injection.

DETERMINATIONS. Methods were as described previously (5). Lactate and malate dehydrogenase and aminopeptidase were measured in the urine using 1mM pyruvate, 0.5mM oxalacetate and 1mM leucine 4-nitroanilide, respectively. Epithelial cells in the urine were counted in a Neubauer haemocytometer.

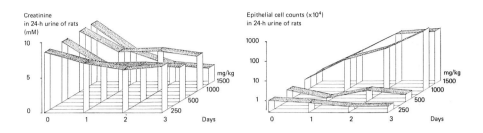

Figure 1. Creatinine and epithelial cells in 24-h urine of rats.

RESULTS IN RATS

URINE ANALYSES. The 24-h urine samples from male rats injected once with 2 g/kg i.v. cefsulodin showed distinct effects: epithelial cells were increased about 1000-fold and contained alkaline phosphatase, demonstrated by histochemical means, indicating their proximal-tubular origin; lactate dehydrogenase was increased up to 20-fold, aminopeptidase 4- to 5-fold and total protein 3-fold. On the other hand, the creatinine content remained unchanged despite a 2- to 3-fold increase in urine volume, indicating that the kidneys reabsorbed water less efficiently after administration of cefsulodin than normally. Once daily injection of different doses of cefsulodin for 3 days led to a progressive, dose-dependent increase in the excretion of epithelial cells (Fig.1) and similarly of malate dehydrogenase (Fig.2), lactate dehydrogenase (Fig.3), aminopeptidase (up to 6-fold) and total protein (up to 10-fold). Moreover, a slight dose-dependent and time-dependent increase in the urine volume was seen, which was already apparent in the 250-mg/kg dose group. Although the creatinine concentration in the urine decreased with ascending doses and the passage of time (Fig.1), the total amount of creatinine excreted was only slightly less than normal. Maximal excretion of any component was found after two injections. The data suggest that 250 mg/kg cefsulodin is well tolerated by rats over a 3-day period of administration without any significant nephrotoxic effect and that maximal nephrotoxic effects are observed after two i.v. injections of 1000 and 1500 mg/kg cefsulodin.

SERUM ANALYSES. Determinations of lactate dehydrogenase and alkaline phosphatase in serum at the time of autopsy revealed no significant changes in rats after 3 days administration of cefsulodin in doses up to 1500 mg/kg. Slight increases in creatinine and urea (170% and 130% of the control with 1500 mg/kg cefsulodin) indicate a nephrotoxic effect of cefsulodin in rats.

KIDNEY HISTOPATHOLOGY. Kidneys of rats were investigated 24h after one or three injections by means of alkaline phosphatase histochemistry in frozen sections (2,6), or after fixation in Bouin solution and PAS staining. The results obtained by the two methods were compatible, except that enzyme histochemistry proved a more sensitive means of detecting changes in the sections than the conventional technique. Results are given in Table 1. Proximal tubules in the outer stripe of the outer medulla showed extensive lesions when animals were treated with 1000 and 1500 mg/kg cefsulodin. The damage increased in tubules of the cortex ascending from the outer medulla in these latter two dose groups. The decrease in enzyme reaction product concomitant with the change in the morphology (Fig.4) is a sign of degeneration and necrosis: damage

TABLE 1. Nephrotoxicity test in rats: Once daily i.v. injection of 10 ml/kg cefsulodin for 3 days: histological evaluation of frozen kidney sections after staining for alkaline phosphatase.*

| Dose (mg/kg) | Tubuli of inner medulla frequency(%) | Damage in proximal tubules | | | |
| | | outer medulla | | cortex | |
		frequency(%)	intensity	frequency(%)	intensity
250	0	4	3	0	-
500	0	40	3	0	-
1000	<1**	90	1-3	5	2-3
1500	3**	100	1-2	20	1-3

*) Stain intensity: negative(0), weak(1), positive(2), strongly positive(3). Frequency: approx.percentage of affected tubules.**)Enzyme containing casts.

TABLE 2. Nephrotoxicity test in rabbits: Once daily i.v. injection of 4 ml/kg cefsulodin for 5 days: histological evaluation of frozen kidney sections after staining for alkaline phosphatase activity.

| Dose (mg/kg) | Tubuli of inner medulla frequency(%) | Damage in proximal tubules | | | |
| | | outer medulla | | cortex | |
		frequency(%)	intensity	frequency(%)	intensity
0	0	5	1	5	1
300	0	0	0	2	1-2
600	0	20*	2	2	1
1200	0	25*	1-2	5**	1-2

*) Wide lumina of tubules. **) At the border between cortex and outer stripe of outer medulla. Symbols as in Table 1.

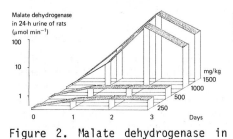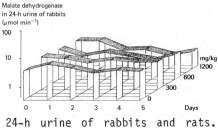

Figure 2. Malate dehydrogenase in 24-h urine of rabbits and rats.

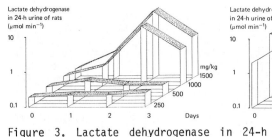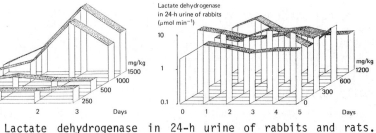

Figure 3. Lactate dehydrogenase in 24-h urine of rabbits and rats.

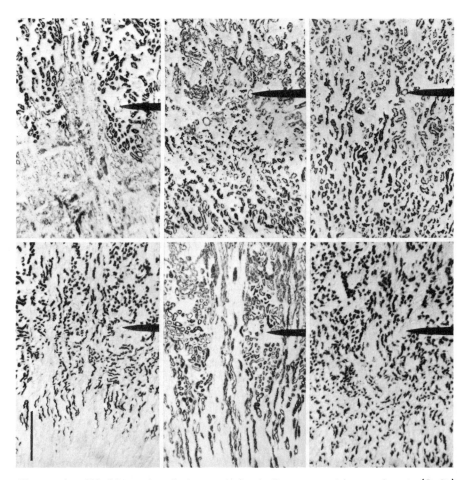

Figure 4. Alkaline phosphatase stained frozen sections of rat (left) and rabbit (right) kidneys. Top: control animals. Middle row: animals 24h after a single i.v. cephaloridine dose (1g/kg in rats, 0.23g/kg in rabbits). Bottom: animals 24h after daily i.v. cefsulodin doses (1g/kg for 3d in rats, 1.2g/kg for 5d in rabbits). Cortex on the left, arrow pointing to the *a. arcuata*, bar = 0.5 mm. Weak and diffuse tubular staining indicates damage of proximal tubules in cortex (middle row) and medulla (bottom, left).

with normal stain intensity is compatible with desquamation in proximal tubules. Whereas after administration of cephaloridine the frequency of damaged cells increased from the cortex to the outer medulla, the opposite was observed after administration of cefsulodin, i.e. the S1 and S2 segments of proximal tubules were affected in the former case (5,6) and the S3 segment in the latter. This effect of cefsulodin was more readily apparent after 3 injections than after a single injection.

EFFECT OF PROBENECID. Rats received 50 mg/kg p.o. probenecid one hour before i.v. injection of 1300 mg/kg cephaloridine or 600, 1200 or 1500mg/kg cefsulodin and were killed 24h later. Up to 98% of the proximal tubules, mainly the S1 and S2 segments, were necrotic after injection of cephaloridine, whereas in the rats given probenecid before the administration of cephaloridine no tubular damage whatever was seen. Cefsulodin, by contrast, caused mainly changes in the S3 segment, and this effect was augmented upon pretreatment with probenecid. Since it has been clearly shown that probenecid inhibits the transport of cephaloridine and prevents the toxicity in the kidney (7), these findings indicate that cephaloridine and cefsulodin act on the proximal tubular cells of rats in different ways.

RESULTS IN RABBITS

URINE ANALYSES. In rabbits injected once daily for two days, no significant effect on epithelial cell counts was noted in 24-h urine samples. In view of the large amount of crystals and calcium phosphate normally present in the urine of rabbits, however, the number of epithelial cells is very difficult to determine and urinary cell counts are therefore unreliable. Cefsulodin (300, 600, 1200 mg/kg) did not significantly increase the urine content of malate dehydrogenase, lactate dehydrogenase, aminopeptidase or total protein in these 2 days. Neither the specific gravity of the urine nor the total amounts of excreted creatinine, sodium and potassium were changed in the 24-h urine samples collected during the application period. These findings were confirmed in a second experiment in which cefsulodin was also injected i.v. once daily, but for 5 days, as exemplified by the contents of malate and lactate dehydrogenase given in Figs.2 and 3. The findings are in contrast to those obtained in rats and confirm earlier results after only one injection (2). Therefore, cefsulodin at doses up to 1200mg/kg, injected either once only or on several consecutive days, does not appear to cause any nephrotoxic effect measurable by urine analyses.

SERUM ANALYSES. No significant changes in creatinine or urea levels were observed in rabbits after administration of cefsulodin for up to 5 days.

KIDNEY HISTOPATHOLOGY. Histological evaluation of frozen kidney sections stained for alkaline phosphatase activity and conventionally stained PAS sections revealed no significant difference between control rabbits and rabbits injected with up to 1200 mg/kg cefsulodin for 5 days. Only marginal changes with increased lumina of the proximal tubules in the outer medulla, i.e. the S3 segment of the tubules, were observed. The amounts of the enzymic reaction product in the S3 cells of controls and treated animals were smaller than those of the S1 and S2 cells (Table 2, Fig.4). The histology was very similar in rabbits treated for two days and for 5 days. Cefsulodin at doses up to 1200 mg/kg causes only marginal changes of proximal tubules in the upper dose groups without any demonstrable cell necrosis. In contrast, cephaloridine at a dose of 100 mg/kg led to cell necrosis in up to 60% of the proximal tubules; mainly the S1 and S2 segments were affected.

DISCUSSION

Cefsulodin is apparently more nephrotoxic in rats than cephaloridine, whereas the reverse is true in rabbits (Table 3). The sites of the nephrotoxic action of the two compounds in the proximal tubule are different. Moreover, probenecid inhibits only the nephrotoxicity of cephaloridine - the nephrotoxicity of cephaloridine being caused by in-

TABLE 3. Synopsis of data from nephrotoxicity tests.

Test compound	Parameters	Rats	Rabbits	Rabbits/rats
cephaloridine	effect level	~1.2 g/kg	~0.2 g/kg	~ 0.15
	site in kidney	cortex	cortex	
	prox.tub.segment	S1, S2	S1, S2	
	with probenecid	protection	protection	
cefsulodin	effect level	~0.5 g/kg	≥1.2 g/kg	~ 2.5
	site in kidney	outer stripe outer medulla	outer stripe outer medulla(?)	
	prox.tub.segment	S3	S3 (?)	
	with probenecid	slight increase	not done	
cefsulodin/cephaloridine		~ 0.4	~ 6	

complete secretion (8,9) - , indicating that tubular secretion does not contribute to the excretion of cefsulodin.The findings suggest that the nephrotoxicity of cefsulodin in rats is provoked by a mechanism distinctly different from that of cephaloridine. One explanation for the species differences might be the morphological differences between the S3 segments of the proximal tubules in rats and rabbits (10-12), e.g. the size of the cells, the density of the microvilli and the basilar interdigitations, whereby the firmest tight junctions are seen in the rat S3. Moreover, the morphology of the S3 segment of the rabbit resembles the human S3 (12,13) more closely than the rat S3 (11), suggesting that in the case of S3 nephrotoxicity the rabbit is perhaps more relevant than the rat to the assessment of possible risks in man.

In CONCLUSION, cephaloridine and cefsulodin differ in their toxic effects in two animal species and also in their site of action. To infere from the effects displayed by cephaloridine in rats that cephsulodin may also be nephrotoxic in man (3) is therefore unjustifiable.

REFERENCES
1. Pharmanual, a comprehensive guide to the therapeutic use of cefsulodin. Karger, Basle, 1981.
2. Wachsmuth ED, Histochemistry 71: 235-248, 1981.
3. Burmann G, Mertens G, Schulz E and Sack K, Infection 5: 233-238, 1981.
4. Balazs T, Jackson B and Hite M, this volume.
5. Wachsmuth ED, Arch.Toxicol. 48: 135-156, 1981.
6. Wachsmuth ED and Wirz H, in Diagnostic Significance of Enzymes and Proteins in Urine. Hans Huber, Bern, pp. 88-104, 1979.
7. Tune BM, Wu KY and Kempson RL, J Pharmacol Exp Ther 202: 466-471, 1977.
8. Tune BM, Fernholt M and Schwartz A, J Pharmacol Exp Ther 191: 311-317, 1974.
9. Tune BM, J Infect Dis 132: 189-194, 1975.
10. Maunsbach AB, J Ultrastruct Res 16: 239-258, 1966.
11. Kriz W, Z Zellforschg 82: 495-535, 1967.
12. Kaissling B and Kriz W, Adv Anat Embryol Cell Biol 56: 1-123, 1979.
13. Tisher CC, Bulger RE, Trump BF, Lab Invest 15: 1357-1394, 1966.

COMPARATIVE PHARMACOLOGY OF THE KIDNEY: IMPLICATIONS FOR DRUG-INDUCED RENAL FAILURE

Gilbert H. Mudge

Departments of Pharmacology and Toxicology and of Medicine, Dartmouth Medical School, Hanover, New Hampshire 03755, USA

ABSTRACT

The questions to which this review is addressed involve the applicability of studies on nephrotoxicity in animal models to the clinical problems encountered in man in relation to drug induced renal failure. These problems involve prophylaxis, diagnosis and treatment, particularly the latter.

Factors may be considered which are either 1) inherent in the experimental design, or 2) biological characteristics, inherent in the animal species themselves. Human disease is most frequently diagnosed after the damage is done. Drug-induced renal failure is often accompanied by circulatory compromise and/or systemic infection. In addition, poly-pharmacy is increasingly the rule rather than the exception. To what extent do such factors alter the application of data obtained from less complicated animal models?

Inherent species differences may be anatomical, physiological, biochemical or pharmacological in nature. Single examples of such differences will be presented without attempting a comprehensive survey. Topics include: size of kidneys and of nephrons, architecture of nephrons, anatomy of papillae, osmolality of urine, tranport of organic compounds, general drug metabolism, renal drug metabolism, drug half-life, mechanisms of drug excretion, patterns of minor metabolites etc.

Although the same pharmacological principles which apply to other organs also apply to the kidney, renal pharmacology nevertheless involves certain unique features. These include the magnitude of the renal circulation as well as its central importance for the principal function of the kidney, e.g. the formation of urine. In addition, unlike most other organs, the kidney can generate local concentrations of solutes, including drugs, which are far different from those which prevail in the circulating blood. The renal mechanisms include drug transport per se as well as those that are secondary to solute and water transport. Both types of function may vary from species to species.

Key Words. Comparative Nephrotoxicity, Prophylaxis, Treatment, Xenobiotic concentration.

INTRODUCTION

This paper is an attempt to provide some answers to the question:
To what extent can animal studies provide new insight into the proper
therapy of nephrotoxicity in man, induced either by drugs or other
chemical agents? As originally formulated the topic was primarily
one of therapeutics but it has without doubt become broader. It
was also originally suggested that some answers might be found in
the field of epidemiology but this has received but little attention.
At first glance comparative nephrotoxicity might be considered a
rather narrow field but it actually is extremely broad if one considers
all the disciplines that are potentially touched upon. The material
has been selected in somewhat arbitrary fashion with emphasis on
organic compounds, the mammalian kidney and mechanisms of pathogenesis.
The therapeutic implications are discussed whenever possible. For
source material several reviews of nephrotoxicity and of comparative
pharmacology are recommended [1-7]. However, comparative nephrotoxicity
as such appears to have attracted little attention.
    It should be noted that comparative pharmacology, like other
comparative disciplines, involves two separate aspects. First, it
describes the observations in different strains or species of animals,
and second, under some circumstances it in itself becomes a productive
research technique. This can happen if the differences between species
are unequivocal. There is little to be gained in the pursuit of minor
differences particularly in a field in which multiple factors are involved,
many of which may be either compensatory or unmeasurable. There is no
example which immediately comes to mind in which comparative observations have played the critical role in the elucidation of mechanisms
of renal toxicity. However the comparative approach was of key importance in the first half of this century in analyzing the nature of
glomerular filtration and tubular transport. Forster [8] has provided
an interesting historical review.

ANATOMY

The comparative anatomy of the kidney has been intensively studied
for many years. Several reviews and monographs are recommended which
have emphasized the relationship of structure to function. These include the classical paper by Sperber [9], several comprehensive texts
[10,11] and recent reviews [12,13].

Nephrons. In going over the extreme range between species there is
an enormous change in body weight as well as in kidney weight (Table
1). However, the number of nephrons normalized to body weight change
to a much lesser extent and, most striking, the dimensions of the
nephron are remarkably constant from one species to another. In Table
1, the radius of the glomeruli and the length and radius of the proximal tubule have been listed as indices of nephron size. In general,
the dimensions of the distal nephron follow the same pattern, with
exceptions related to the conservation of water which will be discussed
separately.
    Clearly the nephron is the functioning architectural unit of the
kidney. The needs of evolution have for the most part been met by
changing the number of nephrons rather than their size or shape. The

Table 1. Comparative anatomy of kidney and nephrons.

	Body wt kg	Kidney wt g	Nephrons per g body wt #	Glom. rad. μ	Prox. length mm	Tubule rad. μ
Mouse	.02	.12	620	37	4	20
Rat	.24	.75	128	61	12	29
Guinea Pig	.57	1.9	134	63	7	28
Rabbit	2.3	6.4	89	71	13	30
Cat	3.0	15	67	70	9	31
Monkey	3.8	9	49	83	-	-
Dog	9.1	31	45	90	20	33
Pig	46	77	26	83	30	35
Man	70	157	16	100	16	36
Elephant	4500	3600	1.7	169	28	38
Whale	32000	40000	6.0	95	13	39

Kidney weight refers to single kidney. Data from [9,10,11,14].

nephrons are arranged in an orderly manner into the next larger anatomical unit, the lobe or renculus, which for practical purposes may be
considered a congregation of nephrons which drain into the same papilla,
or, in the absence of papillary structures, into the same region of
the medullary crest. Oliver [14] has divided mammalian kidneys into
three classes -- unipapillated, compound multirenculated,and discrete
renculated. In compound multirenculated kidneys the separate renculi
have variable anatomical relationships to each other, such as the
medullary crest in the dog or the multilobulated kidney of the cow.
From Oliver's analysis some of these gross anatomical arrangements
may provide functional advantages, but these are quite small.
      Nephron size is probably limited by 1) filtration pressure,
which in addition to counteracting plasma osmotic pressure, must also
be sufficient to overcome the hydrodynamic resistance to flow within
the tubule, 2) the diffusion characteristics of oxygen from the peritubular capillaries, and 3) possibly diffusion of solutes within both the
peritubular and tubular fluids and the consequent relationship to either
reabsorptive or secretory tubular transport. The solution to the challenge of evolution is well illustrated by the whale which possesses two
large bilateral masses of tissue, each consisting of approximately 7,000
renculi arranged in grape-like clusters. Each renculus is a complete
unipyramidal kidney with cortex, medulla and pelvis and its own artery
and vein -- exactly similar to the whole kidney of other animals. Each
renculus weighs about 6 g. This provides a single whale with about
14,000 rabbit kidneys.

Medulla. The most striking intra-species differences involve the
medulla and papilla. As summarized in Table 2 when one runs the gamut
from the fresh water beaver to the desert rodents, the need to conserve
water becomes directly related to the fraction of long loops of Henle
and to the resultant thickness of the medulla. The length of the loops
is more or less directly proportional to the number of sites at which
countercurrent exchange may occur and is thus directly related to the
maximal urinary osmolality which can be generated. Five tube like
structures are involved of which two are vascular and three are part
of the nephron itself -- descending (arterial) vasa recta, ascending
(venous) vasa recta, descending proximal tubule and thin limb, ascending
thin limb, and descending collecting duct. The indispensable prerequisite for a counter-current mechanism is that fluid flows in opposite
directions in closely adjacent structures. There are several patterns
by which the tubular structures are apposed to each other. These differ
somewhat from outer and inner medulla and also to a slight extent between
species. The details have been reviewed by Kriz [13]. In relation to
the problem of toxicity these patterns are probably of significance only
to the extent that they determine final urinary concentrations. The
anatomical location of the tubular structures emphasizes the unique
functional role of the medulla. To emphasize the point, first consider
the cortical portion of the nephron in which the bulk of filtered solute
is reabsorbed. The composition of the fluid which emerges from the proximal tubule is determined by the reabsorptive activity of that individual
nephron. In contrast, the composition of the tubular fluid in the
collecting duct is determined by the activity of multiple adjacent
nephrons which directly contribute to the composition of the medullary
interstitium and thereby indirectly to the reabsorption of solute and
water in nearby nephrons.

Anatomical basis of differences in nephrotoxicity. Beyond the
obvious impact of the medulla on the urinary concentrating mechanism
it is difficult to attribute differences in nephrotoxicity to specific
structural components. Despite the detailed studies that have been
made with electron microscopy and histochemistry there appear to be no
proposals for structure-toxicity correlations. The segmental

Table 2. Relation of structure of medulla to maximal osmolality of
          urine.

	% Long Loops	Relative Medullary Tickness	Maximal Osmolality mOsmol/kg
Beaver	0	1.3	516
Pig	3	1.6	1080
Man	14	3.0	1400
Dog	100	4.3	2610
Cat	100	4.8	3120
Rat	28	5.8	2610
Kangaroo Rat	27	8.5	5590
Jerboa	33	9.3	6450
Psammomys	100	10.7	4950

Data from [15].

distribution of different nephrotoxic lesions has been well summarised
by Darmady and MacIver [45].

The cat has an unusual vasculature in that the renal venous blood
leaves the kidney by two separate routes -- the renal vein in the usual
position in the hilus and a second set of renal veins which flow directly
to the cortex.   Advantage has been taken of this arrangement for physiological studies, but not as far as I know for toxicology.

There is an additional anatomical variant involving specialized
fornices of the renal pelvis which have an extensive vascular network
underlying the epithelium of the parenchyma. This is seen in the dog.
Such a morphological feature would provide a basis for the recycling
of urea from the pelvic urine back into the renal medullary parenchyma
[12]. It is not known whether the same mechanism might also apply
to solutes other than urea, particularly potential nephrotoxins.

PHYSIOLOGY

Undoubtedly the major achievement of renal physiology during the
past century has been the clarification of the separate processes of
filtration, reabsorption and secretion. Two general techniques have
been involved -- the clearance method which can be used either in man
or the experimental animal, and the various modifications of micropuncture which are limited to the experimental animal. Additional
methods have been introduced from biochemistry and cell physiology
but in the final analysis both their validity and applicability has
often depended on the confirmatory data derived with the more classical
approaches.

Excretion of xenobiotics. In the context of nephrotoxicity a central question is the manner in which xenobiotics are handled by the
kidney. This also extends to the non-toxic xenobiotics and to various
metabolites. Indeed it was the renal excretion of foreign rather than
endogenous compounds which established the nature of the basic excretory
mechanisms [8]. When clearance techniques were first developed they
permitted the measurement of the amount of a compound filtered at the
glomerulus. This was based on the measurements of plasma concentration,
protein binding and the filtration rate (GFR). With knowledge of the
amount filtered and of the amount excreted in the voided urine it was
then possible to calculate the amount transported by the tubule in either
the reabsorptive or secretory direction. It should be recognized that
the early calculations of tubular transport assumed, often tacitly,
that transport was unidirectional. While this is still largely correct
for a small number of compounds, e.g. glucose, it is now clear that
the vast majority of compounds, either endogenous or exogenous, are
subject to bidirectional transport and furthermore that multiple
mechanisms may be involved.

With bidirectional transport there arises the possiblity that
compounds may recycle within the kidney and that the prevailing concentrations may be far higher than those in the systemic circulation.
Considered in its simplest terms the mammalian kidney has been faced
by the challenge to solve four separate problems related to a terres-
trial way of life and, in many instaces, to a carnivorous appetite.
These involve the necessity to conserve 1) water, 2) bicarbonate and
3) essential organic compounds such as glucose and amino acids and at

the same time 4) to excrete foreign xenobiotics. The latter need was facilitated in two ways, first by the development of drug metabolizing enzymes, mostly in the liver, capable of converting lipophilic compounds to hydrophilic ones, and second by the development of a secretory system for organic ions in the proximal tubule, capable of introducing into the tubular fluid various compounds in excess of the amounts filtered at the glomerulus. This would expedite their excretion by way of the urine.

The goal of excreting xenobiotics often runs counter to the goal of conserving water and bicarbonate. The metabolites of many xeno-biotics are acidic with pKa's sufficiently within the pH range of the tubular fluid that they may exist in either the protonated or anionic form. Both the reabsorption of water and the acidification of the tubular fluid would increase the tendency for such metabolites to be reabsorbed by non-ionic diffusion. The comparative physiology of renal tubular transport mechanisms has been summarized by Long and Giebisch [16]. The urine pH in carnivorous mammals is far more acid than in herbivourous, but changes in diet such as those that might occure in animal research facilities can readily overcome the natural tendencies.

Torretti and Weiner [17] have summarized the patterns of drug excretion, see Table 3. The examples which are given are probably all valid for man even though the observations are not complete in all in-stances. For all compounds carrier-mediated transport is localized to the proximal tubule. Passive reabsorption may occur throughout the nephron but principally in the distal segments. It is in this region that water reabsorption and acidification produce maximal changes in the concentration of undissociated acids in the tubular fluid. Carrier-mediated transport is specific for either organic acids or organic bases, but within each class there is a wide range in the affinities and capacities of the transport mechanisms.

Table 3. Patterns of Xenobiotic Excretion by Kidney.

1. Filtration only -- inulin
2. Filtration, active secretion -- PAH
3. Filtration, passive reabsorption -- phenacetin, paracetamol
4. Filtration, passive secretion -- ?
5. Filtration, active secretion, passive reabsorption --
     probenecid, some glucuronides / sulfates
6. Filtration, active reabsorption -- glucose, ? xenobiotic
7. Filtration, bidirectional carrier mediated transport --
     PAH in some species, pyrazinoate
8. Filtration, bidirectional carrier mediated transport, passive
     reabsorption -- salicylate
9. Filtration, intracellular sequestration by active transport --
     cephaloridine
10. Filtration, bidirectional passive transport -- urea, ? xenobiotic
11. Metabolism during transtubular transport -- morphine
12. Recycling from pelvis to medullary interstitium --
     urea, ? xenobiotic

Modified from [17]. Pattern #4 with just passive secretion is theoreti-cally possible but has not been demonstrated.

Transport of PAH. On the basis of clearance data for most compounds it is possible to calculate only net tubular transport, i.e. the algebraic sum of transport in both directions, not the magnitude of each unidirectional process. The exception involves those instances in which clearance approaches renal plasma flow so that in the steady state tubular reabsorption must be negligible. This is the case for the clearance of p-aminohippurate (PAH) at low plasma levels. It is generally held that the renal tubule is also impermeable to the reabsorption of PAH at high concentrations and on this basis maximal rates of transport (Tm) have been calculated. In an unanesthetized trained dog we found on repeated determinations over the course of months the standard deviation to be only 15% of the mean Tm. This indicates quite a stable transport mechanism.

In relation to the pathogenesis of renal toxicity, several points warrant comment: 1) As shown in Table 4 the Tm for PAH has considerable species variation. If this were the case for other xenobiotics the resultant concentrations in the tubular fluid could vary widely between species. 2) The presence or absence of tubular secretion varies unpredictably for different compounds. Diatrizoate, iodipamide and methotrexate are secreted in the rabbit but not in the dog and of these only methotrexate is secreted in man [19-21]. To our knowledge systematic studies of putative nephrotoxins are not available. and 3) There is the question of tubular reabsorption of polar conjugates. As indicated above it has usually been assumed that at Tm concentrations PAH is not reabsorbed. However, this lacks rigid proof. For other hydrophilic conjugates whose clearance exceeds the GFR but is less than that of PAH, this finding is usually interpreted to indicate a relatively weak affinity for tubular secretion combined with impermeability to reabsorption. However, tubular reabsorption could account for the same pattern [22]. The question will be considered again in relation to intracellular concentrations. Although this review has been limited to the mammalian kidney, it should be pointed out that the marine teleost kidney offers an unusual opportunity to study mechanisms of organic anion transport. Recent advances in comparative toxicity have been summarized by Pritchard and Miller [23].

Table 4. Tm for PAH in Different Mammalian Species.

	C_{inulin}	Tm_{PAH}	$\dfrac{Tm_{PAH}}{C_{inulin}}$
	ml/min	mg/min	
	per kg body wt		
Rat	6.0	3.0	0.50
Dog	4.3	1.0	0.23
Man	2.0	1.3	0.65
Cebus	2.6	1.5	0.58
Chimpanzee	1.9	2.9	1.52

Data from [10,18].

Recycling of Urea. Although it is generally taught that urea is filtered and then reabsorbed, a secretory mechanism has been detected by micropuncture studies [24]. This results from the fact that the limbs of Henle traverse the medullary interstitium in which there is a high urea concentration so that urea diffuses in a secretory direction from interstitium to tubular fluid. The same forces operate in the reverse direction as the late distal convolution descends from cortex to medulla. This unusual pattern of transport is made possible by the fact that the cortical distal convoluted tubule is virtually impermeable to urea so that as water is reabsorbed from that segment the amount of urea within it remains constant but its concentration rises. To our knowledge the distal tubular impermeability is unique for urea. The possibility warrants consideration that some xenobiotics might have similar characteristics.

Renal circulation. The blood flow to the kidney is unusual for several reasons 1) It is exceptionally high, 2) It varies from one region of the kidney to another, 3) It is essential for glomerular filtration and 4) It is influenced by a large number of vasoactive substances that are produced locally. These include kallikrein-kinin, renin-angiotensin, prostaglandins and the classical autonomic mediators. The activity of these systems is not only influenced by vascular factors such as flow and pressure but also by the composition of the tubular fluid, particularly electrolytes. Between these systems there are many interactions, either inhibitory or stimulatory. This is an active field of investigation and of undoubted importance to the question of nephrotoxicity. Recent symposia provide useful summaries [25,26]. As to the central question of comparative physiology, the findings in laboratory animals appear quite uniform from one species to another and also appear applicable to man.

PHARMACOLOGY

A fundamental tenet of pharmacology and toxicology is that the action of a chemical agent depends on its concentration in the neighborhood of the receptor. "Neighborhood" is used advisedly since it begs the questions which might prevail in the absence of exact measurements. The kidney has an almost unique capacity to expose itself to concentrations of xenobiotics not experienced by other organs or tissues. However, the problem posed in the analysis of nephrotoxic reactions is not so much the renal concentrations themselves as it is the fact that they are influenced by such a large number of different mechanisms. It follows that the concentration of a xenobiotic within the kidney bears no necessary relationship to the administered dose. The processes which generate unique concentrations are those of tubular secretion, isosmotic tubular reabsorption of salt and water and the formation of hypertonic urine. The latter two are separate mechanisms but both may increase the intratubular concentration of a solute.

There is probably no aspect of comparative pharmacology more striking than the differences between species (or strains) in dose-reponse relationships. To a limited extent these depend on specific differences in distribution, metabolism and excretion. An enormous number of factors are involved and few generalizations can be made. In a symposium [1] 47 different variables were listed which should be taken into account for the exact evaluation of comparative toxicity. This did not include those factors peculiar to the kidney. A few examples directly involving

the kidney may be given. Male mice are extremely susceptible to chloroform and develop acute tubular necrosis [27]. Female mice and other
species are far less susceptible. The nephrotoxic dose of cephaloridine
varies almost 20 fold in common laboratory animals. When the degree of
cortical necrosis is correlated with the drug concentration that develops
within the cortex, the sensitivities of the rabbit and guinea pig can
for the most part be attributed to the rates of active uptake [28].

   Renal Concentrations of Drug. Concentrations of drugs within the
kidney are difficult to measure. The kidney is remarkably heterogeneous.
In addition to the usual intra- and extra-cellular compartments of most
tissues it contains an additional compartment, the tubular fluid, which
can vary enormously in composition from its proximal to distal end.
For the interpretation of tissue analyses most workers have used plasma
levels as a reference for samples of cortex and urine concentrations for
medulla. Even so, assignments of drug concentrations are only approximate [28,29]. Only a few micropuncture studies are available, partly
because of analytical problems. Radiochemical techniques are acceptable
only if metabolites and parent compound are clearly separated.
   Most of our current knowledge of tissue concentrations is based on
the physiological mechanisms of excretion. If these are well documented
reasonable extrapolations may be made. However all too often studies
are inadequate. For many pharmacological purposes it may suffice to
determine the total amount excreted in the urine and the major metabolites.
At a minimum a sophisticated analysis of renal mechanisms involves measurements of the effects of pH, urine flow, plasma concentration and standard
inhibitors of transport, along with the determination of inulin clearance
and binding to plasma proteins.
   The stop-flow technique has not been widely accepted for the analysis
of tubular transport because of its quantitative limitations. The
criticism applies mainly to the endogenous solutes such as inorganic
salts and urea. The technique has been quite useful for the localization of the transport of xenobiotics. For some compounds an elevated
intratubular pressure increases tubular permeability [30] and as a
result the stop-flow technique may yield some artifactual results. We
have developed a new technique which determines tubular permeability
to drugs and their interstitial distribution [30]. This involves the
creation of an acute diuresis and the collection of urine samples at
very short intervals. It is patterned after the osmotic diuresis which
results from the bolus injection of urographic contrast agents. High-
ceiling diuretics may also be used. The technique has demonstrated
tubular permeability to the polar phenolic metabolites of paracetamol,
which will be discussed below.

   Renal drug metabolism. The metabolism of drugs by the kidney has
received but relatively little attention. Table 5 summarizes some
of the available data. It is now becoming increasingly clear that the
metabolism of the cortex and medulla should be evaluated separately.
Many enzymes are more active in the cortex and the reverse is also
seen. The cyclo-oxidase enzymes involved in prostaglandin metabolism
are also capable of oxidizing drugs and their activity is highest in the
medulla [33]. Renal drug metabolizing enzymes may be induced and the
pattern may differ considerably from that seen in the liver. In
evaluating the eventual significance of renal drug metabolism it should
be kept in mind that substrate concentrations are apt to be higher than
in other tissues. High cortical concentrations are achieved for those
compounds directly accumulated within the cells by active transport [28].

Renal tubular reabsorption of polar metabolites. In its simplest
form the urinary excretion of lipophilic xenobiotics results from their
conversion to more polar metabolites, principally by the liver, and the
subsequent excretion of these metabolites at high rates in the urine.
It is not clear whether increased polarity per se facilities tubular
secretion. However there is substantial evidence that this decreases
tubular reabsorption.

The possibility of tubular permeability to polar metabolites leads to
a paradoxical situation in which the physiological and toxicological
consequences should be clearly distinguished. The key question is
whether there is complete tubular impermeability, as in the case of
inulin, or whether slight reabsorption is possible. Most polar metabolites have high clearances. If a small amount were to be reabsorbed
this would have a negligible effect on total excretion, but if this were
to occur from a high intraluminal concentration it would generate a
high concentration within the adjacent tubular cells. For the most
compounds the polar metabolites have a low degree of cytotoxicity.
High extracellular concentrations, e.g. within the tubular fluid, are
regarded as non-toxic. The possible significance of their reabsorption
involves three steps: 1) reabsorption of polar metabolite into the
tubular cells, 2) conversion to less polar compounds by enzymatic
deconjugation, and 3) direct cytotoxicity of the deconjugated compounds
or of the reactive intermediates formed from further metabolism. The
mechanism is possibly not subject to absolute proof in vivo. Nevertheless, each step has been separately demonstrated for the polar
phenolic conjugates of paracetamol [31,33]. The point to be emphasized
is that through several sequential processes the kidney has the capacity
to develop high intracellular concentrations of the relevant substrates.
In addition it is of course possible that reactive metabolites might be
formed at extra-renal sites and become directly concentrated within the
kidney.

Table 5. Patterns of renal drug metabolizing enzymes in different species.

	Mixed function oxidase	NADPH-cytochrome c reductase
	Kidney activity as % liver	
Mouse	5	71
Rat	5	48
Hamster	4	22
Guinea Pig	3	25
Rabbit cortex	31	14
medulla outer	ND	11
inner	ND	7
Human	4	15

Data from [32]. ND means none detected.

THE CLINICAL PROBLEM

Nephrotoxicity may be classified by two separate schemes -- either according to the specific etiological agent (e.g. mercuric chloride) or according to the dominant abnormality which is produced. The latter includes ischemia, decreased filtration, cytotoxicity, increased tubular permeability (back leak) and tubular obstruction. There are many examples in which just one of these factors may dominate the picture in its earliest stages. For example, complete occlusion of the renal artery primarily produces ischemia; intraluminal precipita- tion of methotrexate causes tubular obstruction. The most commonly employed experimental procedures have involved ischemia (arterial occlusion vasoconstrictor drugs), cytotoxins (heavy metals), and intratubular obstruction (methotrexate, folic acid) or a combination of several. These animal models have been intensively studied from both a structural and functional point of view. In relation to the present paper, there are two conclusions which are of paramount importance. The first is that the animal models (principally in the rat, rabbit and dog) appear to closely ressemble the disorder as seen in man. Undoubtely there are some minor differences but the general conclusion is valid. The second point is that regardless of the initiating cause there is a common pathophysiological disturbance which characterizes acute renal failure once it is fully developed, that is after 1-3 days have elapsed. With minor exceptions once established the syndrome is characterized by the simultaneous defects of tubular obstruction, increased tubular permeability (back leak) and diminished filtration, all in the presence of essentially normal renal blood flow. It is emphasized that this is the final common picture regardless of the nature of the initial insult [34]. In relation to therapeutics, the effect of this triple abnormality is 1) produce a disorder which results from more than just a single factor, 2) to prevent the further generation of high concentrations of solute within the tubular fluid, and 3) to isolate the renal lesion from substances (either toxins or therapeutic drugs) delivered to the kidney by the circulation.

Ischemia. An inadequate supply of oxygen is an obvious mechanism of renal injury when the renal artery is occluded or high doses of vasoconstrictors are infused directly into it. In addition many nephrotoxins such as heavy metals which are primarily cytotoxic also have vasoconstrictor activity in experimental models. However in each of these instances renal blood flow may subsequently rise to either normal or elevated levels despite the persistence of other signs of renal failure. In established renal failure renal oxygen consumption is reduced approximately proportionately to the reduction in sodium transport, which is the major oxygen consuming activity of the kidney [35]. Thus despite diminished oxygen consumption the kidney does not remain anoxic in the usual sense.

Glomerular Filtration. The GFR falls in response to a sharp drop in intraglomerular pressure regardless of how this is produced. In addition in most models there is a reduction in the ultrafiltration coefficient of the glomerular membrane. This usually persists in extablished renal failure and it, rather than a reduced renal blood flow, is the cause of the persistently low GFR. If tubular obstruction is the dominant primary lesion, there is a rise in intraluminal pressure which counteracts filtration pressure. This lowers GFR. Back leak

proximal to the site of obstruction may eventually reduce intraluminal pressure.

Tubular obstruction. The simplest form of obstruction occurs when
the solubility of a compound within the tubular fluid is exceeded and
the compound precipitates out of solution. Examples include the early
sulfonamides, uric acid and massive doses of methotrexate. Probably
far more common is the obstruction that results from the shedding of
cellular debris into the tubular fluid. This may result from primary
ischemia or from cytotoxins. The obstruction thus produced is of
variable degree since in some instances it may be dislodged by diuresis.
A more complex situation occurs when obstruction involves Tamm-Horsfall
protein. This is a glycoprotein produced by the ascending limb which
can form gels under appropriate conditions of pH and ionic strength
[36]. It is the major constituent of casts. It is probable that
Tamm-Horsfall gels become incorporated to a variable degree into the
obstructive cellular debris described above. Tamm-Horsfall protein
excretion increases in experimental renal failure [37]. Both the
protien and casts are washed out at the onset of the diuretic phase of
renal failure in man in quantities sufficient to indicate prior tubular
obstruction [38]. Coprecipitation of Tamm-Horsfall protein with the
urographic contrast drugs is a likely mechanism for the renal failure
produced by these agents. In addition, recent studies have demonstrated
immunological responses to this protein including an immune-complex
interstitial nephritis [36]. In some patients this might influence the
late course of acute renal failure.
     It has been postulated that acute tubular obstruction can produce
a cascade effect leading to further obstruction. Though difficult to
prove, this is highly likely. While tubular activity is still normal,
any new filtrate delivered to an obstructed nephron will not only be
reabsorbed but probably to a greater extent than in the unobstructed
neprhon. This will increase the intratubular concentration of solutes
and accelerate further precipitation. The effect will be dissipated if
and when tubular permeability increases (back leak).

Prevention of Nephrotoxicity. There are several clear cut indications of therapeutic intervention in order to prevent renal failure.
These involve situations in which one can anticipate the action of the
nephrotoxin in advance. These have been previously outlined [39] and are
briefly summarized: 1) Alkalinization of the urine. This is extremely
effective in preventing the precipitation of sparingly soluble organic
acids. This includes uric acid, particularly when a sudden increase in
its excretion is expected. It should be emphasized that the pH of the
urine should be at its maximum (> 7.5) at the time that the peak excretion of the solute is expected. 2) Reduction of urate production. This
applied primarily to the chemotherapy of malignancy and involves the use
of allopurinol. 3) Inhibition of tubular excretion. The nephrotoxicity
of cephalosporins can be prevented in the experimental animal by probenecid
which inhibts the uptake of the antibiotic by the cells of the proximal
tubule. There is insufficient experience to judge whether this is a
practical clinical approach. and 4) Increase the rate of urine flow.
Loading with saline or mannitol or the administration of high-ceiling
diuretics such as furosemide protect against renal failure in a number
of models which include ischemia, nephrotoxins or obstructive agents as
the dominant initial cause [40]. Such protection is also seen clinically

in the use of cis-platinum or in conjunction with abdominal vascular
surgery. The increased urine flow tends to decrease the intratubular
concentration of putative toxins. Other mechanisms may also be operative. Saline depletes renin stores and furosemide stimulates prostaglandin production, both of which would tend to counteract renal vasoconstriction.

   Treatment of Early Acute Renal Failure. Early diagnosis is an
absolute prerequisite for the treatment of early acute renal failure.
This depends primarily on a high index of suspicion. The patient's
history probably provides the most useful information. It is doubtful
if newly developed types of urine tests will hasten the procedure [41]
although this might be true for subacute or chronic toxicity. It
should be remembered that in its earliest hours, and possibly days,
acute anuria can be completely asymptomatic. It is strongly urged
that once the routine urine analysis has been completed on the intial
urine specimen that the remainder be stored in a refrigerator in case
special studies are subsequently indicated.
   The classical studies on dimercaprol for arsenic and mercury poisoning
are the best examples of successful early treatment. From more recent
studies it is becoming increasingly apparent that measures which are
successful for prevention are usually ineffective for treatment, even
if started early. The early time course of the renal lesions becomes
critical. Lindner et al [42] gave dopamine plus furosemide by infusion
for 6 hours commencing 15 minutes after a nephrotoxic dose of uranyl
acetate. This combination of drugs provided significant protection.
Conger et al [43] induced renal failure with nor-epinephrine and,
starting one hour after the nor-epinephrine had been given, infused
acetylcholine into the renal artery for 6 hours. Renal blood flow
was restored to normal but without any improvement in GFR. Solez et al
[44] studied the model in which the renal artery is clamped and were
able to lessen the degree of renal failure and microvasculature damage
by administering clonidine, an antihypertensive agent that inhibits
renin release and enhances diuresis. This was given 1 hour after the
period of ischemia.
   The above experiments emphasize several points. First the time at
which therapy was intiated was extremely early -- 15 minutes in one
instance, 1 hour in the other two. Second, the duration of the per-
missible delay period has not been systematically studied. And third,
these animal models provide maximal injury to the kidney. It is not
known whether weaker stimuli would permit a longer delay before initiating
therapy.

   Treatment of Established Acute Renal Failure. A large number of
experimental procedures has been tried but almost none with success in
the clinical situation [39]. It is noteworthy that adequate hydration
and high-ceiling diuretics are effective for prophylaxis but have almost
no effect on the established syndrome. It should be exphasized that
this does not refer to general supportive measures but to the specific
effect on the course of the renal disorder. Hyperalimentation appears
to be the one therapeutic regimen which benefits patients with acute
renal failure regardless of etiology.
   In reviewing the specific problem of therapeutic intervention it
is possible that the animal models may suffer from a general defect
in experimental design. It is my impression that the dose of the insult
--be it nephrotoxic drug or vascular insufficiency -- has been deter-

mined by the likelihood that it will produce a predictable physiological defect in essentially all animals. It is readily appreciated that
this is a desireable goal for physiological measurements. However
this may not be the best model for the evaluation of treatment. It
is quite possible that there are therapeutic regimens which would
favorably influence outcome if the initial insult were less and if
it produced a picture of only partial renal failure, perhaps in only
a portion of the animals. This would be a complicated protocol and
might eventually involve the interaction of two different doses, i.e.
the dose of the insult and the dose of the therapeutic agent.

The problem that probably most needs clarification involves the
transition from reversible to non-reversible renal failure. In the
same manner as above, the boundary conditions have been well defined
from a pathophysiological point of view but not, I believe, with
therapeutic goals in mind. This would involve a number of variables,
different drugs, different doses, and most important, different time
schedules. I would think that additional detailed anatomical studies
might be particularly useful in clarifying the time course.

Lastly, there is an enormous problem in collecting valid clinical
data. One is dealing with a moderately unusual clinical problem. It
would be difficult to set up large scale prospective trials even if
done on a cooperative basis. As a first step one might consider a
collaborative retrospective study simply to document experience in a
uniform manner. One can't help but be impressed that even in the largest
series of cases that are reported by individual investigators, the
actual data base for any single clinical entity may be quite skimpy.

REFERENCES

1. Cafruny EJ, Cosmides GJ, Rall DP, Schroeder CR, Weiner IM, eds.
   International Symposium on Comparative Pharmacology, Fed Proc
   26:963-1266, 1967.
2. Mudge GH, Duggin GG eds. Drug Effects on the Kidney. Kid Internat
   18:539-711, 1980.
3. Parke DV, The Biochemistry of Foreign Compounds. Pergamon Press,
   Oxford, 1968, pp 1-269. ISBN 0-08-012202-7.
4. Smith RL, Caldwell J, in Drug Metabolism - from Microbe to Man
   (DV Parke and RL Smith, eds.) Crane Russak Co, New York, 1977
   pp 331-356. ISBN 0-8448-1127-0.
5. Smith JN, in Comparative Biochemistry (M Florkin and HS Mason eds.)
   Academic Press, New York, 1964, 6:403-457. ISBN 0-12-261006-7.
6. Zbinden G, in The Kidney, Morphology, Biochemistry, Physiology
   (C Roviller, AF Muller, eds.) Academic Press, New York, 1969,
   2:401-475. ISBN 0-12-598802-8.
7. Porter G, ed., Nephrotoxic mechanisms of drugs and environmental
   toxins, Plenum Medical, New York and London (in press).
8. Forster RP, Fed Proc 26:1008-1019, 1967.
9. Sperber I, Zoologiska Bidrag Fran Uppsala 22:252-431, 1944.
10. Smith HW, in The Kidney, Structure and Function in Health and
    Disease, Oxford University Press, New York, 1951, pp 520-574.
    ISBN 0-19-501140-6.
11. Roviller C and Muller AF, in The Kidney, Morphology, Biochemistry,
    Physiology. Academic Press, New York, 1969, Vol I pp 1-530.
    ISBN 0-12-598801-X.
12. Bulger RE, Cronin RE, Dobyan DC, Anat Record 194:41-66, 1979.

13. Kriz W, Am J Physiol 241(Regulative Integrative Comp Physiol 10):
    R3-R16, 1981.
14. Oliver J, in Nephrons and Kidneys. Harper and Row, New York, 1968,
    pp 1-116.
15. Schmidt-Nielsen B, O'Dell R, Am J Physiol 200:1119-1124, 1961.
16. Long S, Gietisch G, Yale J Biol Med 52:525-544, 1979.
17. Torretti J, Weiner IM, in Methods in Pharmacology (M Martinez-
    Maldonado, ed.) Plenum Publishing Corp. New York, 1976, 4A:357-379.
    ISBN 0-306-35264-8.
18. Fanelli GM jr, Bohn DL, Reilly SS, Am J Physiol 224:993-996, 1973.
19. Berndt WO, Mudge GH, Invest Radiol 3:414-426, 1968.
20. Liegler DG, Henderson ES, Hahn MA, Oliverio CT, Clin Pharmacol Ther
    10:849-857, 1969.
21. Mudge GH, Berndt WO, Saunders A, Beattie B, Nephron 8:156-172, 1971.
22. Weiner IM, Garlid KD, Romeo JA, Mudge GH, Am J Physiol 200:393-399,
    1961.
23. Pritchard JB, Miller DS, Fed Proc 39:3207-3212, 1980.
24. Lassiter WE, Gottschalk CW, Mylle M, Am J Physiol 200:1139-1147, 1961.
25. Thurau K, ed., Experimental acute renal failure, Kidney Int 10:S1-
    S207, 1976.
26. Frolich JC, Nies AS, Schrier RW, eds., Prostaglandins and the Kidney,
    Kidney Int 19:755-880, 1981.
27. Culliford D, Hewitt HB, J Endocr 14:381-394, 1957.
28. Tune BM, Wu KY, Kempson RL, J Pharmacol Exp Ther 202:466-471, 1977.
29. Duggin GG, Mudge GH, J Pharmacol Exp Ther 199:1-9, 1976.
30. Lorentz WB jr, Lassiter WE, Gottschalk CW, J Clin Invest 51:484-492,
    1972.
31. Duggin GG, Mudge GH, J Pharmacol Exp Ther 207:584-593, 1978.
32. Anders MW, Kidney Int 18:636-647, 1980.
33. Mohandas J, Duggin GG, Horvath JS, Tiller DJ, Toxicol Appl
    Pharmacol (in press).
34. Stein JH, Lifschitz MD, Barnes LD, Am J Physiol 234:F171-F181, 1978.
35. Parekh N, Veith V, Kidney Int 19:306-316, 1981.
36. Hoyer JR, Seiler MW, Kidney Int 16:279-289, 1979.
37. Schwartz RH, Lewis RA, Schenk EA, Lab Invest 27:214-217, 1972.
38. Patel R, McKenzie JK, McQueen EG, Lancet 1:457-461, 1964.
39. Tiller DJ, Mudge GH, Kidney Int 18:700-711, 1980.
40. Thiel G, Brunner F, Wunderlich P, et al., Kidney Int 10:S191-S200,
    1976.
41. Kluwe WM, Toxicol Appl Pharmacol 57:414-424, 1981.
42. Lindner A, Cutler RE, Goodman WG, Kidney Int 16:158-166, 1979.
43. Conger JD, Robinette JB, Guggenheim SJ, Kidney Int 19:399-409, 1981.
44. Solez K, Ideura T, Silvia CB, Hamilton B, Saito H, Kidney Int
    18:309-322, 1980.
45. Darmady EM and McIver A, Renal Pathology, Butterworths, London,
    1980, ISBN 0-407-00119-0.

SUBJECT INDEX

Acetaminophen:- see paracetamol
Acetazolamide 107
Acetylcholine 190,517
Acetylene 409,410
N-Acetyl- -D-glucosamine (NAG)
 7,68,72,73,75,88,120,121,322,
 323,418,419
Acidification of urine 124,125,
346
Acid hydrolases 321,324
Acid phosphatase 36,37,89,90,
 120,121,322,323
Aclofenac 440
Acrodermatitis enteropathica 302
Acute renal failure 1,3,4,75,
 232,233,340-343,415-418,439,
 462,464,466,469,493,494,516,517
  -glomerular filtration 124,
 146,147,149,172,174,179,233,517
  -haemodynamics 124,172,173,
 175-180,233,495,517
  -tubular reabsorbtion 171,172
Adenosine 178-180
Adrenalin 190
Adrenal insufficiency 194,195
Adrenic acid 33,34
Adverse drug reaction 209
Aflatoxin 2,186,192,383
Age differences - in toxicity
 398
Alanine aminopeptidase (ALAT)
 73,88,120,419
Albumin 68,70,71,190,269,328,329
Albuminuria 109,110,373,374,376

Alcohol - nephritis 7,213,438
Aldosterone 42,225,229
Alkaline phosphatase (ALP) 70-
 73,86-90,99,100,312,313,317,
 331,499-502
Allopurinol 516
Alopecia 2,484
Amanita Sp. 379
α-Amanitin 380
Amidopyrine 449
Amikacin 419
Amino acid - cellular uptake
 58,59,68,133,164,264,269,
 284,285,287
Aminoaciduria 124,265,312,374,
 376,418
p-Aminobenzoate 140
Aminoglycoside antibiotics -(see
 also individual compound) 109,
 140,141,418-420
 δ-Aminolevulinic acid 287,292,342
 -dehyratase 342
Aminopeptidase 227,228,499,502
p-Aminophenol (PAP)132,329,330
Ammoniagenesis 35,132
Amoxacillin 415
Amphetamine 64
Amphtericin 69
Ampicillin 415
Amyloidosis 85,442
Anaesthetic agents (see
individual compounds)
Analgesic nephropathy 2,7,8,24,
 75,110,111,125,233,437-439,454,457

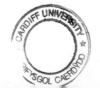